DRUG INTERACTIONS HANDBOOK

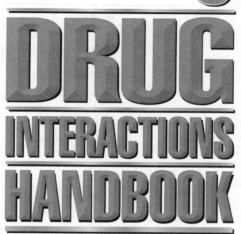

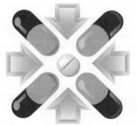

Wolters Kluwer | Lippincott Williams & Wilkins
Health

Philadelphia • Baltimore • New York • London
Buenos Aires • Hong Kong • Sydney • Tokyo

Staff

Executive Publisher
Judith A. Schilling McCann, RN, MSN

Editorial Director
H. Nancy Holmes

Clinical Director
Joan M. Robinson, RN, MSN

Clinical Project Manager
Jennifer Meyering, RN, BSN, MS, CCRN

Senior Art Director
Elaine Kasmer

Editorial Project Managers
Deborah Grandinetti, Ann Houska

Editors
Pat Nale, Russ Sprague

Copy Editors
Kimberly Bilotta (supervisor), Julia M. Catagnus, Amy Furman, Linda Hager, Liz Mooney

Designer
Joseph John Clark (cover)

Digital Composition Services
Diane Paluba (manager), Joyce Rossi Biletz, Donald G. Krauss

Associate Manufacturing Manager
Beth. J. Welsh

Editorial Assistants
Karen J. Kirk, Jeri O'Shea, Linda K. Ruhf

Indexer
Barbara Hodgson

NDIH011108

Library of Congress Cataloging-in-Publication Data

Nursing drug interactions handbook.
  p. ; cm.
  Includes index.
  ISBN-13: 978-0-7817-9281-3 (alk. paper)
  ISBN-10: 0-7817-9281-9 (alk. paper)
  1. Drug interactions—Handbooks, manuals, etc. 2. Nursing—Handbooks, manuals, etc.
I. Lippincott Williams & Wilkins.
  [DNLM: 1. Drug Interactions—Handbooks.
2. Drug Therapy—nursing—Handbooks.
WY 49 N97483 2010]
  RM302.N85 2010
  615'.7045—dc22

                                    2008029183

Contents

How to use this book

Nursing Drug Interactions Handbook is an easy-to-use resource to help you avoid thousands of unintended drug interactions as quickly and conveniently as possible.

You can use this book in two ways. With its A-to-Z organization, you can flip quickly to the generic name of the drug you plan to give. There you'll find, in alphabetical order, the drugs, drug classes, herbs, and foods that may interact with it. Or you can turn first to the book's comprehensive index, find the drug you plan to give, and scan the list of drugs and drug classes it may interact with.

Format

Each entry follows a standard format, making it easy for you to find key information fast. An entry starts with an interacting pair. The pair may be drug-drug, drug-class, drug-herb, or drug-food. Just below the interacting pair, as appropriate, you'll find a selection of common names. If the interacting element is a generic drug, the monograph typically provides common trade names. If the interacting element is a drug class, the monograph provides the generic names of applicable drugs in that class.

Risk rating. The risk rating gives you a quick idea of the overall importance of an interaction. The rating is based on the combined influence of the interaction's severity, onset, and likelihood.

Severity. The severity of a drug interaction may be major, moderate, or minor. A major interaction is one that may be life-threatening or cause permanent damage. A moderate interaction is one that may worsen the patient's condition. A minor interaction may be bothersome or cause little effect.

Onset. A drug interaction with a rapid onset starts within 24 hours of combined use. An interaction with a delayed onset starts days to weeks after the start of combined use.

Likelihood. In this section you'll get an idea of the likelihood that an interaction may occur. An established interaction is one that well-controlled clinical trials have proven can occur. A probable interaction is a very likely possibility but not proven clinically. And a suspected interaction is one that's supported by some reliable evidence but still needs more study. Interactions that are merely possible or unlikely aren't included in this book.

Cause. Next you'll find a brief description of the mechanism by which the interaction occurs.

Effect. This section reviews the main clinical effect of the interaction, usually in a single quick-read sentence.

Nursing considerations.
Finally, each entry includes key
information about drug usage,
patient care, and patient teach-
ing. This section also includes a
special, in-text ⚠ALERT logo to
direct your attention to especially important information.

Index
The comprehensive index for
*Nursing Drug Interactions
Handbook* includes generic
drug names, common trade
names, and drug classes. The
index provides a full, book-wide
look at the potentially dangerous interactions for each drug
included in this handy volume.

Guide to abbreviations

ACE	angiotensin-converting enzyme	DIC	disseminated intravascular coagulation
ADH	antidiuretic hormone	dl	deciliter
AIDS	acquired immunodeficiency syndrome	DNA	deoxyribonucleic acid
ALT	alanine transaminase	ECG	electrocardiogram
APTT	activated partial thromboplastin time	EEG	electroencephalogram
AST	aspartate transaminase	EENT	eyes, ears, nose, throat
AV	atrioventricular	FDA	Food and Drug Administration
b.i.d.	twice daily	g	gram
BPH	benign prostatic hypertrophy	G	gauge
BSA	body surface area	GGT	gamma-glutamyltransferase
BUN	blood urea nitrogen	GI	gastrointestinal
cAMP	cyclic 3′, 5′ adenosine monophosphate	gtt	drops
		GU	genitourinary
CBC	complete blood count	G6PD	glucose-6-phosphate dehydrogenase
CK	creatine kinase	H_1	histamine$_1$
CMV	cytomegalovirus	H_2	histamine$_2$
CNS	central nervous system	HDL	high-density lipoprotein
COPD	chronic obstructive pulmonary disease	HIV	human immunodeficiency virus
CSF	cerebrospinal fluid	HMG-CoA	3-hydroxy-3-methylglutaryl coenzyme A
CV	cardiovascular	5-HT	5-hydroxytryptamine
CYP	cytochrome P-450	I.D.	intradermal
D_5W	dextrose 5% in water	I.M.	intramuscular

INR	International Normalized Ratio	PVC	premature ventricular contraction
IPPB	intermittent positive-pressure breathing	q.i.d.	four times daily
		RBC	red blood cell
IU	international unit	RDA	recommended daily allowance
I.V.	intravenous	REM	rapid eye movement
kg	kilogram		
L	liter	RNA	ribonucleic acid
lb	pound	RSV	respiratory syncytial virus
LDH	lactate dehydrogenase	SA	sinoatrial
LDL	low-density lipoprotein	S.C.	subcutaneous
		sec	second
M	molar	SIADH	syndrome of inappropriate antidiuretic hormone
m^2	square meter		
MAO	monoamine oxidase		
mcg	microgram		
mEq	milliequivalent	S.L.	sublingual
mg	milligram	SSRI	selective serotonin reuptake inhibitor
MI	myocardial infarction	T_3	triiodothyronine
min	minute	T_4	thyroxine
ml	milliliter	t.i.d.	three times daily
mm^3	cubic millimeter	TSH	thyroid-stimulating hormone
NSAID	nonsteroidal anti-inflammatory drug	tsp	teaspoon
OTC	over-the-counter	USP	United States Pharmacopeia
PABA	para-aminobenzoic acid	UTI	urinary tract infection
PCA	patient-controlled analgesia	WBC	white blood cell
P.O.	by mouth	wk	week
P.R.	by rectum		
p.r.n.	as needed		
PT	prothrombin time		
PTT	partial thromboplastin time		

Drug actions, interactions, and reactions

Any drug a patient takes causes a series of physical and chemical events in his body. The first event, when a drug combines with cellular drug receptors, is the drug action. What happens next is the drug effect. Depending on the type of cellular drug receptors affected by a given drug, an effect can be local, systemic, or both. A systemic drug effect can follow a local effect. For example, when you apply a drug to the skin, it causes a local effect. But transdermal absorption of that drug can then produce a systemic effect. A local effect can also follow systemic absorption. For example, the peptic ulcer drug cimetidine produces a local effect after it's swallowed by blocking histamine receptors in the stomach's parietal cells. Diphenhydramine, on the other hand, causes a systemic effect by blocking histamine receptors throughout the body.

Drug properties
Drug absorption, distribution, metabolism, and excretion make up a drug's pharmacokinetics. These parts also describe a drug's onset of action, peak level, duration of action, and bioavailability.

Absorption
Before a drug can act in the body, it must be absorbed into the bloodstream—usually after oral administration, the most common route. Before an oral drug can be absorbed, it must disintegrate into particles small enough to dissolve in gastric juices. Only after dissolving can the drug be absorbed. Most absorption of orally given drugs occurs in the small intestine because the mucosal villi provide extensive surface area. Once absorbed and circulated in the bloodstream, the drug is bioavailable, or ready to produce a drug effect. The speed of absorption and whether absorption is complete or partial depend on the drug's effects, dosage form, administration route, interactions with other substances in the GI tract, and various patient characteristics. Oral solutions and elixirs bypass the need for disintegration and dissolution and are usually absorbed faster. Some tablets have enteric coatings to prevent disintegration in the acidic environment of the stomach; others have coatings of varying thickness that simply delay release of the drug.

Drugs given I.M. must first be absorbed through the muscle into the bloodstream. Rectal suppositories must dissolve to be absorbed through the rectal mucosa. Drugs given I.V. are injected directly into the bloodstream and are bioavailable completely and immediately.

Distribution

After absorption, a drug moves from the bloodstream into the fluids and tissues in the body, a movement known as distribution. All of the area to which a drug is distributed is known as volume of distribution. Individual patient variations can change the amount of drug distributed throughout the body. For example, in an edematous patient, a given dose must be distributed to a larger volume than in a nonedematous patient. Occasionally, a dose is increased to account for this difference. In this case, the dose should be decreased after the edema is corrected. Conversely, a dose given to a dehydrated patient must be decreased to allow for its distribution to a much smaller volume. Patients who are very obese may present another problem when considering drug distribution. Some drugs—such as digoxin, gentamicin, and tobramycin—aren't well-distributed to fatty tissue. Sometimes, doses based on actual body weight may lead to overdose and serious toxicity. In these cases, doses must be based on lean body weight, or adjusted body weight, which may be estimated from actuarial tables that give average weight range for height.

Metabolism

Most drugs are metabolized in the liver. Hepatic diseases may affect the liver's metabolic functions and may increase or decrease a drug's usual metabolism. Closely monitor all patients with hepatic disease for drug effect and toxicity.

The rate at which a drug is metabolized varies from person to person. Some patients metabolize drugs so quickly that the drug levels in their blood and tissues prove therapeutically inadequate. In other patients, the rate of metabolism is so slow that ordinary doses can produce toxicity.

Excretion

The body eliminates drugs by metabolism (usually hepatic) and excretion (usually renal). Drug excretion is the movement of a drug or its metabolites from the tissues back into circulation and from the circulation into the organs of excretion, where they're removed from the body. Most drugs are excreted by the kidneys, but some can be eliminated through the lungs, exocrine glands (sweat, salivary, or mammary), liver, skin, and intestinal tract. Drugs also may be removed artificially by direct mechanical intervention, such as peritoneal dialysis or hemodialysis.

Other modifying factors

One important factor influencing a drug's action and effect is its tendency to bind to plasma proteins, especially albumin, and other tissue components. Because only a free, unbound drug can act in the body, protein binding greatly influences the amount and duration of effect. Malnutrition, renal failure, and the presence of other protein-bound drugs can influence protein binding. When protein binding changes, the drug dose may need to be changed also.

The patient's age is another important factor. Elderly patients usually have decreased hepatic function, less muscle mass, diminished renal function, and lower albumin levels. These patients need lower doses and sometimes longer dosage intervals to avoid toxicity. Neonates have underdeveloped metabolic enzyme systems and inadequate renal function, so they need highly individualized dosages and careful monitoring.

Underlying disease also may affect drug action and effect. For example, acidosis may cause insulin resistance. Genetic diseases, such as G6PD deficiency and hepatic porphyria, may turn drugs into toxins, with serious consequences. Patients with G6PD deficiency may develop hemolytic anemia when given certain drugs, such as sulfonamides. A genetically susceptible patient can develop acute porphyria if given a barbiturate. A patient with a highly active hepatic enzyme system, such as a rapid acetylator, can develop hepatitis when treated with isoniazid because of the quick intrahepatic buildup of a toxic metabolite.

Drug administration issues

How a drug is given can also influence a drug's action in the body. The dosage form of a drug is important. Some tablets and capsules are too large to be easily swallowed by sick patients. An oral solution may be substituted, but it will produce higher drug levels than a tablet because the liquid is more easily and completely absorbed. When a potentially toxic drug (such as digoxin) is given, its increased absorption can cause toxicity. Sometimes a change in dosage form also requires a change in dosage.

Routes of administration aren't interchangeable. For example, diazepam is readily absorbed P.O. but is slowly and erratically absorbed I.M. On the other hand, gentamicin must be given parenterally because oral administration results in drug levels too low for systemic infections.

Improper storage can alter a drug's potency. Store most drugs in tight containers protected from direct sunlight and extremes in temperature and humidity that can cause them to deteriorate. Some drugs require special storage conditions, such as refrigeration. Caution patients not to store drugs in a bathroom because of the constantly changing environment.

The timing of drug administration can be important. Sometimes, giving an oral drug during or shortly after a meal decreases the amount of drug absorbed. In most drugs, this isn't significant and may even be desirable with irritating drugs such as aspirin. But penicillins and tetracyclines shouldn't be taken at mealtimes because certain foods can inactivate them. If in doubt about the effect of food on a certain drug, check with a pharmacist.

Consider the patient's age, height, and weight. The prescriber will need this information when calculating the dosage for many drugs. Record all information accurately on the patient's chart. The chart should also include all current laboratory data, especially renal and liver function studies, so the prescriber can adjust the dosage as needed.

Watch for metabolic changes and physiologic changes (depressed respiratory function, acidosis, or alkalosis) that might alter drug effect.

Know the patient's medical history. Whenever possible, obtain a comprehensive family history from the patient or his family. Ask about past reactions to drugs, possible genetic traits that might affect drug response, and the current use of other prescription, OTC, and illicit drugs, herbal remedies, and vitamin supplements. Multiple drug therapies can cause serious and fatal drug interactions and dramatically change many drugs' effects.

Drug interactions

A drug interaction occurs when a drug given with or shortly after another drug alters the effect of either or both drugs. Usually the effect of one drug is increased or decreased. For instance, one drug may inhibit or stimulate the metabolism or ex-

cretion of the other or free it for further action by releasing the drug from protein-binding sites.

Combination therapy is based on drug interaction. One drug may be given to complement the effects of another. Probenecid, which blocks the excretion of penicillin, is sometimes given with penicillin to maintain an adequate level of penicillin for a longer time. In many cases, two drugs with similar actions are given together precisely because of the additive effect. For instance, aspirin and codeine are commonly given in combination because together they provide greater pain relief than if either is given alone.

Drug interactions are sometimes used to prevent or antagonize certain adverse reactions. The diuretics hydrochlorothiazide and spironolactone are often given together because the former is potassium depleting and the latter potassium-sparing.

Not all drug interactions are beneficial: many drugs interact and decrease efficacy or increase toxicity. An example of decreased efficacy occurs when a tetracycline is given with drugs or foods that contain calcium or magnesium (such as antacids or milk). These bind with tetracycline in the GI tract and cause inadequate drug absorption. An example of increased toxicity can be seen in a patient taking a diuretic and lithium. The diuretic may increase the lithium level, causing lithium toxicity. This drug effect is known as *antagonism*. Avoid drug combinations that produce these effects, if possible.

Adverse reactions

Drugs cause adverse *effects*; patients have adverse *reactions*. An adverse reaction may be tolerated to obtain a therapeutic effect, or it may be hazardous and unacceptable. Some adverse reactions subside with continued use. For example, the drowsiness caused by paroxetine and the orthostatic hypotension caused by prazosin usually subside after several days when the patient develops tolerance. But many adverse reactions are dosage related and lessen or disappear only if the dosage is reduced. Most adverse reactions aren't therapeutically desirable, but a few can be put to clinical use. An outstanding example of this is the drowsiness caused by diphenhydramine, which makes it useful as a mild sedative.

Drug hypersensitivity, or drug allergy, is the result of an antigen-antibody immune reaction that occurs in the body when a drug is given to a susceptible patient. One of the most dangerous of all drug hypersensitivities is penicillin allergy. In its most severe form, penicillin anaphylaxis can rapidly become fatal.

Rarely, idiosyncratic reactions occur. These reactions are highly unpredictable and unusual. One of the best-known idiosyncratic adverse reactions is aplastic anemia caused by the antibiotic chloramphenicol. This reaction may appear in only 1 of 24,000 patients, but when it does occur, it can be fatal. A more common idiosyncratic reaction is extreme sensitivity to very low doses of a drug or insensitivity to higher-than-normal doses.

To deal with adverse reactions correctly, you need to be alert to even minor changes in the patient's clinical status. Such minor changes may be an early warning of pending toxicity. Listen to the patient's complaints about his reactions to a drug, and consider each objectively. You may be able to reduce adverse reactions in several ways. Obviously, dosage reduction can help. But, in many cases, so does a simple rescheduling of the dose. For example, pseudoephedrine may produce stimulation that will be no problem if it's given early in the day. Similarly, drowsiness from antihistamines or tranquilizers can be harmless if these drugs are given at bedtime. Most important, your patient needs to be told which adverse reactions to expect so that he won't become worried or even stop taking the drug on his own. Always advise the patient to report adverse reactions to the prescriber immediately.

Your ability to recognize signs and symptoms of drug allergies or serious idiosyncratic reactions may save your patient's life. Ask each patient about the drugs he's taking currently or has taken in the past and whether he experienced any unusual reactions from taking them. If a patient claims to be allergic to a drug, ask him to tell you exactly what happens when he takes it. He may be calling a harmless adverse reaction, such as upset stomach, an allergic reaction, or he may have a true tendency toward anaphylaxis. In either case, you and the prescriber need to know this. Of course, you must record and report clinical changes throughout the patient's course of treatment. If you suspect a severe adverse reaction, withhold the drug until you can check with the pharmacist and the prescriber.

Toxic reactions

Chronic drug toxicities are usually caused by the cumulative effect and resulting buildup of the drug in the body. These effects may be extensions of the desired therapeutic effect. For example, normal doses of glyburide normalize the glucose level, but higher doses can produce hypoglycemia.

Drug toxicities occur when a drug level rises as a result of impaired metabolism or excretion. For example, hepatic dysfunction impairs the metabolism of theophylline, raising its levels. Similarly, renal dysfunction may cause digoxin toxicity because this drug is eliminated from the body by the kidneys. Of course, excessive dosage can cause toxic levels also. For instance, tinnitus is usually a sign that the safe dose of aspirin has been exceeded.

Most drug toxicities are predictable, dosage-related, and reversible upon dosage adjustment. So, monitor patients carefully for physiologic changes that might alter drug effect. Watch especially for hepatic and renal impairment. Warn the patient about signs of pending toxicity, and tell him what to do if a toxic reaction occurs. Also, make sure to emphasize the importance of taking a drug exactly as prescribed. Warn the patient that serious problems could arise if he changes the dose or schedule or stops taking the drug without his prescriber's knowledge.

acarbose ▶◀ digoxin

Precose   Lanoxin

Risk rating: 2
Severity: Moderate   **Onset: Delayed**   **Likelihood: Probable**

Cause
Absorption of digoxin may be impaired.

Effect
Serum digoxin levels may decrease, thereby decreasing its therapeutic effects.

Nursing considerations
■ Monitor digoxin levels; the therapeutic range is 0.8 to 2 ng/ml.
■ If serum digoxin levels are low, the dose of digoxin may need to be increased or the acarbose dose discontinued.
■ If possible, administer the drugs at least 6 hours apart to avoid the interactions.
■ Instruct the patient to notify the prescriber if he has an irregular or fast heart rate.

acetaminophen ▶◀ alcohol

Acephen, Neopap,
Tylenol

Risk rating: 2
Severity: Moderate   **Onset: Delayed**   **Likelihood: Suspected**

Cause
Long-term alcohol use and acetaminophen-induced hepatotoxicity may induce hepatic microsomal enzymes.

Effect
Risk of liver damage increases.

Nursing considerations
■ Monitor liver function tests as needed.
■ If the patient drinks alcohol often or excessively, urge him to avoid regular or excessive use of acetaminophen.
■ If the patient is an alcoholic, explain that even moderate use of acetaminophen may cause significant hepatotoxicity.
■ Tell the patient to report abdominal pain, yellow skin, or dark urine.

acetaminophen ➤◄ phenytoin
Acephen, Neopap, Tylenol

Dilantin

Risk rating: 2
Severity: Moderate   Onset: Delayed   Likelihood: Suspected

Cause
Phenytoin, a hydantoin, may induce hepatic microsomal enzymes, accelerating acetaminophen metabolism.

Effect
Hepatotoxic metabolites and risk of hepatic impairment may increase. Also, the effect of acetaminophen may be decreased.

Nursing considerations
- Other hydantoins may interact with acetaminophen. If you suspect an interaction, consult the prescriber or pharmacist.
- If the patient takes phenytoin, warn against regular acetaminophen use.
- ⚑ ALERT After acetaminophen overdose, risk of hepatotoxicity is highest in a patient who takes phenytoin regularly.
- At usual therapeutic dosages, no special monitoring or dosage adjustment is needed.
- Tell the patient to notify the prescriber if he has abdominal pain, yellowing of skin or eyes, or dark urine.

acetaminophen ➤◄ sulfinpyrazone
Acephen, Neopap, Tylenol

Anturane

Risk rating: 2
Severity: Moderate   Onset: Delayed   Likelihood: Suspected

Cause
Sulfinpyrazone may induce hepatic microsomal enzymes, accelerating acetaminophen metabolism.

Effect
Hepatotoxic metabolites and risk of hepatic impairment may increase.

Nursing considerations
- If the patient takes sulfinpyrazone, advise against regular use of acetaminophen.
- ⚑ ALERT After acetaminophen overdose, risk of hepatotoxicity is highest in a patient who takes sulfinpyrazone regularly.

- At usual therapeutic dosages, no special monitoring or dosage adjustment is needed.
- Tell the patient to notify the prescriber if he has abdominal pain, yellowing of skin or eyes, or dark urine.

acetaminophen ➤◄ warfarin

Acephen, Neopap,   Coumadin
Tylenol

Risk rating: 2
Severity: Moderate   Onset: Delayed   Likelihood: Suspected

Cause
Acetaminophen or one of its metabolites may antagonize vitamin K.

Effect
Antithrombotic effect of warfarin may increase.

Nursing considerations
ALERT The effects of this interaction seem to be dose related. Daily acetaminophen use at 325 to 650 mg may increase INR 3.5-fold. Daily ingestion of 1,250 mg may increase INR 10-fold.
- At low acetaminophen doses (up to six 325-mg tablets weekly), interaction may have little significance.
- When starting or stopping acetaminophen, monitor coagulation studies once or twice weekly.
- Other risk factors including diarrhea and conditions that affect acetaminophen metabolism, may place the patient at a higher risk.

acetazolamide ➤◄ aspirin

Diamox   Bayer

Risk rating: 2
Severity: Moderate   Onset: Delayed   Likelihood: Suspected

Cause
Aspirin displaces acetazolamide from protein binding sites and also inhibits renal clearance. Also, carbonic anhydrase inhibitors, like acetazolamide, allow increased CNS penetration by salicylates, like aspirin.

Effect
Increased plasma levels and toxicity of acetazolamide may occur, resulting in CNS depression and metabolic acidosis.

Nursing considerations
- Avoid using these drugs together if possible.
- Monitor renal function in patients, especially the elderly, taking acetazolamide.
- If the patient must take both medications together, monitor blood salicylate levels, arterial blood gases, and CNS status.
- Instruct patient to notify the prescriber if he develops lethargy, confusion, urinary incontinence, or other signs of toxicity.

---

acyclovir ▶◀ theophyllines
Zovirax   aminophylline, theophylline

Risk rating: 2
Severity: Moderate   Onset: Delayed   Likelihood: Suspected

Cause
Acyclovir may inhibit oxidative metabolism of theophyllines.

Effect
Theophylline level, adverse effects, and toxicity may increase.

Nursing considerations
- Monitor serum theophylline level closely. Normal therapeutic range is 10 to 20 mcg/ml for adults and 5 to 15 mcg/ml for children.
- Theophylline dosage may need to be decreased while the patient takes acyclovir.
- Watch for increased adverse effects of theophylline, such as tachycardia, anorexia, nausea, vomiting, diarrhea, seizures, restlessness, irritability, and headache.
- Describe adverse effects of theophylline and signs of toxicity, and tell the patient to report them immediately to prescriber.

---

adenosine ▶◀ theophyllines
Adenocard   aminophylline, theophylline

Risk rating: 2
Severity: Moderate   Onset: Rapid   Likelihood: Suspected

Cause
Theophyllines may antagonize the cardiovascular effects of adenosine.

Effect
The exact mechanism is unknown, but it's thought that theophyllines may antagonize the adenosine receptors.

Nursing considerations
- Notify the prescriber of the potential for interaction.
- Larger than normal doses of adenosine may be needed to terminate supraventricular arrhythmias.
- Carefully monitor the patient's electrocardiogram for termination of arrhythmias after receiving adenosine.
- If the patient is scheduled for a pharmacologic stress test with adenosine and has taken a medication that contains theophylline, the test will have to be rescheduled.

aldesleukin ◄►◄ indinavir
Proleukin   Crixivan

Risk rating: 2
Severity: Moderate   **Onset: Delayed**   **Likelihood: Suspected**

Cause
Aldesleukin causes the formation of interleukin-6, an enzyme that inhibits the metabolism of indinavir.

Effect
The plasma concentrations of indinavir may be elevated, along with an increased risk of toxicity.

Nursing considerations
- Aldesleukin taken with other protease inhibitors may cause a similar interaction.
- Monitor the patient and be prepared for adjustments in the dose of indinavir when aldesleukin therapy is initiated or stopped.
- Instruct the patient to notify the prescriber if he develops signs and symptoms of indinavir toxicity, which include hematuria, flank pain, nausea, and vomiting.

alfentanil ◄►◄ azole antifungals
Alfenta   fluconazole, voriconazole

Risk rating: 1
Severity: Major   **Onset: Rapid**   **Likelihood: Suspected**

Cause
Azole antifungals may decrease the metabolism of opioid analgesics.

Effect
The pharmacologic and adverse effects of opioid analgesics may be increased.

Nursing considerations
⚠ **ALERT** Carefully monitor the patient for increased effects of opioid analgesics, including respiratory depression, decreased LOC, and bradycardia.
■ Alert the prescriber to the risk of interaction between the opioid analgesic and the azole antifungal, and discuss a possible decrease in opioid dosage.
■ Keep naloxone available to treat respiratory depression.
■ Monitor the patient's pain level, and administer pain medication as needed to keep him comfortable but without significant adverse effects.

---

alfuzosin ▶◀	azole antifungals
Uroxatral	itraconazole, ketoconazole

Risk rating: 2
Severity: Moderate   **Onset: Delayed**   **Likelihood: Suspected**

Cause
Azole antifungals may inhibit the metabolism of alfuzosin.

Effect
The pharmacologic and adverse effects of alfuzosin may be increased.

Nursing considerations
⚠ **ALERT** Avoid giving alfuzosin and azole antifungals together.
■ Notify the prescriber that the patient is taking an azole antifungal and alfuzosin together and their use together is contraindicated.
■ Monitor the patient for development of adverse effects of alfuzosin, including dizziness, abdominal pain, nausea, and fatigue.

---

alfuzosin ▶◀	tadalafil
Uroxatral	Cialis

Risk rating: 1
Severity: Major   **Onset: Rapid**   **Likelihood: Suspected**

Cause
The cause of the interaction is unknown.

Effect
The hypotensive effects of alpha$_1$-adrenergic blockers may be increased.

Nursing considerations
⚠ **ALERT** Administering tadalafil and an alpha$_1$-adrenergic blocker together is contraindicated.
- If the patient has taken tadalafil and an alpha$_1$-adrenergic blocker, carefully monitor his blood pressure and cardiac output.
- Alert the prescriber that the patient is taking tadalafil and an alpha$_1$-adrenergic blocker together and their use is contraindicated.
- Make sure the patient has readily accessible I.V. access for administration of fluids if needed for hypotension.

---

alfuzosin ━━━►◄━━━ vardenafil
Uroxatral   Levitra

Risk rating: 2
Severity: Moderate   **Onset: Rapid**   **Likelihood: Suspected**

Cause
Vardenafil causes an additive pharmacologic action.

Effect
The risk of hypotension may be increased.

Nursing considerations
⚠ **ALERT** Administering vardenafil and an alpha$_1$-adrenergic blocker together is contraindicated.
- If the patient has taken vardenafil and an alpha$_1$-adrenergic blocker, carefully monitor his blood pressure and cardiac output.
- Alert the prescriber that the patient is taking vardenafil and an alpha$_1$-adrenergic blocker together and their use is contraindicated.
- Make sure the patient has readily accessible I.V. access for administration of fluids if needed for hypotension.

---

allopurinol ━━━►◄━━━ ampicillin
Aloprim, Zyloprim

Risk rating: 2
Severity: Moderate   **Onset: Delayed**   **Likelihood: Suspected**

Cause
The mechanism of this interaction is unknown.

Effect
Risk of ampicillin-induced rash increases.

Nursing considerations
- Allopurinol may increase hypersensitivity to ampicillin, a penicillin.

- Other penicillins may interact with allopurinol. If you suspect an interaction, consult the prescriber or pharmacist.
- **⚠ ALERT** Notify the prescriber if rash appears. The patient may need a lower allopurinol dose or a different drug.
- Instruct the patient to watch for skin changes.

---

allopurinol ━━▶◀━━ thiopurines
Aloprim, Zyloprim   azathioprine, mercaptopurine

Risk rating: 1
Severity: Major   **Onset: Delayed**   **Likelihood: Established**

Cause
Allopurinol inhibits the first-pass metabolism of thiopurines.

Effect
Pharmacologic and toxic effects of orally administered thiopurines increase.

Nursing considerations
- When administering a thiopurine with allopurinol, decrease the dose of the thiopurine by 25% to 33%.
- **⚠ ALERT** Monitor the patient for toxic effects, which include thrombocytopenia and hepatotoxicity.
- Monitor the patient's hematologic and hepatic function tests.
- Advise the patient to report increased bleeding, yellow skin or eyes, or dark-colored urine.

---

almotriptan ━━▶◀━━ azole antifungals
Axert   itraconazole, ketoconazole

Risk rating: 2
Severity: Moderate   **Onset: Delayed**   **Likelihood: Suspected**

Cause
Azole antifungals inhibit CYP3A4 metabolism of certain 5-HT_1 receptor agonists, such as almotriptan.

Effect
Selective 5-HT_1 receptor agonist level and adverse effects may increase.

Nursing considerations
- **⚠ ALERT** Don't give almotriptan within 7 days of itraconazole or ketoconazole.

■ Adverse effects of selective 5-HT$_1$ receptor agonists may include coronary artery vasospasm, dizziness, nausea, paresthesia, and somnolence.

■ To help avoid interactions, urge the patient to tell his prescribers about all drugs and supplements he is taking.

alprazolam ▬▬▶◀▬▬ alcohol
Xanax

Risk rating: 2
Severity: Moderate   **Onset: Rapid**   **Likelihood: Established**

Cause
Alcohol inhibits hepatic enzymes, which decreases clearance and increases peak level of benzodiazepines, such as alprazolam.

Effect
Risk of additive or synergistic effects increases.

Nursing considerations
■ Advise the patient not to consume alcohol while taking alprazolam.
■ Before therapy starts, assess the patient thoroughly for history or evidence of alcohol use.
■ Watch for additive CNS effects, which may suggest benzodiazepine overdose.
■ Other benzodiazepines interact with alcohol. If you suspect an interaction, consult the prescriber or pharmacist.

alprazolam ▬▬▶◀▬▬ azole antifungals
Xanax

fluconazole, itraconazole, ketoconazole, miconazole

Risk rating: 2
Severity: Moderate   **Onset: Rapid**   **Likelihood: Established**

Cause
Azole antifungals decrease CYP3A4 metabolism of certain benzodiazepines such as alprazolam.

Effect
Benzodiazepine effects are increased and prolonged, which may cause CNS depression and psychomotor impairment.

Nursing considerations
■ Various benzodiazepine–azole antifungal combinations may interact. If you suspect an interaction, consult the prescriber or pharmacist.

■ If the patient takes fluconazole or miconazole, talk with the prescriber about giving a lower benzodiazepine dose or a related drug not metabolized by CYP3A4, such as temazepam or lorazepam.
■ Warn the patient that the effects of this interaction may last several days after stopping the azole antifungal.
■ Explain that taking these drugs together may increase sedative effects; tell the patient to report such effects promptly.

alprazolam ■■■■►◄■■■■ carbamazepine
Xanax   Carbatrol, Epitol, Equetro, Tegretol

Risk rating: 2
Severity: Moderate   **Onset: Delayed**   **Likelihood: Suspected**

Cause
Metabolism of benzodiazepines is increased.

Effect
Pharmacologic effects of benzodiazepines may be decreased.

Nursing considerations
■ Carbamazepine may cause decreased effectiveness of benzodiazepines.
■ If the patient is taking carbamazepine and alprazolam together, monitor him for a decreased response to alprazolam.
■ Consult with the prescriber for an increased dose of alprazolam, if needed.

alprazolam ■■■■►◄■■■■ cimetidine
Xanax   Tagamet

Risk rating: 3
Severity: Minor   **Onset: Rapid**   **Likelihood: Probable**

Cause
Hepatic metabolism of benzodiazepines, such as alprazolam, may be decreased.

Effect
Serum levels of alprazolam may be increased, causing increased sedation.

Nursing considerations
◪ **ALERT** Carefully monitor the patient for increased sedation after taking cimetidine and a benzodiazepine.

- Warn the patient about the risk of increased sedation when taking cimetidine and alprazolam together.
- If the patient experiences increased sedation, discuss the possibility of decreasing the dose of alprazolam with the prescriber.
- Monitor serum benzodiazepine levels while the patient is taking cimetidine and a benzodiazepine together.

◘ ALERT Elderly patients are at a higher risk for increased levels of sedation.

---

alprazolam ━━━━◄► macrolide antibiotics

Xanax

clarithromycin, erythromycin, telithromycin

Risk rating: 2
Severity: Moderate   **Onset: Rapid**   **Likelihood: Suspected**

Cause
Macrolide antibiotics may decrease the metabolism of certain benzodiazepines such as alprazolam.

Effect
Sedative effects of benzodiazepines may be increased or prolonged.

Nursing considerations
- Talk with the prescriber about decreasing benzodiazepine dosage during antibiotic therapy.
- Lorazepam, oxazepam, and temazepam probably don't interact with macrolide antibiotics; substitution may be possible.
- Urge the patient to promptly report oversedation.

---

alprazolam ━━━━◄► nonnucleoside reverse-transcriptase inhibitors

Xanax

delavirdine, efavirenz

Risk rating: 2
Severity: Moderate   **Onset: Delayed**   **Likelihood: Suspected**

Cause
Nonnucleoside reverse-transcriptase inhibitors may inhibit CYP3A4 metabolism of certain benzodiazepines such as alprazolam.

Effect
Sedative effects of benzodiazepines may be increased or prolonged, leading to respiratory depression.

Nursing considerations
⚠ **ALERT** Don't combine alprazolam with delavirdine or efavirenz.
■ Other benzodiazepines and nonnucleoside reverse-transcriptase inhibitors may interact. If you suspect an interaction, consult the prescriber or pharmacist.
■ Explain the risk of oversedation and respiratory depression.

---

alprazolam ▰▰▰►◄▰▰▰ protease inhibitors
Xanax   atazanavir, darunavir,
                                         indinavir, nelfinavir, ritonavir,
                                         saquinavir

Risk rating: 1
Severity: Major   **Onset: Delayed**   **Likelihood: Suspected**

Cause
Protease inhibitors may inhibit CYP3A4 metabolism of certain benzodiazepines such as alprazolam.

Effect
Sedative effects of benzodiazepines may be increased and prolonged, leading to severe respiratory depression.

Nursing considerations
⚠ **ALERT** Don't combine alprazolam with protease inhibitors.
■ If the patient takes any benzodiazepine–protease inhibitor combination, notify prescriber. Interaction could involve other drugs in the class.
■ Watch for evidence of oversedation and respiratory depression.
■ Teach the patient and family about the risks of using these drugs together.

---

alprazolam ▰▰▰►◄▰▰▰ St. John's wort
Xanax

Risk rating: 2
Severity: Moderate   **Onset: Delayed**   **Likelihood: Suspected**

Cause
Hepatic and intestinal metabolism of benzodiazepines, such as alprazolam, may be increased.

Effect
Pharmacologic effects of alprazolam may be decreased.

Nursing considerations
- If possible, avoid administering St. John's wort and benzodiazepines together.
- Monitor the patient for a decreased plasma level of benzodiazepines.
- If the patient is taking alprazolam and St. John's wort together, monitor him for a decreased response to the alprazolam.
- Consult with the prescriber about adjusting the dose of alprazolam if a decreased response is noted.
- Tell the patient to inform his health care provider of all nonprescription supplements and prescription drugs he is taking.

alprazolam ◄►◄ theophyllines
Xanax   aminophylline, theophylline

Risk rating: 3
Severity: Minor   **Onset: Rapid**   **Likelihood: Suspected**

Cause
Theophyllines may antagonize the sedative effects of benzodiazepines.

Effect
Sedative effects of alprazolam may be decreased.

Nursing considerations
- Monitor the patient taking a theophylline and a benzodiazepine together for a decreased sedative effect of the benzodiazepine.
- Consult with the prescriber and adjust the dose of alprazolam as needed.

alteplase ◄►◄ heparin
Activase

Risk rating: 1
Severity: Major   **Onset: Rapid**   **Likelihood: Suspected**

Cause
The combined effect of these drugs may be greater than the sum of their individual effects.

Effect
Risk of serious bleeding increases.

Nursing considerations
- **ALERT** Use of heparin with alteplase is contraindicated.

⚠ ALERT Alteplase is contraindicated for acute ischemic stroke when the patient is at risk of bleeding because he was given heparin within 48 hours before onset of stroke or his APTT is elevated. The use of alteplase under these conditions increases the risk of bleeding, disability, and death.

alteplase ▶◀ nitroglycerin
Activase   Minitran, Nitro-Bid, Nitro-Dur, NitroQuick, Nitrostat, NitroTab

Risk rating: 1
Severity: Major   Onset: Rapid   Likelihood: Probable

Cause
Nitroglycerin may enhance hepatic blood flow, thereby increasing alteplase metabolism.

Effect
Alteplase level may decrease, interfering with thrombolytic effect.

Nursing considerations
- Don't use together, if possible.
- If use together is unavoidable, give nitroglycerin at the lowest effective dose.
- Monitor the patient for inadequate thrombolytic effects.

alteplase ▶◀ warfarin
Activase   Coumadin

Risk rating: 1
Severity: Major   Onset: Rapid   Likelihood: Suspected

Cause
The combined effect of these drugs may be greater than the sum of their individual effects.

Effect
Risk of serious bleeding increases.

Nursing considerations
⚠ ALERT Alteplase is contraindicated for acute ischemic stroke when the patient is taking drugs such as oral anticoagulants that increase his risk of bleeding. Adding alteplase increases the risk of bleeding, disability, and death.

■ Alert the prescriber that the patient is also taking warfarin and use together is contraindicated.

---

amikacin ━━━━►◄━━ indomethacin
Amikin   Indocin

Risk rating: 2
Severity: Moderate   Onset: Delayed   Likelihood: Suspected

Cause
NSAIDs may reduce glomerular filtration rate (GFR), causing aminoglycosides, such as amikacin, to accumulate.

Effect
Aminoglycoside levels in premature infants may increase.

Nursing considerations
■ Before NSAID therapy starts, aminoglycoside dose should be reduced.
◣ ALERT Check peak and trough aminoglycoside level after third dose. For peak level, draw blood 30 minutes after I.V. dose or 60 minutes after I.M. dose. For trough level, draw blood just before a dose.
■ Monitor the patient's renal function.
■ Although only indomethacin is known to interact with aminoglycosides, other NSAIDs probably do as well. If you suspect an interaction, consult prescriber or pharmacist.
■ Other drugs cleared by GFR may have a similar interaction.

---

amikacin ━━━━►◄━━ penicillins
Amikin   ampicillin, penicillin G, piperacillin, ticarcillin

Risk rating: 2
Severity: Moderate   Onset: Delayed   Likelihood: Probable

Cause
The mechanism of this interaction is unknown.

Effect
Penicillins may inactivate certain aminoglycosides, such as amikacin, decreasing their therapeutic effects.

Nursing considerations
◣ ALERT Check peak and trough aminoglycoside levels after third dose. For peak level, draw blood 30 minutes after I.V. dose or 60 minutes after I.M. dose. For trough level, draw blood just before a dose.

■ Monitor the patient's renal function.
■ Other aminoglycosides may interact with penicillins. If you suspect an interaction, consult the prescriber or pharmacist.
■ Penicillins affect gentamicin and tobramycin more than amikacin.

amiloride 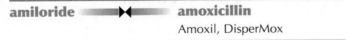 ACE inhibitors

benazepril, captopril, enalapril, fosinopril, lisinopril, moexipril, perindopril, ramipril

Risk rating: 1
Severity: Major   **Onset: Delayed**   **Likelihood: Probable**

Cause
The mechanism of this interaction is unknown.

Effect
Serum potassium level may increase.

Nursing considerations
■ Be cautious about using both with patients at high risk for hyperkalemia, especially those with renal impairment.
■ Monitor BUN, creatinine, and serum potassium levels as needed.
■ Other ACE inhibitors may interact with potassium-sparing diuretics such as amiloride. If you suspect an interaction, consult the prescriber or pharmacist.
■ Urge the patient to immediately report an irregular heart beat, a slow pulse, weakness, and other evidence of hyperkalemia.

amiloride ◄►►► amoxicillin

Amoxil, DisperMox

Risk rating: 3
Severity: Minor   **Onset: Delayed**   **Likelihood: Suspected**

Cause
Amiloride decreases the absorption of amoxicillin.

Effect
Therapeutic activity of amoxicillin may be decreased.

Nursing considerations
■ Monitor the patient for a decreased response to amoxicillin if also taking amiloride.
■ Consult with the prescriber about the need to increase the dose of amoxicillin if decreased therapeutic activity is suspected.

■ This interaction isn't noted with I.V. administration of amoxicillin–only oral administration.

amiloride ◄► eplerenone
Inspira

Risk rating: 1
Severity: **Major** Onset: **Delayed** Likelihood: **Suspected**

Cause
Potassium-sparing diuretics, such as amiloride, decrease renal elimination of potassium ions.

Effect
Serum potassium levels increase.

Nursing considerations
 ALERT Taking eplerenone and potassium-sparing diuretics together is contraindicated.
■ If the patient is taking eplerenone and amiloride together, notify the prescriber that this combination is contraindicated.
■ Monitor the patient for signs of hyperkalemia, such as muscle weakness and cardiac arrhythmias.
■ Monitor serum potassium levels closely.
■ Urge the patient to immediately report an irregular heart beat, a slow pulse, weakness, or other evidence of hyperkalemia.

amiloride ◄► potassium preparations
potassium acetate, potassium chloride, potassium citrate, potassium gluconate, potassium iodine, potassium phosphate

Risk rating: 1
Severity: **Major** Onset: **Delayed** Likelihood: **Established**

Cause
This interaction reduces renal elimination of potassium ions.

Effect
Risk of severe hyperkalemia increases.

Nursing considerations
 ALERT Don't use this combination unless the patient has severe hypokalemia that isn't responding to either drug class alone.

- To avoid hyperkalemia, monitor potassium level when therapy starts and often thereafter.
- Tell the patient to avoid high-potassium foods, such as citrus juices, bananas, spinach, broccoli, beans, potatoes, and salt substitutes.
- Urge the patient to immediately report palpitations, chest pain, nausea, vomiting, paresthesia, muscle weakness, and other signs of potassium overload.

amiloride ━━━▶◀━━━ quinidine

Risk rating: 1
Severity: Major   **Onset: Delayed**   **Likelihood: Suspected**

Cause
This interaction may result from a synergistic increase in myocardial sodium channel blockade.

Effect
Quinidine effects may be reversed, contributing to a proarrhythmic state.

Nursing considerations
- If possible, avoid combining quinidine and amiloride.
- If unavoidable, monitor ECG closely.
- Therapeutic range of quinidine is 2 to 6 mcg/ml. More specific assays have levels of less than 1 mcg/ml.
- Monitor the patient for loss of arrhythmia control.
- Advise the patient to report palpitations, shortness of breath, dizziness or fainting, and chest pain.

aminoglutethimide ▶◀ dexamethasone
Cytadren   Decadron

Risk rating: 2
Severity: Moderate   **Onset: Delayed**   **Likelihood: Suspected**

Cause
The cause of the interaction is unknown.

Effect
Dexamethasone-induced adrenal suppression is decreased. Corticosteroid anti-inflammatory activity may also be decreased.

Nursing considerations
- Tell the prescriber if the patient is taking both drugs together; he may substitute hydrocortisone for dexamethasone.
- Monitor the patient for loss of adrenal suppression from decreased dexamethasone activity.
- If symptoms of decreased adrenal suppression occur, the dose of dexamethasone may need to be increased.

aminoglutethimide ➡◀ warfarin
Cytadren   Coumadin

Risk rating: 2
Severity: Moderate   Onset: Delayed   Likelihood: Suspected

Cause
Liver enzyme activity is increased, resulting in increased warfarin metabolism.

Effect
Warfarin's ability to increase prothrombin time may be reduced.

Nursing considerations
- Carefully monitor the patient's prothrombin time when starting or stopping aminoglutethimide.
- Consult with the prescriber and adjust the dose of warfarin as needed.

aminophylline ➡◀ acyclovir
                              Zovirax

Risk rating: 2
Severity: Moderate   Onset: Delayed   Likelihood: Suspected

Cause
The oxidative metabolism of aminophylline may be inhibited.

Effect
Increased serum theophylline levels along with increased pharmacologic and adverse effects may occur.

Nursing considerations
- Acyclovir taken with aminophylline may cause an increased serum aminophylline level.
- Carefully monitor serum theophylline levels. Therapeutic serum levels are 10 to 20 mcg/ml; toxicity may occur at levels above 20 mcg/ml.

■ If the patient is taking aminophylline and acyclovir together, monitor for increased adverse effects, such as nausea, palpitations, and restlessness.
■ Consult with the prescriber about adjusting the dose of aminophylline if increased serum levels or adverse effects occur.

aminophylline ➤◄ adenosine
Adenocard

Risk rating: 2
Severity: Moderate   **Onset: Rapid**   **Likelihood: Suspected**

Cause
The exact mechanism of the interaction is unknown, but it is thought that theophyllines, such as aminophylline, may antagonize the adenosine receptors.

Effect
The effect of adenosine to terminate supraventricular arrhythmias may be deceased.

Nursing considerations
■ If a patient taking a theophylline needs to receive adenosine to terminate an arrhythmia, be prepared to administer a larger dose, as needed.
■ If the patient taking aminophylline is scheduled for a chemical stress test using adenosine, he would be not able to have the test until the aminophylline has been discontinued.

aminophylline ➤◄ benzodiazepines
alprazolam, diazepam

Risk rating: 3
Severity: Minor   **Onset: Rapid**   **Likelihood: Suspected**

Cause
Theophyllines produce an antagonistic action by competively binding to receptors.

Effect
Sedative effects of the benzodiazepines may be decreased by theophyllines, such as aminophylline.

Nursing considerations
■ Monitor the patient taking a theophylline and a benzodiazepine together for a decreased sedative effect of the benzodiazepine.

■ Consult with the prescriber and adjust the dose of the benzodiazepine as needed.

aminophylline ▬▬►◄▬▬ cimetidine
Tagamet

Risk rating: 2
Severity: Moderate   **Onset: Delayed**   **Likelihood: Established**

Cause
Cimetidine inhibits hepatic metabolism of aminophylline.

Effect
Theophylline level and risk of toxicity may increase.

Nursing considerations
■ Carefully monitor serum theophylline levels. Therapeutic serum
levels are 10 to 20 mcg/ml; toxicity may occur at levels above
20 mcg/ml.
■ Watch for evidence of toxicity, such as tachycardia, anorexia, nausea,
vomiting, diarrhea, seizures, restlessness, irritability, and headache.
■ The aminophylline dosage may need to be decreased by 20% to 40%.
■ Giving ranitidine or famotidine instead of cimetidine for gastric hypersecretion may decrease risk of this interaction.

aminophylline ▬▬►◄▬▬ diltiazem
Cardizem

Risk rating: 2
Severity: Moderate   **Onset: Delayed**   **Likelihood: Suspected**

Cause
Metabolism of theophyllines, such as aminophylline, may be inhibited.

Effect
Theophylline levels and risk of toxicity may increase.

Nursing considerations
■ Carefully monitor serum theophylline levels. Therapeutic serum
levels are 10 to 20 mcg/ml; toxicity may occur at levels above
20 mcg/ml.
■ Watch for evidence of toxicity, such as tachycardia, anorexia, nausea,
vomiting, diarrhea, seizures, restlessness, irritability, and headache.
■ Describe adverse effects of aminophylline and signs of toxicity, and
tell the patient to report them immediately to the prescriber.

aminophylline 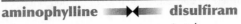 disulfiram
Antabuse

Risk rating: 2
Severity: Moderate   Onset: Delayed   Likelihood: Suspected

Cause
Metabolism of theophyllines, such as aminophylline, may be inhibited.

Effect
Aminophylline effects, including toxic effects, increase.

Nursing considerations
- Carefully monitor serum theophylline levels. Therapeutic serum levels are 10 to 20 mcg/ml; toxicity may occur at levels above 20 mcg/ml.
- Watch for evidence of toxicity, such as tachycardia, anorexia, nausea, vomiting, diarrhea, seizures, restlessness, irritability, and headache.
- Because disulfiram exerts dose-dependent inhibition of aminophylline, aminophylline dosage may need to be adjusted.
- Describe adverse effects of aminophylline and signs of toxicity, and tell the patient to report them immediately to the prescriber.

aminophylline 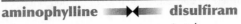 hormonal contraceptives

Risk rating: 2
Severity: Moderate   Onset: Delayed   Likelihood: Suspected

Cause
Oxidative degradation of aminophylline by cytochrome P448 may be decreased.

Effect
Aminophylline toxicity may result from decreased elimination.

Nursing considerations
- Carefully monitor serum theophylline levels. Therapeutic serum levels are 10 to 20 mcg/ml; toxicity may occur at levels above 20 mcg/ml.
- Watch for evidence of toxicity, such as tachycardia, anorexia, nausea, vomiting, diarrhea, seizures, restlessness, irritability, and headache.
- Consult with the prescriber and adjust the dose of aminophylline as indicated
- Describe adverse effects of aminophylline and signs of toxicity, and tell the patient to report them immediately to the prescriber.

aminophylline  levothyroxine
Synthroid

Risk rating: 2
Severity: Moderate   Onset: Delayed   Likelihood: Suspected

Cause
Theophylline levels are related to thyroxine level. Patients who are hyperthyroid or hypothyroid may have varying interactions.

Effect
In hypothyroidism, aminophylline metabolism decreases, and serum level—and risk of toxicity—increase.

Nursing considerations
▪ Carefully monitor serum theophylline levels. Therapeutic serum levels are 10 to 20 mcg/ml; toxicity may occur at levels above 20 mcg/ml.
▪ Adjust dosage of aminophylline as needed to avoid theophylline toxicity.
▪ Watch for evidence of toxicity, such as tachycardia, anorexia, nausea, vomiting, diarrhea, seizures, restlessness, irritability, and headache.
▪ Once a patient becomes euthyroid, aminophylline clearance returns to normal.
▪ Describe adverse effects of aminophylline and signs of toxicity, and tell the patient to report them immediately to the prescriber.

aminophylline  macrolide antibiotics
azithromycin, erythromycin

Risk rating: 2
Severity: Moderate   Onset: Delayed   Likelihood: Established

Cause
Certain macrolides inhibit metabolism of theophyllines such as aminophylline.

Effect
Serum theophylline level and risk of toxicity may increase.

Nursing considerations
▪ Carefully monitor serum theophylline levels. Therapeutic serum levels are 10 to 20 mcg/ml; toxicity may occur at levels above 20 mcg/ml.
▪ Adjust dosage of aminophylline as needed to avoid theophylline toxicity.

■ Watch for evidence of toxicity, such as tachycardia, anorexia, nausea, vomiting, diarrhea, seizures, restlessness, irritability, and headache.
■ If the patient taking aminophylline begins taking a macrolide antibiotic, be prepared to alter aminophylline dosage.
■ Describe adverse effects of aminophylline and signs of toxicity, and tell the patient to report them immediately to the prescriber.

aminophylline 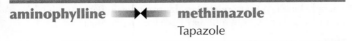 methimazole
Tapazole

Risk rating: 2
Severity: Moderate   Onset: Delayed   Likelihood: Suspected

Cause
Methimazole increases clearance of theophyllines, such as aminophylline, in hyperthyroid patients.

Effect
Theophylline level and effects decrease.

Nursing considerations
■ Watch closely for decreased aminophylline efficacy while abnormal thyroid status continues.
◤ **ALERT** Assess the patient for return to euthyroid state, when interaction no longer occurs.
■ Explain that hyperthyroidism and hypothyroidism can affect aminophylline efficacy and toxicity; tell the patient to immediately report evidence of either one.
■ Urge the patient to have TSH and theophylline levels tested regularly.

aminophylline ▶ mexiletine

Risk rating: 2
Severity: Moderate   Onset: Delayed   Likelihood: Established

Cause
CYP metabolism of theophyllines, such as aminophylline, is inhibited by mexiletine.

Effect
Theophylline level and risk of toxicity may increase.

Nursing considerations
■ Carefully monitor serum theophylline levels. Therapeutic serum levels are 10 to 20 mcg/ml; toxicity may occur at levels above 20 mcg/ml.
■ Adjust dosage of aminophylline as needed to avoid theophylline toxicity.
■ Watch for evidence of toxicity, such as tachycardia, anorexia, nausea, vomiting, diarrhea, seizures, restlessness, irritability, and headache.
■ Interaction usually occurs within 2 days of combining these drugs. Aminophylline dosage may be decreased when mexiletine is started.
■ Describe adverse effects of aminophylline and signs of toxicity, and tell the patient to report them immediately to the prescriber.

aminophylline ➤◀ pancuronium

Risk rating: 2
Severity: Moderate   **Onset: Rapid**   **Likelihood: Suspected**

Cause
These drugs may act antagonistically.

Effect
Neuromuscular blockade may be reversed.

Nursing considerations
■ Monitor the patient receiving nondepolarizing muscle relaxant, such as pancuronium, closely for lack of drug effect.
■ Dosage of nondepolarizing muscle relaxant may need adjustment.
■ This interaction is dose-dependant.
■ Make sure the patient is adequately sedated when receiving pancuronium and aminophylline together.

aminophylline ➤◀ phenytoin
Dilantin

Risk rating: 2
Severity: Moderate   **Onset: Delayed**   **Likelihood: Probable**

Cause
Metabolism of both drugs increases.

Effect
Aminophylline or phenytoin efficacy may decrease.

Nursing considerations
- Monitor levels of both drugs carefully. Normal theophylline level is 10 to 20 mcg/ml for adults and 5 to 15 mcg/ml for children. Normal phenytoin level is 10 to 20 mcg.
- Assess the patient for increased respiratory distress and recurrence of seizures. Report findings to prescriber promptly; dosages may need to be adjusted.
- Interaction typically occurs within 5 days of starting combined use.

aminophylline ➡◀ quinolones
ciprofloxacin, norfloxacin

Risk rating: 2
Severity: Moderate   Onset: Delayed   Likelihood: Established

Cause
Hepatic metabolism of theophyllines, including aminophylline, may be inhibited.

Effect
Increased theophylline levels with toxicity may occur.

Nursing considerations
- Carefully monitor serum theophylline levels. Therapeutic serum levels are 10 to 20 mcg/ml; toxicity may occur at levels above 20 mcg/ml.
- Adjust dosage of aminophylline as needed to avoid theophylline toxicity.
- Watch for evidence of toxicity, such as tachycardia, anorexia, nausea, vomiting, diarrhea, seizures, restlessness, irritability, and headache.
- Describe adverse effects of aminophylline and signs of toxicity, and tell the patient to report them immediately to the prescriber.

aminophylline ➡◀ rifampin
Rifadin, Rimactane

Risk rating: 2
Severity: Moderate   Onset: Delayed   Likelihood: Established

Cause
GI and hepatic metabolism of theophyllines, including aminophylline, may be increased by rifampin.

Effect
Aminophylline efficacy may decrease.

Nursing considerations
■ Carefully monitor serum theophylline levels. Therapeutic serum levels are 10 to 20 mcg/ml; toxicity may occur at levels above 20 mcg/ml.
■ After rifampin is started, watch for increased pulmonary signs and symptoms.
■ Tell the patient to immediately report all concerns about drug efficacy to prescriber; dosage may need adjustment.

aminophylline ▶◀ thiabendazole
Mintezol

Risk rating: 2
Severity: Moderate   **Onset: Delayed**   **Likelihood: Suspected**

Cause
The exact cause of the interaction is unknown, but metabolic inhibition is suspected.

Effect
Theophylline levels may increase with possible toxicity.

Nursing considerations
■ Carefully monitor serum theophylline levels. Therapeutic serum levels are 10 to 20 mcg/ml; toxicity may occur at levels above 20 mcg/ml.
■ Watch for evidence of toxicity, such as tachycardia, anorexia, nausea, vomiting, diarrhea, seizures, restlessness, irritability, and headache.
■ Describe adverse effects of aminophylline and signs of toxicity, and tell the patient to report them immediately to the prescriber.

amiodarone ▶◀ cyclosporine
Cordarone, Pacerone   Gengraf, Neoral, Sandimmune

Risk rating: 2
Severity: Moderate   **Onset: Delayed**   **Likelihood: Suspected**

Cause
Amiodarone probably inhibits cyclosporine metabolism.

Effect
Cyclosporine level and risk of nephrotoxicity may increase.

Nursing considerations
■ Closely monitor cyclosporine level when amiodarone is started, stopped, or the dose is changed.
■ Because amiodarone has a long half-life, monitor cyclosporine level for several weeks after dosage changes.
■ Dosage reductions of cyclosporine (up to 50% in some cases) may be needed to keep cyclosporine level in the desired range.
■ Monitor BUN and creatinine levels and urine output.

---

amiodarone ▶◀ digoxin
Cordarone, Pacerone   Lanoxin

Risk rating: 1
Severity: Major   **Onset: Delayed**   **Likelihood: Probable**

Cause
The mechanism of this interaction is unknown.

Effect
Digoxin level and risk of toxicity may increase.

Nursing considerations
■ Watch for evidence of digoxin toxicity, such as arrhythmias, nausea, vomiting, and agitation.
■ Monitor digoxin level.
■ Digoxin dosage may need to be reduced during amiodarone treatment.
■ Because amiodarone has a long half-life, the effects of the interaction may persist after amiodarone is stopped.

---

amiodarone ▶◀ fentanyl
Cordarone, Pacerone   Sublimaze

Risk rating: 1
Severity: Major   **Onset: Rapid**   **Likelihood: Suspected**

Cause
The mechanism of this interaction is unknown.

Effect
The patient may develop profound bradycardia, sinus arrest, and hypotension.

Nursing considerations
■ It isn't known if these effects are related to fentanyl anesthesia or anesthesia in general; use together cautiously.

- Monitor hemodynamic function.
- Keep inotropic, chronotropic, and pressor support available.
- **ALERT** The bradycardia caused by this interaction usually doesn't respond to atropine.

amiodarone ▶◀ flecainide
Cordarone, Pacerone   Tambocor

Risk rating: 2
Severity: Moderate   Onset: Delayed   Likelihood: Suspected

Cause
Amiodarone decreases the metabolism of flecainide.

Effect
Plasma flecainide levels may be increased.

Nursing considerations
- **ALERT** Monitor the patient for prolonged QRS interval when giving both drugs together.
- Decrease flecainide dosage by 33% to 50% of what's recommended when the patient is also receiving amiodarone.
- The full extent of the interaction may not be seen for up to 2 weeks.
- Patients with heart failure may be at greater risk.

amiodarone ▶◀ macrolide antibiotics
Cordarone, Pacerone   azithromycin, clarithromycin, erythromycin, telithromycin

Risk rating: 1
Severity: Major   Onset: Delayed   Likelihood: Suspected

Cause
An additive increase in the QT interval is seen when administering a macrolide antibiotic and an antiarrhythmic agent such as amiodarone.

Effect
The risk of life-threatening cardiac arrhythmias, including torsades de pointes is increased.

Nursing considerations
- **ALERT** Monitor the patient for prolonged QT interval and torsades de pointes.

- This interaction may be more likely with telithromycin; avoid administering with antiarrhythmics.
- This interaction appears to be dose related.
- Instruct patient to let the prescriber know if he experiences dizziness, palpitations, or light-headedness.
- The QT interval returns to normal within 3 days of stopping the macrolide antibiotic.

---

amiodarone ➤◄ phenytoin
Cordarone, Pacerone   Dilantin

Risk rating: 2
Severity: Moderate   Onset: Delayed   Likelihood: Probable

Cause
Hydantoin metabolism may decrease. Amiodarone metabolism may increase.

Effect
Serum hydantoin level and risk of toxicity increase, and amiodarone level decreases.

Nursing considerations
- The therapeutic range of phenytoin is 10 to 20 mcg/ml. Patients with decreased protein binding may show signs of toxicity despite a "normal" phenytoin level. Free phenytoin level is a better indicator in these patients (range: 1 to 2 mcg/ml).
- **ALERT** Signs and symptoms of toxicity may progress in the following manner: nystagmus, ataxia, slurred speech, nausea, vomiting, lethargy, confusion, seizures, and coma.
- After adjusting dosage of either drug, the patient will need long-term monitoring because effects may be delayed several weeks.
- Watch for loss of amiodarone effect, including palpitations, shortness of breath, dizziness, and chest pain.

---

amiodarone ➤◄ procainamide
Cordarone, Pacerone   Procanbid, Pronestyl

Risk rating: 2
Severity: Moderate   Onset: Rapid   Likelihood: Probable

Cause
The mechanism of the interaction is unknown.

Effect
Amiodarone may increase serum procainamide levels.

Nursing considerations
■ Monitor serum procainamide levels after starting or adjusting amiodarone dosages.
■ Some patients may experience severe nausea and transient hypotension, necessitating a reduction in procainamide dosage.

---

amiodarone ►◄ **protease inhibitors**
Cordarone, Pacerone   atazanavir, indinavir, nelfinavir, ritonavir

Risk rating: 1
Severity: Major   **Onset: Delayed**   **Likelihood: Suspected**

Cause
Protease inhibitors inhibit the CYP3A4 metabolism of amiodarone.

Effect
Amiodarone level increases, raising the risk of toxicity.

Nursing considerations
⚡ **ALERT** Ritonavir and nelfinavir are contraindicated for use with amiodarone because of a large increase in amiodarone level.
■ Use other protease inhibitors cautiously; they may have a similar effect.
■ Increased amiodarone level may prolong the QT interval and cause life-threatening arrhythmias.
■ Monitor ECG and QTc interval closely during combined therapy.
■ Tell the patient to immediately report slowed pulse or fainting.

---

amiodarone ►◄ **quinidine**
Cordarone, Pacerone

Risk rating: 1
Severity: Major   **Onset: Rapid**   **Likelihood: Probable**

Cause
The mechanism of this interaction in unknown.

Effect
Risk of potentially fatal arrhythmias increases.

Nursing considerations
■ If possible, avoid combining quinidine and amiodarone.

■ If unavoidable, monitor ECG closely for prolonged QTc interval, increasing ventricular ectopy, and torsades de pointes.
■ Therapeutic range of quinidine is 2 to 6 mcg/ml. More specific assays have levels of less than 1 mcg/ml.
■ Monitor the patient for signs and symptoms of quinidine toxicity, including GI irritation, arrhythmias, hypotension, vertigo, and rash.
■ Advise the patient to report palpitations, shortness of breath, dizziness or fainting, and chest pain.
■ If amiodarone is stopped in a patient stabilized on combined therapy, the quinidine dosage may need to be increased.

amiodarone ➤◄ quinolones

Cordarone, Pacerone   gatifloxacin, levofloxacin, moxifloxacin, ofloxacin

Risk rating: 1
Severity: Major   **Onset: Delayed**   **Likelihood: Suspected**

Cause
The mechanism of this interaction is unknown.

Effect
Risk of life-threatening arrhythmias, including torsades de pointes, increases.

Nursing considerations
⚡ **ALERT** Use of sparfloxacin with an antiarrhythmic, such as amiodarone, is contraindicated.
■ Quinolones that aren't metabolized by CYP3A4 isoenzymes or that don't prolong the QT interval may be given with antiarrhythmics.
■ Avoid giving class IA or class III antiarrhythmics with gatifloxacin, levofloxacin, and moxifloxacin.
■ Tell the patient to report a rapid heart rate, shortness of breath, dizziness, fainting, and chest pain.

amiodarone ➤◄ thioridazine

Cordarone, Pacerone

Risk rating: 1
Severity: Major   **Onset: Delayed**   **Likelihood: Suspected**

Cause
Synergistic or additive prolongation of the QTc interval may occur.

Effect
Risk of life-threatening arrhythmias, including torsades de pointes, increases.

Nursing considerations
⚠ **ALERT** The use of thioridazine and antiarrhythmic agents together is contraindicated.

■ If the patient is receiving thioridazine and amiodarone, notify the prescriber immediately.

■ Monitor the patient for other risk factors for torsades de pointes, including bradycardia, hypokalemia, and hypomagnesemia.

■ Ask the patient if he or anyone in his family has a history of prolonged QT interval or arrhythmias.

■ Monitor the patient for bradycardia.

---

amiodarone ▬▶◀▬ vardenafil
Cordarone, Pacerone   Levitra

Risk rating: 1
Severity: Major   **Onset: Rapid**   **Likelihood: Suspected**

Cause
The mechanism of this interaction is unknown.

Effect
The QTc interval may be prolonged, particularly in patients with previous QT-interval prolongation, increasing the risk of such life-threatening cardiac arrhythmias as torsades de pointes.

Nursing considerations
⚠ **ALERT** Use of vardenafil with amiodarone or another class IA or class III antiarrhythmic is contraindicated.

■ Monitor the patient's ECG before and periodically after the patient starts taking vardenafil.

■ Urge the patient to report light-headedness, faintness, palpitations, and chest pain or pressure while taking vardenafil.

■ To reduce risk of adverse effects, patients age 65 and older should start with 5 mg vardenafil, half the usual starting dose.

amiodarone ▶◀ **warfarin**
Cordarone, Pacerone   Coumadin

Risk rating: 1
Severity: Major   **Onset: Delayed**   **Likelihood: Established**

Cause
Amiodarone inhibits CYP1A2 and CYP2C9 metabolism of warfarin.

Effect
Anticoagulant effects increase.

Nursing considerations
■ Monitor the patient closely for bleeding. Urge compliance with required blood tests.
◤ ALERT Check INR closely during first 6 to 8 weeks of amiodarone therapy. Warfarin dosage reduction depends on escalating amiodarone dosage. Typically, warfarin dose needs 30% to 50% reduction.
■ If amiodarone is stopped, these effects may persist for up to 4 months, requiring continual warfarin adjustment.
■ Tell the patient and family to watch for signs of bleeding or abnormal bruising and to call prescriber at once if they occur.
■ Advise the use of an electric razor and a soft toothbrush.
■ Tell the patient to wear or carry medical identification that says he is taking an anticoagulant.

amiodarone ▶◀ **ziprasidone**
Cordarone, Pacerone   Geodon

Risk rating: 1
Severity: Major   **Onset: Delayed**   **Likelihood: Suspected**

Cause
The mechanism of this interaction is unknown.

Effect
Risk of life-threatening arrhythmias, including torsades de pointes, increases.

Nursing considerations
◤ ALERT Use of ziprasidone with certain antiarrhythmics is contraindicated.
■ Monitor the patient for other risk factors for torsades de pointes, including bradycardia, hypokalemia, and hypomagnesemia.
■ Ask the patient if he or anyone in his family has a history of prolonged QT interval or arrhythmias.

- Monitor the patient for bradycardia.
- Measure the QTc interval at baseline and throughout therapy.

---

amitriptyline ▶◀ azole antifungals
fluconazole, ketoconazole

Risk rating: 2
Severity: Moderate   **Onset: Delayed**   **Likelihood: Suspected**

Cause
Azole antifungals may inhibit metabolism of tricyclic antidepressants (TCAs) such as amitriptyline.

Effect
Serum TCA level and risk of toxicity may increase.

Nursing considerations
- When starting or stopping an azole antifungal, monitor serum TCA level and adjust dosage as needed.
- After starting an azole antifungal, check sitting and standing blood pressure for changes.
- If the patient takes a TCA and an azole antifungal, assess symptoms and behavior for evidence of adverse reactions, such as increased drowsiness, dizziness, confusion, heart rate or rhythm changes, and urine retention.

---

amitriptyline ▶◀ carbamazepine
Tegretol, Carbatrol, Epitol, Equetro

Risk rating: 2
Severity: Moderate   **Onset: Delayed**   **Likelihood: Probable**

Cause
Tricyclic antidepressants (TCAs), such as amitriptyline, may compete with carbamazepine for hepatic metabolism. Carbamazepine may induce hepatic metabolism.

Effect
TCA level and effects may decrease. Carbamazepine levels and risk of toxicity may increase.

Nursing considerations
- Other TCAs may interact with carbamazepine. If you suspect a drug interaction, consult the prescriber or pharmacist.
- Monitor carbamazepine level; therapeutic range is 4 to 12 mcg/ml.

■ Watch for evidence of carbamazepine toxicity, including dizziness, ataxia, respiratory depression, tachycardia, arrhythmias, blood pressure changes, impaired consciousness, abnormal reflexes, nystagmus, seizures, nausea, vomiting, and urine retention.

amitriptyline ➤◀ cimetidine
Tagamet

Risk rating: 2
Severity: Moderate   **Onset: Rapid**   **Likelihood: Probable**

Cause
Cimetidine may interfere with metabolism of tricyclic antidepressants (TCAs), such as amitriptyline.

Effect
TCA level and bioavailability increase.

Nursing considerations
■ Monitor serum TCA level and adjust dosage as prescribed.
■ If needed, consult prescriber about possible change from cimetidine to ranitidine.
■ Urge the patient and family to watch for—and report— dizziness, drowsiness, psychosis, and increased anticholinergic effects (such as blurred vision, constipation, dry mouth, and difficulty urinating).

amitriptyline ➤◀ fluoxetine
Prozac, Sarafem

Risk rating: 2
Severity: Moderate   **Onset: Delayed**   **Likelihood: Probable**

Cause
Fluoxetine may inhibit hepatic metabolism of tricyclic antidepressants (TCAs) such as amitriptyline.

Effect
Serum TCA level and toxicity may increase.

Nursing considerations
■ Monitor TCA level; watch for evidence of toxicity, such as increased anticholinergic effects (such as blurred vision, constipation, dry mouth and difficulty urinating), along with delirium, dizziness, drowsiness, and psychosis.
■ If a TCA is started when the patient already takes fluoxetine, TCA dosage may need to be decreased by up to 75% to avoid interaction.

■ Other TCAs may interact with fluoxetine. If you suspect an interaction, consult prescriber or pharmacist.

amitriptyline ▸◀ fluvoxamine
Luvox

Risk rating: 2
Severity: Moderate **Onset: Delayed** **Likelihood: Probable**

Cause
Fluvoxamine may inhibit oxidative metabolism of tricyclic antidepressants (TCAs), such as amitriptyline, via the CYP2D6 pathway.

Effect
TCA level and risk of toxicity increase.

Nursing considerations
■ When starting or stopping fluvoxamine, monitor serum TCA level.
■ Inhibitory effects of fluvoxamine may take up to 2 weeks to dissipate after drug is stopped.
■ Using desipramine instead of amitriptyline may avoid this interaction.
■ Urge the patient and family to watch for and report increased anticholinergic effects, and dizziness, drowsiness, and psychosis.

amitriptyline ▸◀ MAO inhibitors
isocarboxazid, phenelzine, tranylcypromine

Risk rating: 1
Severity: Major **Onset: Rapid** **Likelihood: Suspected**

Cause
The mechanism of this interaction is unknown.

Effect
The risk of hyperpyretic crisis, seizures, and death increase.

Nursing considerations
◪ **ALERT** Don't give a tricyclic antidepressant (TCA), such as amitriptyline, with or within 2 weeks of an MAO inhibitor.
■ Watch for adverse effects, including confusion, hyperexcitability, rigidity, seizures, increased temperature, increased pulse, increased respiration, sweating, mydriasis, flushing, headache, coma, and DIC.

amitriptyline 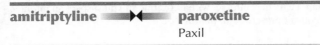 paroxetine
Paxil

Risk rating: 2
Severity: Moderate   Onset: Delayed   Likelihood: Suspected

Cause
Paroxetine may decrease metabolism of tricyclic antidepressants (TCAs), such as amitriptyline, in some people and increase it in others.

Effect
Therapeutic and toxic effects of certain TCAs may increase.

Nursing considerations
■ When starting or stopping paroxetine, monitor TCA level and adjust dosage as needed.
■ If the patient takes a TCA and paroxetine, assess symptoms and behavior for adverse reactions, such as increased drowsiness, dizziness, confusion, heart rate or rhythm changes, and urine retention.
■ Watch closely for evidence of serotonin syndrome, such as delirium, bizarre movements, and tachycardia. Alert the prescriber if they occur.

amitriptyline 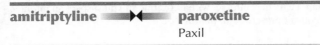 sertraline
Zoloft

Risk rating: 2
Severity: Moderate   Onset: Delayed   Likelihood: Suspected

Cause
Hepatic metabolism of tricyclic antidepressants (TCAs), such as amitriptyline, by CYP2D6 may be inhibited.

Effect
Therapeutic and toxic effects of certain TCAs may increase.

Nursing considerations
■ If possible, avoid this drug combination.
■ If these drugs must be used together, watch for evidence of TCA toxicity and serotonin syndrome.
■ Signs of serotonin syndrome include delirium, bizarre movements, and tachycardia.
■ Monitor serum TCA levels when starting or stopping sertraline.
■ If abnormalities occur, decrease TCA dosage or stop drug.

amitriptyline ━━━━▶◀━━━━ sympathomimetics

epinephrine, norepinephrine, phenylephrine

Risk rating: 2
Severity: Moderate   Onset: Rapid   Likelihood: Established

Cause
Tricyclic antidepressants (TCAs), such as amitriptyline, increase the effects of direct-acting sympathomimetics and decrease the effects of indirect-acting sympathomimetics.

Effect
When sympathomimetic effects increase, the risk of hypertension and arrhythmias increases. When sympathomimetic effects decrease, blood pressure control decreases.

Nursing considerations
■ If possible, avoid using these drugs together.
■ Watch the patient closely for hypertension and heart rhythm changes; they may warrant reduction of sympathomimetic dosage.
■ Other TCAs and sympathomimetics may interact. If you suspect an interaction, consult the prescriber or pharmacist.

amitriptyline ━━━━▶◀━━━━ terbinafine

Lamisil

Risk rating: 2
Severity: Moderate   Onset: Delayed   Likelihood: Suspected

Cause
Hepatic metabolism of tricyclic antidepressants (TCAs), such as amitriptyline, may be inhibited.

Effect
Therapeutic and toxic effects of certain TCAs may increase.

Nursing considerations
■ Check for toxic TCA level, and report abnormal level.
■ TCA dosage may need to be decreased.
■ Adverse effects or toxicity may include vertigo, fatigue, loss of appetite, ataxia, muscle twitching, and trouble swallowing.
■ Terbinafine's inhibitory effects may take several weeks to dissipate after drug is stopped.
■ Describe signs and symptoms the patient should look for.

amitriptyline ━━▶◀━━ valproic acid

divalproex sodium, valproate
sodium, valproic acid

Risk rating: 2
Severity: Moderate   **Onset: Delayed**   **Likelihood: Suspected**

Cause
Valproic acid may inhibit hepatic metabolism of tricyclic antidepressants (TCAs) such as amitriptyline.

Effect
Level and adverse effects of TCAs may increase.

Nursing considerations
- Use these drugs together cautiously.
- If the patient is stable on valproic acid, start TCA at reduced dosage and adjust upward slowly to address symptoms and serum level.
- If the patient is stable on a TCA, monitor serum level and patient status closely when starting or stopping valproic acid.
- Explain signs and symptoms to watch for.
- Other TCAs may interact with valproic acid. If you suspect an interaction, consult the prescriber or pharmacist.

amoxicillin ━━▶◀━━ amiloride

Amoxil

Risk rating: 3
Severity: Minor   **Onset: Delayed**   **Likelihood: Suspected**

Cause
Amiloride interferes with the sodium-hydrogen exchanger, which reduces absorption of amoxicillin.

Effect
Amoxicillin efficacy may be reduced.

Nursing considerations
- Monitor the patient for a decreased response to amoxicillin if also taking amiloride.
- Consult with the prescriber about the need to increase the dose of amoxicillin if decreased therapeutic activity is suspected.
- This interaction isn't noted with I.V. administration of amoxicillin—only oral administration.

amoxicillin 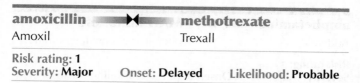 methotrexate
Amoxil   Trexall

Risk rating: 1
Severity: Major   **Onset: Delayed**   **Likelihood: Probable**

Cause
Methotrexate secretion in the renal tubules is inhibited.

Effect
Methotrexate level and risk of toxicity increase.

Nursing considerations
- Monitor the patient for methotrexate toxicity, including renal failure, neutropenia, leukopenia, thrombocytopenia, increased liver function tests, and skin ulcers.
- Monitor the patient for mouth sores. This may be the first outward appearance of methotrexate toxicity; however, in some patients, bone marrow suppression coincides with or precedes mouth sores.
- Obtain methotrexate level twice weekly for the first two weeks.
- Dose and duration of leucovorin rescue may need to be increased.
- Consider using ceftazidime instead of a penicillin if the patient needs broad-spectrum antibiotic.

amoxicillin 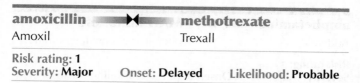 tetracyclines
Amoxil   doxycycline, tetracycline

Risk rating: 1
Severity: Major   **Onset: Delayed**   **Likelihood: Suspected**

Cause
Tetracyclines may disrupt bactericidal activity of penicillins such as amoxicillin.

Effect
Penicillin efficacy may be reduced.

Nursing considerations
- If possible, avoid giving a tetracyclines with a penicillin.
- Monitor the patient closely for lack of penicillin effect.

amphetamine ▸◂ MAO inhibitors

Adderall   phenelzine, tranylcypromine

Risk rating: 1
Severity: Major   **Onset: Rapid**   **Likelihood: Suspected**

Cause
This interaction probably stems from increased norepinephrine level at the synaptic cleft.

Effect
Anorexiant effects increase.

Nursing considerations
■ If possible, avoid giving these drugs together.
■ Headache and severe hypertension may occur rapidly if amphetamine is given to a patient who takes an MAO inhibitor.
⚠ **ALERT** Several deaths have been attributed to this kind of drug-induced hypertensive crisis and the resulting cerebral hemorrhage.
■ Monitor the patient for hypotension, hyperpyrexia, and seizures.
■ Hypertensive reaction may occur for several weeks after stopping an MAO inhibitor.

amphetamine ▸◂ serotonin reuptake inhibitors

Adderall   citalopram, fluoxetine, venlafaxine

Risk rating: 2
Severity: Moderate   **Onset: Rapid**   **Likelihood: Suspected**

Cause
The mechanism of this interaction is unknown.

Effect
Sympathomimetic effects and the risk of serotonin syndrome increase.

Nursing considerations
■ If these drugs must be used together, watch closely for increased CNS effects, such as anxiety, jitteriness, agitation, and restlessness.
■ Mild serotonin-like symptoms may develop, including confusion, diaphoresis, restlessness, tremor, and muscle twitching.
■ Inform the patient of the risk of interaction.

- Make sure the patient can recognize the traits of serotonin syndrome, including confusion, restlessness, incoordination, muscle rigidity, fever, sweating, and tremors.

amphetamine ◼◼◼►◄◼◼◼ urine alkalinizers

Adderall

potassium citrate, sodium acetate, sodium bicarbonate, sodium citrate, sodium lactate, tromethamine

Risk rating: 2
Severity: Moderate   **Onset: Rapid**   **Likelihood: Established**

Cause
When urine is alkaline, amphetamine clearance is prolonged.

Effect
In amphetamine overdose, the toxic period is extended, increasing the risk of injury.

Nursing considerations
◣ **ALERT** Don't administer drugs that may alkalinize the urine, particularly during amphetamine overdose.
- Watch for evidence of amphetamine toxicity, such as dermatoses, marked insomnia, irritability, hyperactivity, and personality changes.
- If the patient takes an anorexiant, advise against excessive use of sodium bicarbonate as an antacid.

ampicillin ◼◼◼►◄◼◼◼ allopurinol

Principen

Aloprim, Zyloprim

Risk rating: 2
Severity: Moderate   **Onset: Delayed**   **Likelihood: Suspected**

Cause
The mechanism of this interaction is unknown.

Effect
Risk of ampicillin-induced rash increases.

Nursing considerations
- Penicillins other than ampicillin may have a similar interaction with allopurinol. Discuss any concerns with the prescriber or pharmacist.
◣ **ALERT** Notify the prescriber if a rash appears. A lower dose of allopurinol or a different drug may be needed.

■ Inform the patient of this interaction so he can watch for—and report—skin changes.

---

ampicillin ▬▬▶◀▬▬ aminoglycosides
Principen   amikacin, gentamicin,
                                                   tobramycin

Risk rating: 2
Severity: Moderate   **Onset: Delayed**   **Likelihood: Probable**

Cause
The mechanism of this interaction is unknown.

Effect
Penicillins, such as ampicillin, may inactivate certain aminoglycosides, decreasing their therapeutic effects.

Nursing considerations
◪ **ALERT** Check peak and trough aminoglycoside levels after third dose. For peak level, draw blood 30 minutes after I.V. dose or 60 minutes after I.M. dose. For trough level, draw blood just before a dose.
■ Monitor the patient's renal function.
■ Other aminoglycosides may interact with penicillins. If you suspect an interaction, consult the prescriber or pharmacist.
■ Penicillins affect gentamicin and tobramycin more than amikacin.

---

ampicillin ▬▬▶◀▬▬ atenolol
Principen   Tenormin

Risk rating: 2
Severity: Moderate   **Onset: Rapid**   **Likelihood: Suspected**

Cause
Ampicillin may impair GI absorption of atenolol.

Effect
Usual blood pressure lowering and antianginal effects of atenolol may be decreased.

Nursing considerations
■ Beta blockers other than atenolol and penicillins other than ampicillin may have this interaction. If you suspect a drug interaction, consult the prescriber or pharmacist.
■ Suggest that the patient separate doses to decrease GI interaction.

■ Notify the prescriber if blood pressure increases; atenolol dosage may be increased or ampicillin broken into smaller, more frequent doses.

■ Teach the patient to report increased episodes or severity of chest pain to the prescriber immediately.

ampicillin ■■■■■▶◀■■■■ food
Principen

Risk rating: 2
Severity: Moderate   Onset: Delayed   Likelihood: Suspected

Cause
Food may delay or reduce GI absorption of certain penicillins such as ampicillin.

Effect
Penicillin efficacy may decrease.

Nursing considerations
■ Food may affect penicillin absorption and peak level.
■ If the patient took ampicillin with food, watch for lack of drug efficacy.
■ Tell the patient to take penicillins 1 hour before or 2 hours after a meal.
■ Other penicillins may interact with food. If you suspect an interaction, consult the prescriber or pharmacist.

amprenavir ■■■■■▶◀■■■■ azole antifungals
Agenerase   fluconazole, itraconazole, ketoconazole

Risk rating: 2
Severity: Moderate   Onset: Delayed   Likelihood: Suspected

Cause
Azole antifungals may inhibit metabolism of protease inhibitors such as amprenavir.

Effect
Protease inhibitor plasma level may increase.

Nursing considerations
■ Protease inhibitor dosage may be decreased when azole antifungal therapy starts.

- Monitor the patient for increased protease inhibitor effects, including hyperglycemia, rash, GI complaints, and altered liver function tests.
- Advise the patient to report increased hunger or thirst, frequent urination, fatigue, and dry, itchy skin.
- Tell the patient not to change dosage or stop either drug without consulting prescriber.
- To help avoid interactions, urge the patient to tell prescribers about all drugs and supplements he is taking.

amprenavir ▶◀ delavirdine
Agenerase   Rescriptor

Risk rating: 2
Severity: Moderate   Onset: Delayed   Likelihood: Suspected

Cause
Amprenavir may induce CYP3A4 metabolism of delavirdine. Delavirdine may inhibit CYP3A4 metabolism of amprenavir.

Effect
Amprenavir level may increase. Delavirdine level may decrease.

Nursing considerations
- Monitor the patient for a decreased response to delavirdine.
- Tell the patient the most common adverse reactions from this interaction are headache, fatigue, rash, and GI complaints.
- Caution the patient to notify the prescriber if adverse effects are bothersome, making it clear he isn't to alter his treatment regimen without medical consent.
- Urge the patient to tell the prescriber about all drugs and supplements he is taking because this will help him avoid dangerous interactions.

amprenavir ▶◀ ergot derivatives
Agenerase   dihydroergotamine, ergonovine, ergotamine, methylergonovine

Risk rating: 1
Severity: Major   Onset: Delayed   Likelihood: Probable

Cause
Protease inhibitors, such as amprenavir, may interfere with CYP3A4 metabolism of ergot derivatives.

Effect
Risk of ergot-induced peripheral vasospasm and ischemia may increase.

Nursing considerations
◼ **ALERT** Use of ergot derivatives with protease inhibitors is contraindicated.
◼ Monitor the patient for evidence of peripheral ischemia, including pain in limb muscles while exercising and later at rest; numbness and tingling of fingers and toes; cool, pale, or cyanotic limbs; red or violet blisters on hands or feet; and gangrene.
◼ Sodium nitroprusside may be used to treat ergot-induced vasospasm.
◼ If the patient takes a protease inhibitor, consult the prescriber and pharmacist about alternative migraine treatments.
◼ Advise the patient to tell the prescriber about all drugs and supplements he is taking and any increase in adverse effects.

amprenavir ◼◼◼◼▶◀◼◼◼ pimozide
Agenerase   Orap

Risk rating: 1
Severity: Major   **Onset: Delayed**   **Likelihood: Suspected**

Cause
Protease inhibitors, such as amprenavir, may inhibit CYP3A4 metabolism of pimozide.

Effect
Risk of life-threatening arrhythmias may increase.

Nursing considerations
◼ **ALERT** Combined use of these drugs is contraindicated.
◼ Arrhythmias are related to prolonged QT interval, a known risk of pimozide.
◼ Interaction warning is based on pharmacokinetics of these drugs, not actual patient studies.

amprenavir ◼◼◼◼▶◀◼◼◼ rifamycins
Agenerase   rifabutin, rifampin

Risk rating: 2
Severity: Moderate   **Onset: Delayed**   **Likelihood: Suspected**

Cause
Amprenavir may decrease CYP3A4 metabolism of rifabutin. Rifampin may increase CYP3A4 metabolism of amprenavir.

Effect
Amprenavir level, effects, and risk of adverse effects may increase.

Nursing considerations
◪ **ALERT** Use of amprenavir with rifampin is contraindicated.
■ If the patient takes amprenavir with rifabutin, watch for adverse reactions.
■ When administering amprenavir and rifabutin, considering decreasing the dose of rifabutin by 50%.
■ Tell the patient he may develop diarrhea, fever, headache, muscle pain, or nausea but not to alter regimen without consulting prescriber.
■ To minimize interactions, urge the patient to tell the prescriber about all drugs and supplements he is taking.

---

amprenavir ▶◀ sildenafil
Agenerase   Viagra

Risk rating: 1
Severity: Major   **Onset: Rapid**   **Likelihood: Suspected**

Cause
Sildenafil metabolism is inhibited.

Effect
Sildenafil level may increase, possibly leading to fatal hypotension.

Nursing considerations
◪ **ALERT** Tell the patient to take sildenafil exactly as prescribed.
■ Dosage of sildenafil may be reduced to 25 mg, and an interval of at least 48 hours between doses may be needed.
■ Warn the patient about potentially fatal low blood pressure if these drugs are taken together.
■ Tell the patient to notify his prescriber if he has dizziness, fainting, or chest pain during use together.

---

amprenavir ▶◀ St. John's wort
Agenerase

Risk rating: 1
Severity: Major   **Onset: Delayed**   **Likelihood: Suspected**

Cause
Hepatic metabolism of protease inhibitors, such as amprenavir, may increase.

Effect
Protease inhibitor level and effects may decrease.

Nursing considerations
⚠ **ALERT** Use of St. John's wort and protease inhibitors together is contraindicated.
■ Tell the patient not to alter HIV regimen without consulting prescriber.
■ To help avoid interactions, urge the patient to tell prescribers about all drugs, supplements, and alternative therapies he uses.

---

aprepitant ■■■■■►◄■■■■■ **corticosteroids**
Emend   dexamethasone,
                               methylprednisolone

Risk rating: 2
Severity: Moderate   **Onset: Delayed**   **Likelihood: Suspected**

Cause
Aprepitant may inhibit first-pass metabolism of certain corticosteroids.

Effect
Corticosteroid level may be increased and the half-life prolonged.

Nursing considerations
■ Corticosteroid dosage may need to be decreased.
■ When starting or stopping aprepitant, adjust corticosteroid dosage as needed.
■ Watch closely for evidence of increased corticosteroid level, such as insomnia, euphoria, increased appetite, mood changes, and increased blood glucose level.
■ Tell the patient to report symptoms of increased blood glucose level, including increased thirst or hunger and increased frequency of urination.

---

aprepitant ■■■■■►◄■■■■ **pimozide**
Emend   Orap

Risk rating: 1
Severity: Major   **Onset: Delayed**   **Likelihood: Suspected**

Cause
Aprepitant may inhibit CYP3A4 metabolism of pimozide.

Effect
Risk of life-threatening arrhythmias may increase.

Nursing considerations
◈ ALERT Combined use of these drugs is contraindicated.
- Arrhythmias are related to prolonged QT interval, a known risk of pimozide.
- Interaction warning is based on pharmacokinetics of these drugs, not actual patient studies.

---

aripiprazole ▸◂ azole antifungals
Abilify   itraconazole, ketoconazole

Risk rating: 2
Severity: Moderate   Onset: Delayed   Likelihood: Suspected

Cause
Azole antifungals may inhibit CYP3A4 metabolism of aripiprazole.

Effect
Plasma concentrations of aripiprazole may be increased, thereby increasing pharmacologic and adverse effects.

Nursing considerations
- When azole antifungals are administered with aripiprazole, reduce the dose of aripiprazole by 50%.
- The dose of aripiprazole will need to be increased when the azole antifungal is discontinued.
- Instruct patient to notify the prescriber of increased adverse effects, such as anxiety, insomnia, nausea and vomiting, and flu-like symptoms.

---

aripiprazole ▸◂ carbamazepine
Abilify   Carbatrol, Epitol, Equetro, Tegretol

Risk rating: 2
Severity: Moderate   Onset: Delayed   Likelihood: Suspected

Cause
Carbamazepine may increase CYP3A4 metabolism of aripiprazole.

Effect
Plasma concentrations of aripiprazole may be decreased, thereby decreasing pharmacologic effects.

Nursing considerations
- When carbamazepine is administered with aripiprazole, double the dose of aripiprazole.

- The dose of aripiprazole may need to be decreased when carbamazepine is discontinued.
- Monitor patient response to aripiprazole. and notify the prescriber if a decreased response to aripiprazole is noticed.
- Instruct the patient to notify the prescriber immediately if he notices a decrease in aripiprazole effects.

aripiprazole ▶◀ quinidine
Abilify

Risk rating: 2
Severity: Moderate   Onset: Delayed   Likelihood: Suspected

Cause
Quinidine may inhibit CYP3A4 metabolism of aripiprazole.

Effect
Plasma concentrations of aripiprazole may be increased, thereby increasing pharmacologic and adverse effects.

Nursing considerations
- When quinidine is administered with aripiprazole, reduce the dose of aripiprazole by 50%.
- The dose of aripiprazole will need to be increased when quinidine is discontinued.
- Instruct the patient to notify the prescriber of increased adverse effects, such as anxiety, insomnia, nausea and vomiting, and flu-like symptoms.

aspirin ▶◀ ACE inhibitors
Bayer   captopril, enalapril,
                       lisinopril, moexipril, ramipril

Risk rating: 2
Severity: Moderate   Onset: Rapid   Likelihood: Suspected

Cause
Salicylates, such as aspirin, inhibit synthesis of prostaglandins, which ACE inhibitors need to lower blood pressure.

Effect
The ACE inhibitor's hypotensive effect is reduced.

Nursing considerations
- This interaction is more likely in people with hypertension, coronary artery disease, or possibly heart failure.

■ At doses less than 100 mg daily, aspirin is less likely to interact.

aspirin ◄►◄ acetazolamide
Bayer   Diamox

Risk rating: 2
Severity: Moderate   Onset: Delayed   Likelihood: Suspected

Cause
Aspirin displaces the carbonic anhydrase inhibitor from protein-binding sites and inhibits renal clearance. As a result, carbonic anhydrase inhibitor accumulates, causing acidosis and increased risk of salicylate penetration into the CNS.

Effect
Carbonic anhydrase inhibitor level and risk of toxicity increase.

Nursing considerations
■ Minimize or avoid using a salicylate, such as aspirin, with a carbonic anhydrase inhibitor.
■ If drugs must be given together, monitor the patient for evidence of toxicity, including lethargy, confusion, fatigue, anorexia, urinary incontinence, tachypnea, and hyperchloremic metabolic acidosis.
■ Chronic salicylate values higher than 15 mg/dl may produce toxicity. Symptoms may appear in days to weeks.
■ Elderly patients and those with renal impairment are at greatest risk of toxic effects.

aspirin ◄►◄ beta blockers
Bayer   carvedilol, pindolol,
                         propranolol

Risk rating: 2
Severity: Moderate   Onset: Rapid   Likelihood: Suspected

Cause
Salicylates, such as aspirin, inhibit synthesis of prostaglandins, which beta blockers need to lower blood pressure. In patients with heart failure, the mechanism of this interaction is unknown.

Effect
Beta blocker effects will decrease.

Nursing considerations
■ Watch the patient closely for signs of heart failure and hypertension.

■ Beta blockers may interact with other salicylates. If you suspect an interaction, consult the prescriber or pharmacist.
■ Explain signs and symptoms of heart failure, and tell the patient when to contact the prescriber.

---

aspirin ▶◀ clopidogrel
Bayer   Plavix

Risk rating: 1
Severity: Major   **Onset: Delayed**   **Likelihood: Probable**

Cause
The exact mechanism of the interaction is unknown, but the effects of aspirin on the GI mucosa may be a risk factor.

Effect
Risk of life-threatening bleeding may be increased in high-risk patients.

Nursing considerations
⚠ ALERT Avoid the use of aspirin and clopidogrel together in high-risk patients with recent ischemic stroke or transient ischemic attack.
■ If the patient is receiving aspirin and clopidogrel together, monitor for signs of GI bleeding or increased intracranial pressure and bleeding.
■ Explain signs and symptoms of bleeding, and tell the patient when to contact the prescriber.
■ The use of aspirin and clopidogrel isn't contraindicated in patients who aren't high risk, but combined use will increase the bleeding time.

---

aspirin ▶◀ corticosteroids
Bayer   dexamethasone, hydrocortisone, methylprednisolone, prednisolone, prednisone

Risk rating: 2
Severity: Moderate   **Onset: Delayed**   **Likelihood: Probable**

Cause
Corticosteroids stimulate hepatic metabolism of salicylates, such as aspirin, and may increase renal excretion.

Effect
Salicylate level and effects decrease.

Nursing considerations
■ Monitor salicylate level; dosage may need adjustment.
⚠ **ALERT** Giving a salicylate while tapering a corticosteroid may result in salicylate toxicity.
■ Watch for evidence of salicylate toxicity, including diaphoresis, nausea, vomiting, tinnitus, hyperventilation, and CNS depression.
■ Patients with renal impairment may be at greater risk.

---

aspirin ➤◄ heparin sodium
Bayer

Risk rating: 1
Severity: Moderate   **Onset: Rapid**   **Likelihood: Probable**

Cause
Aspirin may inhibit platelet aggregation and cause bleeding, adding to heparin's anticoagulation effects.

Effect
Risk of bleeding increases.

Nursing considerations
■ Monitor the patient for signs of bleeding, including bleeding gums, bruises on arms or legs, petechiae, epistaxis, melena, hematuria, and hematemesis.
■ Urge the patient to tell the prescriber about all drugs and supplements he is taking and about any increase in adverse effects.
■ The interaction can persist for up to 24 hours after the discontinuation of heparin.

---

aspirin ➤◄ insulin
Bayer

Risk rating: 2
Severity: Moderate   **Onset: Delayed**   **Likelihood: Probable**

Cause
Basal insulin level is increased; salicylates enhance release of insulin in response to glucose.

Effect
Glucose-lowering effect of insulin may be potentiated.

Nursing considerations
■ Monitor glucose level closely if the patient who takes insulin starts a salicylate.

- Watch for evidence of hypoglycemia: tachycardia, palpitation, anxiety, diaphoresis, nausea, hunger, dizziness, restlessness, headache, confusion, tremors, and speech and motor dysfunction.
- Consult the prescriber if the patient experiences hypoglycemia; insulin dosage may need to be decreased.
- Treat hypoglycemia as needed, such as with fast-acting oral carbohydrates, parenteral glucagon, or I.V. $D_{50}W$ bolus.
- Urge the patient to tell the prescriber about increased adverse effects.
- Make sure the patient and family can recognize hypoglycemia and respond appropriately.

aspirin ▶◀ ketorolac
Bayer   Toradol

Risk rating: 1
Severity: Major   **Onset: Delayed**   **Likelihood: Suspected**

Cause
Aspirin may displace ketorolac from protein-binding sites, increasing the level of unbound ketorolac.

Effect
Risk of serious ketorolac-related adverse effects increases.

Nursing considerations
◾ **ALERT** Ketorolac is contraindicated in patients taking aspirin.
- Watch for adverse effects, such as GI bleeding, neurotoxicity, renal failure, blood dyscrasias, and hepatotoxicity.
- Urge the patient to tell the prescriber and pharmacist about all drugs and supplements he is taking.

aspirin ▶◀ methotrexate
Bayer   Trexall

Risk rating: 1
Severity: Major   **Onset: Rapid**   **Likelihood: Suspected**

Cause
Renal clearance and plasma protein binding of methotrexate may be decreased by salicylates such as aspirin.

Effect
Methotrexate toxicity may occur.

Nursing considerations
■ Monitor the patient for methotrexate toxicity, including renal failure, neutropenia, leukopenia, thrombocytopenia, increased liver function tests, and skin ulcers.
■ Monitor the patient for mouth sores. This may be the first outward appearance of methotrexate toxicity; however, in some patients, bone marrow suppression coincides with or precedes mouth sores.
■ Notify the prescriber if signs of toxicity appear; the methotrexate dose may need to be reduced.

---

aspirin ▶◀	NSAIDs
Bayer	fenoprofen, flurbiprofen, indomethacin, meclofenamate, naproxen, tolmetin

Risk rating: 1
Severity: Major   **Onset: Delayed**   **Likelihood: Suspected**

Cause
Increased metabolism and displaced protein binding of the NSAID may occur.

Effect
Pharmacologic effects of NSAIDs may be decreased. The cardioprotective effect of low-dose, uncoated aspirin may be decreased. Aspirin and NSAIDs are also gastric irritants.

Nursing considerations
■ If possible, use analgesics that don't interfere with the platelet effect for pain control, such as acetaminophen, in place of NSAIDs.
■ If possible, administer the NSAID 8 hours before, or 30 minutes after, immediate-release aspirin.
■ Monitor the patient for signs of bleeding, including bleeding gums, bruises on arms or legs, petechiae, epistaxis, melena, hematuria, and hematemesis.
■ Instruct the patient to notify the prescriber if he notices increased bleeding or bruising.
■ Occasional use of NSAIDs for pain relief won't cause a problematic interaction with aspirin—only regular, long-term use.

aspirin ━━━━▶◀━━━ probenecid
Bayer   Probalan

Risk rating: 2
Severity: Moderate   Onset: Delayed   Likelihood: Probable

Cause
The mechanism of this interaction is unknown. It may stem from altered renal filtration of uric acid.

Effect
Uricosuric action of both drugs is inhibited.

Nursing considerations
■ Typically, giving probenecid with a salicylate, such as aspirin, is contraindicated.
■ Occasional use of aspirin at low doses may not interfere with the uricosuric action of probenecid.
■ Monitor serum urate level; the usual goal of probenecid therapy is about 6 mg/dl.
◪ **ALERT** Remind the patient to carefully read the labels of OTC medicines because many contain salicylates.
■ If an analgesic or antipyretic is needed during probenecid therapy, suggest acetaminophen.
■ Advise adequate fluid intake to prevent uric acid kidney stones.

aspirin ━━━━▶◀━━━ sulfinpyrazone
Bayer   Anturane

Risk rating: 2
Severity: Moderate   Onset: Delayed   Likelihood: Established

Cause
Salicylates, such as aspirin, block the effect of sulfinpyrazone on tubular reabsorption of uric acid, and they displace sulfinpyrazone from plasma protein-binding sites, decreasing sulfinpyrazone level.

Effect
Uricosuric effects of sulfinpyrazone are inhibited.

Nursing considerations
■ Typically, giving sulfinpyrazone with a salicylate is contraindicated.
■ Monitor serum urate level; the usual goal of sulfinpyrazone therapy is about 6 mg/dl.

⚡ **ALERT** Remind the patient to carefully read the labels of OTC medicines because many contain salicylates.
■ Encourage adequate fluid intake to prevent uric acid kidney stones.

aspirin ▶◀ sulfonylureas
Bayer

chlorpropamide, glyburide, tolbutamide

Risk rating: 2
Severity: Moderate   Onset: Delayed   Likelihood: Probable

Cause
Salicylates, such as aspirin, reduce glucose level and promote insulin secretion.

Effect
Hypoglycemic effects of sulfonylureas increase.

Nursing considerations
■ If the patient takes a sulfonylurea, start salicylate carefully, monitoring the patient for hypoglycemia.
■ Consult the prescriber and the patient about possibly replacing a salicylate with acetaminophen or an NSAID.
■ Make sure patient is aware of signs and symptoms of hypoglycemia, including diaphoresis, fatigue, headache, hunger, irritability, malaise, nervousness, rapid heart rate, tension, and trembling.
■ Instruct the patient to eat a small carbohydrate snack or meal if hypoglycemia develops, preferably after checking blood glucose level.

aspirin ▶◀ valproic acid
Bayer

Depakene

Risk rating: 2
Severity: Moderate   Onset: Delayed   Likelihood: Suspected

Cause
Salicylates, such as aspirin, displace valproic acid from its usual binding sites and may alter valproic acid metabolic pathways.

Effect
Toxicity of valproic acid may increase.

Nursing considerations
■ Check serum free fraction and serum valproic acid levels.
■ Hepatotoxic metabolites of valproic acid may be more likely to form.

- Watch for evidence of valproic acid toxicity, such as tremor, drowsiness, ataxia, nystagmus, and personality changes.
- Explain risks of combined use and signs of toxicity.

aspirin ▶◀ warfarin
Bayer   Coumadin

Risk rating: 1
Severity: Moderate   **Onset: Delayed**   **Likelihood: Established**

Cause
Anticoagulant activity increases; platelet aggregation decreases.

Effect
Risk of significant bleeding may increase.

Nursing considerations
⚡ ALERT Use together should be avoided.
- Monitor coagulation values closely.
- Aspirin doses of 500 mg or more daily increase risk of bleeding.
- Tell the patient to report unusual bruising or bleeding.
- Remind the patient that warfarin interacts with many drugs and that he should report any change in drug regimen.
- Explain that interaction can happen with topical or oral salicylates.
⚡ALERT Warfarin dose should be adjusted when aspirin is stopped.

atazanavir ▶◀ amiodarone
Reyataz   Pacerone, Cordarone

Risk rating: 1
Severity: Major   **Onset: Delayed**   **Likelihood: Suspected**

Cause
Protease inhibitors, such as atazanavir, inhibit the CYP3A4 metabolism of amiodarone.

Effect
Amiodarone level increases, increasing the risk of toxicity.

Nursing considerations
- Use other protease inhibitors cautiously; they may have a similar effect.
- Increased amiodarone level may prolong the QT interval and cause life-threatening arrhythmias.
- Monitor ECG and QTc interval closely during combined therapy.
- Tell the patient to immediately report slowed pulse or fainting.

atazanavir ▶◀ benzodiazepines

Reyataz

alprazolam, clorazepate, diazepam, estazolam, flurazepam, midazolam, triazolam

Risk rating: 1
Severity: Major   **Onset: Delayed**   **Likelihood: Suspected**

Cause
Protease inhibitors, such as atazanavir, may inhibit CYP3A4 metabolism of certain benzodiazepines.

Effect
Sedative effects of benzodiazepines may be increased and prolonged, leading to severe respiratory depression.

Nursing considerations
◗ ALERT Don't combine a protease inhibitor with alprazolam, clorazepate, diazepam, estazolam, flurazepam, midazolam, or triazolam.
■ If the patient takes any benzodiazepine–protease inhibitor combination, notify the prescriber. Interaction could involve other drugs in the class.

atazanavir ▶◀ ergot derivatives

Reyataz

dihydroergotamine, ergonovine, ergotamine, methylergonovine

Risk rating: 1
Severity: Major   **Onset: Delayed**   **Likelihood: Probable**

Cause
Protease inhibitors, such as atazanavir, may interfere with CYP3A4 metabolism of ergot derivatives.

Effect
Risk of ergot-induced peripheral vasospasm and ischemia may increase.

Nursing considerations
◗ ALERT Use of ergot derivatives with protease inhibitors is contraindicated.
■ Monitor the patient for evidence of peripheral ischemia, including pain in limb muscles while exercising and later at rest; numbness and

tingling of fingers and toes; cool, pale, or cyanotic limbs; red or violet blisters on hands or feet; and gangrene.
■ Sodium nitroprusside may be given for ergot-induced vasospasm.
■ If the patient takes a protease inhibitor, consult the prescriber or pharmacist about alternative treatments for migraine pain.
■ Advise the patient to tell the prescriber about all drugs and supplements he is taking and any increase in adverse effects.

atazanavir ████████►◄████ lovastatin
Reyataz   Mevacor, Altoprev

Risk rating: 1
Severity: Major   **Onset: Delayed**   **Likelihood: Suspected**

Cause
Protease inhibitors, such as atazanavir, inhibit the CYP3A4 metabolism of lovastatin.

Effect
Lovastatin level may increase.

Nursing considerations
◪ **ALERT** Atazanavir and lovastatin shouldn't be used together.
■ Use other protease inhibitors cautiously; they may have similar effect.
■ If a protease inhibitor is added to a regimen that includes lovastatin, monitor the patient closely.
◪ **ALERT** Watch for evidence of rhabdomyolysis, including dark or red urine, muscle weakness, and myalgia.
■ Urge the patient to immediately report unexplained muscle weakness.

atazanavir ████████►◄████ nonnucleoside reverse transcriptase inhibitors
Reyataz   efavirenz, nevirapine

Risk rating: 2
Severity: Moderate   **Onset: Delayed**   **Likelihood: Suspected**

Cause
The combination increases CYP3A4 metabolism of protease inhibitors, including atazanavir.

Effect
Atazanavir plasma levels and efficacy may be reduced.

Nursing considerations
- Monitor protease inhibitor levels and clinical response when an NNRT inhibitor is started or stopped.
- Adjust atazanavir dosage as needed.
- Tell the patient not to alter HIV regimen without consulting prescriber.

---

atazanavir ▬▬►◄▬▬ opioid analgesics
Reyataz   buprenorphine, fentanyl

Risk rating: 2
Severity: Moderate   Onset: Delayed   Likelihood: Suspected

Cause
Protease inhibitors such as atazanavir inhibit CYP3A4 metabolism of opioid analgesics in the GI tract and liver.

Effect
Adverse reactions of opioid analgesics, including respiratory depression, may increase.

Nursing considerations
- If the patient is receiving an opioid analgesic and atazanavir, monitor him for an extended period of time after receiving the opioid analgesic.
- **ALERT** Closely monitor the patient's respiratory function.
- It may be necessary to decrease the dose of opioid analgesic if the patient is receiving it continuously.
- Other protease inhibitors may have the same interaction.
- If the patient is receiving combination protease inhibitor therapy, the risk of increased adverse reactions increases.
- Adverse reactions improve when the dose of opioid analgesic is decreased.

---

atazanavir ▬▬►◄▬▬ pimozide
Reyataz   Orap

Risk rating: 1
Severity: Major   Onset: Delayed   Likelihood: Suspected

Cause
Protease inhibitors, such as atazanavir, may inhibit CYP3A4 metabolism of pimozide.

Effect
Risk of life-threatening arrhythmias may increase.

Nursing considerations
◀ **ALERT** Combined use of these drugs is contraindicated.
■ Arrhythmias are related to prolonged QT interval, a known risk of pimozide.
■ Other protease inhibitors may have the same interaction.
■ Interaction warning is based on pharmacokinetics of these drugs, not actual patient studies.

---

atazanavir ▬▬▶◀▬▬ **proton pump inhibitors**

Reyataz   esomeprazole, lansoprazole,
                            omeprazole, pantoprazole,
                            rabeprazole

Risk rating: 1
Severity: Major   **Onset: Delayed**   **Likelihood: Suspected**

Cause
GI absorption of protease inhibitors, including atazanavir, may be decreased.

Effect
Antiviral activity of atazanavir may be reduced.

Nursing considerations
■ Use of atazanavir and proton pump inhibitors is not recommended.
■ Monitor the patient for a decrease in antiviral activity.
■ Adjust the dose of the protease inhibitor as needed.

---

atazanavir ▬▬▶◀▬▬ **St. John's wort**

Reyataz

Risk rating: 1
Severity: Major   **Onset: Delayed**   **Likelihood: Suspected**

Cause
Hepatic metabolism of protease inhibitors, such as atazanavir, may increase.

Effect
Protease inhibitor level and effects may decrease.

Nursing considerations
■ If the patient starts or stops taking St. John's wort, monitor protease inhibitor level closely.
■ Monitor CD4+ and T-cell counts; tell prescriber if these counts decrease.
■ Urge the patient to report opportunistic infections.
■ Tell the patient not to change the HIV regimen without consulting prescriber.
■ Urge the patient to tell prescribers about all drugs, supplements, and alternative therapies he uses, to prevent the possibility of a harmful interaction among therapeutic agents.

atenolol ▶◀ aluminum salts
Tenormin

aluminum carbonate, aluminum hydroxide, aluminum phosphate, kaolin

Risk rating: 3
Severity: **Minor**   Onset: **Rapid**   Likelihood: **Suspected**

Cause
Rate of gastric emptying is decreased, leading to reduced bioavailability of atenolol.

Effect
Pharmacologic effects of beta blockers may be decreased.

Nursing considerations
■ Separate administration of aluminium salts and beta blockers by at least 2 hours.
■ Monitor the patient's blood pressure and heart rate.
■ Tell the patient to notify the prescriber if he notices an increase in his heart rate.

atenolol ▶◀ ampicillin
Tenormin

Principen

Risk rating: 2
Severity: **Moderate**   Onset: **Rapid**   Likelihood: **Suspected**

Cause
Ampicillin may impair GI absorption of atenolol.

Effect
Blood pressure-lowering and antianginal effects of atenolol may decrease.

Nursing considerations
■ Beta blockers other than atenolol and penicillins other than ampicillin may interact. If you suspect an interaction, consult the prescriber or pharmacist.
■ Monitor the patient's blood pressure, and assess for anginal symptoms during ampicillin therapy.
■ Suggest that the patient separate doses to decrease GI interaction.
■ Notify the prescriber if blood pressure increases; atenolol dosage may be increased or ampicillin broken into smaller, more frequent doses.
■ Teach the patient to tell the prescriber immediately about increased episodes or severity of chest pain.

---

atenolol ▶◀ clonidine
Tenormin   Catapres

Risk rating: 1
Severity: Major   **Onset: Delayed**   **Likelihood: Suspected**

Cause
The mechanism of this interaction is unclear.

Effect
Potentially life-threatening hypertension may occur.

Nursing considerations
■ Life-threatening hypertension may occur after simultaneously stopping clonidine and a beta blocker.
■ It's unknown whether hypertension is caused by an interaction or withdrawal syndrome linked to each drug.
■ Closely monitor blood pressure after starting or stopping the atenolol or clonidine.
■ When the patient stops combined therapy, gradually withdraw atenolol first to minimize adverse reactions.

---

atenolol ▶◀ lidocaine
Tenormin

Risk rating: 2
Severity: Moderate   **Onset: Rapid**   **Likelihood: Established**

Cause
Beta blockers, such as atenolol, reduce hepatic metabolism of lidocaine.

Effect
Lidocaine level and risk of toxicity may increase.

Nursing considerations
- Check for normal therapeutic level of lidocaine: 2 to 5 mcg/ml.
- Watch closely for evidence of lidocaine toxicity, including dizziness, somnolence, confusion, paresthesia, and seizures.
- Slow the I.V. bolus rate to decrease the risk of high peak level and toxic reactions.
- Explain the warning signs of toxicity to the patient and family, and tell them to contact the prescriber if they have concerns.

---

atenolol	►◄	NSAIDs
Tenormin		ibuprofen, indomethacin, naproxen, piroxicam

Risk rating: 2
Severity: **Moderate**   Onset: **Delayed**   Likelihood: **Probable**

Cause
NSAIDs may inhibit renal prostaglandin synthesis, allowing pressor systems to be unopposed.

Effect
Beta blockers, such as atenolol, may not be able to lower blood pressure.

Nursing considerations
- Avoid using these drugs together if possible.
- Monitor blood pressure and for other evidence of hypertension closely.
- Consult the prescriber about ways to reduce interaction, such as adjusting beta blocker dosage or switching to sulindac as the NSAID.
- Explain the risks of using these drugs together, and teach the patient how to monitor his own blood pressure.
- Other NSAIDs may interact with beta blockers. If you suspect an interaction, consult the prescriber or pharmacist.

---

atenolol	►◄	orange juice
Tenormin		

Risk rating: 2
Severity: **Moderate**   Onset: **Delayed**   Likelihood: **Suspected**

Cause
The mechanism of the interaction is unknown.

Effect
Plasma concentrations and pharmacologic effects of atenolol may be decreased.

Nursing considerations
■ Separate the administration of orange juice and atenolol as much as possible.
■ Monitor the patient's response to atenolol; the dose may need to be adjusted.
■ Monitor the patient's heart rate and blood pressure.
■ Tell the patient to monitor his heart rate and notify the prescriber about any significant increase.

---

atenolol ━━━━━━▶◀━━━━ **quinidine**
Tenormin

Risk rating: 2
Severity: Moderate   **Onset: Rapid**   **Likelihood: Suspected**

Cause
Quinidine may inhibit metabolism of certain beta blockers, such as atenolol, in those who are extensive metabolizers of debrisoquin.

Effect
Beta blocker effects may be increased.

Nursing considerations
■ Monitor pulse and blood pressure more often.
■ If pulse slows or blood pressure falls, consult prescriber. Beta blocker dosage may need to be decreased.
■ Teach the patient how to check blood pressure and pulse rate; tell him to do so regularly.

---

atenolol ━━━━━━▶◀━━━━ **verapamil**
Tenormin   Calan

Risk rating: 1
Severity: Major   **Onset: Rapid**   **Likelihood: Probable**

Cause
Verapamil may inhibit metabolism of beta blockers, such as atenolol.

Effect
Effects of both drugs may increase.

Nursing considerations
- Combination therapy is common in patients with hypertension and unstable angina.
- **⚠ ALERT** Risk of adverse effects increases, including heart failure, conduction disturbances, arrhythmias, and hypotension.
- Monitor the patient for adverse effects, including left ventricular dysfunction and AV conduction defects.
- Risk of interaction is greater when drugs are given I.V.
- Dosages of both drugs may need to be decreased.

---

atomoxetine ▶◀ MAO inhibitors

Strattera   isocarboxazid, phenelzine,
                                       tranylcypromine

Risk rating: 1		
Severity: **Major**	Onset: **Rapid**	Likelihood: **Suspected**

Cause
Level of monoamine in the brain may change.

Effect
Risk of serious or fatal reaction resembling neuroleptic malignant syndrome may increase.

Nursing considerations
- **⚠ ALERT** Use of atomoxetine and an MAO inhibitor together or within 2 weeks of each other is contraindicated.
- Before starting atomoxetine, ask the patient when he last took an MAO inhibitor. Before starting an MAO inhibitor, ask the patient when he last took atomoxetine.
- Monitor the patient for hyperthermia, rapid changes in vital signs, rigidity, muscle twitching, and mental status changes.

---

atorvastatin ▶◀ azole antifungals

Lipitor   fluconazole, itraconazole,
                                       ketoconazole

Risk rating: 1		
Severity: **Major**	Onset: **Rapid**	Likelihood: **Probable**

Cause
Azole antifungals may inhibit hepatic metabolism of HMG-CoA reductase inhibitors such as atorvastatin.

Effect

HMG-CoA reductase inhibitor level and adverse effects may increase.

Nursing considerations

■ If possible, avoid use together.

◆ **ALERT** Use of atorvastatin and itraconazole together is contraindicated.

■ If drugs must be taken together, HMG-CoA reductase inhibitor dosage may need to be decreased.

■ Monitor serum cholesterol and lipid levels to assess the patient's response to therapy.

◆ **ALERT** Assess the patient for evidence of rhabdomyolysis, including fatigue, muscle aches and weakness, joint pain, dark red or cola-colored urine, weight gain, seizures, and greatly increased serum CK level.

■ Pravastatin is least affected by this interaction and may be preferable for use with an azole antifungal, if needed.

---

atorvastatin ◄► cyclosporine

Lipitor   Gengraf, Neoral, Sandimmune

Risk rating: 1
Severity: Major   **Onset: Delayed**   **Likelihood: Probable**

Cause

Metabolism of certain HMG-CoA reductase inhibitors, such as atorvastatin, may decrease.

Effect

HMG-CoA reductase inhibitor level and adverse effects may increase.

Nursing considerations

■ If possible, avoid use together.

■ If used together, HMG-CoA reductase inhibitor dosage may need to be decreased.

■ Monitor serum cholesterol level, lipid level and liver function tests to assess the patient's response to therapy and possible adverse effects.

◆ **ALERT** Assess the patient for evidence of rhabdomyolysis, including fatigue; muscle aches and weakness; joint pain; dark, red, or cola-colored urine; weight gain; seizures; and greatly increased serum CK level.

■ Urge the patient to report unexplained muscle pain, tenderness, or weakness to the prescriber.

atorvastatin 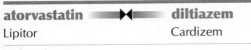 diltiazem
Lipitor   Cardizem

Risk rating: 2
Severity: Moderate   Onset: Delayed   Likelihood: Probable

Cause
CYP3A4 metabolism of certain HMG-CoA reductase inhibitors, such as atorvastatin, may be inhibited.

Effect
HMG-CoA reductase inhibitor level may increase, raising the risk of toxicity, including myositis and rhabdomyolysis.

Nursing considerations
■ If possible, avoid use together.
◩ **ALERT** Assess the patient for evidence of rhabdomyolysis, including fatigue, muscle aches and weakness, joint pain, dark red or cola-colored urine, weight gain, seizures, and greatly increased serum CK level.
■ If the patient may have rhabdomyolysis, notify the prescriber and obtain renal function tests and serum potassium, sodium, calcium, lactic acid, and myoglobin levels.
■ Pravastatin is less likely to interact with diltiazem than other HMG-CoA reductase inhibitors and may be the best choice for combined use.
■ Urge the patient to report unexplained muscle pain, tenderness, or weakness to the prescriber.

atorvastatin 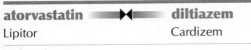 fibric acids
Lipitor   fenofibrate, gemfibrozil

Risk rating: 1
Severity: Major   Onset: Delayed   Likelihood: Suspected

Cause
The mechanism of this interaction is unknown.

Effect
Severe myopathy or rhabdomyolysis may occur.

Nursing considerations
■ Avoid use together.
■ If the patient has severe hyperlipidemia, combined therapy may be an option, but only with careful monitoring.
◩ **ALERT** Assess the patient for evidence of rhabdomyolysis, including fatigue, muscle aches and weakness, joint pain, dark red or cola-

colored urine, weight gain, seizures, and greatly increased serum CK level.

■ Watch for evidence of acute renal failure, including decreased urine output, elevated BUN and creatinine levels, edema, dyspnea, tachycardia, distended neck veins, nausea, vomiting, poor appetite, weakness, fatigue, confusion, and agitation.

■ Urge the patient to report unexplained muscle pain, tenderness, or weakness to the prescriber.

atorvastatin ━━━━▶◀━━━━ grapefruit juice
Lipitor

Risk rating: 2
Severity: Moderate   **Onset: Rapid**   **Likelihood: Probable**

Cause
Grapefruit juice may inhibit CYP3A4 metabolism of certain HMG-CoA reductase inhibitors, such as atorvastatin.

Effect
HMG-CoA reductase inhibitor level may increase, raising the risk of adverse effects.

Nursing considerations
■ Avoid giving atorvastatin with grapefruit juice.
■ Fluvastatin and pravastatin are metabolized by other enzymes and may be less affected by grapefruit juice.
■ Caution the patient to take the drug with a beverage other than grapefruit juice.
■ Urge the patient to report unexplained muscle pain, tenderness, or weakness to the prescriber.

atorvastatin ━━━━▶◀━━━━ macrolide antibiotics
Lipitor   clarithromycin, erythromycin, telithromycin

Risk rating: 1
Severity: Major   **Onset: Delayed**   **Likelihood: Probable**

Cause
CYP3A4 metabolism of certain HMG-CoA reductase inhibitors, such as atorvastatin, may decrease.

Effect
HMG-CoA reductase inhibitor level may increase, raising the risk of severe myopathy or rhabdomyolysis.

Nursing considerations
⧏ ALERT If atorvastatin is given with a macrolide antibiotic, watch for evidence of rhabdomyolysis, especially 5 to 21 days after macrolide is started. Evidence may include fatigue, muscle aches and weakness, joint pain, dark red or cola-colored urine, weight gain, seizures, and greatly increased serum CK level.
- Fluvastatin and pravastatin are metabolized by other enzymes and may be better choices when used with a macrolide antibiotic.
- It may be safe to give atorvastatin with azithromycin.
- Urge the patient to report unexplained muscle pain, tenderness, or weakness to the prescriber.

---

atorvastatin ⧏◀ **protease inhibitors**
Lipitor   ritonavir, saquinavir

Risk rating: 2
Severity: Moderate   **Onset: Delayed**   **Likelihood: Suspected**

Cause
First-pass metabolism of atorvastatin by CYP3A4 in the GI tract may be inhibited.

Effect
Atorvastatin level may increase.

Nursing considerations
- Monitor the patient closely if a protease inhibitor is added to atorvastatin therapy.
⧏ ALERT Watch for evidence of rhabdomyolysis, including fatigue, muscle aches and weakness, joint pain, dark red urine, weight gain, seizures, and greatly increased serum CK level.
- This interaction may be more likely when ritonavir and saquinavir are used together.
- Tell the patient to immediately report unexplained muscle weakness to the prescriber.

---

atorvastatin ⧏◀ **rifampin**
Lipitor   Rifadin, Rimactane

Risk rating: 2
Severity: Moderate   **Onset: Delayed**   **Likelihood: Suspected**

Cause
Rifampin may induce CYP3A4 metabolism of HMG-CoA reductase inhibitors, such as atorvastatin, in the intestine and liver.

Effect

HMG-CoA reductase inhibitor effects may decrease.

Nursing considerations

■ Assess the patient for expected response to therapy. If you suspect an interaction, consult the prescriber or pharmacist; the patient may need a different drug.

■ Check serum cholesterol and lipid levels to monitor the patient's response to therapy.

■ Withhold HMG-CoA reductase inhibitor temporarily if something increases the patient's risk of myopathy or rhabdomyolysis, such as sepsis, hypotension, major surgery, trauma, uncontrolled seizures, or a severe metabolic, endocrine, or electrolyte disorder.

■ Pravastatin is less likely to interact with rifampin and may be the best choice for combined use.

---

atovaquone ▶◀ zidovudine

Mepron   Retrovir

Risk rating: 2
Severity: Moderate   Onset: Delayed   Likelihood: Suspected

Cause

Excretion of zidovudine may be decreased.

Effect

Risk of zidovudine toxicity is increased.

Nursing considerations

■ Monitor the patient for toxic effects of zidovudine, including agranulocytosis, bone marrow suppression, and thrombocytopenia.

■ If an interaction is suspected, a lower dose of zidovudine may be needed.

■ Instruct the patient to notify the prescriber immediately if he notices new or increased bruising or bleeding.

■ Tell the patient not to change his HIV therapy without discussing it with the prescriber.

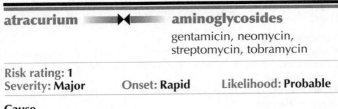

atracurium ►◄ aminoglycosides
gentamicin, neomycin,
streptomycin, tobramycin

Risk rating: 1
Severity: Major   **Onset: Rapid**   **Likelihood: Probable**

Cause
These drugs may be synergistic.

Effect
Effects of nondepolarizing muscle relaxants, such as atracurium, may increase.

Nursing considerations
- Give these drugs together only when needed.
- The nondepolarizing muscle relaxant dose may need adjustment based on neuromuscular response.
- Monitor the patient for prolonged respiratory depression.
- Provide ventilatory support as needed.

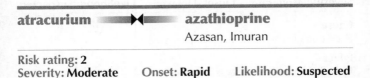

atracurium ►◄ azathioprine
Azasan, Imuran

Risk rating: 2
Severity: Moderate   **Onset: Rapid**   **Likelihood: Suspected**

Cause
Phosphodiesterase is inhibited in the motor nerve terminal.

Effect
Effects of nondepolarizing muscle relaxants, such as atracurium, may decrease.

Nursing considerations
- Closely monitor the patient's respiratory status.
- Dosage reduction may be needed with combination therapy.
- Provide ventilatory support as needed.

atracurium ━━▶◀━━ carbamazepine

Carbatrol, Epitol, Equetro,
Tegretol

Risk rating: 2
Severity: Moderate   **Onset: Rapid**   **Likelihood: Probable**

Cause
The mechanism of this interaction is unknown.

Effect
The effect or duration of atracurium, a nondepolarizing muscle relaxant, may decrease.

Nursing considerations
- Monitor the patient for decreased efficacy of the muscle relaxant.
- Dosage of the nondepolarizing muscle relaxant may need to be increased.
- Make sure the patient is adequately sedated when receiving a nondepolarizing muscle relaxant.

atracurium ━━▶◀━━ inhalation anesthetics

enflurane, isoflurane, nitrous
oxide

Risk rating: 1
Severity: Major   **Onset: Rapid**   **Likelihood: Established**

Cause
These drugs potentiate pharmacologic actions.

Effect
The actions of nondepolarizing muscle relaxants, such as atracurium, are potentiated.

Nursing considerations
- Closely monitor respiratory function.
- The dose of both the inhalation anesthetic and atracurium may need to be adjusted.
- Provide ventilatory support as needed.
- The interaction is dose-dependent.
- If the patient is receiving atracurium continuously, the maintenance dose may need to be decreased 25% to 30%.

atracurium 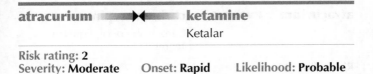 ketamine
Ketalar

Risk rating: 2
Severity: Moderate   **Onset: Rapid**   **Likelihood: Probable**

Cause
Increased acetylcholine release and decreased post-synaptic membrane sensitivity is suspected.

Effect
The actions of nondepolarizing muscle relaxants, including atracurium, are enhanced, leading to profound and severe respiratory depression.

Nursing considerations
- Use these drugs together cautiously.
- The nondepolarizing muscle relaxant dosage may need adjustment.
- Provide ventilatory support as needed.
- The recovery time from atracurium may also be increased.

atracurium 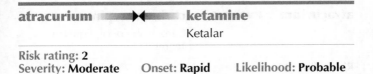 phenytoin
Dilantin

Risk rating: 2
Severity: Moderate   **Onset: Rapid**   **Likelihood: Established**

Cause
Phenytoin has effects at prejunctional sites similar to those of nondepolarizing muscle relaxants.

Effect
Effect or duration of nondepolarizing muscle relaxant may decrease.

Nursing considerations
- Monitor the patient for decreased efficacy of atracurium.
- This interaction may not occur in all patients receiving atracurium and phenytoin.
- The nondepolarizing muscle relaxant dosage may need to increase.
- Make sure the patient is adequately sedated when receiving a nondepolarizing muscle relaxant.

atracurium ◄►◄ polypeptide antibiotics
bacitracin, polymyxin B, vancomycin

Risk rating: 2
Severity: Moderate   **Onset: Rapid**   **Likelihood: Probable**

Cause
Polypeptide antibiotics may act synergistically with nondepolarizing muscle relaxants such as atracurium.

Effect
Neuromuscular blockade may increase.

Nursing considerations
■ If possible, avoid using polypeptide antibiotics with nondepolarizing muscle relaxants.
■ Monitor neuromuscular function closely.
■ Dosage of nondepolarizing muscle relaxant may need adjustment.
■ Make sure the patient is adequately sedated when receiving a nondepolarizing muscle relaxant.

azathioprine ◄►◄ allopurinol
Azasan, Imuran   Aloprim, Zyloprim

Risk rating: 1
Severity: Major   **Onset: Delayed**   **Likelihood: Established**

Cause
Allopurinol reduces the conversion of thiopurines, such as azathioprine, to an inactive form. Allopurinol also inhibits the first-pass metabolism.

Effect
Pharmacologic and toxic effects are increased.

Nursing considerations
■ Reduce the dosage of azathioprine when given with allopurinol.
■ Decrease the initial dose of thiopurines by 25% to 33%.
■ Monitor the patient for toxic effects of azathioprine, including leukopenia, thrombocytopenia, and bone marrow suppression.
■ It is suspected that this interaction is based only on the oral form of azathioprine, not the I.V. form.

azathioprine ━━▶◀━━ mercaptopurine
Azasan, Imuran   Purinethol

Risk rating: 1
Severity: Major   **Onset: Delayed**   **Likelihood: Suspected**

Cause
Additive bone marrow suppression may occur.

Effect
Risk of developing life-threatening myelosuppression may be increased.

Nursing considerations
◪ **ALERT** Avoid administering these drugs together.
▪ Myelosuppression may occur with either drug alone, or in combination.
▪ Monitor the patient for toxic effects of azathioprine, including leukopenia, thrombocytopenia, and bone marrow suppression.

azathioprine ━━▶◀━━ nondepolarizing muscle relaxants
Azasan, Imuran   atracurium, pancuronium

Risk rating: 2
Severity: Moderate   **Onset: Rapid**   **Likelihood: Suspected**

Cause
Phosphodiesterase is inhibited in the motor nerve terminal.

Effect
Effects of nondepolarizing muscle relaxants may decrease.

Nursing considerations
▪ Closely monitor the patient's respiratory status.
▪ Dosage reduction may be needed with combination therapy.
▪ Provide ventilatory support as needed.

azathioprine 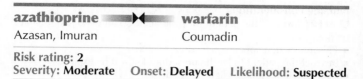 warfarin

Azasan, Imuran   Coumadin

Risk rating: 2
Severity: Moderate   Onset: Delayed   Likelihood: Suspected

Cause
The mechanism of the interaction is unknown. Thiopurines, such as azathioprine, may increase the synthesis of prothrombin and decrease plasma warfarin levels.

Effect
The effects of warfarin may be decreased.

Nursing considerations
- Monitor PT and INR when starting, changing, or stopping azathioprine therapy in the patient who takes warfarin.
- Maintain INR at 2 to 3 for an acute MI, atrial fibrillation, treatment of pulmonary embolism, prevention of systemic embolism, tissue heart valves, valvular heart disease, or prophylaxis or treatment of venous thrombosis. Maintain INR at 3 to 4.5 for mechanical prosthetic valves or recurrent systemic embolism.
- Warfarin dose may need to be adjusted.
- Tell the patient to report unusual bruising or bleeding.
- Remind the patient that warfarin interacts with many drugs and that he should report any change in drug regimen.

azithromycin 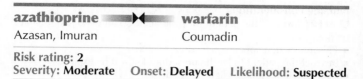 antiarrhythmic agents

Zithromax   amiodarone, bretylium,
                           disopyramide, dofetilide,
                           procainamide, quinidine,
                           sotalol

Risk rating: 1
Severity: Major   Onset: Delayed   Likelihood: Suspected

Cause
An additive increase in the QT interval is seen when administering macrolide antibiotics and antiarrhythmic agents.

Effect
The risk of life-threatening cardiac arrhythmias, including torsades de pointes, is increased.

Nursing considerations
⚡ **ALERT** Monitor the patient for prolonged QT interval and torsades de pointes.
■ This interaction appears to be dose related.
■ Instruct the patient to let the prescriber know if he experiences dizziness, palpitations, or light-headedness.
■ The QT interval returns to normal within 3 days of stopping azithromycin.

---

azithromycin ▬▬▶◀▬ **cyclosporine**
Zithromax   Gengraf, Neoral, Sandimmune

Risk rating: 2
Severity: Moderate   Onset: Delayed   Likelihood: Established

Cause
Macrolide antibiotics, such as azithromycin, interfere with cyclosporine metabolism. The rate and extent of absorption may increase, and the volume of distribution may decrease.

Effect
Elevated cyclosporine levels and increased risk of toxicity may occur.

Nursing considerations
⚡ **ALERT** Monitor the patient carefully for nephrotoxicity or neurotoxicity.
■ Closely monitor BUN and serum creatinine levels.
■ The dose of cyclosporine may need to be decreased.
■ Of all the macrolide antibiotics, azithromycin appears to interact the least with cyclosporine.

---

azithromycin ▬▬▶◀▬ **pimozide**
Zithromax   Orap

Risk rating: 1
Severity: Major   Onset: Delayed   Likelihood: Probable

Cause
Macrolide antibiotics, such as azithromycin, may inhibit CYP3A4 metabolism of pimozide.

Effect
Risk of life-threatening arrhythmias may increase.

Nursing considerations
⚡ **ALERT** Combined use of these drugs is contraindicated.

■ Arrhythmias are related to prolonged QT interval, a known risk of pimozide.

⚠ ALERT People with normal baseline ECG and no history have died from pimozide blood levels 2.5 times the upper limit of normal from this interaction.

---

azithromycin ➤◀ theophyllines
Zithromax   aminophylline, theophylline

Risk rating: 2
Severity: Moderate   Onset: Delayed   Likelihood: Established

Cause
Certain macrolide antibiotics, such as azithromycin, inhibit metabolism of theophyllines.

Effect
Serum theophylline level and risk of toxicity may increase.

Nursing considerations
■ When starting or stopping a macrolide antibiotic, monitor serum theophylline level. Normal therapeutic range is 10 to 20 mcg/ml for adults and 5 to 15 mcg/ml for children.
■ Watch for evidence of toxicity, such as tachycardia, anorexia, nausea, vomiting, diarrhea, seizures, restlessness, irritability, and headache.
■ Describe adverse effects of theophyllines and signs of toxicity, and tell the patient to report them immediately to the prescriber.

---

azithromycin ➤◀ warfarin
Zithromax   Coumadin

Risk rating: 1
Severity: Major   Onset: Delayed   Likelihood: Probable

Cause
Warfarin clearance is reduced.

Effect
Anticoagulant effects and risk of bleeding increase.

Nursing considerations
■ Monitor PT and INR closely when starting or stopping a macrolide antibiotic. The PT may be prolonged within a few days.
■ Warfarin dose adjustment may continue for several days after antibiotic therapy stops.
■ Tell the patient to report unusual bleeding or bruising.

- Remind the patient that warfarin interacts with many drugs and that he should report any changes in drug regimen.
- Advise the patient to keep all follow-up medical appointments for proper monitoring and dosage adjustments.
- Treat excessive anticoagulation with vitamin K.

bacitracin ➤◄	nondepolarizing muscle relaxants
Baci-IM, Baci-Rx	atracurium, pancuronium, vecuronium

Risk rating: 2
Severity: **Moderate**   Onset: **Rapid**   Likelihood: **Probable**

Cause
Polypeptide antibiotics, such as bacitracin, may act synergistically with nondepolarizing muscle relaxants.

Effect
Neuromuscular blockade may increase.

Nursing considerations
- If possible, avoid combining these drugs.
- Monitor neuromuscular function closely.
- Dosage of nondepolarizing muscle relaxant may need adjustment.
- Provide ventilatory support as needed.
- Make sure the patient is adequately sedated when receiving a nondepolarizing muscle relaxant.

benazepril ➤◄	potassium-sparing diuretics
Lotensin	amiloride, spironolactone

Risk rating: 1
Severity: **Major**   Onset: **Delayed**   Likelihood: **Probable**

Cause
The mechanism of this interaction is unknown.

Effect
Serum potassium level may increase.

Nursing considerations
- Use combination cautiously in patients at high risk for hyperkalemia, especially those with renal impairment.
- Monitor BUN, creatinine, and serum potassium levels as needed.

■ ACE inhibitors other than benazepril may interact with potassium-sparing diuretics. If you suspect an interaction, consult the prescriber or pharmacist.
■ Urge the patient to immediately report an irregular heartbeat, a slow pulse, weakness, and other evidence of hyperkalemia.

benztropine ▬▶◀▬ haloperidol
Cogentin   Haldol

Risk rating: 2
Severity: Moderate   **Onset: Delayed**   **Likelihood: Suspected**

Cause
The mechanism of this interaction is unknown. It may involve central cholinergic pathways rather than a true pharmacokinetic interaction.

Effect
Effects may vary. They include decreased haloperidol level, worsened schizophrenic symptoms, and development of tardive dyskinesia.

Nursing considerations
◪ ALERT If the patient takes haloperidol, avoid anticholinergics if possible.
■ Watch for signs of worsening schizophrenia, including delusions, hallucinations, disorganized speech or behavior, inappropriate affect, and abnormal psychomotor activity.
■ Watch for development of tardive dyskinesia—involuntary abnormal repetitive movements, including lip smacking, cheek puffing, chewing motions, tongue thrusting, finger flicking, and trunk twisting.
■ Consult the prescriber if adverse effects occur; benztropine may need to be stopped, or haloperidol dosage may need adjustment.
■ Other anticholinergics may interact with haloperidol. If you suspect an interaction, consult the prescriber or pharmacist.

benztropine ▬▶◀▬ phenothiazines
Cogentin   chlorpromazine, per-
phenazine,   thioridazine

Risk rating: 2
Severity: Moderate   **Onset: Delayed**   **Likelihood: Suspected**

Cause
Anticholinergics, such as benztropine, may antagonize phenothiazines. Also, phenothiazine metabolism may increase.

Effect
Phenothiazine efficacy may decrease.

Nursing considerations
- Data regarding this interaction conflict.
- Monitor the patient for decreased phenothiazine efficacy.
- The phenothiazine dosage may need adjustment.
- Anticholinergic adverse effects may increase.
- Monitor the patient for adynamic ileus, hyperpyrexia, hypoglycemia, and neurologic changes.

---

bisoprolol ━━━━▶◀━━━ rifampin
Zebeta   Rifadin, Rimactane

Risk rating: 2
Severity: Moderate   Onset: Delayed   Likelihood: Suspected

Cause
Rifampin increases hepatic metabolism of beta blockers such as bisoprolol.

Effect
Beta blocker effects decrease.

Nursing considerations
- Monitor blood pressure and heart rate closely to assess beta blocker efficacy.
- If beta blocker effects are decreased, consult the prescriber; dosage may need to be increased.
- Teach the patient how to monitor blood pressure and heart rate, and when to contact the prescriber.
- Other beta blockers may interact with rifampin. If you suspect an interaction, consult the prescriber or pharmacist.

---

bleomycin ━━━━▶◀━━━ phenytoin
Blenoxane   Dilatin

Risk rating: 2
Severity: Moderate   Onset: Delayed   Likelihood: Suspected

Cause
Phenytoin absorption may be decreased or metabolism may be increased.

Effect
Phenytoin level and effects may decrease.

Nursing considerations
- Monitor phenytoin level closely. Dosage may need to be adjusted.
- Therapeutic range for phenytoin is 10 to 20 mcg/ml.
- Toxic effects can occur at therapeutic level. Adjust the measured level for hypoalbuminemia or renal impairment, which can increase free drug level.
- Monitor the patient for seizure activity.
- Carefully monitor phenytoin level between courses of chemotherapy. Phenytoin dose may need to be reduced.
- Signs and symptoms of phenytoin toxicity include nystagmus, slurred speech, ataxia, blurred or double vision, confusion, drowsiness, and lethargy.

---

bosentan ◀▶ **cyclosporine**
Tracleer   Gengraf, Neoral, Sandimmune

Risk rating: 1
Severity: Major   **Onset: Delayed**   **Likelihood: Suspected**

Cause
Bosentan may increase cyclosporine metabolism. Cyclosporine may inhibit bosentan metabolism.

Effect
Bosentan level may increase. Cyclosporine level may decrease.

Nursing considerations
⚑ **ALERT** Use of bosentan with cyclosporine is contraindicated.
- Trough level of bosentan may increase 30 times above normal.
- Cyclosporine level may decrease by 50%.
- Watch for adverse effects from increased bosentan level, such as headache, nausea, vomiting, hypotension, and increased heart rate.

---

bosentan ◀▶ **glyburide**
Tracleer   DiaBeta, Micronase

Risk rating: 1
Severity: Major   **Onset: Delayed**   **Likelihood: Suspected**

Cause
Bosentan increases the CYP3A4 and CYP2C9 metabolism of glyburide.

Effect
Plasma levels of bosentan and glyburide may be decreased. Liver enzymes may be increased, resulting in serious liver injury.

Nursing considerations
⚠ **ALERT** Administration of bosentan and glyburide together is contraindicated.
- Discuss the use of a hypoglycemic agent other than glyburide with the prescriber.
- Monitor the patient's liver enzyme level, and report any increase to the prescriber.
- Monitor the patient for signs of liver damage, including icterus, jaundice, dark urine, and confusion.

---

bosentan ▶◀ hormonal contraceptives
Tracleer

Risk rating: 1
Severity: Major   **Onset: Delayed**   **Likelihood: Suspected**

Cause
Bosentan increases the CYP3A4 and CYP2C9 metabolism of hormonal contraceptives.

Effect
Hormonal contraceptive efficacy may be lost, possibly resulting in unintended pregnancy.

Nursing considerations
- Warn the patient of the risk of contraceptive failure.
- Discuss alternate, nonhormonal, or additional contraceptive use while both drugs are being taken.
- Larger hormonal contraceptive doses may be considered; consult with the prescriber about dosage to prevent breakthrough bleeding.
- Instruct the patient to notify her practitioner immediately if she misses a period or suspects she may be pregnant.

---

bosentan ▶◀ ketoconazole
Tracleer   Nizoral

Risk rating: 2
Severity: Moderate   **Onset: Delayed**   **Likelihood: Suspected**

Cause
Azole antifungals, such as ketoconazole, inhibit CYP3A4 metabolism of bosentan.

Effect
Plasma concentration of bosentan may be increased, thereby increasing pharmacologic and adverse effects.

Nursing considerations
- Closely monitor clinical response to bosentan when starting or stopping ketoconazole.
- Observe the patient for an increase in adverse effects to bosentan.
- An increased number of patients receiving both drugs complained of a headache. Monitor the patient for headache and provide analgesics as ordered.
- Monitor the patient for increased shortness of breath, edema, and heart failure.

---

bosentan ▶◀ warfarin
Tracleer   Coumadin

Risk rating: 2
Severity: Moderate   **Onset: Delayed**   **Likelihood: Suspected**

Cause
Bosentan induces CYP3A4 and CYP2C9 metabolism of warfarin.

Effect
Effects of warfarin may be decreased.

Nursing considerations
- Monitor PT and INR when starting, changing, or stopping bosentan therapy in the patient who takes warfarin.
- Maintain INR at 2 to 3 for an acute MI, atrial fibrillation, treatment of pulmonary embolism, prevention of systemic embolism, tissue heart valves, valvular heart disease, or prophylaxis for, or treatment of, venous thrombosis. Maintain INR at 3 to 4.5 for mechanical prosthetic valves or recurrent systemic embolism.
- Warfarin dose may need to be adjusted.
- Tell the patient to report unusual bruising or bleeding.
- Remind the patient that warfarin interacts with many drugs and that he should report any change in drug regimen.

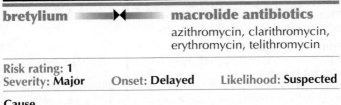

bretylium ◄► macrolide antibiotics

azithromycin, clarithromycin,
erythromycin, telithromycin

Risk rating: 1
Severity: Major   **Onset: Delayed**   **Likelihood: Suspected**

Cause
An additive increase in the QT interval may result.

Effect
Risk of life-threatening arrhythmias, including torsades de pointes,
may increase.

Nursing considerations
■⚠ **ALERT** Administering telithromycin to a patient on a class III an-
tiarrhythmic agent is contraindicated.
■ Monitor ECG for increased QTc interval.
■ Notify the prescriber immediately if the QT interval increases.
■ Tell the patient to report a rapid heartbeat, shortness of breath,
dizziness, fainting, and chest pain.

bretylium ◄► quinolones

gatifloxacin, levofloxacin,
moxifloxacin, ofloxacin

Risk rating: 1
Severity: Major   **Onset: Delayed**   **Likelihood: Suspected**

Cause
The cause of this interaction is unknown.

Effect
Risk of life-threatening arrhythmias, including torsades de pointes,
increases when quinolones are combined with antiarrhythmics, such
as bretylium.

Nursing considerations
■ Avoid giving class III antiarrhythmics with quinolones.
■ Quinolones that aren't metabolized by CYP3A4 isoenzymes or that
don't prolong the QT interval may be given with antiarrhythmics.
■ Monitor ECG for prolonged QTc interval.
■ Tell the patient to report a rapid heartbeat, shortness of breath,
dizziness, fainting, or chest pain.

bretylium 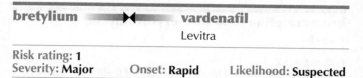 vardenafil
Levitra

Risk rating: 1
Severity: **Major**   Onset: **Rapid**   Likelihood: **Suspected**

Cause
The cause of this interaction is unknown.

Effect
QTc interval may be prolonged, particularly in patients with previous QT-interval prolongation, increasing the risk of such life-threatening arrhythmias as torsades de pointes.

Nursing considerations
◼ **ALERT** Use of vardenafil with a class III antiarrhythmic is contra-indicated.
◼ Monitor ECG before and during vardenafil use.
◼ Urge the patient to report light-headedness, faintness, palpitations, chest pain or pressure while taking vardenafil.
◼ To reduce risk of adverse effects, patients age 65 and older should start with 5 mg vardenafil, half the usual starting dose.

bretylium 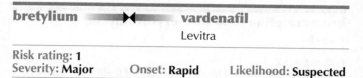 ziprasidone
Geodon

Risk rating: 1
Severity: **Major**   Onset: **Delayed**   Likelihood: **Suspected**

Cause
The cause of this interaction is unknown.

Effect
Risk of life-threatening arrhythmias, including torsades de pointes, increases.

Nursing considerations
◼ **ALERT** Use of ziprasidone with certain antiarrhythmics is contrain-dicated.
◼ Monitor the patient for other risk factors for torsades de pointes, in-cluding bradycardia, hypokalemia, and hypomagnesemia.
◼ Ask the patient if he or anyone in his family has a history of pro-longed QT interval or arrhythmias.
◼ Monitor the patient for bradycardia.
◼ Measure the QTc interval at baseline and throughout therapy.

bromocriptine ▸◂ erythromycin
Parlodel

Risk rating: 2
Severity: Moderate   Onset: Delayed   Likelihood: Suspected

Cause
Erythromycin inhibits hepatic metabolism, resulting in increased bioavailability of bromocriptine.

Effect
Therapeutic and toxic effects of bromocriptine may increase.

Nursing considerations
■ Monitor the patient for increased response to bromocriptine and adjust dose accordingly.
■ Monitor the patient for dizziness and orthostatic hypotension.
■ The most common increased adverse effect is vomiting.
■ Give bromocriptine with food to minimize adverse effects.

budesonide ▸◂ azole antifungals
Pulmicort, Rhinocort   itraconazole, ketoconazole

Risk rating: 2
Severity: Moderate   Onset: Delayed   Likelihood: Suspected

Cause
Budesonide CYP3A4 metabolism may be inhibited, and elimination may decrease.

Effect
Corticosteroid effects and toxicity may be increased.

Nursing considerations
■ Monitor the patient for increased adverse effects to budesonide and adjust dose as needed.
■ Monitor the patient taking a corticosteroid and itraconazole for Cushing syndrome.
■ Carefully monitor the patient for infection, edema, and increased serum glucose level.
■ Instruct the patient not to abruptly stop budesonide; it should gradually be tapered to prevent withdrawal symptoms.

bumetanide ▬▬▶◀▬▬ captopril
Bumex   Capoten

Risk rating: 3
Severity: Minor   **Onset: Delayed**   **Likelihood: Suspected**

Cause
Captopril may inhibit angiotensin II production.

Effect
The effect of loop diuretics, such as bumetanide, may be decreased.

Nursing considerations
- Carefully monitor the patient's fluid status and body weight when starting an ACE inhibitor.
- The dose of bumetanide may need to be altered when starting, changing, or stopping captopril therapy.
- Instruct the patient to weight himself at the same time everyday, in the same clothes, and to notify the prescriber if he gains more than 2 pounds overnight, or 5 pounds in 1 week.

bumetanide ▬▬▶◀▬▬ cisplatin
Bumex   Platinol

Risk rating: 2
Severity: Moderate   **Onset: Rapid**   **Likelihood: Suspected**

Cause
The mechanism of this interaction is unknown.

Effect
Interaction may cause additive ototoxicity.

Nursing considerations
- If possible, avoid giving a loop diuretic, such as bumetanide, and cisplatin together.
- Obtain hearing tests to detect early hearing loss.
- These drugs may cause ototoxicity much more severe than that caused by either drug alone.
- Ototoxicity may be permanent.
- Tell the patient to report ringing in the ears, change in balance, or muffled sounds. Also, ask family members to watch for changes.

bumetanide ▰▰▰▶◀▰▰▰ digoxin
Bumex   Lanoxin

Risk rating: 1
Severity: Major   **Onset: Delayed**   **Likelihood: Probable**

Cause
Urinary excretion of potassium and magnesium is increased.

Effect
Electrolyte disturbances may predispose the patient to digitalis-induced arrhythmias.

Nursing considerations
■ Monitor serum potassium and magnesium levels; decreased levels may predispose the patient to arrhythmias.
■ Carefully monitor the patient's ECG while receiving digoxin and a loop diuretic.
■ If the patient develops hypomagnesemia or hypokalemia, be prepared to administer supplements.
■ Monitor the patient for increased serum sodium level.
■ Changing the patient from a loop diuretic to a potassium-sparing diuretic will minimize the risk of arrhythmias.
■ This interaction appears to be dose-related.

bumetanide ▰▰▰▶◀▰▰▰ lithium
Bumex   Eskalith

Risk rating: 2
Severity: Moderate   **Onset: Delayed**   **Likelihood: Suspected**

Cause
The mechanism of this interaction is unknown.

Effect
Increased lithium levels and risk of toxicity may occur.

Nursing considerations
■ Monitor serum lithium levels. Steady state lithium level should be 0.6 to 1.2 mEq/L.
■ Adjust lithium dose as needed.
■ Monitor the patient for evidence of lithium toxicity, such as diarrhea, vomiting, dehydration, drowsiness, muscle weakness, tremor, fever, and ataxia.
■ Despite this interaction, lithium and loop diuretics may be used together safely, with close monitoring of lithium level.

bumetanide ▶◀ thiazide diuretics

Bumex

chlorothiazide, hydrochlorothiazide, indapamide, methyclothiazide, metolazone, poly-
thiazide, trichlormethiazide

Risk rating: 2
Severity: Moderate   **Onset: Rapid**   **Likelihood: Probable**

Cause
The mechanism of this interaction is likely a renal tubular mechanism.

Effect
Because these drugs work synergistically, they may cause profound
diuresis and serious electrolyte abnormalities.

Nursing considerations
- This combination may be used for therapeutic benefit.
- Expect increased sodium, potassium, and chloride excretion and
greater diuresis during combined therapy.
- Monitor the patient for dehydration and electrolyte abnormalities.

buprenorphine ▶◀ diazepam

Buprenex, Subutex   Valium

Risk rating: 2
Severity: Moderate   **Onset: Rapid**   **Likelihood: Suspected**

Cause
Additive or synergistic effects are involved.

Effect
Buprenorphine strength and drug effects are increased.

Nursing considerations
- Monitor the patient for increased sedation.
- Instruct the patient not to perform such tasks as driving or operating machinery.
- The interaction appears to be dose and time related, with the greatest increase in adverse effects occurring 1 to 2 hours after taking the
diazepam.

buprenorphine ◄►◄ protease inhibitors
Buprenex, Subutex   atazanavir, ritonavir, saquinavir

Risk rating: 2
Severity: Moderate   **Onset: Delayed**   **Likelihood: Suspected**

Cause
Using both together may inhibit metabolism of opioid analgesics, such as buprenorphine, in the GI tract and liver.

Effect
Buprenorphine level may increase; half-life lengthens.

Nursing considerations
⚑ ALERT If the patient is taking a protease inhibitor, watch closely for respiratory depression if buprenorphine is added.
■ Because buprenorphine half-life is prolonged, monitoring period should be extended, even after buprenorphine is stopped.
■ Keep naloxone available to treat respiratory depression.
■ If buprenorphine is continuously infused, dose should be decreased.
■ Decreasing dose of buprenorphine may decrease adverse effects.

bupropion ◄►◄ carbamazepine
Wellbutrin, Zyban   Carbatrol, Epitol, Equetro, Tegretol

Risk rating: 2
Severity: Moderate   **Onset: Delayed**   **Likelihood: Suspected**

Cause
Carbamazepine increases hepatic metabolism of bupropion.

Effect
Bupropion level may decrease.

Nursing considerations
⚑ ALERT Bupropion is contraindicated in patients with a seizure disorder.
■ Monitor the patient's response to bupropion.
■ Bupropion dosage may need adjustment.
■ The risk of bupropion-related seizures may be reduced by keeping the daily dose below 450 mg (400 mg SR; 450 mg XL); giving the daily dose b.i.d. or t.i.d. (depending on preparation) to avoid high peak levels; and increasing doses gradually.

■ Urge the patient to tell the prescriber about all drugs and supplements he is taking.

---

bupropion ►◄ MAO inhibitors
Wellbutrin, Zyban

isocarboxazid, phenelzine, selegiline, tranylcypromine

Risk rating: 1
Severity: Major   **Onset: Delayed**   **Likelihood: Suspected**

Cause
The cause of this interaction is unknown.

Effect
Risk of acute bupropion toxicity is increased.

Nursing considerations
◄ **ALERT** Administration of bupropion and an MAO inhibitor together is contraindicated.
■ Allow at least 14 days between discontinuing an MAO inhibitor and starting bupropion.
■ Interaction warning is based on animal trials, not actual patient studies.

---

bupropion ►◄ ritonavir
Wellbutrin, Zyban

Norvir

Risk rating: 2
Severity: Moderate   **Onset: Delayed**   **Likelihood: Suspected**

Cause
Ritonavir may inhibit bupropion metabolism.

Effect
Large increases in serum bupropion level may occur.

Nursing considerations
◄ **ALERT** Use together is contraindicated.
■ If used together, risk of seizures due to bupropion toxicity increases.
■ To minimize the risk of interactions, urge the patient to tell prescribers about all drugs and supplements he is taking.

buspirone 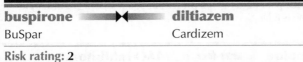 diltiazem
BuSpar   Cardizem

Risk rating: 2
Severity: Moderate   Onset: Delayed   Likelihood: Suspected

Cause
CYP3A4 metabolism of buspirone may decrease.

Effect
Buspirone level and adverse effects may increase.

Nursing considerations
■ During buspirone therapy, monitor the patient closely if diltiazem is started or stopped, or if its dosage is changed.
■ Monitor the patient for signs of buspirone toxicity, including increased CNS effects (such as dizziness, drowsiness, and headache), vomiting, and diarrhea.
■ An antianxiety drug not metabolized by CYP3A4 (such as lorazepam) should be considered as alternative therapy if the patient takes the calcium channel blocker diltiazem.
■ Dihydropyridine calcium channel blockers (such as amlodipine and felodipine) that don't inhibit CYP3A4 metabolism probably wouldn't interfere with buspirone metabolism.
■ Other calcium channel blockers may also have this interaction. If you suspect a drug interaction, consult the prescriber or pharmacist.

buspirone 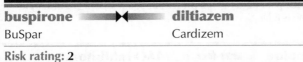 erythromycin
BuSpar   E-Mycin

Risk rating: 2
Severity: Moderate   Onset: Delayed   Likelihood: Suspected

Cause
CYP3A4 metabolism of buspirone may be inhibited by macrolide antibiotics such as erythromycin.

Effect
Buspirone level and adverse effects may increase.

Nursing considerations
◪ **ALERT** Use of other macrolide antibiotics (such as azithromycin or dirithromycin) should be considered because they probably don't interact with buspirone. Consult the prescriber or pharmacist.
■ During buspirone therapy, monitor the patient closely if a macrolide antibiotic is started or stopped, or if its dosage is changed.

- If the patient takes a macrolide antibiotic, starting buspirone dose should be conservative.
- Monitor the patient for signs of buspirone toxicity, including increased CNS effects (such as dizziness, drowsiness, and headache), vomiting, and diarrhea.
- Adjust buspirone dose as needed.

---

buspirone ▶◀ fluvoxamine
BuSpar   Luvox

Risk rating: 3
Severity: Minor   **Onset: Delayed**   **Likelihood: Suspected**

Cause
CYP3A4 metabolism of buspirone may be inhibited by fluvoxamine.

Effect
Buspirone level may increase.

Nursing considerations
- Monitor the patient's clinical response to buspirone while taking fluvoxamine.
- The dose of buspirone may need to be adjusted.

---

buspirone ▶◀ grapefruit juice
BuSpar

Risk rating: 2
Severity: Moderate   **Onset: Delayed**   **Likelihood: Probable**

Cause
CYP3A4 metabolism of buspirone may be inhibited by grapefruit juice.

Effect
Buspirone level and adverse effects may increase.

Nursing considerations
- If buspirone and grapefruit juice are taken together, buspirone adverse effects may increase, including dizziness, drowsiness, headache, vomiting, and diarrhea.
- Advise the patient to take buspirone with liquids other than grapefruit juice.
- Urge the patient to tell the prescriber about all drugs and supplements he is taking and about any increase in adverse effects.

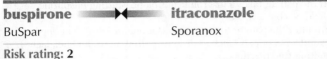

buspirone ━━━▶◀━━━ itraconazole
BuSpar   Sporanox

Risk rating: 2
Severity: Moderate   Onset: Delayed   Likelihood: Probable

Cause
Azole antifungals such as itraconazole may inhibit the CYP3A4 isoenzyme responsible for buspirone metabolism.

Effect
Plasma buspirone level may increase.

Nursing considerations
■ If the patient is taking buspirone, monitor him closely when an
azole antifungal is started or stopped or its dosage is changed.
■ If the patient is taking itraconazole, initial buspirone dose should be
conservative.
■ Monitor the patient for signs of buspirone toxicity, including increased CNS effects (such as dizziness, drowsiness, and headache),
vomiting, and diarrhea.
■ Urge the patient to tell the prescriber about all drugs and supplements he takes and about any increase in adverse effects.

buspirone ━━━▶◀━━━ rifampin
BuSpar   Rifadin, Rimactane

Risk rating: 2
Severity: Moderate   Onset: Delayed   Likelihood: Probable

Cause
Buspirone metabolism may be increased via induction of CYP3A4
metabolism by rifamycins.

Effect
Buspirone effects may decrease.

Nursing considerations
■ Other rifamycins (such as rifaximin) may interact. If you suspect an
interaction, consult the prescriber or pharmacist.
■ Watch for expected buspirone effects when you start, stop, or
change the dose of a rifamycin antibiotic.
■ Advise the patient to report increases or changes in anxiety if a rifamycin antibiotic is started.
■ Urge the patient to tell the prescriber about all drugs and supplements he takes and about any increase in adverse effects.

buspirone ━━━━▶◀━━━━ verapamil
BuSpar   Calan

Risk rating: 2
Severity: Moderate   Onset: Delayed   Likelihood: Suspected

Cause
CYP3A4 metabolism of buspirone may decrease.

Effect
Buspirone level and adverse effects may increase.

Nursing considerations
- Calcium channel blockers other than verapamil may interact with buspirone. If you suspect an interaction, consult the prescriber or pharmacist.
- During buspirone therapy, monitor the patient closely if verapamil is started or stopped or the dosage changes.
- Monitor the patient for signs of buspirone toxicity, which include vomiting, diarrhea, and increased CNS effects, such as dizziness, drowsiness, and headache.
- An antianxiety drug not metabolized by CYP3A4 (such as lorazepam) should be considered as an alternative therapy if the patient takes verapamil.
- Dihydropyridine calcium channel blockers (such as amlodipine and felodipine) that don't inhibit CYP3A4 metabolism probably wouldn't interfere with buspirone metabolism. Consult the prescriber or pharmacist.

busulfan ━━━━▶◀━━━━ itraconazole
Myleran   Sporanox

Risk rating: 2
Severity: Moderate   Onset: Delayed   Likelihood: Suspected

Cause
The mechanism of the interaction is unknown.

Effect
Itraconazole may increase plasma busulfan levels, increasing the risk of toxicity.

Nursing considerations
- Monitor the patient taking busulfan and itraconazole for increased toxicity.

- If a patient taking busulfan is started on itraconazole, the busulfan dose may need to decrease.
- Monitor the patient for persistent cough, labored breathing, thrombocytopenia, and signs of infection.
- Tell the patient to call the prescriber if he notices increased bleeding or bruising, jaundice, or fever, sore throat, or fatigue.
- Fluconazole may be used as a safe alternative instead of itraconazole.

---

busulfan ◢◤ metronidazole
Myleran   Flagyl

Risk rating: 1
Severity: Major   **Onset: Delayed**   **Likelihood: Suspected**

Cause
The mechanism of the interaction is unknown.

Effect
Busulfan trough level may be elevated, increasing the risk of serious toxicity, including veno-occlusive disease and hemorrhagic cystitis.

Nursing considerations
⚠ ALERT The use of these two drugs together is contraindicated.
- Monitor the patient for persistent cough, labored breathing, thrombocytopenia, and signs of infection.
- Tell the patient to call the prescriber if he notices increased bleeding or bruising, jaundice, fever, sore throat, or fatigue.

---

cabergoline ◢◤ clarithromycin
Dostinex   Biaxin

Risk rating: 2
Severity: Moderate   **Onset: Delayed**   **Likelihood: Suspected**

Cause
Clarithromycin inhibits the CYP3A4 metabolism of cabergoline.

Effect
Cabergoline plasma levels may be increased, increasing the risk of toxicity.

Nursing considerations
- If possible, avoid administering these drugs together.
- Carefully monitor the clinical response of patients taking this combination of drugs.

- This interaction may be increased in a patient with a history of levodopa-induced psychosis or dyskinesia.
- Cabergoline may interact with any macrolide antibiotic.

---

candesartan ▶◀ lithium
Atacand   Eskalith

Risk rating: 2
Severity: Moderate   **Onset: Delayed**   **Likelihood: Suspected**

Cause
Angiotensin II receptor antagonists may decrease lithium excretion.

Effect
Lithium level, effects, and risk of toxicity may increase.

Nursing considerations
- If the patient takes lithium, consider an antihypertensive other than an angiotensin II receptor antagonist.
- Monitor lithium level. Steady state lithium level should be 0.6 to 1.2 mEq/L.
- Adjust lithium dose as needed.
- Monitor the patient for evidence of lithium toxicity, such as diarrhea, vomiting, dehydration, drowsiness, muscle weakness, tremor, fever, and ataxia.

---

candesartan ▶◀ spironolactone
Atacand   Aldactone

Risk rating: 1
Severity: Major   **Onset: Delayed**   **Likelihood: Suspected**

Cause
Both angiotensin II receptor antagonists, such as candesartan, and potassium-sparing diuretics may increase serum potassium level.

Effect
Risk of hyperkalemia may increase, especially among high-risk patients.

Nursing considerations
- High-risk patients include elderly people and those with renal impairment or type 2 diabetes; monitor these patients closely.
- Check serum potassium, BUN, and creatinine levels regularly. If they increase, notify the prescriber.

■ Advise the patient to report an irregular heartbeat, slow pulse, weakness, or other evidence of hyperkalemia immediately.
■ Give the patient a list of foods high in potassium; stress the need to eat only moderate amounts.

capecitabine ▶◀ warfarin
Xeloda   Coumadin

Risk rating: 1
Severity: Major   **Onset: Delayed**   **Likelihood: Suspected**

Cause
May inhibit warfarin metabolism, clotting factor synthesis, and possibly, protein displacement.

Effect
Anticoagulant effects increase.

Nursing considerations
■ Monitor PT and INR closely during and after chemotherapy.
■ Tell the patient to report unusual bruising or bleeding.
■ Remind the patient that warfarin interacts with many drugs and that he should report any change in drug regimen.

captopril ▶◀ aspirin
Capoten   Bayer, Ecotrin

Risk rating: 2
Severity: Moderate   **Onset: Rapid**   **Likelihood: Suspected**

Cause
Salicylates such as aspirin inhibit synthesis of prostaglandins, which ACE inhibitors need to lower blood pressure.

Effect
The hypotensive effect of captopril will be reduced.

Nursing considerations
■ This interaction is more likely in people with hypertension, coronary artery disease, or possibly heart failure.
■ At doses less than 100 mg daily, aspirin is less likely to interact.

captopril ━━━━━━►◄━━━━━━ food
Capoten

Risk rating: 2
Severity: Moderate   **Onset: Rapid**   **Likelihood: Suspected**

Cause
Food decreases GI absorption of captopril.

Effect
Antihypertensive effectiveness may be reduced.

Nursing considerations
◤ **ALERT** Give captopril 1 hour before meals.
- This interaction may occur with ACE inhibitors other than captopril. If you suspect a drug interaction, consult the prescriber or pharmacist.
- Food doesn't reduce absorption of enalapril or lisinopril.

captopril ━━━━━━►◄━━━━━━ indomethacin
Capoten   Indocin

Risk rating: 2
Severity: Moderate   **Onset: Rapid**   **Likelihood: Probable**

Cause
Indomethacin inhibits synthesis of prostaglandins, which captopril and other ACE inhibitors need to lower blood pressure.

Effect
ACE inhibitor's hypotensive effect will decrease.

Nursing considerations
◤ **ALERT** Monitor blood pressure closely. Severe hypertension may persist until indomethacin is stopped.
- The patient taking indomethacin may need an alternate antihypertensive.
- Other ACE inhibitors may interact with indomethacin. If you suspect an interaction, consult the prescriber or pharmacist.
- Remind the patient that hypertension commonly causes no physical symptoms but sometimes may cause headache and dizziness.

captopril ━━━━▶◀ loop diuretics
Capoten   bumetanide, furosemide

Risk rating: 3
Severity: Minor   **Onset: Delayed**   **Likelihood: Suspected**

Cause
Captopril may inhibit angiotensin II production.

Effect
The effects of loop diuretics may be decreased.

Nursing considerations
■ Monitor fluid status and body weight in the patient taking a loop diuretic when captopril therapy is started, stopped, or the dosage is adjusted.
■ Weigh the patient daily.
■ Monitor the patient for expected loop diuretic effects: reduction in peripheral edema, resolution of pulmonary edema, or decreased blood pressure in hypertensive patients.

captopril ━━━━▶◀ potassium-sparing diuretics
Capoten   amiloride, spironolactone

Risk rating: 1
Severity: Major   **Onset: Delayed**   **Likelihood: Probable**

Cause
The mechanism of this interaction is unknown.

Effect
Serum potassium level may increase.

Nursing considerations
■ Use cautiously in patients at high risk for hyperkalemia, especially those with renal impairment.
■ Monitor BUN, creatinine, and serum potassium levels as needed.
■ ACE inhibitors other than captopril may interact with potassium-sparing diuretics. If you suspect an interaction, consult the prescriber or pharmacist.
■ Urge the patient to report an irregular heartbeat, a slow pulse, weakness, and other evidence of hyperkalemia immediately

carbamazepine ➤◀ aripiprazole
Carbatrol, Epitol,
Equetro, Tegretol

Abilify

Risk rating: 2
Severity: Moderate   **Onset: Delayed**   **Likelihood: Suspected**

Cause
Carbamazepine may increase CYP3A4 metabolism of aripiprazole.

Effect
Plasma concentrations of aripiprazole may be decreased; drug may exhibit decreased pharmacologic effects.

Nursing considerations
- When carbamazepine is administered with aripiprazole, double the dose of aripiprazole.
- The dose of aripiprazole may need to be decreased when carbamazepine is discontinued.
- Monitor the patient's response to aripiprazole, and notify the prescriber if you notice a decreased response to aripiprazole.
- Instruct the patient to notify the prescriber immediately if he notices a decrease in aripiprazole effects.

carbamazepine ➤◀ azole antifungals
Carbatrol, Epitol,
Equetro, Tegretol

fluconazole, itraconazole,
ketoconazole

Risk rating: 2
Severity: Moderate   **Onset: Delayed**   **Likelihood: Suspected**

Cause
Azole antifungals may inhibit CYP3A4 metabolism of carbamazepine.

Effect
Carbamazepine effects, including adverse effects, may increase.

Nursing considerations
- Monitor the patient's response when an azole antifungal is started or stopped.
- Monitor carbamazepine level; therapeutic range is 4 to 12 mcg/ml.
- **◤ ALERT** Watch for signs of anorexia or subtle appetite changes, which may indicate an excessive carbamazepine level.
- Monitor the patient for signs of carbamazepine toxicity, including dizziness, ataxia, respiratory depression, tachycardia, arrhythmias,

blood pressure changes, impaired consciousness, abnormal reflexes, nystagmus, seizures, nausea, vomiting, and urine retention.
■ Other azole antifungals may interact with carbamazepine. If you suspect an interaction, consult the prescriber or pharmacist.

carbamazepine ➤◄ benzodiazepines
Carbatrol, Epitol,
Equetro, Tegretol

alprazolam, midazolam

Risk rating: 2
Severity: Moderate   **Onset: Delayed**   **Likelihood: Suspected**

Cause
The metabolism of benzodiazepines is increased.

Effect
The pharmacologic effects of benzodiazepines may be decreased.

Nursing considerations
■ Carbamazepine may cause decreased effectiveness of benzodiazepines.
■ If the patient is taking carbamazepine and a benzodiazepine together, monitor the patient for a decreased response to the benzodiazepine.
■ Consult with the prescriber for an increased dose of the benzodiazepine if needed.

carbamazepine ➤◄ bupropion
Carbatrol, Epitol,
Equetro, Tegretol

Wellbutrin, Zyban

Risk rating: 2
Severity: Moderate   **Onset: Delayed**   **Likelihood: Suspected**

Cause
Carbamazepine increases hepatic metabolism of bupropion.

Effect
Bupropion level may decrease.

Nursing considerations
⚡ **ALERT** Bupropion is contraindicated in patients with a seizure disorder.
■ Monitor the patient's response to bupropion.
■ Bupropion dosage may need adjustment.

- The risk of bupropion-related seizures may be reduced by keeping the daily dose below 450 mg (400 mg SR; 450 mg XL); giving the daily dose b.i.d. or t.i.d. (depending on preparation used) to avoid high peak levels; and increasing doses gradually.
- Urge the patient to tell the prescriber about all drugs and supplements he takes.

carbamazepine ■■■►◄■■■ cimetidine

Carbatrol, Epitol,
Equetro, Tegretol

Tagamet

Risk rating: 2
Severity: Moderate   Onset: Delayed   Likelihood: Suspected

Cause
Cimetidine may inhibit hepatic metabolism of carbamazepine.

Effect
Carbamazepine plasma level and risk of toxicity may increase.

Nursing considerations
- Monitor the patient's response when cimetidine starts (especially during the first 4 weeks of therapy) or stops.
- Monitor carbamazepine level; therapeutic range is 4 to 12 mcg/ml.
- ◩ ALERT Watch for signs of anorexia or subtle appetite changes, which may indicate an excessive carbamazepine level.
- Monitor the patient for signs of carbamazepine toxicity, including dizziness, ataxia, respiratory depression, tachycardia, arrhythmias, blood pressure changes, impaired consciousness, abnormal reflexes, nystagmus, seizures, nausea, vomiting, and urine retention.
- Carbamazepine dosage may need adjustment.

carbamazepine ■■■►◄■■■ cyclosporine

Carbatrol, Epitol,
Equetro, Tegretol

Gengraf, Neoral, Sandimmune

Risk rating: 2
Severity: Moderate   Onset: Delayed   Likelihood: Suspected

Cause
Carbamazepine may induce hepatic metabolism of cyclosporine.

Effect
Cyclosporine level and effects may decrease.

Nursing considerations
- Monitor cyclosporine level; dosage may need adjustment.
- Watch for signs of rejection if carbamazepine therapy starts.
- Watch for signs of cyclosporine toxicity if carbamazepine therapy is stopped; signs of toxicity include hepatotoxicity, nephrotoxicity, nausea, vomiting, tremors, and seizures.

carbamazepine ━━▶◀━━ danazol
Carbatrol, Epitol,
Equetro, Tegretol

Risk rating: 2
Severity: **Moderate**   Onset: **Delayed**   Likelihood: **Suspected**

Cause
Danazol inhibits carbamazepine metabolism.

Effect
Carbamazepine level and toxicity may increase.

Nursing considerations
⚠ ALERT Avoid this combination if possible.
- Monitor carbamazepine level; therapeutic range is 4 to 12 mcg/ml.
- Carbamazepine dosage may need adjustment if danazol is started or stopped.
⚠ ALERT Watch for signs of anorexia or subtle appetite changes, which may indicate an excessive carbamazepine level.
- Monitor the patient for evidence of carbamazepine toxicity, including dizziness, ataxia, respiratory depression, tachycardia, arrhythmias, blood pressure changes, impaired consciousness, abnormal reflexes, nystagmus, seizures, nausea, vomiting, and urine retention.

carbamazepine ━━▶◀━━ diltiazem
Carbatrol, Epitol,   Cardizem
Equetro, Tegretol

Risk rating: 2
Severity: **Moderate**   Onset: **Delayed**   Likelihood: **Suspected**

Cause
Diltiazem, a calcium channel blocker, may inhibit carbamazepine metabolism.

Effect

Carbamazepine level and risk of toxicity may increase.

Nursing considerations

■ Monitor carbamazepine level; therapeutic range is 4 to 12 mcg/ml.
■ If diltiazem therapy starts, watch for signs of carbamazepine toxicity, including dizziness, ataxia, respiratory depression, tachycardia, arrhythmias, blood pressure changes, impaired consciousness, abnormal reflexes, nystagmus, seizures, nausea, vomiting, and urine retention.
■ If diltiazem therapy stops, watch for loss of carbamazepine effects (loss of seizure control). Carbamazepine dose may need to be increased.
■ Urge the patient to tell the prescriber about all drugs and supplements he takes.
■ Other calcium channel blockers may have this interaction. If you suspect an interaction, consult the prescriber or pharmacist.

---

carbamazepine ■━▶◀■ doxycycline

Carbatrol, Epitol,   Monodox, Oracea
Equetro, Tegretol

Risk rating: 2
Severity: Moderate   Onset: Delayed   Likelihood: Suspected

Cause

Carbamazepine increases the hepatic metabolism of doxycycline, a tetracycline.

Effect

The serum levels and therapeutic efficacy of doxycycline decreases.

Nursing considerations

■ Dose of doxycycline may need to be increased during carbamazepine administration.
■ Monitor the patient for resolving infection. If the infection doesn't resolve, discuss the interaction with the prescriber.
■ If possible, consider the use of another tetracycline; the interaction isn't seen in other tetracyclines.

carbamazepine ━▶◀━ felbamate

Carbatrol, Epitol,   Felbatol
Equetro, Tegretol

Risk rating: 2
Severity: Moderate   Onset: Delayed   Likelihood: Suspected

Cause
The mechanism of this interaction is unknown. Carbamazepine metabolism may increase, or conversion of carbamazepine metabolites may decrease. Also, felbamate metabolism may increase.

Effect
Carbamazepine and felbamate levels and effects may decrease.

Nursing considerations
◧ **ALERT** Monitor the patient for loss of seizure control.
▪ Monitor carbamazepine level; therapeutic range is 4 to 12 mcg/ml.
▪ Dosage may need adjustment when felbamate starts.
▪ Urge the patient to tell the prescriber about all drugs and supplements he takes.

carbamazepine ━▶◀━ felodipine

Carbatrol, Epitol,   Plendil
Equetro, Tegretol

Risk rating: 2
Severity: Moderate   Onset: Delayed   Likelihood: Suspected

Cause
The mechanism of this interaction is unknown. Carbamazepine may increase felodipine metabolism and decrease its availability.

Effect
Felodipine effects may decrease.

Nursing considerations
▪ Felodipine dose may need to be increased.
▪ If carbamazepine starts, watch for loss of blood pressure control, and urge the patient to have his blood pressure monitored.
▪ If carbamazepine is stopped, watch for evidence of felodipine toxicity, such as peripheral vasodilation, hypotension, bradycardia, and palpitations.
▪ Remind the patient that hypertension commonly has no symptoms, although it may cause headache and dizziness.

carbamazepine ⬛▶◀⬛ fluoxetine
Carbatrol, Epitol,
Equetro, Tegretol

Prozac

Risk rating: 2
Severity: Moderate   **Onset: Delayed**   **Likelihood: Suspected**

Cause
The mechanism of this interaction is unknown. Fluoxetine may inhibit carbamazepine metabolism.

Effect
Carbamazepine level and risk of toxicity may increase.

Nursing considerations
■ Monitor carbamazepine level; therapeutic range is 4 to 12 mcg/ml.
◤ ALERT Watch for signs of anorexia or subtle appetite changes, which may indicate excessive carbamazepine level.
■ Monitor the patient for evidence of carbamazepine toxicity, including dizziness, ataxia, respiratory depression, tachycardia, arrhythmias, blood pressure changes, impaired consciousness, abnormal reflexes, nystagmus, seizures, nausea, vomiting, and urine retention.
■ Carbamazepine dosage may need adjustment if fluoxetine is started or stopped.
■ If fluoxetine starts during stabilized carbamazepine therapy, advise the patient to report nausea, vomiting, dizziness, visual disturbances, difficulty balancing, tremors, or any new adverse effects.
■ SSRIs other than fluoxetine may interact with carbamazepine. If you suspect a drug interaction, consult the prescriber or pharmacist.

carbamazepine ⬛▶◀⬛ grapefruit juice
Carbatrol, Epitol,
Equetro, Tegretol

Risk rating: 2
Severity: Moderate   **Onset: Delayed**   **Likelihood: Suspected**

Cause
CYP3A4 metabolism of carbamazepine may be inhibited.

Effect
Carbamazepine level and adverse effects may increase.

Nursing considerations
◤ ALERT Don't give carbamazepine with grapefruit juice.

- Carbamazepine's adverse effects may be increased, including dizziness, ataxia, arrhythmias, impaired consciousness, worsening seizures, nausea, and vomiting.
- Therapeutic carbamazepine level is 4 to 12 mcg/ml.
- Advise the patient to tell the prescriber about all drugs and supplements he takes and any increase in adverse effects.

carbamazepine ▶◀ haloperidol
Carbatrol, Epitol,   Haldol
Equetro, Tegretol

Risk rating: 2
Severity: Moderate   Onset: Delayed   Likelihood: Suspected

Cause
Carbamazepine may increase haloperidol hepatic metabolism; haloperidol may inhibit carbamazepine metabolism.

Effect
Haloperidol effects may decrease; carbamazepine effects, including adverse effects, may increase.

Nursing considerations
- Monitor haloperidol level; therapeutic range is 5 to 20 ng/ml.
- Monitor carbamazepine level; therapeutic range is 4 to 12 mcg/ml.
- Watch for loss of haloperidol effects, including symptoms of psychomotor agitation, obsessive-compulsive rituals, withdrawn behavior, auditory hallucinations, delusions, and delirium.
- **✷ ALERT** Watch for signs of anorexia or subtle appetite changes, which may indicate an excessive carbamazepine level.
- Watch for signs of carbamazepine toxicity, including dizziness, ataxia, respiratory depression, tachycardia, arrhythmias, blood pressure changes, impaired consciousness, abnormal reflexes, nystagmus, seizures, nausea, vomiting, and urine retention.

carbamazepine ▶◀ hormonal contraceptives
Carbatrol, Epitol,   Ortho-Novum
Equetro, Tegretol

Risk rating: 1
Severity: Major   Onset: Delayed   Likelihood: Suspected

Cause
Hepatic metabolism of hormonal contraceptives may increase.

Effect

Contraceptive effectiveness may decrease.

Nursing considerations

■ Other hormonal contraceptives may interact with carbamazepine. If you suspect a drug interaction, consult the prescriber or pharmacist.

■ Urge the patient to use an alternative method of birth control to avoid unintended pregnancy.

■ Larger hormonal contraceptive doses may be considered; consult the prescriber about the right dosage to prevent breakthrough bleeding.

carbamazepine ▬►◄▬ isoniazid

Carbatrol, Epitol,   Nydrazid
Equetro, Tegretol

Risk rating: 2

Severity: Moderate   **Onset: Delayed**   **Likelihood: Suspected**

Cause

Isoniazid may inhibit carbamazepine metabolism. Carbamazepine may increase isoniazid hepatotoxicity.

Effect

Risk of carbamazepine toxicity and isoniazid hepatotoxicity increases.

Nursing considerations

■ Monitor carbamazepine level; therapeutic range is 4 to 12 mcg/ml.

■ Watch for signs of carbamazepine toxicity, including dizziness, ataxia, respiratory depression, tachycardia, arrhythmias, blood pressure changes, impaired consciousness, abnormal reflexes, nystagmus, seizures, nausea, vomiting, and urine retention.

■ Monitor liver function tests.

■ Advise the patient to report signs of hepatotoxicity, including abdominal pain, loss of appetite, fatigue, yellow skin or eyes, and dark urine.

carbamazepine ▬►◄▬ lamotrigine

Carbatrol, Epitol,   Lamictal
Equetro, Tegretol

Risk rating: 2

Severity: Moderate   **Onset: Delayed**   **Likelihood: Probable**

Cause

Lamotrigine metabolism may increase. Lamotrigine may increase carbamazepine toxicity.

Effect
Lamotrigine effects may decrease. Carbamazepine metabolite level and risk of toxicity may increase.

Nursing considerations
■ Watch for expected lamotrigine effects when starting it in a patient who takes carbamazepine.
■ Lamotrigine dosage may need adjustment when starting or stopping carbamazepine or changing its dosage.
■ Monitor carbamazepine level when adding lamotrigine; therapeutic range is 4 to 12 mcg/ml.
■ Monitor the patient for evidence of carbamazepine toxicity, including dizziness, ataxia, respiratory depression, tachycardia, arrhythmias, blood pressure changes, impaired consciousness, abnormal reflexes, nystagmus, seizures, nausea, vomiting, and urine retention.
■ Carbamazepine dosage may need reduction.

carbamazepine ►◄ lithium
Carbatrol, Epitol,   Eskalith
Equetro, Tegretol

Risk rating: 2
Severity: **Moderate**   Onset: **Delayed**   Likelihood: **Suspected**

Cause
The mechanism of this interaction is unknown.

Effect
Interaction increases risk of adverse CNS effects, including lethargy, muscle weakness, ataxia, tremor, and hyperreflexia.

Nursing considerations
■ The combination may be beneficial in treating bipolar depression and may be justified if benefits outweigh risks.
■ Some patients can tolerate the combination without adverse effects.

carbamazepine ►◄ macrolide antibiotics
Carbatrol, Epitol,   clarithromycin, erythromycin
Equetro, Tegretol

Risk rating: 1
Severity: **Major**   Onset: **Rapid**   Likelihood: **Established**

Cause
CYP3A4 metabolism of carbamazepine is inhibited, decreasing carbamazepine clearance.

Effect
Carbamazepine level and toxicity may increase.

Nursing considerations
ALERT If possible, avoid use together.

■ Consult the prescriber or pharmacist about an alternative macrolide antibiotic (such as azithromycin) or an alternative anti-infective drug unlikely to interact with carbamazepine.

■ If using a macrolide antibiotic, monitor carbamazepine level; therapeutic range is 4 to 12 mcg/ml.

■ Monitor the patient for evidence of carbamazepine toxicity, including dizziness, ataxia, respiratory depression, tachycardia, arrhythmias, blood pressure changes, impaired consciousness, abnormal reflexes, nystagmus, seizures, nausea, vomiting, and urine retention.

■ Carbamazepine dosage may need adjustment.

---

carbamazepine ➤◀ MAO inhibitors
Carbatrol, Epitol, Equetro, Tegretol

isocarboxazid, phenelzine, tranylcypromine

Risk rating: 1
Severity: Major   **Onset: Delayed**   **Likelihood: Suspected**

Cause
The mechanism of this interaction is unknown.

Effect
Risk of severe adverse effects, including hyperpyrexia, hyperexcitability, muscle rigidity, and seizures, may increase.

Nursing considerations
ALERT Use of carbamazepine with an MAO inhibitor is contraindicated.

ALERT Carbamazepine is structurally related to tricyclic antidepressants, which may cause hypertensive crisis, seizures, and death when given with MAO inhibitors.

■ MAO inhibitor should be stopped at least 14 days before carbamazepine starts.

■ Urge the patient to tell the prescriber about all drugs and supplements he takes and about any increase in adverse effects.

carbamazepine ▬▬►◄▬▬ nefazodone

Carbatrol, Epitol,
Equetro, Tegretol

Risk rating: 1
Severity: Major   **Onset: Delayed**   **Likelihood: Suspected**

Cause
Nefazodone may inhibit CYP3A4 hepatic metabolism of carbamazepine. Carbamazepine may induce nefazodone metabolism.

Effect
Carbamazepine level and risk of adverse effects may increase. Nefazodone level and effects may decrease.

Nursing considerations
■ **ALERT** Use of carbamazepine with nefazodone is contraindicated.
■ If drugs are combined for any reason, monitor carbamazepine serum level; therapeutic range is 4 to 12 mcg/ml.
■ Monitor the patient for evidence of carbamazepine toxicity, including dizziness, ataxia, respiratory depression, tachycardia, arrhythmias, blood pressure changes, impaired consciousness, abnormal reflexes, nystagmus, seizures, nausea, vomiting, and urine retention.
■ Urge the patient to tell the prescriber about all drugs and supplements he takes and about any increase in adverse effects.

carbamazepine ▬▬►◄▬▬ nondepolarizing muscle relaxants

Carbatrol, Epitol,
Equetro, Tegretol

atracurium, cisatracurium,
pancuronium, rocuronium,
vecuronium

Risk rating: 2
Severity: Moderate   **Onset: Rapid**   **Likelihood: Probable**

Cause
The mechanism of this interaction is unknown.

Effect
Effect or duration of nondepolarizing muscle relaxant may decrease.

Nursing considerations
■ Monitor the patient for decreased efficacy of muscle relaxant.
■ Dosage of muscle relaxant may need to be increased.
■ Make sure the patient is adequately sedated when receiving a nondepolarizing muscle relaxant.

carbamazepine ▶◀ olanzapine

Carbatrol, Epitol,
Equetro, Tegretol

Zyprexa

Risk rating: 3
Severity: Minor   **Onset: Delayed**   **Likelihood: Suspected**

Cause
Carbamazepine increases hepatic metabolism.

Effect
Olanzapine level and effects decrease.

Nursing considerations
■ Observe the patient's clinical response to olanzapine.
■ If an interaction is suspected, adjust the dose of olanzapine as needed.
■ Monitor the patient for increased agitation, manic or depressed episodes, or schizophrenic activity.

carbamazepine ▶◀ phenytoin

Carbatrol, Epitol,
Equetro, Tegretol

Dilantin

Risk rating: 2
Severity: Moderate   **Onset: Delayed**   **Likelihood: Suspected**

Cause
Carbamazepine metabolism may increase. Carbamazepine also may decrease phenytoin availability.

Effect
Carbamazepine level and effects decrease. The effect of carbamazepine on phenytoin is variable.

Nursing considerations
■ Monitor serum levels of both drugs as appropriate, especially when starting or stopping either one.
■ Therapeutic carbamazepine level is 4 to 12 mcg/ml.
■ Therapeutic phenytoin level is 10 to 20 mcg/ml.
■ Dosage adjustments may be needed to maintain therapeutic effects and avoid toxicity.
■ Monitor the patient for loss of drug effect (loss of seizure control).

carbamazepine ▶◀ primidone

Carbatrol, Epitol,
Equetro, Tegretol

Mysoline

Risk rating: 2
Severity: Moderate   Onset: Delayed   Likelihood: Suspected

Cause
The combination may alter hepatic metabolism.

Effect
Carbamazepine and primidone levels may decrease.

Nursing considerations
- Monitor serum levels of both drugs as appropriate, especially when starting or stopping either one.
- Therapeutic carbamazepine level is 4 to 12 mcg/ml.
- Dosage adjustments may be needed to maintain therapeutic effects.
- Monitor the patient for loss of drug effect (loss of seizure control).

carbamazepine ▶◀ propoxyphene

Carbatrol, Epitol,
Equetro, Tegretol

Darvon

Risk rating: 2
Severity: Moderate   Onset: Rapid   Likelihood: Suspected

Cause
Hepatic metabolism of carbamazepine is inhibited, decreasing drug clearance.

Effect
Carbamazepine level and risk of toxicity may increase.

Nursing considerations
- ⚠ ALERT Avoid combined use if possible.
- Monitor carbamazepine level; therapeutic range is 4 to 12 mcg/ml.
- Monitor the patient for evidence of carbamazepine toxicity, including dizziness, ataxia, respiratory depression, tachycardia, arrhythmias, blood pressure changes, impaired consciousness, abnormal reflexes, nystagmus, seizures, nausea, vomiting, and urine retention.
- Consult the prescriber or pharmacist about alternative analgesics to propoxyphene.

carbamazepine ▶◀ protease inhibitors

Carbatrol, Epitol,
Equetro, Tegretol

indinavir, lopinavir/ritonavir,
nelfinavir, ritonavir, saquinavir

Risk rating: 2
Severity: Moderate   **Onset: Rapid**   **Likelihood: Suspected**

Cause
Inhibition of CYP3A4 metabolism of carbamazepine. Carbamazepine
may also induce CYP3A4 metabolism of protease inhibitors.

Effect
Carbamazepine level and risk of toxicity increase. Protease inhibitor
levels may decrease, resulting in antiretroviral treatment failure.

Nursing considerations
■ Closely monitor carbamazepine level when starting, stopping, or
changing the dose of the protease inhibitor.
■ Therapeutic carbamazepine level is 4 to 12 mcg/ml.
■ Dosage adjustments may be needed to maintain therapeutic effects
and avoid toxicity.
■ Monitor the clinical response to the protease inhibitor therapy.
■ Monitor the patient for evidence of carbamazepine toxicity, including dizziness, ataxia, respiratory depression, tachycardia, arrhythmias,
blood pressure changes, impaired consciousness, abnormal reflexes,
nystagmus, seizures, nausea, vomiting, and urine retention.
■ Monitor lab values for increased CD4+ T-cell count and a decreased HIV-1 RNA level.

carbamazepine ▶◀ sertraline

Carbatrol, Epitol,
Equetro, Tegretol

Zoloft

Risk rating: 2
Severity: Moderate   **Onset: Delayed**   **Likelihood: Suspected**

Cause
Increased CYP3A4 metabolism of sertraline.

Effect
Carbamazepine may decrease or reverse therapeutic effect of sertraline.

Nursing considerations
■ If patient is receiving carbamazepine, considering administering an antidepressant such as paroxetine, which isn't affected by CYP3A4 metabolism.
■ Closely monitor the patient's response to sertraline.
■ Be prepared to adjust the dose of sertraline when starting, stopping, or changing the carbamazepine dose.
■ Increasing the dose of sertraline may help decrease the interaction.

---

carbamazepine ▶◀ simvastatin
Carbatrol, Epitol,   Zocor
Equetro, Tegretol

Risk rating: 2
Severity: Moderate   Onset: Delayed   Likelihood: Suspected

Cause
Carbamazepine may increase CYP3A4 metabolism of HMG-CoA reductase inhibitors such as simvastatin.

Effect
Simvastatin effects may be reduced.

Nursing considerations
■ If possible, avoid using together.
■ If that can't be avoided, monitor serum cholesterol and lipid levels to assess the patient's response to therapy.
■ If hypercholesterolemia increases, notify the prescriber.
■ Pravastatin and rosuvastatin may be less likely to interact with carbamazepine and may be better choices than other HMG-CoA reductase inhibitors.

---

carbamazepine ▶◀ tricyclic antidepressants
Carbatrol, Epitol,   amitriptyline, desipramine,
Equetro, Tegretol   doxepin, imipramine,
                                      nortriptyline

Risk rating: 2
Severity: Moderate   Onset: Delayed   Likelihood: Probable

Cause
Tricyclic antidepressants (TCAs) may compete with carbamazepine for hepatic metabolism. Carbamazepine may induce hepatic TCA metabolism.

Effect
Carbamazepine level and risk of toxicity may increase. TCA level and effects may decrease.

Nursing considerations
■ Other TCAs may interact with carbamazepine. If you suspect a drug interaction, consult the prescriber or pharmacist.
■ Monitor carbamazepine level; therapeutic range is 4 to 12 mcg/ml.
■ Watch for evidence of carbamazepine toxicity, including dizziness, ataxia, respiratory depression, tachycardia, arrhythmias, blood pressure changes, impaired consciousness, abnormal reflexes, nystagmus, seizures, nausea, vomiting, and urine retention.

carbamazepine ➤◀ valproic acid
Carbatrol, Epitol,
Equetro, Tegretol

Risk rating: 2
Severity: Moderate   Onset: Delayed   Likelihood: Established

Cause
Metabolism of valproic acid may be altered by carbamazepine. Conversion of valproic acid to a hepatotoxic and teratogenic metabolite may increase.

Effect
Valproic acid level decreases, with possible loss of seizure control. Also, carbamazepine levels may change.

Nursing considerations
■ These drugs have been used safely together in many patients to help manage epilepsy and psychiatric disorders.
■ Monitor seizure control and toxicity for at least 1 month after starting or stopping combined use.
■ Check levels of both drugs during use and for 1 month after either drug is stopped.
■ Although rare, pancreatitis and acute psychosis may arise because of slow excretion after combined use has stopped.

carbamazepine ━━►◄━━ verapamil
Carbatrol, Epitol,   Calan
Equetro, Tegretol

Risk rating: 2
Severity: Moderate   Onset: Delayed   Likelihood: Suspected

Cause
Verapamil, a calcium channel blocker, may decrease hepatic metabolism of carbamazepine.

Effect
Carbamazepine level, effects, and toxic effects may increase.

Nursing considerations
■ Monitor carbamazepine level; therapeutic range is 4 to 12 mcg/ml.
■ Watch for evidence of carbamazepine toxicity, including dizziness, ataxia, respiratory depression, tachycardia, arrhythmias, blood pressure changes, impaired consciousness, abnormal reflexes, nystagmus, seizures, nausea, vomiting, and urine retention.
■ Carbamazepine dose may need to be reduced by 40% to 50%.
■ If verapamil is stopped, watch for loss of carbamazepine effect.
■ Other calcium channel blockers may interact with carbamazepine. If you suspect a drug interaction, consult the prescriber or pharmacist.

carbamazepine ━━►◄━━ voriconazole
Carbatrol, Epitol,   Vfend
Equetro, Tegretol

Risk rating: 1
Severity: Major   Onset: Delayed   Likelihood: Suspected

Cause
Carbamazepine may increase CYP3A4 metabolism of voriconazole.

Effect
Voriconazole effects may decrease.

Nursing considerations
⚡ **ALERT** Use of these drugs together is contraindicated.
■ Instruct the patient to avoid carbamazepine while taking voriconazole; consult the prescriber about alternative therapies.

carbamazepine ➤◀ warfarin
Carbatrol, Epitol,
Equetro, Tegretol

Coumadin

Risk rating: 2
Severity: Moderate   **Onset: Delayed**   **Likelihood: Suspected**

Cause
Carbamazepine may increase hepatic metabolism of warfarin.

Effect
Anticoagulant effect of warfarin decreases.

Nursing considerations
■ If the patient takes warfarin, monitor PT and INR when starting or stopping carbamazepine or changing its dosage.
■ For an acute MI, atrial fibrillation, treatment of pulmonary embolism, prevention of systemic embolism, tissue heart valves, valvular heart disease, or prophylaxis or treatment of venous thrombosis, maintain INR at 2 to 3. For mechanical prosthetic valves or recurrent systemic embolism, maintain INR at 3 to 4.5.

carbamazepine ➤◀ ziprasidone
Carbatrol, Epitol,
Equetro, Tegretol

Geodon

Risk rating: 2
Severity: Moderate   **Onset: Delayed**   **Likelihood: Suspected**

Cause
Carbamazepine induces increased CYP3A4 metabolism of ziprasidone.

Effect
Ziprasidone levels and effects may be decreased.

Nursing considerations
■ Monitor the patient's response to ziprasidone when starting, stopping, or changing the dose of carbamazepine.
■ Be prepared to change the dose of ziprasidone as needed.
■ Monitor the patient for increased schizophrenic symptoms, agitation, mania, or acute depression.

124 carboplatin–phenytoin

carboplatin ━━━▶◀━━━ phenytoin
Paraplatin   Dilantin

Risk rating: 2
Severity: Moderate   **Onset: Delayed**   **Likelihood: Suspected**

Cause
Phenytoin absorption may be decreased or metabolism may be increased.

Effect
Phenytoin level and effects may decrease.

Nursing considerations
- Monitor phenytoin level closely. Dosage may need to be adjusted.
- Therapeutic range for phenytoin is 10 to 20 mcg/ml.
- Toxic effects can occur at therapeutic level. Adjust the measured level for hypoalbuminemia or renal impairment, which can increase free drug level.
- Monitor the patient for seizure activity.
- Carefully monitor phenytoin level between courses of chemotherapy. Phenytoin may need to be decreased.
- Signs and symptoms of phenytoin toxicity include nystagmus, slurred speech, ataxia, blurred or double vision, confusion, drowsiness, and lethargy.

carboplatin ━━━▶◀━━━ warfarin
Paraplatin   Coumadin

Risk rating: 1
Severity: Major   **Onset: Delayed**   **Likelihood: Suspected**

Cause
Warfarin metabolism, clotting factor synthesis, and possibly protein displacement may be inhibited.

Effect
Anticoagulant effects increase.

Nursing considerations
- Monitor PT and INR closely during and after chemotherapy.
- Tell the patient to report unusual bruising or bleeding.
- Remind the patient that warfarin interacts with many drugs and that he should report any change in drug regimen.

carmustine ▶◀ cimetidine
BiCNU   Tagamet

Risk rating: 1
Severity: Major   **Onset: Delayed**   **Likelihood: Suspected**

Cause
The mechanism of interaction is unknown, but may involve additive bone marrow suppression or decreased carmustine metabolism.

Effect
Carmustine myelosuppressive effects increase.

Nursing considerations
⚠ ALERT Avoid combined use if possible.
■ Monitor CBC, WBC, and platelet counts if used together.
■ Be prepared to provide supportive measures, such as blood components and granulocyte-colony stimulating factor, as ordered.
■ Consult the prescriber or pharmacist for an alternative drug to avoid severe myelosuppression.
■ H_2-receptor antagonists other than cimetidine may interact with carmustine. If you suspect an interaction, consult the prescriber or pharmacist.

carmustine ▶◀ phenytoin
BiCNU   Dilantin

Risk rating: 2
Severity: Moderate   **Onset: Delayed**   **Likelihood: Suspected**

Cause
Phenytoin absorption may be decreased or metabolism may be increased.

Effect
Phenytoin level and effects may decrease.

Nursing considerations
■ Monitor phenytoin level closely. Dosage may need to be adjusted.
■ Therapeutic range for phenytoin is 10 to 20 mcg/ml.
■ Toxic effects can occur at therapeutic level. Adjust the measured level for hypoalbuminemia or renal impairment, which can increase free drug level.
■ Carefully monitor phenytoin level between courses of chemotherapy. Phenytoin may need to be decreased.

■ Signs and symptoms of phenytoin toxicity include nystagmus, slurred speech, ataxia, blurred or double vision, confusion, drowsiness, and lethargy.

carvedilol ━━━►◄━━ aspirin
Coreg   Bayer, Ecotrin

Risk rating: 2
Severity: Moderate   **Onset: Rapid**   **Likelihood: Suspected**

Cause
Salicylates such as aspirin inhibit synthesis of prostaglandins, which carvedilol and other beta blockers need to lower blood pressure. In patients with heart failure, the mechanism of this interaction is unknown.

Effect
Beta blocker effects decrease.

Nursing considerations
■ Watch closely for signs of heart failure and hypertension, and notify the prescriber if they occur.
■ Consult the prescriber about switching the patient to a different antihypertensive or antiplatelet drug.
■ Other beta blockers may interact with salicylates. If you suspect an interaction, consult the prescriber or pharmacist.
■ Explain signs and symptoms of heart failure, and tell the patient when to contact the prescriber.

carvedilol ━━━►◄━━ cyclosporine
Coreg   Gengraf, Neoral, Sandimmune

Risk rating: 2
Severity: Moderate   **Onset: Delayed**   **Likelihood: Suspected**

Cause
Carvedilol may interfere with cyclosporine metabolism.

Effect
Cyclosporine level and risk of toxicity may increase.

Nursing considerations
■ Beta blockers other than carvedilol may interact with cyclosporine.
■ Watch for evidence of cyclosporine toxicity, such as nephrotoxicity and neurotoxicity.
■ Monitor serum creatinine level.

■ Monitor cyclosporine level.

carvedilol ▬▬▬►◄▬▬ digoxin
Coreg   Lanoxin

Risk rating: 2
Severity: Moderate   **Onset: Rapid**   **Likelihood: Probable**

Cause
Carvedilol increases digoxin bioavailability. Renal excretion of digoxin may be decreased and additive depression of myocardial conduction may occur.

Effect
Digoxin level and risk of toxicity may occur. Synergistic bradycardia may occur.

Nursing considerations
■ **ALERT** Carefully monitor patients receiving carvedilol and digoxin for bradycardia.
■ Monitor digoxin level. Therapeutic range is 0.8 to 2 nanograms/ml.
■ Watch for evidence of digoxin toxicity. These include arrhythmias (bradycardia, AV block, and ventricular ectopy); along with lethargy, drowsiness, confusion, hallucinations, headaches, syncopes, visual disturbances, nausea, anorexia, vomiting, and diarrhea.
■ Digoxin dosage may need to be decreased.
■ Patients with higher serum digoxin levels have an increased risk of toxicity.

ceftazidime ▬▬▬►◄▬▬ aminoglycosides
Fortaz   gentamicin, tobramycin

Risk rating: 2
Severity: Moderate   **Onset: Delayed**   **Likelihood: Suspected**

Cause
The mechanism of this interaction is unknown.

Effect
Bactericidal activity may increase against some organisms, but the risk of nephrotoxicity may also increase.

Nursing considerations
■ **ALERT** Check peak and trough aminoglycoside level after third dose. For peak level, draw blood 30 minutes after I.V. or 60 minutes after I.M. dose. For trough dose, draw blood just before a dose.

- Assess BUN and creatinine levels.
- Monitor urine output, and check urine for increased protein, cell, or cast levels.
- If renal insufficiency develops, notify the prescriber. Dosage may need to be reduced, or drugs may need to be stopped.
- Other cephalosporins may interact with aminoglycosides. If you suspect an interaction, consult the prescriber or pharmacist.

cephalosporins ➤◄ warfarin

cefoperazone, cefotetan, cefoxitin, ceftriaxone   Coumadin

Risk rating: 2
Severity: Moderate   **Onset: Delayed**   **Likelihood: Suspected**

Cause
The mechanism of this interaction is unknown.

Effect
Anticoagulant effects increase.

Nursing considerations
- Warfarin dose may need to be reduced if given with a parenteral cephalosporin.
- Monitor PT and INR closely.
- Patients with renal insufficiency may be at greater risk.
- Monitor the patient for signs of bleeding.
- Tell the patient to report unusual bleeding or bruising.
- Remind the patient that warfarin interacts with many drugs and that he should report any change in drug regimen to the prescriber or pharmacist.

chloramphenicol ➤◄ hydantoins

Chloromycetin   fosphenytoin, phenytoin

Risk rating: 2
Severity: Moderate   **Onset: Delayed**   **Likelihood: Suspected**

Cause
Hydantoin metabolism is altered.

Effect
Phenytoin level and risk of toxicity increases. Chloramphenicol concentration may also change.

Nursing considerations
- Monitor drug levels closely. Dosage may need to be adjusted.
- The therapeutic range for phenytoin is 10 to 20 mcg/ml.
- Toxic effects of phenytoin can occur at therapeutic level. Adjust the measured level for hypoalbuminia or renal impairment.
- Signs and symptoms of phenytoin toxicity include nystagmus, slurred speech, ataxia, blurred or double vision, confusion, drowsiness, and lethargy.

chloramphenicol ➤◄ iron salts

Chloromycetin

ferrous fumarate, ferrous gluconate, ferrous sulfate, iron dextran

Risk rating: 2
Severity: Moderate   **Onset: Delayed**   **Likelihood: Suspected**

Cause
Chloramphenicol causes bone marrow toxicity, which leads to decreased iron clearance and erythropoiesis.

Effect
Iron levels may increase.

Nursing considerations
- If the patient shows signs of bone marrow suppression, use an alternative antimicrobial agent, if possible.
- Carefully monitor iron stores, and adjust the iron dosage as needed.
- Serum iron levels may begin to increase within 5 to 7 days of beginning chloramphenicol.
- Assess the patient for evidence of iron deficiency, including fatigue, dyspnea, tachycardia, palpitations, dizziness, and orthostatic hypotension.

chloramphenicol ➤◄ sulfonylureas

Chloromycetin

acetohexamide, chlorpropamide, glipizide, glyburide, tolazamide, tolbutamide

Risk rating: 2
Severity: Moderate   **Onset: Delayed**   **Likelihood: Suspected**

Cause
Chloramphenicol reduces hepatic clearance of sulfonylureas.

Effect
Because sulfonylurea level is prolonged, hypoglycemia may occur.

Nursing considerations
- Monitor the patient for hypoglycemia.
- Describe signs and symptoms of hypoglycemia, including diaphoresis, fatigue, headache, hunger, irritability, malaise, nervousness, rapid heart rate, tension, and trembling.
- Instruct the patient to eat a small carbohydrate snack or meal if hypoglycemia develops, preferably after checking blood glucose level.

chloramphenicol ➤◀ warfarin
Chloromycetin   Coumadin

Risk rating: 2
Severity: Moderate   Onset: Delayed   Likelihood: Suspected

Cause
Hepatic metabolism of warfarin is inhibited.

Effect
Anticoagulant effects may increase.

Nursing considerations
- Monitor coagulation values carefully.
- A lower warfarin dose may be needed if the patient is taking chloramphenicol.
- Tell the patient to report unusual bleeding or bruising.
- Remind the patient that warfarin interacts with many drugs and that he should report any change in drug regimen.

chlordiazepoxide ➤◀ alcohol
Librium

Risk rating: 2
Severity: Moderate   Onset: Rapid   Likelihood: Established

Cause
Alcohol inhibits hepatic enzymes, which decreases clearance and increases peak level of benzodiazepines such as chlordiazepoxide.

Effect
Combining a benzodiazepine with alcohol may have additive or synergistic effects.

Nursing considerations
- Advise against consuming alcohol while taking a benzodiazepine.
- Before benzodiazepine therapy starts, assess the patient thoroughly for history or evidence of alcohol use.
- Watch for additive CNS effects, which may suggest benzodiazepine overdose.
- Other benzodiazepines interact with alcohol. If you suspect an interaction, consult the prescriber or pharmacist.
- When a patient starts a benzodiazepine, stress the high risks of consuming alcohol.

---

chlordiazepoxide ➡◀ azole antifungals
Librium   fluconazole, itraconazole,
                                         ketoconazole, voriconazole

Risk rating: 2
Severity: Moderate   Onset: Delayed   Likelihood: Established

Cause
Azole antifungals decrease CYP3A4 metabolism of certain benzodiazepines such as chlordiazepoxide.

Effect
Benzodiazepine effects are increased and prolonged, which may cause CNS depression and psychomotor impairment.

Nursing considerations
- If the patient takes fluconazole, consult the prescriber about giving a lower benzodiazepine dose or a drug not metabolized by CYP3A4, such as temazepam or lorazepam.
- Caution that the effects of this interaction may last several days after stopping the azole antifungal.
- Various benzodiazepine–azole antifungal combinations may interact. If you suspect an interaction, consult the prescriber or pharmacist.

---

chlordiazepoxide ➡◀ phenytoin
Librium   Dilantin

Risk rating: 2
Severity: Moderate   Onset: Delayed   Likelihood: Suspected

Cause
Metabolism of phenytoin and benzodiazepines such as chlordiazepoxide, may be altered.

Effect
Phenytoin level and risk of toxicity may increase, but data is not conclusive.

Nursing considerations
■ Monitor phenytoin level closely. Dosage may need to be adjusted.
■ The therapeutic range for phenytoin is 10 to 20 mcg/ml.
■ Toxic effects can occur at therapeutic level. Adjust the measured level for hypoalbuminemia or renal impairment, which can increase free drug level.
■ Signs and symptoms of phenytoin toxicity include nystagmus, slurred speech, ataxia, blurred or double vision, confusion, drowsiness, and lethargy.
■ Monitor the patient's response to chlordiazepoxide; a larger dose may be needed.

chloroquine ▶◀ cimetidine
Aralen   Tagamet

Risk rating: 3
Severity: Minor   Onset: Delayed   Likelihood: Suspected

Cause
Cimetidine inhibits hepatic metabolism of chloroquine.

Effect
Pharmacologic effects of chloroquine may be increased.

Nursing considerations
■ Monitor clinical response to chloroquine.
■ Dose of chloroquine may need to be decreased.
■ Monitor the patient when starting, stopping, or changing dose of cimetidine.

chlorothiazide ▶◀ lithium
Diuril   Eskalith

Risk rating: 2
Severity: Moderate   Onset: Delayed   Likelihood: Established

Cause
Thiazide diuretics such as chlorothiazide may decrease lithium clearance.

Effect
Lithium level, effects, and risk of toxicity may increase.

Nursing considerations
■ Despite this interaction, lithium and thiazide diuretics may be used together safely with close monitoring of the lithium level.
■ Reduction in lithium clearance may depend on chlorothiazide dose.
■ Monitor lithium level and adjust dose as needed.
■ Monitor the patient for evidence of lithium toxicity, such as diarrhea, vomiting, dehydration, drowsiness, muscle weakness, tremor, fever, and ataxia.

chlorothiazide ➤◄ sulfonylureas
Diuril   chlorpropamide, tolbutamide

Risk rating: 2
Severity: Moderate   Onset: Delayed   Likelihood: Probable

Cause
Chlorothiazide, a thiazide diuretic, may decrease insulin secretion and tissue sensitivity to insulin, and it may increase sodium loss.

Effect
Risk of hyperglycemia and hyponatremia may increase.

Nursing considerations
■ Use these drugs together cautiously.
■ Monitor blood glucose and sodium levels regularly, and consult the prescriber about dosage adjustments to maintain stable levels.
■ This interaction may occur several days to many months after dual therapy starts but is readily reversible when the diuretic stops.
■ Describe signs and symptoms of hypoglycemia, including diaphoresis, fatigue, headache, hunger, irritability, malaise, nervousness, rapid heart rate, tension, and trembling.
■ Instruct the patient to eat a small carbohydrate snack or meal if hypoglycemia develops, preferably after checking blood glucose level.

chlorpromazine ➤◄ alcohol
Thorazine

Risk rating: 2
Severity: Moderate   Onset: Rapid   Likelihood: Probable

Cause
The mechanism of this interaction is unknown. It may be that these substances produce CNS depression by working on different sites in the brain. Also, alcohol may lower resistance to neurotoxic effects of phenothiazines such as chlorpromazine.

Effect
CNS depression may increase.

Nursing considerations
■ Watch for extrapyramidal reactions, such as dystonic reactions and acute akathisia or restlessness.
■ If the patient takes a phenothiazine, warn that alcohol may worsen CNS depression and impair psychomotor skills.
■ Discourage the patient from drinking alcohol when taking a phenothiazine.

chlorpromazine ➤◀ anticholinergics

Thorazine

benztropine, orphenadrine
procyclidine, trihexyphenidyl

Risk rating: 2
Severity: Moderate   Onset: Delayed   Likelihood: Suspected

Cause
While the data is not conclusive, anticholinergics may antagonize phenothiazines such as chlorpromazine. Also, phenothiazine metabolism may increase.

Effect
Phenothiazine efficacy may decrease.

Nursing considerations
■ Monitor the patient for decreased phenothiazine efficacy.
■ Phenothiazine dosage may need adjustment.
■ Anticholinergic side effects may increase.
■ Monitor the patient for adynamic ileus, hyperpyrexia, hypoglycemia, and neurologic changes.

chlorpromazine ➤◀ beta blockers

Thorazine

pindolol, propranolol

Risk rating: 1
Severity: Major   Onset: Delayed   Likelihood: Probable

Cause
Chlorpromazine may inhibit first-pass hepatic metabolism of beta blockers.

Effect
Effects of both drugs and the risk of serious adverse reactions may increase.

Nursing considerations
■ If a beta blocker and chlorpromazine must be used together, monitor blood pressure and pulse rate regularly; beta blocker dosage may need to be decreased.

■ Assess the patient for adverse reactions to beta blockers, such as fatigue, lethargy, dizziness, nausea, heart failure, and agranulocytosis.

■ Explain to the patient and his family the expected and adverse effects of these drugs and the risk of interaction.

■ Other beta blockers may interact with phenothiazines such as chlorpromazine. If you suspect an interaction, consult the prescriber or pharmacist.

---

chlorpromazine ➡◄ fluoxetine
Thorazine   Prozac

Risk rating: 1
Severity: Major   **Onset: Delayed**   **Likelihood: Suspected**

Cause
Fluoxetine inhibits the metabolism of phenothiazines such as chlorpromazine.

Effect
Chlorpromazine level and risk of life-threatening arrhythmias (such as torsades de pointes) may increase.

Nursing considerations
■ Closely monitor the ECG and QTc interval when administering chlorpromazine and fluoxetine together.

■ The risk of arrhythmias increases if the patient is taking any other drugs that increase the QTc interval.

■ Ask the patient if he or any member of his family has a history of prolonged QTc interval.

---

chlorpromazine ➡◄ meperidine
Thorazine   Demerol

Risk rating: 2
Severity: Moderate   **Onset: Rapid**   **Likelihood: Probable**

Cause
Additive CNS depressant and cardiovascular effects may occur.

Effect
Excessive sedation and hypotension may occur.

Nursing considerations
- Avoid using meperidine with phenothiazines such as chlorpromazine.
- These drugs have been used together to minimize opioid dosage and control nausea and vomiting, but risks may outweigh benefits.
- Monitor the patient for more severe and extended respiratory depression.

chlorpromazine ➤◀ tricyclic antidepressants

Thorazine

desipramine, imipramine, nortriptyline

Risk rating: 3
Severity: Minor   **Onset: Delayed**   **Likelihood: Probable**

Cause
Competitive inhibition of TCA metabolism may occur.

Effect
TCA levels may increase.

Nursing considerations
- Monitor the patient's clinical response to TCAs, and decrease the dose if needed.
- No toxic effects were noted from this interaction.

chlorpromazine ➤◀ ziprasidone

Thorazine

Geodon

Risk rating: 1
Severity: Major   **Onset: Delayed**   **Likelihood: Suspected**

Cause
Prolongation of the QT interval occurs, possibly due to an additive effect of both drugs.

Effect
Risk of life-threatening arrhythmias, including torsades de pointes, increases.

Nursing considerations
- **ALERT** Use of ziprasidone with a phenothiazine, such as chlorpromazine, is contraindicated.
- Monitor the patient with other risk factors for torsades de pointes, including bradycardia, hypokalemia, and hypomagnesemia.

- Ask the patient if he or anyone in his family has a history of prolonged QT interval or arrhythmias.
- Monitor the patient for bradycardia.
- Measure the QTc interval at baseline and throughout therapy.

chlorpropamide ▬►◄▬ alcohol
Diabinese

Risk rating: 2
Severity: Moderate   **Onset: Rapid**   **Likelihood: Established**

Cause
Chronic alcohol use may interact with chlorpropamide by an unknown mechanism.

Effect
A disulfiram-like reaction may occur.

Nursing considerations
- Alcohol also interacts with sulfonylureas other than chlorpropamide.
- Naloxone may be used to antagonize a disulfiram-like reaction.
- Tell the patient who takes an oral antidiabetic to avoid alcohol as a rule; however, the occasional single drink is okay.
- Describe the signs of a disulfiram-like reaction, including facial flushing and possible burning that spreads to the neck, headache, nausea, and tachycardia. Explain that it typically occurs within 20 minutes of alcohol intake and lasts for 1 to 2 hours.
- Urge the patient to have regular follow-up blood tests to monitor diabetes and decrease episodes of hyperglycemia and hypoglycemia.

chlorpropamide ▬►◄▬ aspirin
Diabinese   Ecotrin, Bayer

Risk rating: 2
Severity: Moderate   **Onset: Delayed**   **Likelihood: Probable**

Cause
Salicylates reduce blood glucose level and prompt insulin secretion.

Effect
Hypoglycemic effects of chlorpropamide and other sulfonylureas increase.

Nursing considerations
- Monitor the patient for hypoglycemia.

■ Consult the prescriber and the patient about possibly replacing a salicylate with acetaminophen or an NSAID.
■ Describe signs and symptoms of hypoglycemia, including diaphoresis, fatigue, headache, hunger, irritability, malaise, nervousness, rapid heart rate, tension, and trembling.
■ Instruct the patient to eat a small carbohydrate snack or meal if hypoglycemia develops, preferably after checking blood glucose level.

chlorpropamide ▬►◄▬ chloramphenicol
Diabinese   Chloromycetin

Risk rating: 2
Severity: Moderate   **Onset: Delayed**   **Likelihood: Suspected**

Cause
Chloramphenicol reduces hepatic clearance of sulfonylureas such as chlorpropamide.

Effect
Because sulfonylurea level is prolonged, hypoglycemia may occur.

Nursing considerations
▣ If patient takes a sulfonylurea, start chloramphenicol carefully, and monitor the patient for hypoglycemia.
■ Describe signs and symptoms of hypoglycemia, including diaphoresis, fatigue, headache, hunger, irritability, malaise, nervousness, rapid heart rate, tension, and trembling.
■ Instruct the patient to eat a small carbohydrate snack or meal if hypoglycemia develops, preferably after checking blood glucose level.

chlorpropamide ▬►◄▬ MAO inhibitors
Diabinese   phenelzine, tranylcypromine

Risk rating: 2
Severity: Moderate   **Onset: Rapid**   **Likelihood: Suspected**

Cause
The mechanism of this interaction is unknown.

Effect
MAO inhibitors increase the hypoglycemic effects of sulfonylureas such as chlorpropamide.

Nursing considerations
■ If the patient takes a sulfonylurea, start an MAO inhibitor carefully, monitoring the patient for hypoglycemia.

■ Consult the prescriber about adjustments to either drug to control glucose level and mental state.

■ Describe signs and symptoms of hypoglycemia, including diaphoresis, fatigue, headache, hunger, irritability, malaise, nervousness, rapid heart rate, tension, and trembling.

■ Instruct the patient to eat a small carbohydrate snack or meal if hypoglycemia develops, preferably after checking blood glucose level.

---

chlorpropamide ■■▶◀■■ rifampin
Diabinese   Rifadin, Rimactane

Risk rating: 2
Severity: Moderate   **Onset: Delayed**   **Likelihood: Probable**

Cause
Rifampin may increase hepatic metabolism of certain sulfonylureas such as chlorpropamide.

Effect
The risk of hyperglycemia increases.

Nursing considerations
■ Use these drugs together cautiously.

■ Monitor the patient's blood glucose level regularly; consult the prescriber about adjustments to either drug to maintain stable glucose level.

■ Teach the patient to use a self-monitoring glucose meter and to report significant changes to the prescriber.

■ Tell the patient to stay alert for increased fatigue, thirst, eating, or urination and possible blurred vision or dry skin and mucous membranes as evidence of high blood glucose level.

---

chlorpropamide ■■▶◀■■ thiazide diuretics
Diabinese   chlorothiazide,
                               hydrochlorothiazide

Risk rating: 2
Severity: Moderate   **Onset: Delayed**   **Likelihood: Probable**

Cause
Thiazide diuretics may decrease insulin secretion and tissue sensitivity to insulin, and they may increase sodium loss.

Effect
The risk of hyperglycemia and hyponatremia may increase.

Nursing considerations
- Use these drugs together cautiously.
- Monitor the patient's blood glucose and sodium levels regularly; consult the prescriber about adjustments to either drug to maintain stable levels.
- This interaction may occur several days to many months after dual therapy starts but is readily reversible when the diuretic stops.
- Describe to the patient the signs and symptoms of hypoglycemia, such as diaphoresis, fatigue, headache, hunger, irritability, malaise, nervousness, rapid heart rate, tension, and trembling.
- Instruct the patient to eat a small carbohydrate snack or meal if hypoglycemia develops, preferably after checking blood glucose level.

chlorthalidone ▶◀ lithium
Thalitone   Eskalith

Risk rating: 2
Severity: Moderate   Onset: Delayed   Likelihood: Established

Cause
Thiazide diuretics, such as chlorthalidone, may decrease lithium clearance.

Effect
Lithium level, effects, and risk of toxicity may increase.

Nursing considerations
- Despite this interaction, lithium and thiazide diuretics may be used together safely, with close monitoring of lithium level.
- Reduction in lithium clearance may depend on chlorthalidone dose.
- Monitor lithium level and adjust dose as needed.
- Monitor the patient for evidence of lithium toxicity, such as diarrhea, vomiting, dehydration, drowsiness, muscle weakness, tremor, fever, and ataxia.

chlorzoxazone ▶◀ disulfiram
Parafon Forte DSC   Antabuse

Risk rating: 2
Severity: Moderate   Onset: Delayed   Likelihood: Probable

Cause
Disulfiram inhibits hepatic metabolism of chlorzoxazone.

Effect
CNS depressant effects of chlorzoxazone may increase.

Nursing considerations
- Monitor the patient for increased CNS adverse effects including dizziness, drowsiness, headache, and light-headedness.
- Signs of more severe toxicity include nausea, vomiting, diarrhea, loss of muscle tone, decreased or absent deep tendon reflexes, respiratory depression, and hypotension.
- Advise the patient to avoid hazardous activities that require alertness or physical coordination until CNS depressant effects are determined.
- Chlorzoxazone dose may need to be reduced during combined therapy.

---

chlorzoxazone ◄►◄ **isoniazid**
Parafon Forte DSC   Nydrazid

Risk rating: 2
Severity: Moderate   **Onset: Delayed**   **Likelihood: Suspected**

Cause
Isoniazid inhibits the CYP2E1 hepatic metabolism of chlorzoxazone.

Effect
Chlorzoxazone levels and its therapeutic and adverse effects may increase.

Nursing considerations
- Monitor the patient for increased CNS adverse effects, including dizziness, drowsiness, headache, and light-headedness.
- Signs of more severe toxicity include nausea, vomiting, diarrhea, loss of muscle tone, decreased or absent deep tendon reflexes, respiratory depression, and hypotension.
- Advise the patient to avoid hazardous activities that require alertness or physical coordination until CNS depressant effects are determined.
- Chlorzoxazone dose may need to be reduced during combined therapy.

chlorzoxazone ━━▶◀━━ watercress
Parafon Forte DSC

Risk rating: 2
Severity: Moderate   **Onset: Rapid**   **Likelihood: Suspected**

Cause
Watercress may inhibit the CYP2E1 hepatic metabolism of chlorzoxazone.

Effect
Chlorzoxazone levels and its therapeutic and adverse effects may increase.

Nursing considerations
■ Monitor the patient for increased CNS adverse effects including dizziness, drowsiness, headache, and light-headedness.
■ Signs of more severe toxicity include nausea, vomiting, diarrhea, loss of muscle tone, decreased or absent deep tendon reflexes, respiratory depression, and hypotension.
■ Advise the patient to avoid hazardous activities that require alertness or physical coordination until CNS depressant effects are determined.

cholestyramine ━━▶◀━━ digoxin
LoCHOLEST, Prevalite,   Lanoxin
Questran

Risk rating: 2
Severity: Moderate   **Onset: Delayed**   **Likelihood: Probable**

Cause
Cholestyramine may decrease digoxin absorption by binding to it. It also may interrupt digoxin metabolism in the liver.

Effect
Digoxin bioavailability and effects may be reduced.

Nursing considerations
■ Monitor digoxin level.
■ Monitor the patient for decreased digoxin effects.
■ Adjust digoxin dose as needed.
■ Consider using digoxin capsules because the interaction may be minimized.
■ Give cholestyramine 8 hours before or after digoxin to minimize the effects of the interaction.

cholestyramine ➤◀ fluvastatin

LoCHOLEST, Prevalite,
Questran

Lescol

Risk rating: 4
Severity: Moderate   **Onset: Delayed**   **Likelihood: Possible**

Cause
GI absorption of fluvastatin may decrease.

Effect
Fluvastatin effects may decrease.

Nursing considerations
◪ **ALERT** Separate doses of fluvastatin and cholestyramine, a bile acid sequestrant, by at least 4 hours.

■ If possible, give cholestyramine before meals and fluvastatin in the evening.

■ Monitor serum cholesterol and lipid levels to assess the patient's response to therapy.

■ Help the patient develop a daily plan to ensure proper intervals between drug doses.

cholestyramine ➤◀ furosemide

LoCHOLEST, Prevalite,
Questran

Lasix

Risk rating: 2
Severity: Moderate   **Onset: Rapid**   **Likelihood: Suspected**

Cause
Cholestyramine may bind to furosemide, inhibiting furosemide absorption.

Effect
Furosemide effects may decrease.

Nursing considerations
■ Cholestyramine should be taken at least 2 hours after furosemide.

■ Monitor the patient for expected furosemide effects, including reduction in peripheral edema, resolution of pulmonary edema, and decreased blood pressure in hypertensive patients.

■ If furosemide is needed, consult the prescriber or pharmacist about alternative cholesterol-lowering therapy.

■ Bile acid sequestrants other than cholestyramine may interact with furosemide. If you suspect a drug interaction, consult the prescriber or pharmacist.

---

cholestyramine ➡◀ hydrocortisone

LoCHOLEST, Prevalite,   Cortef
Questran

Risk rating: 2
Severity: Moderate   Onset: Delayed   Likelihood: Suspected

Cause
Bile acid sequestrants, such as cholestyramine, interfere with GI absorption of hydrocortisone.

Effect
Hydrocortisone effects may decrease.

Nursing considerations
■ If the patient needs hydrocortisone, consider a different cholesterol-lowering drug.
■ If drugs must be taken together, separate doses to help improve hydrocortisone absorption, even though doing so has no proven effect.
■ Check for expected hydrocortisone effects.
■ If needed, consult the prescriber about increasing hydrocortisone dosage to achieve desired effect.
■ Help the patient develop a daily plan to ensure proper intervals between drug doses.

---

cholestyramine ➡◀ levothyroxine

LoCHOLEST, Prevalite,   Levoxyl, Synthroid
Questran

Risk rating: 2
Severity: Moderate   Onset: Delayed   Likelihood: Suspected

Cause
Cholestyramine may prevent GI absorption of thyroid hormones.

Effect
Effects of exogenous thyroid hormone may be lost, and hypothyroidism may recur.

Nursing considerations
■ Separate doses by 6 hours.

- Monitor the patient for evidence of hypothyroidism, including weakness, fatigue, weight gain, coarse dry hair and skin, cold intolerance, muscle aches, constipation, depression, irritability, and memory loss.
- Monitor thyroid function tests during combined therapy (TSH, 0.2 to 5.4 microunits/ml; T_3, 80 to 200 nanograms/dl; T_4, 5.4 to 11.5 mcg/dl).
- Other thyroid hormones may interact with cholestyramine. If you suspect a drug interaction, consult the prescriber or pharmacist.

cholestyramine ◄ NSAIDs

LoCHOLEST, Prevalite, Questran

diclofenac, piroxicam, sulindac

Risk rating: 3
Severity: Minor   **Onset: Delayed**   **Likelihood: Probable**

Cause
Absorption of NSAIDs in the GI tract is decreased.

Effect
Pharmacologic effects of NSAIDs may be decreased.

Nursing considerations
- If an interaction is suspected, increase the dose of the NSAID during administration of cholestyramine.
- Monitor the patient for clinical response to the NSAID.
- Tell the patient to notify the prescriber if he experiences increased pain or discomfort, suggesting a decreased effect of the NSAID.

cholestyramine ◄ valproic acid

LoCHOLEST, Prevalite, Questran

divalproex sodium, valproate sodium, valproic acid

Risk rating: 2
Severity: Moderate   **Onset: Rapid**   **Likelihood: Suspected**

Cause
Cholestyramine may prevent GI absorption of valproic acid.

Effect
Valproic acid effects may decrease.

Nursing considerations
- Give valproic acid at least 3 hours before or 3 hours after cholestyramine.

- Watch for loss of seizure control.
- Valproic acid dosage may need adjustment.

cholestyramine ◼◼◼►◄◼◼◼ warfarin
LoCHOLEST, Prevalite,   Coumadin
Questran

Risk rating: 2
Severity: Moderate   Onset: Delayed   Likelihood: Probable

Cause
Warfarin absorption may decrease and elimination increase.

Effect
Anticoagulant effects may decrease.

Nursing considerations
- Tell the patient to separate warfarin dose from cholestyramine by at least 3 hours.
- Advise the patient of the risk of reduced anticoagulant effects.
- Help the patient develop a plan to ensure proper dosage intervals.
- Tell the patient to report unusual bleeding or bruising.
- Remind the patient that warfarin interacts with many drugs and that he should report any change in drug regimen.

cilostazol ◼◼◼►◄◼◼◼ erythromycin
Pletal   E-Mycin

Risk rating: 2
Severity: Moderate   Onset: Delayed   Likelihood: Suspected

Cause
Certain macrolide antibiotics such as erythromycin inhibit CYP3A4 metabolism of cilostazol.

Effect
Cilostazol effects, including adverse effects, may increase.

Nursing considerations
- Cilostazol dose may need to be decreased during combined therapy; consider cilostazol 50 mg b.i.d.
- Watch for evidence of cilostazol toxicity, including severe headache, diarrhea, hypotension, tachycardia, and arrhythmias.
- Urge the patient to tell the prescriber about all drugs and supplements he takes and about any increase in adverse effects.

■ Other macrolide antibiotics may interact with cilostazol. If you suspect a drug interaction, consult the prescriber or pharmacist.

cilostazol ━━━━▶◀━━━━ omeprazole
Pletal   Prilosec

Risk rating: 2
Severity: Moderate   **Onset: Delayed**   **Likelihood: Suspected**

Cause
Omeprazole may inhibit CYP2C19 metabolism of cilostazol.

Effect
Cilostazol effects, including adverse effects, may increase.

Nursing considerations
■ Cilostazol dose may need to be decreased during combined therapy; consider cilostazol 50 mg b.i.d.
■ Watch for evidence of cilostazol toxicity, including severe headache, diarrhea, hypotension, tachycardia, and arrhythmias.
■ Urge the patient to tell the prescriber about all drugs and supplements he takes and about any increase in adverse effects.

cimetidine ━━━━▶◀━━━━ azole antifungals
Tagamet   itraconazole, ketoconazole

Risk rating: 2
Severity: Moderate   **Onset: Delayed**   **Likelihood: Suspected**

Cause
Azole antifungal availability may decrease because elevated gastric pH may reduce tablet dissolution.

Effect
Azole antifungal effects may decrease.

Nursing considerations
■ If possible, don't administer an azole antifungal with an H2 antagonist.
■ If combined use is needed, give 680 mg of glutamic acid hydrochloride 15 minutes before ketoconazole.
■ Watch for expected antifungal effects.
■ Explain that other drugs that increase gastric pH, such as antacids, may also decrease azole antifungal absorption.

cimetidine ◄► benzodiazepines

Tagamet

alprazolam, clorazepate, diazepam, flurazepam, midazolam, triazolam

Risk rating: 3
Severity: Minor   **Onset: Rapid**   **Likelihood: Probable**

Cause
Hepatic metabolism of benzodiazepines may be decreased.

Effect
Serum levels of benzodiazepines may be increased, causing increased sedation.

Nursing considerations
▷ **ALERT** Carefully monitor the patient for increased sedation after taking cimetidine and a benzodiazepine.
■ Warn the patient about the risk of increased sedation when taking cimetidine and a benzodiazepine together.
■ If this occurs, discuss the possibility of decreasing the dose of the benzodiazepine with the prescriber.
■ Monitor serum benzodiazepine levels while the patient is taking cimetidine and a benzodiazepine together.
▷ **ALERT** Elderly patients are at a higher risk for increased levels of sedation.

cimetidine ◄► beta blockers

Tagamet

metoprolol, propranolol, timolol

Risk rating: 2
Severity: Moderate   **Onset: Rapid**   **Likelihood: Probable**

Cause
By inhibiting the CYP pathway, cimetidine reduces the first-pass metabolism of certain beta blockers.

Effect
Beta blocker clearance is decreased, increasing their action.

Nursing considerations
■ Monitor the patient for severe bradycardia and hypotension.
■ If interaction occurs, notify the prescriber; beta blocker dosage may be decreased.

- Teach the patient to monitor pulse rate. If it's significantly lower than usual, tell him to withhold the beta blocker and to contact the prescriber.
- Instruct the patient to change positions slowly to reduce effects of orthostatic hypotension.
- Other beta blockers may interact with cimetidine. If you suspect an interaction, consult the prescriber or pharmacist.

cimetidine ▬▬▬►◄▬▬▬ carbamazepine
Tagamet   Carbatrol, Epitol, Equetro, Tegretol

Risk rating: 2
Severity: Moderate   **Onset: Delayed**   **Likelihood: Suspected**

Cause
Cimetidine may inhibit hepatic carbamazepine metabolism.

Effect
Carbamazepine plasma level and risk of toxicity may increase.

Nursing considerations
- Monitor the patient's response, especially during the first 4 weeks after cimetidine is started, or when it is stopped.
- Monitor carbamazepine level; therapeutic range is 4 to 12 mcg/ml.
- **ALERT** Watch for signs of anorexia or subtle appetite changes, which may indicate an excessive carbamazepine level.
- Monitor the patient for signs of carbamazepine toxicity, including dizziness, ataxia, respiratory depression, tachycardia, arrhythmias, blood pressure changes, impaired consciousness, abnormal reflexes, nystagmus, seizures, nausea, vomiting, and urine retention.
- Carbamazepine dosage adjustment may be needed.

cimetidine ▬▬▬►◄▬▬▬ carmustine
Tagamet   BiCNU

Risk rating: 1
Severity: Major   **Onset: Delayed**   **Likelihood: Suspected**

Cause
The mechanism of this interaction is unknown, but may involve additive bone marrow suppression or decreased carmustine metabolism by cimetidine.

Effect
Carmustine myelosuppressive effects increase.

Nursing considerations
◼ **ALERT** Avoid combined use if possible.
■ Monitor CBC, WBC, and platelet counts.
■ Be prepared to provide supportive measures, such as blood components and granulocyte-colony stimulating factor.
■ H$_2$-receptor antagonists other than cimetidine may interact with carmustine. If you suspect an interaction, consult the prescriber or pharmacist.
■ Consult the prescriber for alternative drug therapy to avoid severe myelosuppression.

---

cimetidine ▶◀ chloroquine
Tagamet   Aralen

Risk rating: 3
Severity: Minor   **Onset: Delayed**   **Likelihood: Suspected**

Cause
Cimetidine inhibits hepatic metabolism of chloroquine.

Effect
Pharmacologic effects of chloroquine may be increased.

Nursing considerations
■ Monitor clinical response to chloroquine.
■ Dose of chloroquine may need to be decreased.
■ Monitor the patient when starting, stopping, or changing the dose of cimetidine.

---

cimetidine ▶◀ dofetilide
Tagamet   Tikosyn

Risk rating: 1
Severity: Major   **Onset: Delayed**   **Likelihood: Suspected**

Cause
Dofetilide renal elimination may be inhibited.

Effect
Dofetilide level and risk of ventricular arrhythmias, including torsades de pointes, may increase.

Nursing considerations
◪ ALERT Use of dofetilide with cimetidine is contraindicated.
- Monitor ECG for excessive prolongation of QTc interval and development of ventricular arrhythmias.
- Omeprazole, ranitidine, and aluminum and magnesium antacids don't affect dofetilide elimination. Consult the prescriber for alternative therapy.
- Monitor renal function and QTc interval every 3 months during dofetilide therapy.
- Urge the patient to tell the prescriber about all drugs and supplements he takes and about any increase in adverse effects.

---

cimetidine ▬▬◤◥▬ lidocaine
Tagamet   Xylocaine

Risk rating: 2
Severity: Moderate   **Onset: Rapid**   **Likelihood: Established**

Cause
Hepatic lidocaine metabolism may decrease.

Effect
Risk of lidocaine toxicity increases.

Nursing considerations
- Monitor the patient for lidocaine toxicity: dizziness, somnolence, confusion, tremors, paresthesias, seizures, hypotension, arrhythmias, respiratory depression, and coma.
- Adjust lidocaine dosage as ordered.
- Consult the prescriber or pharmacist for a safer H_2-receptor antagonist, such as ranitidine or famotidine, as an alternative to cimetidine. Monitor serum lidocaine level; therapeutic range is 1.5 to 6 mcg/ml.
- Other H_2-receptor antagonists interact with lidocaine. If you suspect a drug interaction, consult the prescriber or pharmacist.

---

cimetidine ▬▬◤◥▬ nifedipine
Tagamet   Procardia

Risk rating: 2
Severity: Moderate   **Onset: Delayed**   **Likelihood: Suspected**

Cause
The exact mechanism of this interaction is unknown; hepatic metabolism of nifedipine may be reduced.

Effect
Nifedipine effects, including adverse effects, may increase.

Nursing considerations
■ Monitor the patient for increased adverse effects, including hypotension, dizziness, light-headedness, syncope, peripheral edema, flushing, and nausea.
■ Adjust the nifedipine dose as ordered.
■ H_2-receptor antagonists other than cimetidine may interact with nifedipine. Calcium channel blockers other than nifedipine may interact with cimetidine. If you suspect an interaction, consult the prescriber or pharmacist.

---

cimetidine ━━▶◀━━ phenytoin
Tagamet   Dilantin

Risk rating: 2
Severity: Moderate   Onset: Delayed   Likelihood: Established

Cause
The hepatic metabolism of phenytoin is inhibited.

Effect
Phenytoin level and risk of toxicity may increase.

Nursing considerations
■ Hydantoins other than phenytoin may have a similar interaction with cimetidine.
■ Monitor phenytoin level closely. Dosage may need to be adjusted.
■ The therapeutic range for phenytoin is 10 to 20 mcg/ml.
■ Toxic effects can occur at therapeutic level. Adjust the measured level for hypoalbuminemia or renal impairment, which can increase free drug level.
■ Signs and symptoms of phenytoin toxicity include nystagmus, slurred speech, ataxia, blurred or double vision, confusion, drowsiness, and lethargy.
■ Ranitidine and feldopine may be better alternatives to use than cimetidine.

cimetidine ▶◀ praziquantel
Tagamet
Biltricide

Risk rating: 2
Severity: Moderate **Onset: Delayed** **Likelihood: Probable**

Cause
Cimetidine may inhibit first-pass metabolism of praziquantel.

Effect
Praziquantel levels and effects, including adverse effects, may be increased.

Nursing considerations
- Observe for increased effects of praziquantel, which may include fever, hives, or GI upset.
- Praziquantel dosage may need adjustment.
- Ranitidine may be a better alternative to use than cimetidine.

cimetidine ▶◀ procainamide
Tagamet
Pronestyl

Risk rating: 2
Severity: Moderate **Onset: Rapid** **Likelihood: Established**

Cause
Cimetidine may reduce procainamide renal clearance.

Effect
Procainamide level and risk of toxicity may increase.

Nursing considerations
- **ALERT** Avoid combined use if possible.
- If drugs are used together, monitor procainamide level and its active metabolite, NAPA. Therapeutic range for procainamide is 4 to 8 mcg/ml; therapeutic level of NAPA is 10 to 30 mcg/ml.
- Monitor the patient for increased adverse effects, including severe hypotension, widening QRS complex, arrhythmias, seizures, oliguria, confusion, lethargy, nausea, and vomiting.
- Procainamide dosage may need adjustment.
- H_2-receptor antagonists other than cimetidine may interact with procainamide. If you suspect a drug interaction, consult the prescriber or pharmacist.

cimetidine ▶◀ quinidine
Tagamet

Risk rating: 2
Severity: Moderate   Onset: Delayed   Likelihood: Probable

Cause
Interaction may result from increased quinidine absorption, decreased quinidine metabolism, or both.

Effect
Quinidine effects and risk of toxicity increase.

Nursing considerations
- If possible, use of quinidine with cimetidine should be avoided.
- Monitor quinidine level closely; dose may need to be reduced.
- Therapeutic range of quinidine is 2 to 6 mcg/ml. More specific assays have levels of less than 1 mcg/ml.
- ◪ ALERT Monitor the patient for evidence of quinidine toxicity, including GI irritation, arrhythmias, hypotension, vertigo, and rash.
- Advise the patient to report palpitations, shortness of breath, dizziness or fainting, and chest pain.

cimetidine ▶◀ theophyllines
Tagamet   aminophylline, theophylline

Risk rating: 2
Severity: Moderate   Onset: Delayed   Likelihood: Established

Cause
Cimetidine inhibits hepatic metabolism of theophyllines.

Effect
Theophylline level and risk of toxicity may increase.

Nursing considerations
- Monitor serum theophylline level closely. Normal therapeutic range is 10 to 20 mcg/ml for adults and 5 to 15 mcg/ml for children.
- Watch for evidence of toxicity, such as tachycardia, anorexia, nausea, vomiting, diarrhea, seizures, restlessness, irritability, and headache.
- The theophylline dosage may need to be decreased by 20% to 40%.
- Describe adverse effects of theophylline and signs of toxicity, and tell the patient to report them immediately to the prescriber.
- Giving ranitidine or famotidine instead of cimetidine for gastric hypersecretion may decrease risk of this interaction.

cimetidine ▶◀ tricyclic antidepressants
Tagamet

amitriptyline, desipramine, doxepin, imipramine, nortriptyline

Risk rating: 2
Severity: Moderate   **Onset: Rapid**   **Likelihood: Probable**

Cause
Cimetidine may interfere with metabolism of tricyclic antidepressants (TCAs).

Effect
TCA level and bioavailability increase.

Nursing considerations
■ Monitor serum TCA level and adjust dosage as prescribed.
■ If needed, consult the prescriber about a possible change from cimetidine to ranitidine.
■ Urge the patient and his family to watch for and report increased anticholinergic effects such as dizziness, drowsiness, and psychosis.

cimetidine ▶◀ warfarin
Tagamet

Coumadin

Risk rating: 1
Severity: Major   **Onset: Delayed**   **Likelihood: Established**

Cause
Hepatic metabolism of warfarin is inhibited.

Effect
Anticoagulant effects increase.

Nursing considerations
■ Suggest the use of an H2 antagonist other than cimetidine because famotidine, ranitidine, and nizatidine are unlikely to interact with warfarin.
■ Avoid using these drugs together. If unavoidable, monitor coagulation values closely.
■ Tell the patient to report unusual bleeding or bruising.
■ Remind the patient that warfarin interacts with many drugs and that he should report any change in drug regimen.

ciprofloxacin ➤◄ didanosine
Cipro   Videx

Risk rating: 2
Severity: Moderate   **Onset: Rapid**   **Likelihood: Suspected**

Cause
Buffers in didanosine chewable tablets and pediatric powder for oral solution decrease GI absorption of ciprofloxacin.

Effect
Ciprofloxacin effects decrease.

Nursing considerations
■ Avoid use together. If it's unavoidable, give ciprofloxacin at least 2 hours before or 6 hours after didanosine.
■ The unbuffered form of didanosine doesn't affect ciprofloxacin absorption.
■ Help the patient develop a daily plan to ensure proper intervals between drug doses.
■ To help prevent interactions, urge the patient to tell the prescriber about all drugs and supplements he takes.

ciprofloxacin ➤◄ iron salts
Cipro   ferrous fumarate, ferrous gluconate, ferrous sulfate

Risk rating: 2
Severity: Moderate   **Onset: Rapid**   **Likelihood: Probable**

Cause
Formation of an iron-quinolone complex decreases GI absorption of ciprofloxacin.

Effect
Effects of quinolones, such as ciprofloxacin, decrease.

Nursing considerations
■ Tell the patient to separate ciprofloxacin from iron by at least 2 hours.
■ Help the patient develop a daily plan to ensure proper intervals between drug doses.
■ Other quinolones may interact with iron.

ciprofloxacin ◆ milk
Cipro

Risk rating: 2
Severity: Moderate   **Onset: Rapid**   **Likelihood: Suspected**

Cause
GI absorption of some quinolones (such as ciprofloxacin) decreases.

Effect
Quinolone effects may decrease.

Nursing considerations
- Advise the patient not to take the drug with milk and to allow as much time as possible between milk ingestion and the quinolone dose.
- This interaction doesn't affect all quinolones.
- Monitor the patient for quinolone efficacy.

ciprofloxacin ◆ procainamide
Cipro   Pronestyl

Risk rating: 2
Severity: Moderate   **Onset: Rapid**   **Likelihood: Suspected**

Cause
Tubular secretion of procainamide decreases.

Effect
Procainamide levels may increase.

Nursing considerations
- Monitor levels of procainamide and its active metabolite, NAPA. Therapeutic range for procainamide is 4 to 8 mcg/ml; therapeutic level of NAPA is 10 to 30 mcg/ml.
- Monitor the patient for increased adverse effects, including severe hypotension, widening QRS complex, arrhythmias, seizures, oliguria, confusion, lethargy, nausea, and vomiting.
- Procainamide dosage may need adjustment.

ciprofloxacin ━━▶◀━━ sevelamer

Cipro   Renagel

Risk rating: 2
Severity: Moderate   **Onset: Rapid**   **Likelihood: Suspected**

Cause
Decreased GI absorption of ciprofloxacin is suspected.

Effect
Ciprofloxacin effects decrease.

Nursing considerations
■ Tell the patient to separate ciprofloxacin from sevelamer by at least
4 hours.
■ Help the patient develop a daily plan to ensure proper intervals be-
tween drug dosages.
■ Realize that other quinolones may interact with sevelamer.

ciprofloxacin ━━▶◀━━ sucralfate

Cipro   Carafate

Risk rating: 2
Severity: Moderate   **Onset: Rapid**   **Likelihood: Probable**

Cause
Sucralfate decreases GI absorption of ciprofloxacin.

Effect
Ciprofloxacin effects decrease.

Nursing considerations
■ Avoid use together. If it's unavoidable, give sucralfate at least
6 hours after ciprofloxacin.
■ Monitor the patient for resolving infection.
■ Help the patient develop a daily plan to ensure proper intervals be-
tween drug doses.
■ To help avoid interactions, urge the patient to tell the prescriber
about all drugs and supplements he takes.

ciprofloxacin ➤◄ theophyllines
Cipro   aminophylline, theophylline

Risk rating: 2
Severity: Moderate   Onset: Delayed   Likelihood: Established

Cause
Hepatic metabolism of theophyllines is decreased.

Effect
Theophylline levels may increase, causing toxicity.

Nursing considerations
- Monitor theophylline level closely. Therapeutic range is 10 to 20 mcg/ml for adults and 5 to 15 mcg/ml for children.
- Interaction doesn't appear to affect ciprofloxacin or other quinolones.
- Watch for evidence of toxicity, such as ventricular tachycardia, anorexia, nausea, vomiting, diarrhea, seizures, restlessness, irritability, and headache.
- Describe adverse effects of theophylline and signs of toxicity, and tell the patient to report them immediately to the prescriber.

ciprofloxacin ➤◄ warfarin
Cipro   Coumadin

Risk rating: 2
Severity: Moderate   Onset: Delayed   Likelihood: Suspected

Cause
The mechanism of the interaction is unknown.

Effect
Anticoagulant effects may increase.

Nursing considerations
- Monitor PT and INR closely.
- Tell the patient to report unusual bleeding or bruising.
- Remind the patient that warfarin interacts with many drugs and that he should report any change in his drug regimen.

cisatracurium ▰▰◀▶▰▰ carbamazepine

Nimbex   Carbatrol, Epitol, Equetro,
                                Tegretol

Risk rating: 2
Severity: Moderate   **Onset: Rapid**   **Likelihood: Probable**

Cause
The mechanism of this interaction is unknown.

Effect
Effect or duration of cisatracurium, a nondepolarizing muscle relaxant, may decrease.

Nursing considerations
- Monitor the patient for decreased efficacy of muscle relaxant.
- Cisatracurium dosage may need to be increased.
- Make sure the patient is adequately sedated when receiving a nondepolarizing muscle relaxant.

cisatracurium ▰▰◀▶▰▰ phenytoin

Nimbex   Dilantin

Risk rating: 2
Severity: Moderate   **Onset: Rapid**   **Likelihood: Established**

Cause
Phenytoin has effects at prejunctional sites similar to those of nondepolarizing muscle relaxants such as cisatracurium.

Effect
Nondepolarizing muscle relaxant effect or duration may decrease.

Nursing considerations
- Monitor the patient for decreased efficacy of the muscle relaxant.
- Cisatracurium dosage may need to be increased.
- Atracurium may be a suitable alternative because this interaction may not occur in all patients.
- Make sure the patient is adequately sedated when receiving a nondepolarizing muscle relaxant.

cisplatin ◄► loop diuretics
Platinol

bumetanide, ethacrynic acid, furosemide

Risk rating: 2
Severity: Moderate   **Onset: Rapid**   **Likelihood: Suspected**

Cause
The mechanism of this interaction is unknown.

Effect
Interaction may cause additive ototoxicity.

Nursing considerations
- If possible, avoid giving loop diuretics and cisplatin together.
- If drugs are given together, obtain hearing tests to detect early hearing loss.
- Combined therapy may cause ototoxicity much more severe than therapy with either drug alone.
- Ototoxicity caused by combined therapy may be permanent.
- Tell the patient to report ringing in the ears, a change in balance, or muffled sounds. Also, ask his family members to watch for changes.

cisplatin ◄► phenytoin
Platinol

Dilantin

Risk rating: 2
Severity: Moderate   **Onset: Delayed**   **Likelihood: Suspected**

Cause
Phenytoin absorption may be decreased or metabolism may be increased.

Effect
Phenytoin level and effects may decrease.

Nursing considerations
- Monitor phenytoin level closely. Dosage may need to be adjusted.
- Therapeutic range for phenytoin is 10 to 20 mcg/ml.
- Toxic effects can occur at therapeutic level. Adjust the measured level for hypoalbuminemia or renal impairment, which can increase free drug level.
- Monitor the patient for seizure activity.
- Carefully monitor phenytoin level between courses of chemotherapy. Phenytoin dose may need to be reduced.

■ Signs and symptoms of phenytoin toxicity include nystagmus, slurred speech, ataxia, blurred or double vision, confusion, drowsiness, and lethargy.

citalopram ━━━━►◄━━━━ clozapine
Celexa   Clozaril

Risk rating: 1
Severity: Major   **Onset: Delayed**   **Likelihood: Established**

Cause
Serotonin reuptake inhibitors, such as citalopram, inhibit hepatic metabolism of clozapine.

Effect
Clozapine level and risk of toxicity increase.

Nursing considerations
■ Not all serotonin reuptake inhibitors share this interaction. If you suspect an interaction, consult the prescriber or pharmacist.
■ Monitor serum clozapine level.
■ Assess the patient for increased adverse effects or toxicity, including agranulocytosis, ECG changes, and seizures.
■ Adjust clozapine dose as needed when adding or withdrawing a serotonin reuptake inhibitor.

citalopram ━━━━►◄━━━━ linezolid
Celexa   Zyvox

Risk rating: 1
Severity: Major   **Onset: Delayed**   **Likelihood: Suspected**

Cause
Serotonin may accumulate rapidly in the CNS.

Effect
The risk of serotonin syndrome increases.

Nursing considerations
◪ **ALERT** Don't use these drugs together.
■ Allow 2 weeks after stopping linezolid and administering citalopram.
■ Allow 2 weeks after stopping an SSRI such as citalopram and administering linezolid.
■ Make sure that the patient is aware of the signs of serotonin syndrome, including confusion, restlessness, uncoordination, muscle tremors and rigidity, fever, and sweating.

■ Explain that serotonin-induced symptoms can be fatal if not treated immediately.

citalopram ◀▶ MAO inhibitors
Celexa

isocarboxazid, phenelzine, selegiline, tranylcypromine

Risk rating: 1
Severity: Major   **Onset: Rapid**   **Likelihood: Probable**

Cause
Serotonin may accumulate rapidly in the CNS.

Effect
The risk of serotonin syndrome increases.

Nursing considerations
◤ ALERT Don't use these drugs together.
■ Allow 2 weeks after stopping citalopram before giving an MAO inhibitor.
■ Allow 2 weeks after stopping an MAO inhibitor before giving an SSRI such as citalopram.
■ Make sure that patient is aware of signs of serotonin syndrome, including confusion, restlessness, uncoordination, muscle tremors and rigidity, fever, and sweating.
■ Explain that serotonin-induced symptoms can be fatal if not treated immediately.

citalopram ◀▶ pimozide
Celexa

Orap

Risk rating: 1
Severity: Major   **Onset: Delayed**   **Likelihood: Suspected**

Cause
The mechanism of this interaction is unknown.

Effect
Risk of life-threatening arrhythmias, including torsades de pointes, may increase.

Nursing considerations
◤ ALERT Combined use of these drugs is contraindicated.
■ Arrhythmias are related to prolonged QT interval, a known risk of pimozide.

■ Interaction warning is based on actual patient experience with these drugs as well as pharmacokinetics.

citalopram ►◄ sympathicomimetics
Celexa   amphetamine, dextroampheta-
                            mine, phentermine

Risk rating: 2
Severity: Moderate   Onset: Rapid   Likelihood: Suspected

Cause
The mechanism of this interaction is unknown.

Effect
Sympathicomimetic effects and risk of serotonin syndrome increase.

Nursing considerations
■ Watch closely for increased CNS effects, such as anxiety, jitteriness, agitation, and restlessness.
■ Mild serotonin-like symptoms may develop, including anxiety, dizziness, restlessness, nausea, and vomiting.
■ Explain the risk of interaction and the need to avoid sympathomimetics.
■ Describe traits of serotonin syndrome: CNS irritability, motor weakness, shivering, myoclonus, and altered consciousness.

citalopram ►◄ tramadol
Celexa   Ultram

Risk rating: 1
Severity: Major   Onset: Delayed   Likelihood: Suspected

Cause
The combination may result in additive serotonergic effects.

Effect
Serotonin syndrome may occur.

Nursing considerations
■ Watch closely for increased CNS effects, such as anxiety, jitteriness, agitation, and restlessness.
■ If serotonin syndrome occurs, stop the citalopram, and obtain immediate medical attention for the patient.
■ Make sure the patient knows the signs of serotonin syndrome: CNS irritability, motor weakness, shivering, myoclonus, and altered consciousness.

■ Urge the patient to report adverse effects immediately.

clarithromycin ➤◀ antiarrhythmic agents

Biaxin

amiodarone, bretylium, disopyramide, Dofetilide, procainamide, quinidine, sotalol

Risk rating: 1
Severity: Major   **Onset: Delayed**   **Likelihood: Suspected**

Cause
An additive increase in the QT interval is seen when administering clarithromycin, a macrolide antibiotic, and antiarrhythmic agents.

Effect
The risk of life-threatening cardiac arrhythmias, including torsades de pointes, is increased.

Nursing considerations
◪ ALERT Monitor the patient for prolonged QT interval and torsades de pointes.
■ This interaction also appears with other macrolide antibiotics.
■ This interaction appears to be dose related.
■ Instruct the patient to let the prescriber know if he experiences dizziness, palpitations, or light-headedness.
■ The QT interval returns to normal within 3 days of stopping the medications.

clarithromycin ➤◀ benzodiazepines

Biaxin

alprazolam, diazepam, midazolam, triazolam

Risk rating: 2
Severity: Moderate   **Onset: Rapid**   **Likelihood: Suspected**

Cause
Macrolide antibiotics, such as clarithromycin, may decrease metabolism of certain benzodiazepines.

Effect
Sedative effects of benzodiazepines may be increased or prolonged.

Nursing considerations
■ Consult the prescriber about decreasing benzodiazepine dosage during antibiotic therapy.

■ Lorazepam, oxazepam, and temazepam probably don't interact with macrolide antibiotics; substitution may be possible.
■ Urge the patient to report oversedation immediately.

---

clarithromycin ▶◀ cabergoline
Biaxin   Dostinex

Risk rating: 2
Severity: Moderate   **Onset: Delayed**   **Likelihood: Suspected**

Cause
Clarithromycin inhibits the CYP3A4 metabolism of cabergoline.

Effect
Cabergoline plasma levels may be increased, increasing the risk of toxicity.

Nursing considerations
■ If possible, avoid administering these drugs together.
■ Carefully monitor the clinical response of patients taking this drug combination.
■ This interaction may be increased in patients with a history of levodopa-induced psychosis or dyskinesia.
■ Cabergoline may interact with any macrolide antibiotic.

---

clarithromycin ▶◀ carbamazepine
Biaxin   Carbatrol, Epitol, Equestro, Tegretol

Risk rating: 1
Severity: Major   **Onset: Rapid**   **Likelihood: Established**

Cause
CYP3A4 metabolism of carbamazepine is inhibited, decreasing carbamazepine clearance.

Effect
Carbamazepine level and toxicity may increase.

Nursing considerations
⚠ **ALERT** If possible, avoid using together.
■ Consult the prescriber or pharmacist about an alternative macrolide antibiotic (such as azithromycin) or an alternative anti-infective drug unlikely to interact with carbamazepine.
■ If using a macrolide antibiotic, monitor carbamazepine level; therapeutic range is 4 to 12 mcg/ml.

■ Monitor the patient for evidence of carbamazepine toxicity, including dizziness, ataxia, respiratory depression, tachycardia, arrhythmias, blood pressure changes, impaired consciousness, abnormal reflexes, nystagmus, seizures, nausea, vomiting, and urine retention.
■ Carbamazepine dosage may need adjustment.

clarithromycin ━━▶◀━━ colchicine
Biaxin

Risk rating: 1
Severity: Major   **Onset: Delayed**   **Likelihood: Suspected**

Cause
Metabolism of colchicine is inhibited.

Effect
Colchicine levels and risk of toxicity increase.

Nursing considerations
■ Monitor the serum levels of colchicine.
■ If using colchicine and a macrolide antibiotic such as clarithromycin, it may be necessary to decrease the dose of colchicine.
■ Monitor the patient for fever, diarrhea, abdominal pain, myalgia, convulsions, and hair loss.
■ Patients with hepatic or renal impairment are more at risk for toxicity.

clarithromycin ━━▶◀━━ conivaptan
Biaxin   Vaprisol

Risk rating: 1
Severity: Major   **Onset: Delayed**   **Likelihood: Suspected**

Cause
Macrolide antibiotics such as clarithromycin may inhibit the CYP3A4 metabolism of conivaptan.

Effect
Conivaptan levels and adverse effects may be increased.

Nursing considerations
⚡ **ALERT** Administration of macrolide antibiotics and conivaptan together is contraindicated.
■ The risk of increased conivaptan levels is unknown.
■ Further studies are needed to determine the total extent of this interaction.

clarithromycin ➡◀ cyclosporine
Biaxin   Gengraf, Neoral, Sandimmune

Risk rating: 2
Severity: Moderate   Onset: Delayed   Likelihood: Established

Cause
Macrolide antibiotics such as clarithromycin interfere with cyclosporine metabolism. The rate and extent of absorption may increase, and the volume of distribution may decrease.

Effect
Elevated cyclosporine levels and increased risk of toxicity may occur.

Nursing considerations
◼ **ALERT** Monitor the patient carefully for nephrotoxicity or neurotoxicity.
◼ Closely monitor BUN and serum creatinine levels.
◼ The dose of cyclosporine may need to be decreased.
◼ Of all the macrolide antibiotics, azithromycin appears to interact the least with cyclosporine.

clarithromycin ➡◀ digoxin
Biaxin   Lanoxin

Risk rating: 1
Severity: Major   Onset: Delayed   Likelihood: Established

Cause
Macrolide antibiotics may alter GI flora and increase digoxin absorption. Clarithromycin may inhibit renal clearance of digoxin.

Effect
Digoxin level and risk of toxicity may increase.

Nursing considerations
◼ Monitor digoxin level. Therapeutic range is 0.8 to 2 ng/ml.
◼ Watch for evidence of digoxin toxicity: lethargy, drowsiness, confusion, hallucinations, headaches, syncope, visual disturbances, nausea, anorexia, vomiting, diarrhea, and arrhythmias (bradycardia, AV blocks, and ventricular ectopy).
◼ Digoxin dosage may need reduction.
◼ **ALERT** Clarithromycin doesn't affect the serum level of digoxin given I.V. Capsule form of digoxin may increase digoxin availability and decrease risk of interaction.

■ Other macrolide antibiotics may interact with digoxin. If you suspect an interaction, consult the prescriber or pharmacist.

clarithromycin ▬▬◄▬▬ eplerenone
Biaxin   Inspira

Risk rating: 1
Severity: Major   **Onset: Delayed**   **Likelihood: Suspected**

Cause
Macrolide antibiotics such as clarithromycin inhibit the CYP3A4 metabolism of eplerenone.

Effect
Eplerenone level increases, which may increase risk of hyperkalemia and serious arrhythmias.

Nursing considerations
◤ **ALERT** Administration of clarithromycin and eplerenone is contraindicated.
■ The basis for this interaction is the risk of hyperkalemia from eplerenone therapy.
■ The interaction is based on pharmacodynamics, not actual patient studies.

clarithromycin ▬▬◄▬▬ ergot derivatives
Biaxin   dihydroergotamine, ergotamine

Risk rating: 1
Severity: Major   **Onset: Rapid**   **Likelihood: Probable**

Cause
Macrolide antibiotics such as clarithromycin interfere with hepatic metabolism of ergotamine, although the exact mechanism of this interaction is unknown.

Effect
The patient may develop symptoms of acute ergotism.

Nursing considerations
■ Monitor the patient for evidence of peripheral ischemia, including pain in limb muscles while exercising and later at rest; numbness and tingling of fingers and toes; cool, pale, or cyanotic limbs; red or violet blisters on hands or feet; and gangrene.
■ Dosage of ergot drug may need to be decreased, or both drugs may need to be stopped.

■ Consult the prescriber about a different anti-infective drug that's less likely to interact with ergot derivatives.
⚡ **ALERT** Sodium nitroprusside may be used to treat macrolide–ergot-induced vasospasm.
■ Explain evidence of ergot-induced peripheral ischemia. Urge the patient to report it promptly to the prescriber.

---

clarithromycin ▶◀ food

Biaxin   food, grapefruit juice

Risk rating: 1
Severity: Major   **Onset: Delayed**   **Likelihood: Suspected**

Cause
Grapefruit may inhibit metabolism of clarithromycin and other macrolide antibiotics.

Effect
With food, efficacy of clarithromycin may decrease. With grapefruit, clarithromycin level and adverse effects may increase.

Nursing considerations
■ Enteric-coated tablets aren't affected by food and may be taken without regard to meals.
■ Advise the patient to take clarithromycin with a beverage other than grapefruit juice.

---

clarithromycin ▶◀ HMG-CoA reductase inhibitors

Biaxin   atorvastatin, lovastatin, simvastatin

Risk rating: 1
Severity: Major   **Onset: Delayed**   **Likelihood: Probable**

Cause
CYP3A4 metabolism of certain HMG-CoA reductase inhibitors may decrease.

Effect
HMG-CoA reductase inhibitor level may increase, raising the risk of severe myopathy or rhabdomyolysis.

Nursing considerations
⚡ **ALERT** If atorvastatin, lovastatin, or simvastatin is given with a macrolide antibiotic, such as clarithromycin, watch for evidence of

rhabdomyolysis, especially 5 to 21 days after macrolide starts. Evidence may include fatigue; muscle aches and weakness; joint pain; dark, red, or cola-colored urine; weight gain; seizures; and greatly increased serum CK level.

■ Fluvastatin and pravastatin are metabolized by other enzymes and may be better choices when used with a macrolide antibiotic.

■ Urge the patient to report unexplained muscle pain, tenderness, or weakness to the prescriber.

clarithromycin ➤◄ methylprednisolone
Biaxin   Medrol

Risk rating: 2
Severity: Moderate   Onset: Delayed   Likelihood: Established

Cause
The mechanism of this interaction is unclear.

Effect
Methylprednisolone effects, including toxic effects, may increase.

Nursing considerations
■ This interaction may be used for therapeutic benefit because it may be possible to reduce methylprednisolone dosage.

■ Methylprednisolone dosage may need adjustment.

■ Monitor the patient for adverse or toxic effects, such as euphoria, insomnia, peptic ulceration, and cushingoid effects.

clarithromycin ➤◄ omeprazole
Biaxin   Prilosec

Risk rating: 3
Severity: Minor   Onset: Delayed   Likelihood: Suspected

Cause
Clarithromycin inhibits the metabolism of omeprazole. Omeprazole increases clarithromycin absorption.

Effect
Omeprazole and clarithromycin levels may increase. Gastric mucus concentration of clarithromycin may increase.

Nursing considerations
■ This interaction may be beneficial in the treatment of *Helicobacter pylori* infections.

■ No special action is needed with this interaction.

clarithromycin ▬▶◀▬ pimozide
Biaxin   Orap

Risk rating: 1
Severity: Major   **Onset: Delayed**   **Likelihood: Suspected**

Cause
Macrolide antibiotics such as clarithromycin may inhibit CYP3A4 metabolism of pimozide.

Effect
Risk of life-threatening arrhythmias may increase.

Nursing considerations
◪ **ALERT** Combined use of these drugs is contraindicated.
▪ Arrhythmias are related to prolonged QT interval, a known risk of pimozide.
◪ **ALERT** People with normal baseline ECG and no history have died from pimozide blood levels 2.5 times the upper limit of normal from this interaction.

clarithromycin ▬▶◀▬ proton pump inhibitors
Biaxin   esomeprazole, lansoprazole

Risk rating: 2
Severity: Moderate   **Onset: Delayed**   **Likelihood: Suspected**

Cause
Clarithromycin inhibits the CYP3A metabolism of certain proton pump inhibitors.

Effect
Proton pump inhibitors levels and the risk of adverse effects increase.

Nursing considerations
▪ Monitor the patient for adverse reactions.
▪ Watch the patient for headache, abdominal pain, constipation, diarrhea, dry mouth, nausea, and vomiting.
▪ Teach the patient to watch for adverse reactions and to notify the prescriber if adverse reactions increase.
▪ Administration of clarithromycin with other proton pump inhibitors may not cause this interaction.

clarithromycin ━━▶◀━━ repaglinide
Biaxin   Prandin

Risk rating: 2
Severity: Moderate   Onset: Delayed   Likelihood: Suspected

Cause
Certain macrolide antibiotics such as clarithromycin may inhibit metabolism of repaglinide.

Effect
Repaglinide level and effects, including adverse effects, may increase.

Nursing considerations
■ Monitor blood glucose level closely.
■ Repaglinide dose should be adjusted as needed.
■ Monitor the patient for evidence of hypoglycemia, including hunger, dizziness, shakiness, sweating, confusion, and light-headedness.
■ Advise the patient to carry glucose tablets or another simple sugar in case of hypoglycemia.
■ Make sure the patient and his family know what to do if hypoglycemia occurs.

clarithromycin ━━▶◀━━ rifabutin
Biaxin   Mycobutin

Risk rating: 2
Severity: Moderate   Onset: Delayed   Likelihood: Probable

Cause
Metabolism of rifabutin may be inhibited. Metabolism of macrolide antibiotics such as clarithromycin may be increased.

Effect
Adverse effects of rifabutin may increase. Antimicrobial effects of macrolide antibiotic may decrease.

Nursing considerations
■ Monitor the patient for increased rifabutin adverse effects, such as abdominal pain, anorexia, nausea, vomiting, diarrhea, and rash.
■ Monitor the patient for decreased response to clarithromycin.
■ Rifabutin and clarithromycin usually cause nausea, vomiting, or diarrhea. This interaction doesn't occur with azithromycin; this drug may be a better choice.

- Giving clarithromycin with rifabutin may increase the risk of neutropenia.

---

clarithromycin ◼▶◀ tacrolimus
Biaxin   Prograf

Risk rating: 2
Severity: Moderate   **Onset: Delayed**   **Likelihood: Suspected**

Cause
Certain macrolide antibiotics, such as clarithromycin, inhibit CYP3A4 metabolism of tacrolimus.

Effect
Tacrolimus level and risk of toxicity may increase.

Nursing considerations
- If possible, use a different class of antibiotics.
- Monitor tacrolimus level and renal function test results. Expected trough level of tacrolimus is 6 to 10 mcg/L.
- This effect occurs in children and adults.
- Tacrolimus may need to be stopped temporarily because reduced dosages may not prevent renal changes.
- Other macrolide antibiotics may interact.

---

clarithromycin ◼▶◀ warfarin
Biaxin   Coumadin

Risk rating: 1
Severity: Major   **Onset: Delayed**   **Likelihood: Probable**

Cause
Warfarin clearance is reduced.

Effect
Anticoagulant effects and risk of bleeding increase.

Nursing considerations
- Monitor PT and INR closely when starting or stopping a macrolide antibiotic. The PT may be prolonged within a few days.
- Warfarin dose adjustment may continue for several days after antibiotic therapy stops.
- Treat excessive anticoagulation with vitamin K.
- Tell the patient to report unusual bleeding or bruising.
- Remind the patient that warfarin interacts with many drugs and that he should report any change in drug regimen.

■ Advise the patient to keep all follow-up medical appointments for proper monitoring and dosage adjustments.

---

clindamycin ▶◀ pancuronium
Cleocin

Risk rating: 2
Severity: Moderate   **Onset: Rapid**   **Likelihood: Suspected**

Cause
Clindamycin may potentiate the actions of pancuronium.

Effect
Pancuronium effects may increase.

Nursing considerations
■ If possible, avoid using clindamycin and other lincosamides with pancuronium.
■ Monitor the patient for respiratory depression.
■ Provide ventilatory support as needed.
■ Cholinesterase inhibitors or calcium may be useful in reversing drug effects.
■ Make sure the patient is adequately sedated when receiving pancuronium.

---

clomipramine ▶◀ fluvoxamine
Anafranil   Luvox

Risk rating: 2
Severity: Moderate   **Onset: Delayed**   **Likelihood: Probable**

Cause
Fluvoxamine may inhibit oxidative metabolism of tricyclic antidepressants (TCAs) such as clomipramine by CYP2D6 pathway.

Effect
TCA level and risk of toxicity increase.

Nursing considerations
■ If combined use can't be avoided, TCA dosage may need to be decreased.
■ Monitor TCA level.
■ Report evidence of toxicity or increased TCA level.
■ Inhibitory effects of fluvoxamine may take up to 2 weeks to dissipate after drug is stopped.
■ Using the TCA desipramine may avoid this interaction.

■ Urge the patient and his family to watch for and report increased anticholinergic effects, dizziness, drowsiness, and psychosis.

---

clomipramine ▶◀ MAO inhibitors

Anafranil

isocarboxazid, phenelzine, tranylcypromine

Risk rating: 1
Severity: Major   **Onset: Rapid**   **Likelihood: Suspected**

Cause
The mechanism of this interaction is unknown.

Effect
Risk of hyperpyretic crisis, seizures, and death increases.

Nursing considerations
🖎 **ALERT** Don't give a tricyclic antidepressant (TCA), such as clomipramine, with or within 2 weeks of an MAO inhibitor.
■ Clomipramine and imipramine may be more likely than other TCAs to interact with MAO inhibitors.
■ Watch for adverse effects, including confusion, hyperexcitability, rigidity, seizures, increased temperature, increased pulse, increased respiration, sweating, mydriasis, flushing, headache, coma, and DIC.

---

clomipramine ▶◀ valproic acid

Anafranil

divalproex sodium, valproate sodium, valproic acid

Risk rating: 2
Severity: Moderate   **Onset: Delayed**   **Likelihood: Suspected**

Cause
Valproic acid may inhibit hepatic metabolism of tricyclic antidepressants (TCAs) such as clomipramine.

Effect
TCA level and adverse effects may increase.

Nursing considerations
■ Use these drugs together cautiously.
■ If the patient is stable on valproic acid, start TCA at reduced dosage and adjust upward slowly to address symptoms and serum level.
■ If the patient is stable on a TCA, monitor serum level and patient status closely when starting or stopping valproic acid.

- Explain signs and symptoms to watch for when these drugs are combined.
- Other TCAs may interact with valproic acid. If you suspect an interaction, consult the prescriber or pharmacist.

---

clonidine ▶◀ beta blockers
Catapres · atenolol, propranolol, timolol

Risk rating: 1
Severity: Major **Onset: Delayed** **Likelihood: Suspected**

Cause
The mechanism of this interaction is unclear.

Effect
Potentially life-threatening hypertension may occur.

Nursing considerations
- Life-threatening hypertension may occur after simultaneously stopping clonidine and a beta blocker.
- It's unknown whether hypertension is caused by an interaction or withdrawal syndrome linked to each drug.
- Closely monitor blood pressure after starting or stopping the beta blocker or clonidine.
- When stopping combined therapy, gradually withdraw the beta blocker first to minimize adverse reactions.

---

clonidine ▶◀ tricyclic antidepressants
Catapres · desipramine, imipramine

Risk rating: 1
Severity: Major **Onset: Rapid** **Likelihood: Probable**

Cause
Tricyclic antidepressants (TCAs) inhibit alpha$_2$-adrenergic receptors, which clonidine stimulates for blood pressure control.

Effect
Clonidine efficacy in reducing blood pressure decreases.

Nursing considerations
- Life-threatening increases in blood pressure may occur.
- The intensity of this effect depends on the dosage of both drugs.
- **ALERT** Tell the prescriber that the patient takes a TCA.
- Tell the patient to keep an up-to-date list of all drugs he takes, so the prescriber can avoid possible interactions.

■ Other types of antidepressants can be used as an alternative treatment without this potential interaction.

---

clopidogrel ━━▶◀━━ aspirin
Plavix   Bayer, Ecotrin

Risk rating: 1
Severity: Major   **Onset: Delayed**   **Likelihood: Probable**

Cause
The exact mechanism of the interaction is unknown, but the effects of aspirin on the GI mucosa may be a risk factor.

Effect
Risk of life-threatening bleeding may be increased in high-risk patients.

Nursing considerations
🔰 **ALERT** Avoid the use of aspirin and clopidogrel together in high-risk patients with recent ischemic stroke or transient ischemic attack.
■ If the patient is receiving aspirin and clopidogrel together, monitor for signs of GI bleeding or increased intracranial pressure and bleeding.
■ Explain signs and symptoms of bleeding, and tell the patient when to contact the prescriber.
■ The use of aspirin and clopidogrel in patients who aren't high risk isn't contraindicated, but will increase the bleeding time.

---

clorazepate ━━▶◀━━ cimetidine
Tranxene   Tagamet

Risk rating: 3
Severity: Minor   **Onset: Rapid**   **Likelihood: Probable**

Cause
Hepatic metabolism of benzodiazepines such as clorazepate may be decreased.

Effect
Serum levels of benzodiazepines may be increased, causing increased sedation.

Nursing considerations
🔰 **ALERT** Carefully monitor the patient for increased sedation after taking cimetidine and a benzodiazepine.

- Warn the patient about the risk of increased sedation when taking cimetidine and a benzodiazepine together.
- If the patient has increased sedation, discuss the possibility of decreasing the dose of the benzodiazepine with the prescriber.
- Monitor serum benzodiazepine levels while the patient is taking cimetidine and a benzodiazepine together.

⚡ ALERT Elderly patients are at a higher risk for increased levels of sedation.

---

clorazepate ━━◄►━━ protease inhibitors

Tranxene

atazanavir, darunavir indinavir, nelfinavir, ritonavir, saquinavir

Risk rating: 1
Severity: Major   **Onset: Delayed**   **Likelihood: Suspected**

Cause
Protease inhibitors may inhibit CYP3A4 metabolism of certain benzodiazepines such as clorazepate.

Effect
Sedative effects of benzodiazepines may be increased and prolonged, leading to severe respiratory depression.

Nursing considerations
⚡ ALERT Don't combine clorazepate with a protease inhibitor.
- If the patient takes any benzodiazepine–protease inhibitor combination, notify the prescriber. Interaction could involve other drugs in the class.
- Watch for evidence of oversedation and respiratory depression.
- Teach the patient and his family about the risks of using these drugs together.

---

cloxacillin ━━◄►━━ food

Cloxapen

Risk rating: 2
Severity: Moderate   **Onset: Delayed**   **Likelihood: Suspected**

Cause
Food may delay or reduce GI absorption of penicillins such as cloxacillin.

Effect
Cloxacillin efficacy may decrease.

Nursing considerations
■ Food may affect cloxacillin absorption and peak level.
■ Other penicillins, such as Penicillin V and amoxicillin, don't have this interaction and may be given without regard to meals.
■ Tell the patient to take cloxacillin 1 hour before or 2 hours after a meal.
■ If the patient took cloxacillin with food, watch for lack of drug efficacy.

---

clozapine ➤◀ **ritonavir**

Clozaril   Norvir

Risk rating: 1
Severity: Major   **Onset: Delayed**   **Likelihood: Suspected**

Cause
Ritonavir may inhibit clozapine metabolism.

Effect
Clozapine level and risk of toxicity may increase.

Nursing considerations
⚠ **ALERT** Use of clozapine with ritonavir is contraindicated.
■ Increased clozapine dose may increase risk of seizures.
■ Watch for evidence of clozapine toxicity, including agranulocytosis, ECG changes, and seizures.
■ Monitor ECG. Clozapine-induced ECG changes should normalize after drug is stopped.

---

clozapine ➤◀ **serotonin reuptake inhibitors**

Clozaril   citalopram, fluoxetine, fluvoxamine, sertraline

Risk rating: 1
Severity: Major   **Onset: Delayed**   **Likelihood: Established**

Cause
Serotonin reuptake inhibitors inhibit hepatic metabolism of clozapine.

Effect
Clozapine level and risk of toxicity increase.

Nursing considerations
- Not all serotonin reuptake inhibitors share this interaction. If you suspect an interaction, consult the prescriber or pharmacist.
- Monitor serum clozapine level.
- Assess the patient for increased adverse effects or toxicity, including agranulocytosis, ECG changes, and seizures.
- Adjust clozapine dose as needed when adding or withdrawing a serotonin reuptake inhibitor.

colchicine ◀ cyclosporine
Gengraf, Neoral, Sandimmune

Risk rating: 2
Severity: **Moderate**   Onset: **Delayed**   Likelihood: **Suspected**

Cause
The mechanism of this interaction is unknown.

Effect
Severe adverse effects, including toxicity, may occur.

Nursing considerations
- Watch for GI, hepatic, renal, and neuromuscular adverse effects.
- Check cyclosporine level.
- Monitor LDH, liver enzyme, bilirubin, and creatinine levels.
- If an interaction is suspected and both drugs must be used, adjust cyclosporine dose as needed.
- Adverse effects should quickly subside once either drug is stopped.

colchicine ◀ macrolide antibiotics
clarithromycin, erythromycin

Risk rating: 1
Severity: **Major**   Onset: **Delayed**   Likelihood: **Suspected**

Cause
Metabolism of colchicine is inhibited.

Effect
Colchicine levels and risk of toxicity increase.

Nursing considerations
- Monitor the serum levels of colchicine.
- If using a macrolide antibiotic and colchicine together, it may be necessary to decrease the dose of colchicine.

■ Monitor the patient for fever, diarrhea, abdominal pain, myalgia, convulsions, and hair loss.
■ Patients with hepatic or renal impairment are more at risk for toxicity.

colestipol ━━━▶◀━━━ digoxin
Colestid   Lanoxin

Risk rating: 2
Severity: Moderate   Onset: Rapid   Likelihood: Suspected

Cause
Colestipol may bind with digoxin and decrease its GI absorption. Colestipol also may interfere with normal recycling of digoxin between the liver and intestines.

Effect
Digoxin effects may decrease.

Nursing considerations
■ Colestipol may be useful in treating digoxin toxicity.
■ If the patient is taking colestipol routinely, monitor serum digoxin level. Therapeutic range is 0.8 to 2 ng/ml.
■ Assess the patient for expected digoxin effects, including decreased heart rate, arrhythmia conversion, maintenance of converted rhythm, and improvement of heart failure symptoms.
■ Bile acid sequestrants other than colestipol may also have this interaction. If you suspect a drug interaction, consult the prescriber or pharmacist.

colestipol ━━━▶◀━━━ furosemide
Colestid   Lasix

Risk rating: 2
Severity: Moderate   Onset: Rapid   Likelihood: Suspected

Cause
Colestipol may bind to furosemide, inhibiting furosemide absorption.

Effect
Furosemide effects may decrease.

Nursing considerations
■ Separate doses; colestipol should be taken at least 2 hours after furosemide.

- Monitor the patient for expected furosemide effects, including reduction in peripheral edema, resolution of pulmonary edema, and decreased blood pressure in hypertensive patients.
- Monitor urine output and blood pressure to assess diuretic effect.
- If furosemide must be used, consult the prescriber or pharmacist about alternative cholesterol-lowering therapy.
- Help the patient develop a daily plan to ensure proper intervals between drug doses.
- Bile acid sequestrants other than colestipol may interact with furosemide. If you suspect an interaction, consult the prescriber or pharmacist.

colestipol ◄► hydrocortisone
Colestid   Cortef

Risk rating: 2
Severity: Moderate   Onset: Delayed   Likelihood: Suspected

Cause
Bile acid sequestrants, such as colestipol, interfere with GI absorption of hydrocortisone.

Effect
Hydrocortisone effects may decrease.

Nursing considerations
- If the patient needs hydrocortisone, consider a different cholesterol-lowering drug as an alternative to colestipol.
- Check for expected hydrocortisone effects.
- Help the patient develop a daily plan to ensure proper intervals between drug doses.

conivaptan ◄► azole antifungals
Vaprisol   itraconazole, ketoconazole

Risk rating: 1
Severity: Major   Onset: Delayed   Likelihood: Suspected

Cause
Azole antifungals may inhibit the CYP3A4 metabolism of conivaptan.

Effect
Conivaptan levels and risk of adverse reactions may increase.

Nursing considerations
⚠ **ALERT** Use of conivaptan and azole antifungals together is contra-indicated.
- The basis for this interaction is pharmacodynamics, not actual patient studies.

---

conivaptan ■■■■▶◀■■■■ clarithromycin
Vaprisol   Biaxin

Risk rating: 1
Severity: Major   **Onset: Delayed**   **Likelihood: Suspected**

Cause
Macrolide antibiotics such as clarithromycin may inhibit the CYP3A4 metabolism of conivaptan.

Effect
Conivaptan levels and adverse effects may be increased.

Nursing considerations
⚠ **ALERT** Administration of macrolide antibiotics and conivaptan together is contraindicated.
- The risk of increased conivaptan levels is unknown.
- Further studies are needed to determine the total extent of this interaction.

---

conivaptan ■■■■▶◀■■■■ protease inhibitors
Vaprisol   indinavir, ritonavir

Risk rating: 1
Severity: Major   **Onset: Delayed**   **Likelihood: Suspected**

Cause
Protease inhibitors may inhibit the CYP3A4 metabolism of conivaptan.

Effect
Conivaptan levels and adverse effects may be increased.

Nursing considerations
⚠ **ALERT** Administration of protease inhibitors and conivaptan together is contraindicated.
- The risk of increased conivaptan levels is unknown.
- Further studies are needed to determine the total extent of this interaction.

corticotropin ◄► cholinesterase inhibitors
neostigmine, pyridostigmine

Risk rating: 1
Severity: Major   **Onset: Delayed**   **Likelihood: Probable**

Cause
In myasthenia gravis, corticotropin and other corticosteroids antagonize the effects of cholinesterase inhibitors by an unknown mechanism.

Effect
The patient may develop severe muscular depression refractory to cholinesterase inhibitor.

Nursing considerations
- Corticosteroid therapy may have long-term benefits in myasthenia gravis.
- Combined therapy may be attempted under strict supervision.
- Monitor the patient with myasthenia gravis for severe muscle deterioration.
- **⬆ ALERT** Be prepared to provide respiratory support and mechanical ventilation if needed.
- Consult the prescriber or pharmacist about safe corticosteroid delivery to maximize improvement in muscle strength.

cortisone ◄► cholinesterase inhibitors
neostigmine, pyridostigmine

Risk rating: 1
Severity: Major   **Onset: Delayed**   **Likelihood: Probable**

Cause
In myasthenia gravis, cortisone and other corticosteroids antagonize the effects of cholinesterase inhibitors by an unknown mechanism.

Effect
The patient may develop severe muscular depression refractory to cholinesterase inhibitor.

Nursing considerations
- Corticosteroid therapy may have long-term benefits in myasthenia gravis.
- Combined therapy may be attempted under strict supervision.
- If the patient has myasthenia gravis, watch for severe muscle deterioration.

ALERT Be prepared to provide respiratory support and mechanical ventilation if needed.
- Consult the prescriber or pharmacist about safe corticosteroid delivery to maximize improvement in muscle strength.

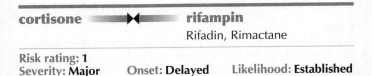

cortisone ━━━►◄━━━ **rifampin**
Rifadin, Rimactane

Risk rating: 1
Severity: Major   **Onset: Delayed**   **Likelihood: Established**

Cause
Rifamycins such as rifampin increase hepatic metabolism of corticosteroids such as cortisone.

Effect
Corticosteroid effects may be decreased.

Nursing considerations
- If possible, avoid giving rifamycins with corticosteroids.
- Monitor the patient for decreased corticosteroid effects, including loss of disease control.
- Monitor the patient closely for symptom control after increasing rifamycin dose. Drug may need to be stopped to regain control of disease.
- Corticosteroid effects may decrease within days of starting rifampin and may stay decreased 2 to 3 weeks after it stops.
- Corticosteroid dose may need to be doubled after adding rifampin.

cyclophosphamide ━━►◄━━ **azole antifungals**
Cytoxan   fluconazole, itraconazole

Risk rating: 2
Severity: Moderate   **Onset: Delayed**   **Likelihood: Suspected**

Cause
Inhibition of cyclophosphamide hepatic metabolism is suspected.

Effect
Cyclophosphamide exposure and its metabolites may be increased, increasing the risk of adverse effects.

Nursing considerations
- Monitor the patient for increased adverse effects.
- Monitor liver and renal function tests.

■ Watch the patient for hemorrhagic cystitis, infection, cardiotoxicity, and anemia.
■ Teach the patient adverse effects of cyclophosphamide, and instruct him to call the prescriber immediately if any occur.

cyclophosphamide ➡◀ succinylcholine
Cytoxan   Anectine

Risk rating: 2
Severity: Moderate   **Onset: Rapid**   **Likelihood: Probable**

Cause
Cyclophosphamide decreases succinylcholine metabolism by inhibiting cholinesterase activity.

Effect
Prolonged neuromuscular blockade caused by succinylcholine may occur.

Nursing considerations
■ If possible, avoid giving succinylcholine to a patient who has been receiving cyclophosphamide.
■ Effect of cyclophosphamide on plasma cholinesterase level is dose dependent.
■ If succinylcholine is given, measure plasma cholinesterase level.
■ If cholinesterase level declines, succinylcholine dosage may need to be reduced.
■ Monitor the patient for prolonged neuromuscular blockade.

cyclophosphamide ➡◀ warfarin
Cytoxan   Coumadin

Risk rating: 1
Severity: Major   **Onset: Delayed**   **Likelihood: Suspected**

Cause
Warfarin metabolism, clotting factor synthesis, and possible protein displacement may be inhibited.

Effect
Anticoagulant effects increase.

Nursing considerations
■ Monitor PT and INR closely during and after chemotherapy.
■ Tell the patient to report unusual bleeding or bruising.

■ Remind the patient that warfarin interacts with many drugs and that he should report any change in drug regimen.

cyclosporine ➤◀ amiodarone
Gengraf, Neoral, Sandimmune

Cordarone, Pacerone

Risk rating: 2
Severity: Moderate   Onset: Delayed   Likelihood: Suspected

Cause
Amiodarone may inhibit cyclosporine metabolism.

Effect
Cyclosporine level and risk of nephrotoxicity may increase.

Nursing considerations
■ Closely monitor cyclosporine level when amiodarone is started or stopped or its dosage is changed.
■ Because of amiodarone's long half-life, monitor cyclosporine level for several weeks after any dose alterations.
■ Cyclosporine dosage may need reduction (up to 50% in some cases) to keep cyclosporine level in the desired range.
■ Monitor the patient for signs of nephrotoxicity.
■ Monitor BUN and creatinine levels and urine output.
■ Check urine for increased proteins, cells, or casts.
■ If renal insufficiency develops, notify the prescriber.

cyclosporine ➤◀ androgens
Gengraf, Neoral, Sandimmune

danazol, methyltestosterone

Risk rating: 2
Severity: Moderate   Onset: Delayed   Likelihood: Suspected

Cause
Cyclosporine metabolism is inhibited.

Effect
Cyclosporine level and risk of toxicity may increase.

Nursing considerations
■ Monitor the patient for signs and symptoms of cyclosporine toxicity, such as nephrotoxicity and neurotoxicity.
■ Monitor BUN and creatinine levels and urine output.
■ Monitor cyclosporine level.

- Adjust cyclosporine dosage as needed. It may need to be reduced 20% to 50%.
- Check urine for increased proteins, cells, or casts.
- If renal insufficiency develops, notify the prescriber.

---

cyclosporine ▶◀ azole antifungals

Gengraf, Neoral, Sandimmune

fluconazole, itraconazole, ketoconazole, voriconazole

Risk rating: 2
Severity: Moderate   Onset: Delayed   Likelihood: Established

Cause
Azole antifungals decrease cyclosporine metabolism.

Effect
Cyclosporine level and toxicity may increase.

Nursing considerations
- Cyclosporine level may increase 1 to 3 days after starting an azole antifungal and persist for more than 1 week after stopping it.
- Monitor cyclosporine level.
- Adjust cyclosporine dosage to maintain therapeutic level.
- Cyclosporine dose may need to be decreased by 68% to 97%.
- Monitor the patient for hepatotoxicity and nephrotoxicity.

---

cyclosporine ▶◀ bosentan

Gengraf, Neoral, Sandimmune

Tracleer

Risk rating: 1
Severity: Major   Onset: Delayed   Likelihood: Suspected

Cause
Bosentan may increase cyclosporine metabolism. Cyclosporine may inhibit bosentan metabolism.

Effect
Bosentan level may increase. Cyclosporine level may decrease.

Nursing considerations
- ⚠ ALERT Use of bosentan with cyclosporine is contraindicated.
- Trough level of bosentan may increase 30 times over normal.
- Cyclosporine level may decrease by 50%.
- Watch for adverse effects from increased bosentan level, such as headache, nausea, vomiting, hypotension, and increased heart rate.

cyclosporine ▬▬▶◀▬▬ carbamazepine

Gengraf, Neoral,
Sandimmune

Carbatrol, Epitol, Equetro,
Tegretol

Risk rating: 2
Severity: Moderate   **Onset: Delayed**   **Likelihood: Suspected**

Cause
Carbamazepine may induce hepatic metabolism of cyclosporine.

Effect
Cyclosporine level and effects may decrease.

Nursing considerations
■ Monitor cyclosporine level.
■ If carbamazepine therapy is started, observe the patient for signs of rejection or decreased clinical effect.
■ If carbamazepine therapy is stopped, observe the patient for signs of cyclosporine toxicity, such as hepatotoxicity, nephrotoxicity, nausea, vomiting, tremors, and seizures.
■ Cyclosporine dosage may need adjustment.
■ Advise the patient to report signs of organ rejection; for example, decreased urine output in kidney transplant patients or shortness of breath and decreased stamina in heart transplant patients.

cyclosporine ▬▬▶◀▬▬ carvedilol

Gengraf, Neoral,
Sandimmune

Coreg

Risk rating: 2
Severity: Moderate   **Onset: Delayed**   **Likelihood: Suspected**

Cause
Carvedilol, a beta blocker, may disrupt cyclosporine metabolism.

Effect
Cyclosporine level and risk of toxicity may increase.

Nursing considerations
■ Monitor the patient for signs and symptoms of cyclosporine toxicity, such as nephrotoxicity and neurotoxicity.
■ Monitor serum creatinine level.
■ Monitor cyclosporine level.
■ Adjust cyclosporine dosage to maintain therapeutic level.
■ Other beta blockers may interact with cyclosporine.

cyclosporine ◄►►◄ colchicine

Gengraf, Neoral,
Sandimmune

Risk rating: 2
Severity: Moderate   **Onset: Delayed**   **Likelihood: Suspected**

Cause
The mechanism for this interaction is unknown.

Effect
Severe adverse effects, including toxicity, may occur.

Nursing considerations
- Watch for GI, hepatic, renal, and neuromuscular adverse effects.
- Monitor cyclosporine level.
- Monitor LDH, liver enzyme, bilirubin, and creatinine levels.
- If an interaction is suspected and both drugs must be used, adjust cyclosporine dose as needed.
- Adverse reactions should quickly subside once either drug stops.

cyclosporine ◄►►◄ diltiazem

Gengraf, Neoral,   Cardizem
Sandimmune

Risk rating: 2
Severity: Moderate   **Onset: Delayed**   **Likelihood: Established**

Cause
Diltiazem may inhibit cyclosporine metabolism in the liver.

Effect
Cyclosporine level and risk of toxicity may increase.

Nursing considerations
- Monitor cyclosporine level when adding or stopping diltiazem.
- Adjust cyclosporine dosage as needed. It may need to be reduced by 20% to 50%.
- Monitor the patient for arthralgia and encephalopathy, which may occur when cyclosporine and diltiazem are given together.
- Adverse reactions should subside when diltiazem is stopped.
- **⚡ ALERT** Rejection episodes may increase when diltiazem stops because cyclosporine level may be reduced. Monitor the patient closely.

cyclosporine ◀▶ etoposide

Gengraf, Neoral,
Sandimmune

VePesid

Risk rating: 2
Severity: Moderate   **Onset: Delayed**   **Likelihood: Established**

Cause
Cyclosporine may decrease etoposide clearance and inhibit its metabolism.

Effect
Etoposide level and risk of toxicity may increase.

Nursing considerations
- Monitor the patient for evidence of etoposide toxicity, including myelosuppression, nausea, vomiting, and diarrhea.
- Monitor CBC for evidence of leukopenia and thrombocytopenia.
- Adjust etoposide dosage as needed.

cyclosporine ◀▶ ezetimibe

Gengraf, Neoral,
Sandimmune

Zetia

Risk rating: 2
Severity: Moderate   **Onset: Delayed**   **Likelihood: Suspected**

Cause
The mechanism of the interaction is unknown.

Effect
Exposure to cyclosporine and ezetimibe may be increased, increasing therapeutic and adverse effects.

Nursing considerations
- Monitor cyclosporine level.
- Adjust the dose of cyclosporine as needed.
- Carefully monitor cyclosporine level when starting, stopping, or adjusting ezetimibe therapy.
- Monitor the patient for adverse effects, including shakiness, headache, tremor, hypertension, and fatigue.
- Monitor serum cholesterol and lipid levels to assess the patient's response to therapy.

cyclosporine ■■■■►◄■■■ food

Gengraf, Neoral,
Sandimmune

grapefruit juice, high-fat food

Risk rating: 2
Severity: Moderate   **Onset: Rapid**   **Likelihood: Probable**

Cause
Some foods may inhibit the intestinal enzyme responsible for cyclosporine metabolism.

Effect
Cyclosporine level may increase.

Nursing considerations
■ Despite dosage reduction, cyclosporine level may increase when taken with grapefruit juice.
■ Monitor cyclosporine level.
■ Advise the patient to avoid taking cyclosporine with grapefruit juice.
■ If the patient drinks grapefruit juice, watch for cyclosporine toxicity, including hepatotoxicity, nephrotoxicity, nausea, vomiting, tremors, and seizures.
■ Advise the patient that high-fat meals may increase cyclosporine level.

cyclosporine ■■■■►◄■■■ foscarnet

Gengraf, Neoral,
Sandimmune

Foscavir

Risk rating: 1
Severity: Major   **Onset: Delayed**   **Likelihood: Suspected**

Cause
Foscarnet and cyclosporine may work synergistically to cause nephrotoxicity.

Effect
Risk of renal failure may be increased.

Nursing considerations
■ Individualize foscarnet dosage based on renal function.
■ Monitor renal function carefully.
■ If nephrotoxicity occurs, consider stopping foscarnet.
■ Nephrotoxicity should resolve when foscarnet is stopped.

cyclosporine ▬▬►◄▬▬ HMG-CoA reductase inhibitors

Gengraf, Neoral
Sandimmune

atorvastatin, lovastatin,
pravastatin, rosuvastatin,
simvastatin

Risk rating: 1
Severity: Major   **Onset: Delayed**   **Likelihood: Probable**

Cause
Metabolism of some HMG-CoA reductase inhibitors may decrease,
and bioavailability may increase.

Effect
HMG-CoA reductase inhibitor level and adverse effects may increase.

Nursing considerations
- If possible, avoid use together.
- HMG-CoA reductase inhibitor dosage may need to be decreased.
- Monitor serum cholesterol and lipid levels to assess the patient's re-
sponse to therapy.
- **⚡ ALERT** Assess the patient for evidence of rhabdomyolysis: fatigue;
muscle aches and weakness; joint pain; dark, red, or cola-colored
urine; weight gain; seizures; and greatly increased serum CK level.
- Urge the patient to report unexplained muscle pain, tenderness, or
weakness to the prescriber.

cyclosporine ▬▬►◄▬▬ imipenem-cilastatin

Gengraf, Neoral,
Sandimmune

Primaxin

Risk rating: 2
Severity: Moderate   **Onset: Rapid**   **Likelihood: Suspected**

Cause
Additive or synergistic toxicity may occur.

Effect
Adverse CNS effects of both drugs may increase.

Nursing considerations
- Monitor the patient for adverse CNS effects, including confusion,
agitation, and tremors.
- Decreasing cyclosporine dose may decrease risk of adverse effects.

- Consider giving an alternative antibiotic if an interaction is suspected.
- Adverse effects should improve after stopping imipenem-cilastatin.

---

cyclosporine ▶◀ macrolide antibiotics

Gengraf, Neoral,
Sandimmune

azithromycin, clarithromycin,
erythromycin

Risk rating: 2
Severity: Moderate   Onset: Delayed   Likelihood: Established

Cause
Macrolide antibiotics interfere with cyclosporine metabolism. The rate and extent of absorption may increase, and the volume of distribution may decrease.

Effect
Elevated cyclosporine levels and increased risk of toxicity may occur.

Nursing considerations
⚡ ALERT Monitor the patient carefully for nephrotoxicity or neurotoxicity.
- Closely monitor BUN and serum creatinine levels.
- The dose of cyclosporine may need to be decreased.
- Of all the macrolide antibiotics, azithromycin appears to interact the least with cyclosporine.

---

cyclosporine ▶◀ methotrexate

Gengraf, Neoral,
Sandimmune

Trexall

Risk rating: 2
Severity: Moderate   Onset: Delayed   Likelihood: Suspected

Cause
Cyclosporine blocks the metabolism of methotrexate.

Effect
Methotrexate levels and pharmacologic and adverse effects increase.

Nursing considerations
- Closely monitor clinical response to methotrexate when starting or stopping cyclosporine.
- Adjust the dose of methotrexate as needed.
- No effect is seen on cyclosporine.

■ Monitor the patient for methotrexate toxicity, including renal failure, neutropenia, leukopenia, thrombocytopenia, increased liver function tests, and skin ulcers.
■ Monitor the patient for mouth sores. This may be the first outward appearance of methotrexate toxicity; however, in some patients, bone marrow suppression coincides with or precedes mouth sores.

cyclosporine ➤◄ metoclopramide
Gengraf, Neoral, Sandimmune   Reglan

Risk rating: 2
Severity: Moderate   Onset: Delayed   Likelihood: Suspected

Cause
Metoclopramide increases gastric emptying time, which may increase cyclosporine absorption.

Effect
Cyclosporine level and risk of toxicity may increase.

Nursing considerations
■ Monitor cyclosporine level closely.
■ Watch for cyclosporine toxicity, including hepatotoxicity, nephrotoxicity, nausea, vomiting, tremors, and seizures.
■ Consider decreasing cyclosporine dose as needed.
■ It isn't known whether altering dosage or schedule of metoclopramide would decrease risk or severity of interaction.

cyclosporine ➤◄ micafungin
Gengraf, Neoral, Sandimmune   Mycamine

Risk rating: 2
Severity: Moderate   Onset: Delayed   Likelihood: Suspected

Cause
Micafungin inhibits CYP3A metabolism of cyclosporine.

Effect
Cyclosporine level and risk of adverse reactions may increase.

Nursing considerations
■ Cyclosporine dose may need to be adjusted when starting or stopping micafungin therapy.
■ Monitor cyclosporine level closely.

- Watch for signs and symptoms of toxicity, including shakiness, headaches, tremor, hypertension, and fatigue.
- Decrease cyclosporine dose as needed.

cyclosporine ◄► nefazodone
Gengraf, Neoral,
Sandimmune

Risk rating: 2
Severity: Moderate   Onset: Delayed   Likelihood: Probable

Cause
Nefazodone, an antidepressant, may inhibit cyclosporine metabolism.

Effect
Cyclosporine level and risk of toxicity may increase.

Nursing considerations
- For a patient taking cyclosporine, consider another antidepressant.
- Monitor cyclosporine level closely.
- Signs and symptoms of toxicity may include shakiness, headaches, tremor, hypertension, and fatigue.
- Decrease cyclosporine dose as needed.

cyclosporine ◄► nicardipine
Gengraf, Neoral,   Cardene
Sandimmune

Risk rating: 2
Severity: Moderate   Onset: Delayed   Likelihood: Suspected

Cause
Nicardipine may inhibit cyclosporine metabolism in the liver.

Effect
Cyclosporine level and risk of renal toxicity may increase.

Nursing considerations
- Monitor cyclosporine level. Trough level may be elevated.
- Assess renal function.
- Monitor the patient for signs and symptoms of toxicity.
- Adjust cyclosporine dose as needed.
- If nicardipine is stopped, consider increasing the cyclosporine dose to prevent rejection.

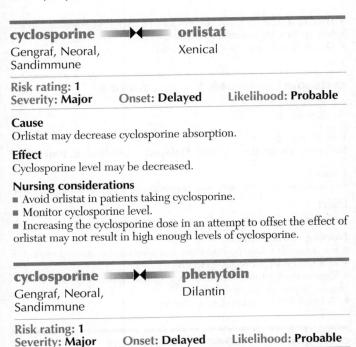

cyclosporine ▶◀ orlistat
Gengraf, Neoral,
Sandimmune

Xenical

Risk rating: 1
Severity: Major   **Onset: Delayed**   **Likelihood: Probable**

Cause
Orlistat may decrease cyclosporine absorption.

Effect
Cyclosporine level may be decreased.

Nursing considerations
- Avoid orlistat in patients taking cyclosporine.
- Monitor cyclosporine level.
- Increasing the cyclosporine dose in an attempt to offset the effect of orlistat may not result in high enough levels of cyclosporine.

cyclosporine ▶◀ phenytoin
Gengraf, Neoral,
Sandimmune

Dilantin

Risk rating: 1
Severity: Major   **Onset: Delayed**   **Likelihood: Probable**

Cause
Cyclosporine absorption may decrease or metabolism may increase.

Effect
Cyclosporine level may decrease.

Nursing considerations
- Patients may be at risk for transplant rejection when cyclosporine is given with phenytoin.
- Cyclosporine level decreases within 48 hours of phenytoin treatment and returns to normal within 1 week of stopping phenytoin.
- Monitor cyclosporine level closely.
- Adjust cyclosporine dose as needed.

cyclosporine ▬▬►◄▬▬ repaglinide
Gengraf, Neoral,   Prandin
Sandimmune

Risk rating: 2
Severity: Moderate   **Onset: Delayed**   **Likelihood: Suspected**

Cause
Cyclosporine may inhibit repaglinide metabolism.

Effect
The combination may increase repaglinide level and effects, including adverse effects.

Nursing considerations
- Monitor blood glucose level closely.
- Adjust repaglinide dose as needed.
- Monitor the patient for evidence of hypoglycemia, including hunger, dizziness, shakiness, sweating, confusion, and light-headedness.
- Advise the patient to carry glucose tables or another simple sugar in case of hypoglycemia.
- Make sure the patient and his family know what to do if hypoglycemia occurs.

cyclosporine ▬▬►◄▬▬ rifamycins
Gengraf, Neoral,   rifabutin, rifampin
Sandimmune

Risk rating: 1
Severity: Major   **Onset: Delayed**   **Likelihood: Probable**

Cause
Rifamycins increase CYP3A4 cyclosporine metabolism.

Effect
Immunosuppressive effects of cyclosporine may decrease.

Nursing considerations
- Avoid using rifamycins during cyclosporine treatment if possible.
- Cyclosporine effects may decrease within 2 days after starting a rifamycin and may continue 1 to 3 weeks after it's stopped.
- Monitor cyclosporine level often during and after rifamycin treatment.
- Adjust cyclosporine dose as needed.
- Cyclosporine level may remain decreased despite dosage increases.

■ Assess the patient for signs and symptoms of rejection.
■ Monitor creatinine level during and after rifamycin treatment.

---

cyclosporine ➤◀ serotonin reuptake inhibitors

Gengraf, Neoral,
Sandimmune

fluoxetine, fluvoxamine

Risk rating: 2
Severity: Moderate   **Onset: Delayed**   **Likelihood: Suspected**

Cause
Serotonin reuptake inhibitors inhibit cyclosporine metabolism.

Effect
Cyclosporine level and risk of toxicity may increase.

Nursing considerations
■ Consider using citalopram as an alternative to these serotonin reuptake inhibitors to prevent this effect.
■ When the patient is on both, monitor cyclosporine level when adding or stopping a serotonin reuptake inhibitor.
■ Adjust cyclosporine dose as needed.

---

cyclosporine ➤◀ sirolimus

Gengraf, Neoral,
Sandimmune

Rapamune

Risk rating: 2
Severity: Moderate   **Onset: Delayed**   **Likelihood: Probable**

Cause
The mechanism of this interaction is unknown.

Effect
Sirolimus level and risk of toxicity may increase.

Nursing considerations
■ Administer sirolimus 4 hours after cyclosporine.
■ Monitor the patient for evidence of sirolimus toxicity, such as anxiety, headache, hypertension, and thrombocytopenia.
■ Sirolimus level may decrease when cyclosporine is stopped.
■ Anticipate need for increased sirolimus dosage if cyclosporine is stopped.

cyclosporine ━━◄►━━ St. John's wort
Gengraf, Neoral,
Sandimmune

Risk rating: 1
Severity: Major   **Onset: Delayed**   **Likelihood: Probable**

Cause
St. John's wort may increase cyclosporine metabolism.

Effect
Cyclosporine level and efficacy may decrease.

Nursing considerations
- Discourage use of St. John's wort with cyclosporine.
- Monitor the patient for signs and symptoms of transplant rejection.
- Warn the patient to consult the prescriber before taking OTC or herbal products.

cyclosporine ━━◄►━━ sulfonamides
Gengraf, Neoral,   sulfadiazine, sulfamethoxazole,
Sandimmune   trimethoprim-sulfamethoxazole

Risk rating: 2
Severity: Moderate   **Onset: Delayed**   **Likelihood: Suspected**

Cause
The mechanism of this interaction is unknown.

Effect
Effect of cyclosporine may be decreased. Oral sulfonamides increase the risk of nephrotoxicity.

Nursing considerations
- Frequently monitor cyclosporine levels.
- Adjust cyclosporine level as needed.
- Monitor the patient for signs and symptoms of transplant rejection.
- Monitor creatinine level.
- Watch the patient for decreased urine output, increased weight, crackles, and other signs of fluid retention.

cyclosporine ▬▶◀ terbinafine
Gengraf, Neoral,
Sandimmune

Lamisil

Risk rating: 2
Severity: Moderate   **Onset: Delayed**   **Likelihood: Suspected**

Cause
Terbinafine may increase cyclosporine metabolism.

Effect
Cyclosporine level may decrease.

Nursing considerations
■ Monitor cyclosporine level.
■ Adjust cyclosporine dose as needed.
■ Closely monitor the patient for signs and symptoms of transplant rejection when terbinafine is started or stopped.

cyclosporine ▬▶◀ ticlopidine
Gengraf, Neoral,
Sandimmune

Ticlid

Risk rating: 2
Severity: Moderate   **Onset: Delayed**   **Likelihood: Suspected**

Cause
The mechanism of this interaction is unknown.

Effect
Cyclosporine level may decrease.

Nursing considerations
■ Monitor cyclosporine level.
■ Adjust cyclosporine dose as needed.
■ Closely monitor the patient for signs and symptoms of transplant rejection when ticlopidine is started or stopped.

cyclosporine ━━━━▶◀━━━━ verapamil

Gengraf, Neoral,
Sandimmune

Calan

Risk rating: 2
Severity: Moderate   **Onset: Delayed**   **Likelihood: Established**

Cause
Hepatic and gut wall metabolism of cyclosporine is inhibited.

Effect
Cyclosporine levels and risk of nephrotoxicity may increase.

Nursing considerations
- Monitor cyclosporine level.
- Decrease cyclosporine dose as needed.
- Assess renal function.
- Signs and symptoms of toxicity may include shakiness, headaches, tremor, hypertension, and fatigue.
- Administering verapamil before cyclosporine may be nephroprotective.
- This interaction is generally seen within 7 days of starting verapamil and decreases within 1 week of discontinuation.

cyproheptadine ━━━━▶◀━━━━ metyrapone

Metopirone

Risk rating: 2
Severity: Moderate   **Onset: Rapid**   **Likelihood: Probable**

Cause
Cyproheptadine decreases the expected ACTH secretion seen after administering metyrapone.

Effect
Combining both decreases pituitary-adrenal response to metyrapone.

Nursing considerations
🔊 **ALERT** Discontinue cyproheptadine before assessing pituitary-adrenal axis with metyrapone.
- Make the patient aware of how important it is to tell his practitioners about all the drugs he is taking.

cyproheptadine ➤◀ serotonin reuptake inhibitors

fluoxetine, paroxetine

Risk rating: 2
Severity: Moderate   **Onset: Rapid**   **Likelihood: Suspected**

Cause
Because cyproheptadine is a serotonin antagonist, the interaction is thought to occur at the receptor level.

Effect
Pharmacologic effects of SSRIs decrease.

Nursing considerations
■ Monitor the patient's clinical response to his serotonin reuptake inhibitor.
■ If loss of antidepressant efficacy occurs, consider eliminating cyproheptadine from the patient's drug regimen.
■ Depressive symptoms may resolve within 5 days of discontinuing this combination.

danazol ➤◀ carbamazepine

Danocrine   Carbatrol, Epitol, Equetro, Tegretol

Risk rating: 2
Severity: Moderate   **Onset: Delayed**   **Likelihood: Suspected**

Cause
Danazol inhibits carbamazepine metabolism.

Effect
Carbamazepine level and toxicity may increase.

Nursing considerations
⚠ ALERT Avoid this combination if possible.
■ Monitor carbamazepine level; the therapeutic range is 4 to 12 mcg/ml.
■ If danazol is started or stopped, carbamazepine dosage may need adjustment.
⚠ ALERT Watch for signs of anorexia or subtle appetite changes, which may indicate excessive carbamazepine level.
■ Watch for carbamazepine toxicity: dizziness, ataxia, respiratory depression, tachycardia, arrhythmias, blood pressure changes, impaired consciousness, abnormal reflexes, nystagmus, seizures, nausea, vomiting, and urine retention.

danazol ▸◂ cyclosporine
Danocrine   Gengraf, Neoral, Sandimmune

Risk rating: 2
Severity: Moderate   **Onset: Delayed**   **Likelihood: Suspected**

Cause
Cyclosporine metabolism is inhibited.

Effect
Cyclosporine level and risk of toxicity may increase.

Nursing considerations
- Monitor the patient for signs and symptoms of cyclosporine toxicity, such as nephrotoxicity and neurotoxicity.
- Monitor BUN and creatinine levels and urine output.
- Monitor cyclosporine level.
- Adjust cyclosporine dosage as needed. It may need to be reduced 20% to 50%.
- Check urine for increased proteins, cells, or casts.
- If renal insufficiency develops, notify the prescriber.

danazol ▸◂ warfarin
Danocrine   Coumadin

Risk rating: 1
Severity: Major   **Onset: Delayed**   **Likelihood: Probable**

Cause
The mechanism of this interaction is unknown.

Effect
Anticoagulant effects increase.

Nursing considerations
- Avoid this combination if possible.
- Monitor coagulation values carefully. Warfarin dosage will be decreased.
- Tell the patient to report unusual bleeding or bruising.
- Remind the patient that warfarin interacts with many drugs and that he should report any change in drug regimen.

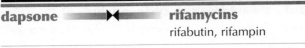

dapsone ▶◀ rifamycins
rifabutin, rifampin

Risk rating: 2
Severity: Moderate   **Onset: Delayed**   **Likelihood: Suspected**

Cause
Rifamycins increase the metabolism of dapsone.

Effect
Pharmacologic effects of dapsone may be decreased.

Nursing considerations
- Monitor for clinical failure of dapsone.
- Dosage of dapsone may need to be increased.
- If the patient is taking a rifamycin, consider using an alternative *Pneumocystis carinii* pneumonia prophylaxis.

dapsone ▶◀ trimethoprims
trimethoprim, trimethoprim-sulfamethoxazole

Risk rating: 2
Severity: Moderate   **Onset: Delayed**   **Likelihood: Suspected**

Cause
Mechanism is unknown; it's possible that dapsone and trimethoprims decrease the elimination of each other.

Effect
Levels of dapsone and trimethoprim may increase, along with pharmacologic and toxic effects.

Nursing considerations
- Monitor the patient for dapsone toxicity.
- Watch the patient for signs and symptoms of toxicity, including shortness of breath, cyanosis, mental status changes, headache, fatigue, and dizziness.
- No adverse effects from increased trimethoprim levels have been noted.
- Patients taking trimethoprim-sulfamethoxazole have increased toxicity compared to patients taking trimethoprim.

darunavir ►◄ benzodiazepines

Prezista

alprazolam, clorazepate, diazepam, estazolam, flurazepam, midazolam, triazolam

Risk rating: 1
Severity: Major   **Onset: Delayed**   **Likelihood: Suspected**

Cause
Protease inhibitors, such as darunavir, may inhibit CYP3A4 metabolism of benzodiazepines.

Effect
Sedative effects of benzodiazepines may be increased and prolonged, leading to severe respiratory depression.

Nursing considerations
◣ ALERT Don't combine darunavir with a benzodiazepine.
- If the patient takes any benzodiazepine–protease inhibitor combination, notify the prescriber. Interaction could involve other drugs in the class.
- Watch the patient for evidence of oversedation and respiratory depression.
- Teach the patient and his family about the risks of using these drugs together.

darunavir ►◄ ergot derivatives

Prezista

dihydroergotamine, ergonovine, ergotamine, methylergonovine

Risk rating: 1
Severity: Major   **Onset: Delayed**   **Likelihood: Probable**

Cause
Protease inhibitors, such as darunavir, may interfere with CYP3A4 metabolism of ergot derivatives.

Effect
Combining darunavir with an ergot derivative may increase risk of ergot-induced peripheral vasospasm and ischemia.

Nursing considerations
◣ ALERT Use of ergot derivatives with protease inhibitors is contraindicated.

■ Monitor the patient for evidence of peripheral ischemia, including pain in limb muscles while exercising and later at rest; numbness and tingling of fingers and toes; cool, pale, or cyanotic limbs; red or violet blisters on hands or feet; and gangrene.

■ Sodium nitroprusside may be used to treat ergot-induced vasospasm.

■ If the patient takes a protease inhibitor, consult the prescriber and the pharmacist about alternative migraine treatments.

■ Advise the patient to tell the prescriber about all drugs and supplements he takes and any increase in adverse effects.

---

darunavir ▶◀ lovastatin
Prezista   Mevacor

Risk rating: 1
Severity: Major   **Onset: Delayed**   **Likelihood: Suspected**

Cause
Protease inhibitors, such as darunavir, inhibit the CYP3A4 metabolism of lovastatin.

Effect
Lovastatin level may increase.

Nursing considerations
◣ ALERT Darunavir and lovastatin should not be used together.

■ Use other protease inhibitors cautiously; they may have similar effects.

■ If a protease inhibitor is added to a regimen that includes lovastatin, monitor the patient closely.

◣ ALERT Watch for evidence of rhabdomyolysis, including dark or red urine, muscle weakness, and myalgia.

■ Urge the patient to report unexplained muscle weakness immediately.

---

darunavir ▶◀ pimozide
Prezista   Orap

Risk rating: 1
Severity: Major   **Onset: Delayed**   **Likelihood: Suspected**

Cause
Protease inhibitors, such as darunavir, may inhibit CYP3A4 metabolism of pimozide.

Effect
Risk of life-threatening arrhythmias may increase.

Nursing considerations
▶ **ALERT** Combined use of these drugs is contraindicated.
- Arrhythmias are related to prolonged QT interval, a known risk of pimozide.
- Other protease inhibitors may have the same interaction.
- Interaction warning is based on pharmacokinetics of these drugs, not actual patient studies.

---

darunavir ◀▶ **St. John's wort**
Prezista

Risk rating: 1
Severity: Major   **Onset: Delayed**   **Likelihood: Suspected**

Cause
Hepatic metabolism of a protease inhibitor, such as darunavir, may increase.

Effect
Protease inhibitor level and effects may decrease.

Nursing considerations
- If the patient starts or stops taking St. John's wort, monitor protease inhibitor level closely.
- Monitor CD4+ and T-cell counts; tell the prescriber if they decrease.
- Urge the patient to report opportunistic infections.
- Tell the patient not to change an HIV regimen without consulting his prescriber.
- To help prevent interactions, urge the patient to tell his prescribers about all drugs, supplements, and alternative therapies he uses.

---

darunavir ◀▶ **simvastatin**
Prezista   Zocor

Risk rating: 1
Severity: Major   **Onset: Delayed**   **Likelihood: Suspected**

Cause
The combination may inhibit first-pass metabolism of simvastatin by CYP3A4 in the GI tract.

Effect
Simvastatin level may increase.

Nursing considerations
ALERT Combined use of these drugs is contraindicated.

■ If a protease inhibitor is added to simvastatin, monitor the patient closely.

ALERT Watch for evidence of rhabdomyolysis, including dark or red urine, muscle weakness, and myalgia.

■ Urge the patient to report unexplained muscle weakness immediately.

---

delavirdine ▬▬►◄▬▬ amprenavir
Rescriptor   Agenerase

Risk rating: 2
Severity: Moderate   Onset: Delayed   Likelihood: Suspected

Cause
Amprenavir may induce CYP3A4 metabolism of delavirdine; while delavirdine may *inhibit* CYP3A4 metabolism of amprenavir.

Effect
Amprenavir level may increase. Delavirdine level may decrease.

Nursing considerations
■ If the patient is started on amprenavir, watch for decreased delavirdine effects.

■ Review common adverse reactions caused by this interaction: headache, fatigue, rash, and GI complaints.

■ Caution the patient to report bothersome effects but not to alter regimen without consulting his prescriber.

---

delavirdine ▬▬►◄▬▬ benzodiazepines
Rescriptor   alprazolam, midazolam,
                                    triazolam

Risk rating: 2
Severity: Moderate   Onset: Delayed   Likelihood: Suspected

Cause
Nonnucleoside reverse-transcriptase inhibitors, such as delavirdine, may inhibit CYP3A4 metabolism of some benzodiazepines.

Effect
Sedative effects of benzodiazepines may be increased or prolonged, leading to respiratory depression.

Nursing considerations
⚠ ALERT Don't combine alprazolam, midazolam, or triazolam with delavirdine.

■ Other benzodiazepines and nonnucleoside reverse-transcriptase inhibitors may interact. If you suspect an interaction, consult the prescriber or pharmacist.

■ Make the patient aware of the risk of oversedation and respiratory depression.

■ Urge the patient to promptly report any suspected interaction.

---

delavirdine ▶◀ ergot derivatives
Rescriptor   dihydroergotamine, ergotamine

Risk rating: 1
Severity: Major   **Onset: Delayed**   **Likelihood: Suspected**

Cause
Nonnucleoside reverse-transcriptase inhibitors, such as delavirdine, may decrease CYP3A4 metabolism of ergot derivatives.

Effect
The risk of ergot-induced peripheral vasospasm and ischemia may increase.

Nursing considerations
⚠ ALERT Use of ergot derivatives with delavirdine is contraindicated.

■ Watch for evidence of peripheral ischemia: pain in limb muscles while exercising and later at rest; numbness and tingling of fingers and toes; cool, pale, or cyanotic limbs; red or violet blisters on hands or feet; and gangrene.

■ Ergot toxicity may cause nausea, vomiting, lassitude, impaired mental function, delirium, severe dyspnea, hypotension, hypertension, rapid or weak pulse, unconsciousness, limb spasms, seizures, and shock.

■ Give vasodilators for vasospasm and diazepam for seizures.

■ Other nonnucleoside reverse-transcriptase inhibitors, such as nevirapine, may interact with ergot derivatives. If you suspect an interaction, consult the prescriber or pharmacist.

delavirdine ▰▰▰▶◀▰▰▰ indinavir
Rescriptor   Crixivan

Risk rating: 2
Severity: Moderate   **Onset: Delayed**   **Likelihood: Probable**

Cause
Decreased metabolism and clearance of indinavir.

Effect
Indinavir level, effects, and risk of adverse effects may increase.

Nursing considerations
■ Watch for increased indinavir adverse effects, including nausea, vomiting, diarrhea, and adverse renal effects.
■ Monitor the patient for nephrolithiasis; the patient may experience pain and hematuria.
■ The indinavir dose may need to be decreased.

delavirdine ▰▰▰▶◀▰▰▰ rifamycins
Rescriptor   rifabutin, rifampin

Risk rating: 2
Severity: Moderate   **Onset: Delayed**   **Likelihood: Suspected**

Cause
Rifamycins increase the metabolism of delavirdine.

Effect
Delavirdine levels decrease.

Nursing considerations
◖ **ALERT** Avoid concurrent use of delavirdine and rifamycins.
■ Monitor the patient for fever, fatigue, headache, nausea, abdominal pain, or cough.
■ Tell the patient not to alter drug regimen without notifying the prescriber or practitioner.

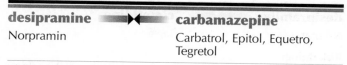

desipramine ▶◀ carbamazepine
Norpramin

Carbatrol, Epitol, Equetro,
Tegretol

Risk rating: 2
Severity: Moderate   **Onset: Delayed**   **Likelihood: Probable**

Cause
Tricyclic antidepressants (TCAs), such as desipramine, may compete
with carbamazepine for hepatic metabolism. Carbamazepine may induce hepatic TCA metabolism.

Effect
Carbamazepine level and risk of toxicity may increase. Desipramine
and effects may decrease.

Nursing considerations
■ Other TCAs may interact with carbamazepine. If you suspect a drug
interaction, consult prescriber or pharmacist.
■ Monitor carbamazepine level; therapeutic range is 4 to 12 mcg/ml.
■ Watch for evidence of carbamazepine toxicity, including dizziness,
ataxia, respiratory depression, tachycardia, arrhythmias, blood pressure changes, impaired consciousness, abnormal reflexes, nystagmus,
seizures, nausea, vomiting, and urine retention.

desipramine ▶◀ chlorpromazine
Norpramin

Thorazine

Risk rating: 3
Severity: Minor   **Onset: Delayed**   **Likelihood: Probable**

Cause
Competitive inhibition of tricyclic antidepressant (TCA) metabolism
may occur.

Effect
The combination leads to increased levels of TCAs.

Nursing considerations
■ Monitor the patient's clinical response to TCAs, and decrease the
dose if needed.
■ No toxic effects are noted from this interaction.

desipramine ◄►◄ cimetidine
Norpramin   Tagamet

Risk rating: 2
Severity: Moderate   **Onset: Rapid**   **Likelihood: Probable**

Cause
Cimetidine may interfere with metabolism of tricyclic antidepressants (TCAs) such as desipramine.

Effect
TCA level and bioavailability increase.

Nursing considerations
■ When starting or stopping cimetidine, monitor serum TCA level and adjust dosage as needed.
■ Tell the prescriber if TCA level or effect increases; dosage may need to be decreased.
■ If needed, consult the prescriber about possible change from cimetidine to ranitidine.
■ Urge the patient and his family to watch for and report increased anticholinergic effects, dizziness, drowsiness, and psychosis.

desipramine ◄►◄ clonidine
Norpramin   Catapres

Risk rating: 1
Severity: Major   **Onset: Rapid**   **Likelihood: Probable**

Cause
Tricyclic antidepressants (TCAs), such as desipramine, inhibit alpha$_2$-adrenergic receptors, which clonidine stimulates for blood pressure control.

Effect
Clonidine efficacy in reducing blood pressure decreases.

Nursing considerations
■ Life-threatening increases in blood pressure may occur.
■ The intensity of this effect depends on the dosage of both drugs.
■ Tell prescriber that the patient takes a TCA.
■ Tell the patient to keep an up-to-date list of all drugs he takes so the prescriber can avoid possible interactions.
■ Other types of antidepressants can be used as an alternative treatment without this potential interaction.

desipramine ━━━▶◀━━━ fluoxetine
Norpramin   Prozac, Sarafem

Risk rating: 2
Severity: Moderate   **Onset: Delayed**   **Likelihood: Probable**

Cause
Fluoxetine may inhibit hepatic metabolism of tricyclic antidepressants (TCAs) such as desipramine.

Effect
Serum TCA level and toxicity may increase.

Nursing considerations
▪ Monitor serum TCA level, and watch closely for evidence of toxicity, such as increased anticholinergic effects, delirium, dizziness, drowsiness, and psychosis.
▪ Report evidence of increased TCA level or toxicity; dosage may need to be decreased.
▪ If a patient on fluoxetine starts on TCA, the TCA dosage may need to be decreased by up to 75% to avoid interaction.
▪ Other TCAs may interact with fluoxetine. If you suspect an interaction, consult the prescriber or pharmacist.

desipramine ━━━▶◀━━━ MAO inhibitors
Norpramin   isocarboxazid, phenelzine,
                             tranylcypromine

Risk rating: 1
Severity: Major   **Onset: Rapid**   **Likelihood: Suspected**

Cause
The mechanism of this interaction is unknown.

Effect
The risk of hyperpyretic crisis, seizures, and death increases.

Nursing considerations
🔌 **ALERT** Don't give a tricyclic antidepressant, such as desipramine, with or within 2 weeks of an MAO inhibitor.
▪ Watch for adverse effects, including confusion, hyperexcitability, rigidity, seizures, increased temperature, increased pulse, increased respiration, sweating, mydriasis, flushing, headache, coma, and DIC.

desipramine ━━━▶◀━━━ paroxetine
Norpramin   Paxil

Risk rating: 2
Severity: Moderate   Onset: Delayed   Likelihood: Suspected

Cause
Paroxetine may decrease desipramine metabolism in some people and increase it in others.

Effect
Therapeutic and toxic effects of certain tricyclic antidepressants (TCAs), such as desipramine, may increase.

Nursing considerations
■ When starting or stopping paroxetine, monitor TCA level and adjust dosage as needed.
■ Watch for adverse reactions, such as increased drowsiness, dizziness, confusion, heart rate or rhythm changes, and urine retention.
■ Watch closely for evidence of serotonin syndrome, such as delirium, bizarre movements, and tachycardia. Alert the prescriber if they occur; TCA may need to be stopped.
■ Symptoms of serotonin syndrome may resolve within 24 hours of stopping a TCA and starting a short course of cyproheptadine.
◤ **ALERT** TCAs other than desipramine may have this interaction.

desipramine ━━━▶◀━━━ sertraline
Norpramin   Zoloft

Risk rating: 2
Severity: Moderate   Onset: Delayed   Likelihood: Suspected

Cause
This combination may inhibit the hepatic metabolism, by CYP2D6, of a tricyclic antidepressant (TCA) such as desipramine.

Effect
Therapeutic and toxic effects of certain TCAs may increase.

Nursing considerations
■ Avoid this drug combination if possible.
■ Watch for evidence of TCA toxicity and serotonin syndrome, including delirium, bizarre movements, and tachycardia.
■ Monitor serum TCA levels when starting or stopping sertraline.
■ If abnormalities occur, decrease TCA dosage or stop the drug.

desipramine ◄►► sympathomimetics
Norpramin

epinephrine, norepinephrine,
phenylephrine

Risk rating: 2
Severity: Moderate   **Onset: Rapid**   **Likelihood: Established**

Cause
Tricyclic antidepressants (TCAs), such as desipramine, increase the
effects of direct-acting sympathomimetics and decrease the effects of
indirect-acting sympathomimetics.

Effect
When sympathomimetic effects increase, the risk of hypertension
and arrhythmias increases. When sympathomimetic effects decrease,
blood pressure control decreases.

Nursing considerations
- Avoid using these drugs together if possible.
- Watch closely for hypertension and heart rhythm changes; they may
warrant reduction of sympathomimetic dosage.
- If the patient takes a mixed-acting sympathomimetic, watch for neg-
ative effects; dosage may need to be altered.
- Other TCAs and sympathomimetics may interact. If you suspect an
interaction, consult the prescriber or pharmacist.

desipramine ◄►► terbinafine
Norpramin

Lamisil

Risk rating: 2
Severity: Moderate   **Onset: Delayed**   **Likelihood: Suspected**

Cause
Hepatic metabolism of tricyclic antidepressants (TCAs), such as desipramine, may be inhibited.

Effect
Therapeutic and toxic effects of certain TCAs may increase.

Nursing considerations
- Check for abnormal TCA levels; report them to the prescriber.
- TCA dosage may be decreased while the patient takes terbinafine.
- Interaction may cause vertigo, fatigue, loss of appetite, ataxia, mus-
cle twitching, and trouble swallowing.
- Terbinafine's inhibitory effects may take several weeks to dissipate
after drug is stopped.
- Describe signs and symptoms of interaction.

dexamethasone ⧓ aminoglutethimide

Decadron | Cytadren

Risk rating: 2
Severity: Moderate **Onset: Delayed** **Likelihood: Suspected**

Cause
The cause of the interaction is unknown.

Effect
Dexamethasone-induced adrenal suppression is decreased. Corticosteroid anti-inflammatory activity may also be decreased.

Nursing considerations
- Tell the prescriber if the patient is taking both drugs together; he may substitute hydrocortisone for dexamethasone.
- Monitor the patient for loss of adrenal suppression from decreased dexamethasone activity.
- If symptoms of decreased adrenal suppression occur, the dose of dexamethasone may need to be increased.

dexamethasone ⧓ aprepitant

Decadron | Emend

Risk rating: 2
Severity: Moderate **Onset: Delayed** **Likelihood: Suspected**

Cause
Aprepitant may inhibit first-pass metabolism of certain corticosteroids such as dexamethasone.

Effect
Corticosteroid level may be increased and half-life prolonged.

Nursing considerations
- Corticosteroid dosage may need to be decreased.
- When starting or stopping aprepitant, adjust corticosteroid dosage as needed.
- Watch closely for evidence of increased corticosteroid level, such as insomnia, euphoria, increased appetite, mood changes, and increased blood glucose level.
- Tell the patient to report any symptoms reflecting an increased blood glucose level, including increased thirst or hunger and frequent urination.

dexamethasone ━━►◄━━ azole antifungals
Decadron
itraconazole, ketoconazole

Risk rating: 2
Severity: Moderate   **Onset: Delayed**   **Likelihood: Suspected**

Cause
Metabolism of corticosteroids, such as dexamethasone, is inhibited; elimination is decreased.

Effect
Corticosteroid pharmacologic effects and risk of toxicity may be increased.

Nursing considerations
- Corticosteroid dosage may need to be decreased by up to 50%.
- When starting or stopping an azole antifungal, adjust corticosteroid dosage as needed.
- Watch closely for evidence of increased corticosteroid level, such as insomnia, euphoria, increased appetite, mood changes, and increased blood glucose level.
- Tell the patient to report symptoms of increased blood glucose level, including increased thirst or hunger and frequent urination.

dexamethasone ━━►◄━━ barbiturates
Decadron
pentobarbital, phenobarbital, primidone

Risk rating: 2
Severity: Moderate   **Onset: Delayed**   **Likelihood: Established**

Cause
Barbiturates induce liver enzymes, which stimulate metabolism of corticosteroids such as dexamethasone.

Effect
Corticosteroid effects may be decreased.

Nursing considerations
- Avoid giving barbiturates with corticosteroids.
- If the patient takes a corticosteroid, watch for worsening symptoms when a barbiturate is started or stopped.
- During barbiturate treatment, corticosteroid dosage may need to be increased.

dexamethasone ▨▶◀▨ phenytoin

Decadron   Dilantin

Risk rating: 2
Severity: Moderate   Onset: Delayed   Likelihood: Established

Cause
Hydantoins induce liver enzymes, which stimulate metabolism of corticosteroids such as dexamethasone. Dexamethasone may enhance hepatic clearance of phenytoin.

Effect
Corticosteroid effects may decrease.

Nursing considerations
■ Avoid giving hydantoins with corticosteroids if possible.
■ Watch for decreased corticosteroid effects, monitor phenytoin level, and adjust dosage of either drug as needed.
■ Dosage of either or both drugs may need to be increased.
■ The effects of a corticosteroid may decrease within days after starting the patient on phenytoin and remain at that reduced level until 3 weeks after the phenytoin is discontinued.

dexamethasone ▨▶◀▨ salicylates

Decadron   aspirin, choline salicylate,
                            sodium salicylate

Risk rating: 2
Severity: Moderate   Onset: Delayed   Likelihood: Probable

Cause
Dexamethasone and other corticosteroids stimulate hepatic metabolism of salicylates and may increase their renal excretion.

Effect
Salicylate level and effects decrease.

Nursing considerations
■ Monitor salicylate level and efficacy; dosage may need adjustment.
⚡ **ALERT** Giving a salicylate while tapering a corticosteroid may result in salicylate toxicity.
■ Watch for evidence of salicylate toxicity, including diaphoresis, nausea, vomiting, tinnitus, hyperventilation, and CNS depression.
■ Patients with renal impairment may be at greater risk.

dexmethylphenidate ►◄ tranylcypromine
Focalin   Parnate

Risk rating: 1
Severity: Major   **Onset: Delayed**   **Likelihood: Suspected**

Cause
The mechanism of this interaction is unknown.

Effect
The risk of hypertensive crisis increases.

Nursing considerations
⚑ **ALERT** Use of dexmethylphenidate with MAO inhibitors is contra-indicated.
■ Don't use dexmethylphenidate within 14 days after stopping an MAO inhibitor.
■ Monitor blood pressure closely if methylphenidate is given with an MAO inhibitor.
■ Teach the patient and his family to monitor and record blood pressure.

dextroamphetamine ►◄ MAO inhibitors
Dexedrine   phenelzine, tranylcypromine

Risk rating: 1
Severity: Major   **Onset: Rapid**   **Likelihood: Suspected**

Cause
This interaction probably stems from increased norepinephrine levels at the synaptic cleft.

Effect
Anorexiant effects increase.

Nursing considerations
■ Avoid giving these drugs together if possible.
■ Headache and severe hypertension may occur rapidly if an amphetamine, such as dextroamphetamine, is given to the patient who takes an MAO inhibitor.
⚑ **ALERT** Death may result from hypertensive crisis and resulting cerebral hemorrhage.
■ Monitor the patient for hypotension, hyperpyrexia, and seizures.
■ Hypertensive reaction may occur for several weeks after stopping an MAO inhibitor.

dextroamphetamine ➡◀ SSRIs

Dexedrine

citalopram, fluoxetine,
venlafaxine

Risk rating: 2
Severity: Moderate   **Onset: Rapid**   **Likelihood: Suspected**

Cause
The mechanism of this interaction is unknown.

Effect
Sympathomimetic effects and risk of serotonin syndrome increase.

Nursing considerations
- If these drugs must be used together, watch closely for increased CNS effects, such as anxiety, jitteriness, agitation, and restlessness.
- Mild serotonin-like symptoms may develop, including anxiety, dizziness, restlessness, nausea, and vomiting.
- Counsel the patient about the risk of this interaction; make sure he knows to avoid amphetamines such as dextroamphetamine.
- Familiarize the patient with the traits of serotonin syndrome, including CNS irritability, motor weakness, shivering, myoclonus, and altered consciousness, so he can report any such symptoms.

dextroamphetamine ➡◀ urine acidifiers

Dexedrine

Risk rating: 3
Severity: Minor   **Onset: Rapid**   **Likelihood: Established**

Cause
Urinary elimination of amphetamines, such as dextroamphetamine, is increased by the acidification of urine.

Effect
Amphetamine duration of action is decreased.

Nursing considerations
- There are no special precautions necessary with this interaction.
- This interaction has been used for therapeutic purposes in amphetamine poisoning.

dextroamphetamine ➡◀ urine alkalinizers

Dexedrine

potassium citrate, sodium acetate, sodium bicarbonate, sodium citrate, sodium lactate, tromethamine

Risk rating: 2
Severity: Moderate   **Onset: Rapid**   **Likelihood: Established**

Cause
When urine is alkaline, amphetamine clearance is prolonged.

Effect
In amphetamine overdose, the toxic period will be extended, increasing the risk of injury.

Nursing considerations
■ **ALERT** Avoid drugs that may alkalinize the urine, particularly during overdose with an amphetamine such as dextroamphetamine.
■ Watch for evidence of amphetamine toxicity, such as dermatoses, marked insomnia, irritability, hyperactivity, and personality changes.
■ If the patient takes an anorexiant, advise against excessive use of sodium bicarbonate as an antacid.

dextromethorphan ➡◀ MAO inhibitors

Robitussin DM

isocarboxazid, phenelzine

Risk rating: 1
Severity: Major   **Onset: Rapid**   **Likelihood: Suspected**

Cause
MAO inhibitor may decrease serotonin metabolism. Dextromethorphan may decrease synaptic reuptake of serotonin.

Effect
Risk of serotonin syndrome increases.

Nursing considerations
■ Avoid giving these drugs together if possible.
■ **ALERT** Combined use may cause hyperpyrexia, abnormal muscle movement, hypotension, coma, and death.
■ If the patient takes an MAO inhibitor, caution against taking OTC cough and cold medicines that contain dextromethorphan.

dextromethorphan ➤◀ sibutramine
Robitussin DM   Meridia

Risk rating: 1
Severity: Major   **Onset: Rapid**   **Likelihood: Suspected**

Cause
Additive serotonergic effects of both agents may occur.

Effect
Risk of serotonin syndrome increases.

Nursing considerations
■ Avoid giving these drugs together if possible.
■ **ALERT** Combined use may cause hyperpyrexia, abnormal muscle movement, hypotension, coma, and death.
■ This interaction is based on pharmacokinetics, not actual patient studies.

diazepam ➤◀ alcohol
Valium

Risk rating: 2
Severity: Moderate   **Onset: Rapid**   **Likelihood: Established**

Cause
Alcohol inhibits hepatic enzymes, which decreases clearance and increases peak levels of benzodiazepines such as diazepam.

Effect
Effects may be additive or synergistic.

Nursing considerations
■ Tell the patient to avoid alcohol while taking a benzodiazepine.
■ Assess the patient thoroughly for history or evidence of alcohol use before starting him on benzodiazepine therapy.
■ Watch for additive CNS effects, which may suggest benzodiazepine overdose.
■ Other benzodiazepines interact with alcohol. If you suspect an interaction, consult the prescriber or pharmacist.

diazepam ◄► cimetidine
Valium   Tagamet

Risk rating: 3
Severity: Minor   **Onset: Rapid**   **Likelihood: Probable**

Cause
Hepatic metabolism of benzodiazepines, such as diazepam, may be decreased.

Effect
Serum levels of benzodiazepines may be increased, causing increased sedation.

Nursing considerations
■ **ALERT** Carefully monitor the patient for increased sedation after taking cimetidine and a benzodiazepine.
■ Warn the patient about the risk of increased sedation when taking cimetidine and diazepam together.
■ If the patient has increased sedation, discuss the possibility of decreasing the dose of diazepam with the prescriber.
■ Monitor serum benzodiazepine levels while the patient is taking cimetidine and a benzodiazepine together.
■ **ALERT** Elderly patients are at a higher risk for increased levels of sedation.

diazepam ◄► diltiazem
Valium   Cardizem

Risk rating: 2
Severity: Moderate   **Onset: Rapid**   **Likelihood: Probable**

Cause
Diltiazem may decrease metabolism of some benzodiazepines such as diazepam.

Effect
Benzodiazepine effects may increase.

Nursing considerations
■ Watch for signs of increased CNS depression: sedation, dizziness, confusion, asthenia, ataxia, altered level of consciousness, hypoactive reflexes, hypotension, bradycardia, and respiratory depression.
■ Lower diazepam dose may be needed.
■ Explain the risk of increased and prolonged CNS effects to the patient.

■ Warn the patient to avoid hazardous activities until effects of this combination are clear.
■ Other benzodiazepines may interact with diltiazem. If you suspect an interaction, consult the prescriber or pharmacist.

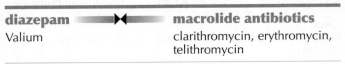

diazepam ◀ macrolide antibiotics
Valium   clarithromycin, erythromycin,
                                telithromycin

Risk rating: 2
Severity: Moderate   **Onset: Rapid**   **Likelihood: Suspected**

Cause
Macrolide antibiotics may decrease the metabolism of certain benzodiazepines such as diazepam.

Effect
Sedative effects of benzodiazepines may be increased or prolonged.

Nursing considerations
■ Consult the prescriber about decreasing benzodiazepine dosage.
■ Lorazepam, oxazepam, and temazepam probably don't interact with macrolide antibiotics; substitution may be possible.
■ Urge the patient to report oversedation promptly.

diazepam ◀ omeprazole
Valium   Prilosec

Risk rating: 3
Severity: Minor   **Onset: Delayed**   **Likelihood: Suspected**

Cause
Metabolism of benzodiazepines, such as diazepam, may be decreased.

Effect
Half-life of diazepam may be increased, leading to increased levels. Sedation or ataxia may be enhanced.

Nursing considerations
■ Monitor the patient for increased sedation or CNS impairment.
■ Consult the prescriber about reducing diazepam dosage.
■ Other benzodiazepines may not have this interaction.

diazepam ▰▰▰▶◀▰▰▰ opioid analgesics
Valium   buprenorphine, methadone

Risk rating: 2
Severity: Moderate   **Onset: Rapid**   **Likelihood: Suspected**

Cause
Additive or synergistic effects are involved.

Effect
Buprenorphine strength and drug effects are increased.

Nursing considerations
- Monitor the patient for increased sedation.
- Instruct the patient not to drive, operate machinery, or perform other tasks that may be hazardous if he is not fully alert.
- The interaction appears to be dose-and time-related, with the greatest increase in adverse effects typically occurring 1 to 2 hours after taking the diazepam.

diazepam ▰▰▰▶◀▰▰▰ phenytoin
Valium   Dilantin

Risk rating: 2
Severity: Moderate   **Onset: Delayed**   **Likelihood: Suspected**

Cause
Metabolism of phenytoin and benzodiazepines, such as diazepam, is altered.

Effect
Phenytoin levels and risk of toxicity may increase.

Nursing considerations
- Monitor phenytoin level closely. Dosage may need to be adjusted. Therapeutic range for phenytoin is 10 to 20 mcg/ml.
- Toxic effects can occur at therapeutic level. Adjust the measured level for hypoalbumenia or renal impairment, which can increase free drug level.
- Signs and symptoms of phenytoin toxicity include nystagmus, slurred speech, ataxia, blurred or double vision, confusion, drowsiness, and lethargy.
- In some cases, the efficacy of diazepam may decrease, resulting in the need for a larger dose.

diazepam ▰▰▰◀▶ protease inhibitors
Valium   atazanavir, darunavir, indinavir,
                          nelfinavir, ritonavir, saquinavir

Risk rating: 1
Severity: Major   **Onset: Delayed**   **Likelihood: Suspected**

Cause
Protease inhibitors may inhibit CYP3A4 metabolism of certain benzodiazepines such as diazepam.

Effect
Sedative effects of benzodiazepines may be increased and prolonged, leading to severe respiratory depression.

Nursing considerations
■ If the patient takes any benzodiazepine–protease inhibitor combination, notify the prescriber. Other drugs in this class can also give rise to this kind of interaction.
■ Watch for evidence of oversedation and respiratory depression.
■ Teach the patient and his family about the risks of combined use.

diazepam ▰▰▰◀▶ rifampin
Valium   Rifadin, Rimactane

Risk rating: 2
Severity: Moderate   **Onset: Delayed**   **Likelihood: Suspected**

Cause
Rifampin may increase CYP3A4 metabolism of benzodiazepines such as diazepam.

Effect
Antianxiety, sedative, and sleep-inducing effects of benzodiazepines may be decreased.

Nursing considerations
■ Watch for the expected benzodiazepine effects and any lack of efficacy.
■ If benzodiazepine efficacy is reduced, dosage may be increased.
■ Other benzodiazepines may interact with rifampin. If you suspect an interaction, consult the prescriber or pharmacist.
■ Temazepam may be more effective for patients with insomnia because it doesn't undergo CYP3A4 metabolism.

diazepam ◄►◄ theophyllines
Valium
aminophylline, theophylline

Risk rating: 3
Severity: Minor   **Onset: Rapid**   **Likelihood: Suspected**

Cause
Theophyllines produce an antagonistic action by competitively binding to receptors.

Effect
The sedative effects of the benzodiazepines may be decreased by theophyllines such as aminophylline.

Nursing considerations
- If a patient is taking theophyllines and benzodiazepines, monitor him for a decreased sedative effect of the benzodiazepine.
- Consult with the prescriber, and adjust the dose of the benzodiazepine as needed.

dicloxacillin ◄►◄ food

Risk rating: 2
Severity: Moderate   **Onset: Delayed**   **Likelihood: Suspected**

Cause
Food may delay or reduce GI absorption of penicillins such as dicloxacillin.

Effect
Penicillin efficacy may decrease.

Nursing considerations
- Food may affect penicillin absorption and peak level.
- Penicillin V and amoxicillin don't have this interaction and may be given without regard to meals.
- If the patient takes penicillin with food, watch for lack of drug efficacy.
- Tell the patient to take penicillin 1 hour before or 2 hours after a meal.

dicloxacillin ➤◄ warfarin
Coumadin

Risk rating: 2
Severity: Moderate   Onset: Delayed   Likelihood: Suspected

Cause
Warfarin induces hypoprothrombinemia, and dicloxacillin inhibits platelet aggregation.

Effect
Bleeding time is prolonged. Warfarin resistance may also occur.

Nursing considerations
- Monitor PT and INR closely during combined use.
- Risk of interaction increases with large doses of I.V. penicillins.
- Monitor coagulation values before starting dicloxacillin and for at least 3 weeks after stopping to check for warfarin resistance.
- Tell the patient to report unusual bleeding or bruising.
- Remind the patient that warfarin interacts with many drugs and that he should report any change in drug regimen.
- Advise the patient to keep all follow-up medical appointments for proper monitoring and dosage adjustments.

didanosine ➤◄ azole antifungals
Videx   itraconazole, ketoconazole

Risk rating: 2
Severity: Moderate   Onset: Rapid   Likelihood: Suspected

Cause
Inert ingredients in chewable didanosine tablets decrease absorption of azole antifungals.

Effect
Efficacy of azole antifungals may decrease.

Nursing considerations
- To minimize interaction, instruct the patient to take the antifungal drug 2 hours before didanosine.
- Monitor the patient for lack of response to antifungal drug.
- Help the patient develop a plan to ensure proper dosage intervals.
- Other azole antifungals may interact with didanosine. If you suspect an interaction, consult the prescriber or pharmacist.

didanosine ━━━━▶◀━━━━ ciprofloxacin
Videx   Cipro

Risk rating: 2
Severity: Moderate   **Onset: Rapid**   **Likelihood: Suspected**

Cause
Buffers in didanosine chewable tablets and pediatric powder for oral solution decrease GI absorption of quinolones such as ciprofloxacin.

Effect
Quinolone effects decrease.

Nursing considerations
■ Avoid this combination. If it's unavoidable, give the quinolone at least 2 hours before or 6 hours after didanosine.
■ Monitor the patient for improvement in infection.
■ Unbuffered didanosine doesn't affect quinolone absorption.
■ Help the patient develop a plan to ensure proper dosage intervals.

didanosine ━━━━▶◀━━━━ indinavir
Videx   Crixivan

Risk rating: 2
Severity: Moderate   **Onset: Rapid**   **Likelihood: Suspected**

Cause
Indinavir absorption may be decreased by buffers in didanosine.

Effect
Indinavir effects may decrease.

Nursing considerations
◣ ALERT Give indinavir and didanosine at least 1 hour apart on an empty stomach.
■ Watch for expected therapeutic effects of indinavir, including improvement in HIV symptoms.
■ Monitor laboratory values for an increased CD4+ T-cell count and a decreased HIV-1 RNA level.
■ Help the patient develop a plan to ensure proper dosage intervals.

didanosine ━━━▶◀━━━ tenofovir
Videx   Viread

Risk rating: 1
Severity: Major   **Onset: Delayed**   **Likelihood: Suspected**

Cause
The mechanism of this interaction is unknown.

Effect
Didanosine levels and risk of adverse effects may be increased.

Nursing considerations
- Carefully monitor the patient for adverse effects, such as lactic acidosis, pancreatitis, and neuropathy.
- Monitor the patient for abdominal pain, nausea, vomiting, or diarrhea.
- Dosage of didanosine may need to be decreased.
- Instruct the patient to call the prescriber if he experiences numbness or tingling in the extremities.
- Patients with renal insufficiency are at a higher risk for this interaction.

digoxin ━━━▶◀━━━ acarbose
Lanoxin   Precose

Risk rating: 2
Severity: Moderate   **Onset: Delayed**   **Likelihood: Probable**

Cause
Absorption of digoxin may be impaired.

Effect
Serum digoxin levels may decrease, thereby decreasing its therapeutic effects.

Nursing considerations
- Monitor digoxin levels; the therapeutic range is 0.8 to 2 ng/ml.
- If serum digoxin levels are low, the dose of digoxin may need to be increased or the acarbose dose discontinued.
- If possible, administer the drugs at least 6 hours apart to avoid the interactions.
- Instruct the patient to notify the prescriber if he has an irregular or fast heart rate.

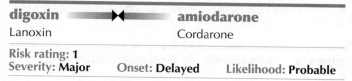

digoxin
Lanoxin

amiodarone
Cordarone

Risk rating: 1
Severity: Major   **Onset: Delayed**   **Likelihood: Probable**

Cause
The mechanism for this interaction is unknown.

Effect
Digoxin level and risk of toxicity may increase.

Nursing considerations
- Watch for evidence of digoxin toxicity, such as arrhythmias, nausea, vomiting, and agitation.
- Monitor digoxin level; digoxin dosage may need to be reduced during amiodarone treatment.
- Higher amiodarone doses cause greatest increase in digoxin level.
- Because amiodarone has a long half-life, effects of interaction may persist after amiodarone is stopped.

digoxin
Lanoxin

beta-adrenergic blockers
carvedilol, propranolol

Risk rating: 2
Severity: Moderate   **Onset: Rapid**   **Likelihood: Probable**

Cause
Carvedilol increases digoxin bioavailability. Renal excretion of digoxin may be decreased and additive depression of myocardial conduction may occur.

Effect
Digoxin level and risk of toxicity may occur. Synergistic bradycardia may occur.

Nursing considerations
- **ALERT** Carefully monitor patients receiving beta-adrenergic blockers and digoxin for bradycardia.
- Monitor digoxin level. Therapeutic range is 0.8 to 2 nanograms/ml.
- Watch for evidence of digoxin toxicity: lethargy, drowsiness, confusion, hallucinations, headaches, syncopes, visual disturbances, nausea, anorexia, vomiting, diarrhea, and arrhythmias (bradycardia, AV block, and ventricular ectopy).
- Digoxin dosage may need to be decreased.

■ Patients with higher serum digoxin levels have an increased risk of toxicity.

---

digoxin ▶◀ **cholestyramine**

Lanoxin

LoCHOLEST, Prevalite, Questran

Risk rating: 2
Severity: Moderate   **Onset: Delayed**   **Likelihood: Probable**

Cause
Cholestyramine may decrease digoxin absorption by binding to it. Cholestyramine may also interrupt digoxin metabolism in the liver.

Effect
Digoxin bioavailability and effects may decrease.

Nursing considerations
■ Monitor digoxin level.
■ Watch for decreased digoxin effects; dosage may need adjustment.
■ Digoxin capsules may minimize the interaction.
■ Give cholestyramine 8 hours before or after digoxin.
■ Cholestyramine may be useful in treating digoxin toxicity.

---

digoxin ▶◀ **colestipol**

Lanoxin

Colestid

Risk rating: 2
Severity: Moderate   **Onset: Rapid**   **Likelihood: Suspected**

Cause
Colestipol may bind with digoxin and decrease its GI absorption. Colestipol also may interfere with normal recycling of digoxin between liver and intestine.

Effect
Digoxin effects may decrease.

Nursing considerations
■ Colestipol may be useful in treating digoxin toxicity.
■ If you suspect an interaction, consult the prescriber or pharmacist.
■ If the patient takes colestipol routinely, monitor digoxin level. Therapeutic range for digoxin is 0.8 to 2 nanograms/ml.
■ Monitor the patient for expected digoxin effects, including decreased heart rate, arrhythmia conversion, maintenance of converted rhythm, and improvement of heart failure symptoms.

■ If digoxin level or effects decrease, dosage may need adjustment.

---

digoxin ►◄ diltiazem
Lanoxin   Cardizem

Risk rating: 2
Severity: Moderate   **Onset: Delayed**   **Likelihood: Suspected**

Cause
Diltiazem decreases the clearance of digoxin.

Effect
Digoxin level and risk of toxicity may increase.

Nursing considerations
■ Monitor digoxin level and clinical status. Therapeutic range is 0.8 to 2 nanograms/ml.
■ Watch for evidence of digoxin toxicity: arrhythmias (bradycardia, AV block, and ventricular ectopy), lethargy, drowsiness, confusion, hallucinations, headaches, syncope, visual disturbances, nausea, anorexia, vomiting, and diarrhea.
■ Digoxin dosage may need reduction.

---

digoxin ►◄ indomethacin
Lanoxin   Indocin

Risk rating: 2
Severity: Moderate   **Onset: Delayed**   **Likelihood: Suspected**

Cause
Indomethacin may reduce renal digoxin elimination.

Effect
Digoxin level and risk of toxicity may increase.

Nursing considerations
■ This interaction may not occur in patients with normal renal function.
◪ **ALERT** Use cautiously in preterm infants with decreased renal function; digoxin dose may need to be reduced by half when indomethacin starts.
■ Monitor digoxin level. Therapeutic range is 0.8 to 2 nanograms/ml.
■ Check renal function tests and urine output.
■ Watch for evidence of digoxin toxicity: lethargy, drowsiness, confusion, hallucinations, headaches, syncope, visual disturbances, nausea, vomiting, diarrhea, anorexia, failure to thrive, and arrhythmias (such

as bradycardia and AV blocks, which are more common in children; and ventricular ectopy, which is more common in adults).

digoxin ◄─►◄ itraconazole
Lanoxin   Sporanox

Risk rating: 2
Severity: Moderate   **Onset: Delayed**   **Likelihood: Established**

Cause
Renal digoxin clearance may decrease and absorption increase.

Effect
Digoxin level and risk of toxicity may increase.

Nursing considerations
■ Monitor digoxin level. Therapeutic range is 0.8 to 2 ng/ml.
■ Watch for evidence of digoxin toxicity: arrhythmias (bradycardia, AV block, and ventricular ectopy), lethargy, drowsiness, confusion, hallucinations, headaches, syncope, visual disturbances, nausea, anorexia, vomiting, and diarrhea.
■ Digoxin dosage may need reduction.
■ Azole antifungals other than itraconazole may interact with digoxin. If you suspect an interaction, consult the prescriber or pharmacist.

digoxin ◄─►◄ loop diuretics
Lanoxin   bumetanide, ethacrynic acid, furosemide

Risk rating: 1
Severity: Major   **Onset: Delayed**   **Likelihood: Probable**

Cause
Urinary excretion of potassium and magnesium is increased.

Effect
Electrolyte disturbances may predispose the patient to digoxin-induced arrhythmias.

Nursing considerations
■ Monitor serum potassium and magnesium levels; decreased levels may predispose the patient to arrhythmias.
■ Carefully monitor the patient's ECG while receiving digoxin and a thiazide diuretic.
■ If the patient develops hypomagnesemia or hypokalemia, be prepared to administer supplements.

- Monitor the patient for increased serum sodium.
- Changing the patient from a loop-diuretic to a potassium-sparing diuretic will minimize the risk of arrhythmias.
- This interaction appears to be dose related.

---

digoxin ▸◂ macrolide antibiotics

Lanoxin

clarithromycin, erythromycin, telithromycin

Risk rating: 1
Severity: Major   **Onset: Delayed**   **Likelihood: Established**

Cause
Macrolide antibiotics may alter GI flora and increase digoxin absorption. Clarithromycin may inhibit renal clearance of digoxin.

Effect
Digoxin level and risk of toxicity may increase.

Nursing considerations
- Monitor digoxin level. Therapeutic range is 0.8 to 2 ng/ml.
- Watch for evidence of digoxin toxicity: lethargy, drowsiness, confusion, hallucinations, headaches, syncope, visual disturbances, nausea, anorexia, vomiting, diarrhea, and arrhythmias (bradycardia, AV blocks, and ventricular ectopy).
- Digoxin dose may need to be reduced.
- **⚡ ALERT** Neither clarithromycin nor erythromycin affects the serum level of digoxin given by I.V.
- The capsule form of digoxin may increase its availability and decrease risk of interaction.
- Other macrolide antibiotics may interact with digoxin. If you suspect an interaction, consult the prescriber or pharmacist.

---

digoxin ▸◂ metoclopramide

Lanoxin

Reglan

Risk rating: 2
Severity: Moderate   **Onset: Delayed**   **Likelihood: Probable**

Cause
Increased GI motility may decrease digoxin absorption.

Effect
Digoxin level and effects may decrease.

Nursing considerations
- Monitor the patient for decreased digoxin level; therapeutic range is 0.8 to 2 ng/ml.
- Watch for expected digoxin effects: decreased heart rate, arrhythmia conversion, maintenance of converted rhythm, and improvement of heart failure symptoms.
- If digoxin level or effects decrease, dosage may need adjustment.
- ⚡ **ALERT** This interaction may not occur with high-bioavailability digoxin forms, including capsules, elixir, and tablets with a high dissolution rate.
- Urge the patient to tell the prescriber about increased adverse effects.

---

digoxin ▶◀ **paroxetine**
Lanoxin   Paxil

Risk rating: 1
Severity: Major   **Onset: Delayed**   **Likelihood: Suspected**

Cause
Renal excretion of digoxin is inhibited.

Effect
Digoxin level and risk of toxicity may increase.

Nursing considerations
- Monitor digoxin level. Therapeutic range is 0.8 to 2 ng/ml.
- Check ECG for digoxin toxicity: arrhythmias, such as bradycardia and AV blocks, ventricular ectopy, and shortened QTc interval.
- Watch for other evidence of digoxin toxicity: lethargy, drowsiness, confusion, hallucinations, headaches, syncope, visual disturbances, nausea, anorexia, failure to thrive, vomiting, and diarrhea.
- If paroxetine starts or stops during digoxin therapy, digoxin dosage may need adjustment.
- Citalopram and venlafaxine don't have this interaction with digoxin and may be better alternatives than paroxetine.

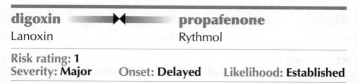

digoxin ▶◀ propafenone
Lanoxin   Rythmol

Risk rating: 1
Severity: Major   **Onset: Delayed**   **Likelihood: Established**

Cause
Digoxin distribution and renal and nonrenal digoxin clearance may decrease.

Effect
Digoxin level and risk of toxicity may increase.

Nursing considerations
- Monitor digoxin level. Therapeutic range is 0.8 to 2 ng/ml.
- Check ECG for digoxin toxicity: arrhythmias, such as bradycardia and AV blocks, ventricular ectopy, and shortened QTc interval.
- Watch for other evidence of digoxin toxicity: lethargy, drowsiness, confusion, hallucinations, headaches, syncope, visual disturbances, nausea, anorexia, failure to thrive, vomiting, and diarrhea.
- If propafenone starts or stops during digoxin therapy, digoxin dosage may need adjustment.

digoxin ▶◀ quinidine
Lanoxin

Risk rating: 1
Severity: Major   **Onset: Delayed**   **Likelihood: Established**

Cause
Total renal and biliary digoxin clearance decreases.

Effect
Digoxin level and risk of toxicity may increase.

Nursing considerations
- Monitor digoxin level. Therapeutic range is 0.8 to 2 ng/ml.
- Some patients may have toxicity even with serum digoxin levels in therapeutic range.
- Watch for signs of digoxin toxicity: arrhythmias (bradycardia, AV blocks, and ventricular ectopy); lethargy; drowsiness; confusion; hallucinations; headaches; syncope; visual disturbances; nausea; anorexia; vomiting; and diarrhea.
- If the patient is started on quinidine, digoxin dosage may need reduction of up to 50%.

digoxin 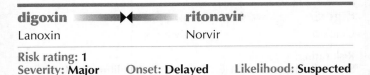 ritonavir
Lanoxin   Norvir

Risk rating: 1
Severity: Major   **Onset: Delayed**   **Likelihood: Suspected**

Cause
Renal clearance of digoxin in the proximal tubules is decreased.

Effect
Digoxin level and risk of toxicity may increase.

Nursing considerations
- Monitor digoxin level. Therapeutic range is 0.8 to 2 ng/ml.
- Some patients may have toxicity even with serum digoxin level in therapeutic range.
- Watch for signs of digoxin toxicity: arrhythmias (bradycardia, AV blocks, and ventricular ectopy); lethargy; drowsiness; confusion; hallucinations; headaches; syncope; visual disturbances; nausea; anorexia; vomiting; and diarrhea.
- If the patient is started on ritonavir, his digoxin dosage may need to be reduced.

digoxin 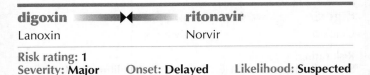 spironolactone
Lanoxin   Aldactone

Risk rating: 2
Severity: Moderate   **Onset: Rapid**   **Likelihood: Suspected**

Cause
Spironolactone may lessen digoxin's ability to strengthen myocardial contraction. It also may decrease renal clearance of digoxin.

Effect
Digoxin level may increase; positive inotropic effect may decrease.

Nursing considerations
- Watch for expected digoxin effects, especially in heart failure.
- Monitor digoxin level. Therapeutic range is 0.8 to 2 ng/ml.
- **⚡ ALERT** Spironolactone may interfere with determination of serum digoxin level, causing a falsely elevated level.
- During spironolactone therapy, digoxin dosage may need adjustment.

digoxin ➤◀ St. John's wort
Lanoxin

Risk rating: 2
Severity: Moderate   **Onset: Delayed**   **Likelihood: Suspected**

Cause
St. John's wort may decrease absorption and availability of digoxin.

Effect
Digoxin level and effects may decrease.

Nursing considerations
- Watch for decreased digoxin level. Therapeutic range is 0.8 to 2 ng/ml.
- Monitor the patient for expected digoxin effects: decreased heart rate; arrhythmia conversion; maintenance of converted rhythm; and improvement of heart failure symptoms.
- Advise the patient to avoid taking St. John's wort with digoxin.
- If a patient stabilized on combined use stops taking St. John's wort, monitor digoxin level and adjust dosage as needed.

digoxin ➤◀ tetracycline
Lanoxin   Sumycin

Risk rating: 1
Severity: Major   **Onset: Delayed**   **Likelihood: Suspected**

Cause
Tetracyclines may alter GI flora and increase digoxin absorption.

Effect
Digoxin level and risk of toxicity may increase.

Nursing considerations
- **⚠ ALERT** Effects of tetracyclines on digoxin may persist for several months after the antibiotic is stopped.
- Monitor digoxin level. Therapeutic range is 0.8 to 2 ng/ml.
- Watch for signs of digoxin toxicity: lethargy; drowsiness; confusion; hallucinations; headaches; syncope; visual disturbances; nausea; anorexia; vomiting; diarrhea; and arrhythmias (bradycardia, AV block, and ventricular ectopy).
- Digoxin dosage may need reduction.
- Capsule form may increase digoxin availability and decrease the risk of interaction.

digoxin ━━━━▶◀━━━━ thyroid hormones
Lanoxin   levothyroxine, liothyronine

Risk rating: 2
Severity: Moderate   Onset: Delayed   Likelihood: Established

Cause
Digoxin level may decrease in hyperthyroidism or when a hypothyroid patient becomes euthyroid.

Effect
Digoxin effects may decrease.

Nursing considerations
■ Monitor digoxin level. Therapeutic range is 0.8 to 2 ng/ml.
■ Watch for expected digoxin effects: decreased heart rate, arrhythmia conversion, maintenance of converted rhythm, and improvement of heart failure symptoms.
■ Monitor thyroid function tests (TSH, 0.2 to 5.4 microunits/ml; T_3, 80 to 200 ng/dl; and T_4, 5.4 to 11.5 mcg/dl).
■ If a hypothyroid patient becomes euthyroid, digoxin dosage may need to be increased.
■ If the patient is euthyroid and taking a thyroid hormone when digoxin starts, no special precautions are needed.

digoxin ━━━━▶◀━━━━ verapamil
Lanoxin   Calan

Risk rating: 1
Severity: Major   Onset: Delayed   Likelihood: Established

Cause
Verapamil decreases digoxin elimination. Verapamil and digoxin have additive effects that decrease AV conduction.

Effect
Digoxin level, effects, and risk of toxicity may increase.

Nursing considerations
■ Monitor digoxin level. Therapeutic range is 0.8 to 2 ng/ml.
■ Watch for signs of digoxin toxicity: arrhythmias (bradycardia, AV block, and ventricular ectopy); lethargy; drowsiness; confusion; hallucinations; headaches; syncope; visual disturbances; nausea; anorexia; vomiting; and diarrhea.
■ Digoxin dosage may need reduction.
■ Urge the patient to report adverse reactions that may suggest toxicity: nausea, vomiting, diarrhea, appetite loss, and visual disturbances.

dihydroergotamine ▇◀ azole antifungals

D.H.E. 45

itraconazole, ketoconazole, voriconazole

Risk rating: 1
Severity: **Major**   Onset: **Delayed**   Likelihood: **Suspected**

Cause
Itraconazole may inhibit CYP3A4 metabolism of ergot derivatives such as dihydroergotamine.

Effect
Risk of ergot toxicity may increase.

Nursing considerations
⚑ ALERT Use of these drugs together is contraindicated.
▪ Signs of ergot toxicity include peripheral vasospasm and ischemia.

dihydroergotamine ▇◀ macrolide antibiotics

D.H.E. 45

clarithromycin, erythromycin, telithromycin

Risk rating: 1
Severity: **Major**   Onset: **Rapid**   Likelihood: **Probable**

Cause
Macrolide antibiotics interfere with hepatic metabolism of ergotamine, although exact mechanism is unknown.

Effect
The patient may develop symptoms of acute ergotism, mainly peripheral ischemia.

Nursing considerations
▪ Watch for evidence of peripheral ischemia: pain in limb muscles while exercising and later at rest; numbness and tingling of fingers and toes; cool, pale, or cyanotic limbs; red or violet blisters on hands or feet; and gangrene.
▪ Dosage of ergot derivative, such as dihydroergotamine, may need to be decreased, or both drugs may need to be stopped.
▪ Consider a different anti-infective drug that's less likely to interact with an ergot derivative.
⚑ ALERT Sodium nitroprusside may be given for macrolide-ergot–induced vasospasm.
▪ Explain evidence of ergot-induced peripheral ischemia. Urge the patient to report it promptly.

dihydroergotamine ⇥⇤ nitrates

D.H.E. 45

isosorbide dinitrate,
nitroglycerin

Risk rating: 2
Severity: Moderate   **Onset: Rapid**   **Likelihood: Suspected**

Cause
Dihydroergotamine metabolism decreases, increasing the drug's
availability and antagonizing nitrate-induced coronary vasodilation.

Effect
Increased dihydroergotamine availability may increase systolic blood
pressure and decrease antianginal effects.

Nursing considerations
- Use these drugs together cautiously in patients with angina.
- Monitor the patient for evidence of ergotism: peripheral ischemia,
paresthesia, headache, nausea, and vomiting.
- Urge the patient to report immediately possible peripheral ischemia: numbness or tingling in fingers and toes, red blisters on
hands or feet. Dihydroergotamine dosage may need to be decreased.

dihydroergotamine ⇥⇤ nonnucleoside reverse-
transcriptase inhibitors

D.H.E. 45

delavirdine, efavirenz

Risk rating: 1
Severity: Major   **Onset: Delayed**   **Likelihood: Suspected**

Cause
Nonnucleoside reverse-transcriptase inhibitors may decrease
CYP3A4 metabolism of ergot derivatives such as dihydroergotamine.

Effect
Risk of ergot-induced peripheral vasospasm and ischemia may increase.

Nursing considerations
- **⚑ ALERT** Use of ergot derivatives with delavirdine or efavirenz is
contraindicated.
- Watch for evidence of peripheral ischemia: pain in limb muscles
while exercising and later at rest; numbness and tingling of fingers
and toes; cool, pale, or cyanotic limbs; red or violet blisters on hands
or feet; and gangrene.
- Ergot toxicity also may cause nausea, vomiting, lassitude, impaired
mental function, delirium, severe dyspnea, hypotension, hyperten-

sion, rapid or weak pulse, unconsciousness, limb spasms, seizures, and shock.

■ Give a vasodilator for vasospasm and diazepam for seizures as needed.

■ Other nonnucleoside reverse-transcriptase inhibitors, such as nevirapine, may interact with ergot derivatives. If you suspect an interaction, consult the prescriber or pharmacist.

dihydroergotamine ►◄ propranolol
D.H.E. 45   Inderal

Risk rating: 2
Severity: Moderate   **Onset: Delayed**   **Likelihood: Suspected**

Cause
Vasoconstriction and blockade of peripheral beta$_2$ receptors allow unopposed ergot action.

Effect
Vasoconstrictive effects of ergot derivatives, such as dihydroergotamine, increase.

Nursing considerations
■ Watch for evidence of peripheral ischemia, cold extremities, and possible gangrene.

■ If needed, stop the beta-adrenergic blocker, and adjust the ergot derivative.

■ Other ergot derivatives may interact with beta-adrenergic blockers. If you suspect an interaction, consult the prescriber or pharmacist.

dihydroergotamine ►◄ protease inhibitors
D.H.E. 45   amprenavir, atazanavir,
                                   darunavir, indinavir, lopinavir-
                                   ritonavir, nelfinavir, ritonavir,
                                   saquinavir

Risk rating: 1
Severity: Major   **Onset: Delayed**   **Likelihood: Probable**

Cause
Protease inhibitors may interfere with CYP3A4 metabolism of ergot derivatives such as dihydroergotamine.

Effect
The risk of ergot-induced peripheral vasospasm and ischemia may increase.

Nursing considerations
◊ ALERT Use of ergot derivatives with protease inhibitors is contra-indicated.
■ Watch for evidence of peripheral ischemia: pain in limb muscles while exercising and later at rest; numbness and tingling of fingers and toes; cool, pale, or cyanotic limbs; red or violet blisters on hands or feet; and gangrene.
◊ ALERT Sodium nitroprusside may be given for ergot-induced va-sospasm.
■ If the patient takes a protease inhibitor, consult the prescriber and pharmacist about alternative treatments for migraine pain.
◊ ALERT Urge the patient to tell the prescriber about increased adverse effects.

---

dihydroergotamine ■◄ selective 5-HT$_1$ receptor agonists

D.H.E. 45

eletriptan, frovatriptan, naratriptan, rizatriptan, sumatriptan, zolmitriptan

Risk rating: 1
Severity: Major   **Onset: Rapid**   **Likelihood: Suspected**

Cause
Combined use may have additive effects.

Effect
The risk of vasospastic effects increases.

Nursing considerations
◊ ALERT Use of these drugs or any two selective 5-HT$_1$ receptor agonists within 24 hours of each other is contraindicated.
■ Combined use may cause severe vasospastic effects, including sustained coronary artery vasospasm that triggers MI.
■ Warn the patient not to mix migraine drugs within 24 hours of each other; advise him to call the prescriber if a drug isn't effective.

---

dihydroergotamine ■◄ sibutramine
D.H.E. 45

Risk rating: 1
Severity: Major   **Onset: Rapid**   **Likelihood: Suspected**

Cause
Drugs may have additive serotonergic effects.

Effect
Risk of serotonin syndrome increases.

Nursing considerations
⚠ **ALERT** If possible, avoid giving an ergot derivative with sibutramine.

■ Watch for evidence of serotonin syndrome, including excitement, hypomania, restlessness, loss of consciousness, confusion, disorientation, anxiety, agitation, motor weakness, myoclonus, tremor, hemiballismus, hyperreflexia, ataxia, dysarthria, incoordination, hyperthermia, shivering, papillary dilation, diaphoresis, emesis, hypertension, and tachycardia. If serotonin syndrome occurs, stop these drugs and provide supportive care as needed.

■ Other ergot derivatives may interact with sibutramine. If you suspect an interaction, consult the prescriber or pharmacist.

■ Advise the patient to tell the prescriber about increased adverse effects.

---

diltiazem ━━━━━▶◀━━━━ **benzodiazepines**
Cardizem   diazepam, midazolam, triazolam

Risk rating: 2
Severity: Moderate   **Onset: Rapid**   **Likelihood: Probable**

Cause
Diltiazem may decrease metabolism of some benzodiazepines.

Effect
Benzodiazepine effects may increase.

Nursing considerations
■ Watch for signs of increased CNS depression: sedation, dizziness, confusion, asthenia, ataxia, altered level of consciousness, hypoactive reflexes, hypotension, bradycardia, and respiratory depression.

■ Lower benzodiazepine dose may be needed.

■ Explain the risk of increased and prolonged CNS effects.

■ Warn the patient to avoid hazardous activities until effects of this combination are clear.

■ Other benzodiazepines may interact with diltiazem. If you suspect an interaction, consult the prescriber or pharmacist.

diltiazem ▶◀ buspirone
Cardizem   BuSpar

Risk rating: 2
Severity: Moderate   Onset: Delayed   Likelihood: Suspected

Cause
CYP3A4 metabolism of buspirone may decrease.

Effect
Buspirone level and adverse effects may increase.

Nursing considerations
- If the patient takes buspirone, watch closely when the calcium channel blocker diltiazem starts or stops or when its dosage changes.
- Watch for signs of buspirone toxicity: increased CNS effects (dizziness, drowsiness, and headache); vomiting; and diarrhea.
- Adjust buspirone dose as needed.
- If the patient takes diltiazem, the prescriber may consider an antianxiety drug not metabolized by CYP3A4 such as lorazepam.
- Dihydropyridine calcium channel blockers that don't inhibit CYP3A4 metabolism, such as amlodipine and felodipine, probably won't disrupt buspirone metabolism.
- Other calcium channel blockers may have this interaction. If you suspect an interaction, consult the prescriber or pharmacist.

diltiazem ▶◀ carbamazepine
Cardizem   Carbatrol, Epitol, Equetro, Tegretol

Risk rating: 2
Severity: Moderate   Onset: Delayed   Likelihood: Suspected

Cause
Diltiazem may inhibit carbamazepine metabolism.

Effect
Carbamazepine level and risk of toxicity may increase.

Nursing considerations
- Monitor carbamazepine level; therapeutic range is 4 to 12 mcg/ml.
- If diltiazem therapy starts, watch for signs of carbamazepine toxicity: dizziness, ataxia, respiratory depression, tachycardia, arrhythmias, blood pressure changes, impaired consciousness, abnormal reflexes, nystagmus, seizures, nausea, vomiting, and urine retention.
- If diltiazem therapy stops, watch for loss of carbamazepine effects (loss of seizure control). Dosage may need to be increased.

■ Calcium channel blockers other than diltiazem may have this interaction. If you suspect an interaction, consult the prescriber or pharmacist.

diltiazem ▶◀ cyclosporine
Cardizem | Gengraf, Neoral, Sandimmune

Risk rating: 2
Severity: Moderate   **Onset: Delayed**   **Likelihood: Established**

Cause
Diltiazem may inhibit cyclosporine metabolism in the liver.

Effect
Cyclosporine level and risk of toxicity may increase.

Nursing considerations
■ When starting or stopping diltiazem, monitor cyclosporine level.
■ Cyclosporine dosage may need to be reduced by 20% to 50%.
■ Watch for arthralgia and encephalopathy.
■ Adverse reactions typically subside when diltiazem stops.
◪ ALERT Rejection episodes may increase when diltiazem is stopped
because cyclosporine level may be reduced.

diltiazem ▶◀ digoxin
Cardizem | Lanoxin

Risk rating: 2
Severity: Moderate   **Onset: Delayed**   **Likelihood: Suspected**

Cause
Diltiazem decreases the clearance of digoxin.

Effect
Digoxin level and risk of toxicity may increase.

Nursing considerations
■ Monitor digoxin level and clinical status. Therapeutic range is 0.8 to
2 ng/ml.
■ Watch for evidence of digoxin toxicity: arrhythmias (bradycardia, AV
block, and ventricular ectopy); lethargy; drowsiness; confusion; hallucinations; headaches; syncope; visual disturbances; nausea; anorexia;
vomiting; and diarrhea.
■ Digoxin dosage may need reduction.

diltiazem ━━━━▶◀ HMG-CoA reductase inhibitors

Cardizem

atorvastatin, lovastatin, simvastatin

Risk rating: 2
Severity: Moderate   Onset: Delayed   Likelihood: Probable

Cause
CYP3A4 metabolism of certain HMG-CoA reductase inhibitors may be inhibited.

Effect
HMG-CoA reductase inhibitor level may increase, raising the risk of toxicity, including myositis and rhabdomyolysis.

Nursing considerations
- If possible, avoid use together.
- Assess the patient for evidence of rhabdomyolysis: fatigue; muscle aches and weakness; joint pain; dark, red, or cola-colored urine; weight gain; seizures; and greatly increased serum CK level.
- ⚠ ALERT If the patient may have rhabdomyolysis, notify the prescriber, and obtain renal function tests and serum potassium, sodium, calcium, lactic acid, and myoglobin levels.
- Pravastatin is less likely to interact with diltiazem than other HMG-CoA reductase inhibitors and may be the best choice for combined use.
- Urge the patient to report unexplained muscle pain, tenderness, or weakness to the prescriber.

diltiazem ━━━━▶◀ methylprednisolone

Cardizem

Medrol

Risk rating: 2
Severity: Moderate   Onset: Delayed   Likelihood: Suspected

Cause
Methylprednisolone CYP3A4 metabolism may be inhibited.

Effect
Methylprednisolone effects and risk of toxicity may increase.

Nursing considerations
- Monitor the patient for appropriate response to methylprednisolone.

■ Watch for signs of methylprednisolone toxicity: nervousness, sleepiness, depression, psychoses, weakness, decreased hearing, lower leg edema, skin disorders, hypertension, muscle weakness, and seizures.
■ Methylprednisolone dosage may need adjustment.
■ Advise the patient to report increased adverse effects.
■ Corticosteroids other than methylprednisolone may interact with diltiazem. If you suspect an interaction, consult the prescriber or pharmacist.

---

diltiazem ◄► moricizine

Cardizem   Ethmozine

Risk rating: 2
Severity: Moderate   Onset: Delayed   Likelihood: Suspected

Cause
Moricizine metabolism may decrease; diltiazem metabolism may increase.

Effect
Moricizine effects (including adverse effects) may increase; diltiazem effects may decrease.

Nursing considerations
■ Watch for expected effects of diltiazem.
■ Urge the patient to report increased angina or symptoms of hypertension, including headache, dizziness, and blurred vision.
■ Watch for increased adverse moricizine effects, particularly headache, dizziness, and paresthesia.
■ Caution the patient to avoid hazardous activities if adverse CNS reactions or blurred vision occurs. These adverse effects may be more common with increased moricizine level.
■ Dosage adjustment may be needed when either drug starts, stops, or changes dosage. Consult the prescriber or pharmacist.

---

diltiazem ◄► nifedipine

Cardizem   Procardia

Risk rating: 3
Severity: Minor   Onset: Rapid   Likelihood: Suspected

Cause
Possible reduction of hepatic clearance.

Effect
Levels, effects, and risk of toxicity of digoxin and nifedipine increase.

Nursing considerations
■ Monitor the patient for increased adverse effects, including hypotension and dizziness.
■ Dosage of nifedipine or diltiazem may need to be decreased.
■ Diltiazem may interact with other calcium channel blockers in the same way.

---

diltiazem ━━━━▶◀━━━━ quinidine
Cardizem

Risk rating: 2
Severity: Moderate   Onset: Delayed   Likelihood: Suspected

Cause
Hepatic metabolism of quinidine may be inhibited.

Effect
Quinidine effects and risk of toxicity may increase.

Nursing considerations
■ Monitor quinidine level. Therapeutic range is 2 to 6 mcg/ml.
■ Watch ECG for widened QRS complexes, prolonged QT and PR intervals, and ventricular arrhythmias, including torsades de pointes.
■ Monitor the patient for signs of quinidine toxicity: hypotension, seizures, ataxia, anuria, respiratory distress, irritability, and hallucinations.
■ Explain that adverse GI effects, especially diarrhea, may signal quinidine toxicity. Tell the patient to alert the prescriber if these effects occur.
■ Adjust quinidine dosage if needed.

---

diltiazem ━━━━▶◀━━━━ sirolimus
Cardizem   Rapamune

Risk rating: 2
Severity: Moderate   Onset: Delayed   Likelihood: Suspected

Cause
First-pass metabolism of sirolimus is inhibited.

Effect
Sirolimus level and side effects may increase.

Nursing considerations
■ Monitor sirolimus levels when starting, stopping, or changing diltiazem therapy.

- Adjust the dose of sirolimus as needed.
- The effects of diltiazem are not affected in this interaction.

---

diltiazem ━━━━▶◀ tacrolimus
Cardizem   Prograf

Risk rating: 2
Severity: Moderate   Onset: Delayed   Likelihood: Suspected

Cause
Hepatic metabolism of tacrolimus by CYP3A4 may be inhibited.

Effect
Tacrolimus level and risk of toxicity may increase.

Nursing considerations
- Diltiazem may have similar effects on cyclosporine and sirolimus.
- Monitor tacrolimus level. Therapeutic range for liver transplants is 5 to 20 ng/ml and for kidney transplants is 7 to 20 ng/ml for the first 3 months, 5 to 15 ng/ml through 1 year.
- Monitor the patient for tacrolimus toxicity: delirium, confusion, agitation, tremor, adverse GI effects, and abnormal renal function tests.
- Tacrolimus dosage may need adjustment when diltiazem starts, stops, or changes dosage.

---

diltiazem ━━━━▶◀ theophyllines
Cardizem   aminophylline, theophylline

Risk rating: 2
Severity: Moderate   Onset: Delayed   Likelihood: Suspected

Cause
Theophylline metabolism may be inhibited.

Effect
Theophylline level and risk of toxicity may increase.

Nursing considerations
- Watch for evidence of toxicity, such as tachycardia, anorexia, nausea, vomiting, diarrhea, seizures, restlessness, irritability, and headache.
- Monitor serum theophylline level closely. Normal therapeutic range is 10 to 20 mcg/ml for adults and 5 to 15 mcg/ml for children.
- Describe adverse effects of theophylline and signs of toxicity, and tell the patient to report them to the prescriber immediately.

disopyramide ▸◂ macrolide antibiotics

Norpace

azithromycin, clarithromycin, erythromycin, telithromycin

Risk rating: 1
Severity: Major   **Onset: Delayed**   **Likelihood: Suspected**

Cause
An additive increase in the QT interval is seen when administering macrolide antibiotics and antiarrhythmic agents such as disopyramide.

Effect
The risk of life-threatening cardiac arrhythmias, including torsades de pointes, is increased.

Nursing considerations
◣ **ALERT** Monitor the patient for prolonged QT interval and torsades de pointes.
■ This interaction appears to be dose related.
■ Instruct the patient to let the prescriber know if he experiences dizziness, palpitations, or light-headedness.
■ The QT interval returns to normal within 3 days of stopping the medications.

disopyramide ▸◂ phenytoin

Norpace

Dilantin

Risk rating: 2
Severity: Moderate   **Onset: Delayed**   **Likelihood: Suspected**

Cause
Hepatic metabolism of disopyramide is increased.

Effect
Disopyramide levels and effects may be decreased. Anticholinergic actions may be increased.

Nursing considerations
■ Monitor the clinical response to disopyramide. The dose may need to be increased.
■ This interaction may continue for several days after discontinuing phenytoin.
■ Monitor the patient for increase or return of arrhythmias.
■ If increased anticholinergic effects are seen, consider using another antiarrhythmic agent besides disopyramide.

disopyramide ━━▶◀━━ quinolones

Norpace

gatifloxacin, levofloxacin,
moxifloxacin, ofloxacin

Risk rating: 1
Severity: Major   **Onset: Delayed**   **Likelihood: Suspected**

Cause
The mechanism of this interaction is unknown.

Effect
Risk of life-threatening arrhythmias, including torsades de pointes,
increases.

Nursing considerations
■ Use of sparfloxacin with an antiarrhythmic such as disopyramide is
contraindicated.
■ Avoid giving a class IA or class III antiarrhythmic with gatifloxacin,
levofloxacin, or moxifloxacin.
■ Quinolones that aren't metabolized by CYP3A4 isoenzymes or that
don't prolong the QT interval may be given with antiarrhythmics.
■ Monitor ECG for prolonged QTc interval.
■ Tell the patient to report a rapid heartbeat, shortness of breath,
dizziness, fainting, and chest pain.

disopyramide ━━▶◀━━ rifampin

Norpace

Rimactane, Rifadin

Risk rating: 2
Severity: Moderate   **Onset: Delayed**   **Likelihood: Suspected**

Cause
Hepatic metabolism of disopyramide is increased.

Effect
Disopyramide levels are decreased. Levels of an active metabolite
may be increased, so it isn't known if decreased effects occur.

Nursing considerations
■ Monitor the patient's ECG while taking rifampin.
■ An increase in disopyramide dose may be necessary.

disopyramide ━━▶◀━━ thioridazine
Norpace

Risk rating: 1
Severity: Major   **Onset: Delayed**   **Likelihood: Suspected**

Cause
Synergistic or additive prolongation of the QTc interval.

Effect
Risk of life-threatening arrhythmias, including torsades de pointes, increases.

Nursing considerations
- The use of thioridazine and antiarrhythmic agents together is contraindicated.
- If the patient is receiving thioridazine and disopyramide, notify the prescriber immediately.
- Monitor the patient for other risk factors for torsades de pointes, including bradycardia, hypokalemia, and hypomagnesemia.
- Ask the patient if he or anyone in his family has a history of prolonged QT interval or arrhythmias.
- Monitor the patient for bradycardia.

disopyramide ━━▶◀━━ vardenafil
Norpace   Levitra

Risk rating: 1
Severity: Major   **Onset: Rapid**   **Likelihood: Suspected**

Cause
The mechanism of this interaction is unknown.

Effect
QTc interval may be prolonged, particularly in patients with previous QT-interval prolongation and those taking certain antiarrhythmics such as disopyramide. This increases the risk of such life-threatening arrhythmias as torsades de pointes.

Nursing considerations
- Use of vardenafil with a class IA or class III antiarrhythmic is contraindicated.
- Monitor ECG before and periodically after the patient starts vardenafil.
- Urge the patient to report light-headedness, faintness, palpitations, and chest pain or pressure while taking vardenafil.

2577

- To reduce risk of adverse effects, patients age 65 and older should start with 5 mg vardenafil, half the usual starting dose.

disopyramide ◄━━► ziprasidone
Norpace   Geodon

Risk rating: 1
Severity: Major   **Onset: Delayed**   **Likelihood: Suspected**

Cause
The mechanism of this interaction is unknown.

Effect
Risk of life-threatening arrhythmias, including torsades de pointes, increases.

Nursing considerations
◤ **ALERT** Use of ziprasidone with certain antiarrhythmics is contraindicated.
- Monitor the patient for other risk factors for torsades de pointes, including bradycardia, hypokalemia, and hypomagnesemia.
- Ask the patient if he or anyone in his family has a history of prolonged QT interval or arrhythmias.
- Monitor the patient for bradycardia.
- Measure the QTc interval at baselines and throughout therapy.

disulfiram ◄━━► alcohol
Antabuse

Risk rating: 1
Severity: Major   **Onset: Rapid**   **Likelihood: Established**

Cause
Disulfiram inhibits alcohol metabolism, which causes acetaldehyde—a toxic metabolite—to accumulate.

Effect
A disulfiram reaction occurs.

Nursing considerations
◤ **ALERT** Patients taking disulfiram shouldn't be exposed to, or consume, any products containing alcohol, including back rub preparations, cough syrups, liniments, and shaving lotion.
◤ **ALERT** Disulfiram should be taken only if the patient has abstained from alcohol for at least 12 hours. Make sure the patient understands the consequences of disulfiram use and consents to its use.

- Disulfiram reaction may cause flushing, throbbing headache, dyspnea, nausea, copious vomiting, diaphoresis, thirst, chest pain, palpitations, hyperventilation, hypotension, syncope, anxiety, weakness, blurred vision, confusion, and arthropathy. More severe reactions may include respiratory depression, cardiovascular collapse, arrhythmias, MI, acute heart failure, seizures, unconsciousness, or death.
- Mild reactions may occur in sensitive patients at a blood alcohol level of 5 to 10 mg/dl; symptoms are fully developed at 50 mg/dl; unconsciousness typically occurs at 125 to 150 mg/dl level. Reaction may last 30 minutes to several hours or as long as alcohol stays in the blood.
- Caution the patient's family not to give disulfiram to him without his knowledge; severe reaction or death could result if the patient drinks alcohol.

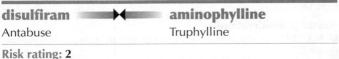

disulfiram ▸◂ aminophylline
Antabuse   Truphylline

Risk rating: 2
Severity: Moderate   Onset: Delayed   Likelihood: Suspected

Cause
Disulfiram inhibits aminophylline metabolism.

Effect
Aminophylline effects, including toxic effects, increase.

Nursing considerations
- Watch for evidence of toxicity, such as tachycardia, anorexia, nausea, vomiting, diarrhea, seizures, restlessness, irritability, and headache.
- Monitor serum aminophylline level closely. Normal therapeutic range is 10 to 20 mcg/ml for adults and 5 to 15 mcg/ml for children.
- Because disulfiram exerts dose-dependent inhibition of aminophylline, aminophylline dosage may need adjustment.
- Describe adverse effects of aminophylline and signs of toxicity, and tell the patient to report them immediately to the prescriber.

disulfiram ▸◂ chlorzoxazone
Antabuse   Parafon Forte DSC

Risk rating: 2
Severity: Moderate   Onset: Delayed   Likelihood: Probable

Cause
Disulfiram inhibits the hepatic metabolism of chlorzoxazone.

Effect
The CNS depressant effects of chlorzoxazone may increase.

Nursing considerations
- Watch for increased adverse CNS effects including dizziness, drowsiness, headache, and light-headedness.
- Signs of more severe toxicity include nausea, vomiting, diarrhea, loss of muscle tone, decreased or absent deep tendon reflexes, respiratory depression, and hypotension.
- Advise the patient to avoid hazardous activities until CNS depressant effects are known.
- Chlorzoxazone dose may need to be reduced.
- Urge the patient to tell the prescriber about increased adverse effects.

---

disulfiram ◄► metronidazole
Antabuse   Flagyl

Risk rating: 2
Severity: Moderate   **Onset: Delayed**   **Likelihood: Suspected**

Cause
Interaction may stem from excess dopaminergic activity.

Effect
Risk of acute psychosis or confusion increases.

Nursing considerations
- **ALERT** Avoid use together.
- Disulfiram given alone may cause acute encephalopathy, paranoid ideas, disorientation, impaired memory, ataxia, and confusion.
- Monitor the patient for acute psychosis and confusion.
- If adverse effects occur, consult the prescriber; one or both drugs may need to be stopped.
- Urge the patient to tell the prescriber about increased adverse effects.

---

disulfiram ◄► phenytoin
Antabuse   Dilantin

Risk rating: 2
Severity: Moderate   **Onset: Rapid**   **Likelihood: Established**

Cause
Disulfiram inhibits hepatic metabolism of phenytoin and may interfere with elimination.

Effect
Phenytoin level, effects, and risk of toxicity may increase.

Nursing considerations
■ Monitor phenytoin level; therapeutic range is 10 to 20 mcg/ml.
■ Watch for evidence of phenytoin toxicity: drowsiness, nausea, vomiting, nystagmus, ataxia, dysarthria, tremor, slurred speech, hypotension, arrhythmias, respiratory depression, and coma.
■ If disulfiram is stopped, assess the patient for loss of phenytoin effects (loss of seizure control).
■ Adjust phenytoin dose as ordered.
■ Hydantoins other than phenytoin may interact with disulfiram. If you suspect an interaction, consult the prescriber or pharmacist.

---

disulfiram ━━━▶◀━━━ **warfarin**
Antabuse   Coumadin

Risk rating: 2
Severity: Moderate   **Onset: Delayed**   **Likelihood: Probable**

Cause
The mechanism of this interaction is unknown.

Effect
Anticoagulant effects may increase.

Nursing considerations
■ Monitor coagulation values.
■ Disulfiram's effects on warfarin may be dose-dependent. If disulfiram dose decreases, warfarin dose may need to be increased.
■ Monitor the patient for signs of bleeding.
■ Tell the patient to report unusual bruising or bleeding.
■ Remind the patient that warfarin interacts with many drugs and that he should report any change in drug regimen.

---

divalproex sodium ■▶◀■ **tricyclic antidepressants**
Depakote   amitriptyline, clomipramine

Risk rating: 2
Severity: Moderate   **Onset: Delayed**   **Likelihood: Suspected**

Cause
Valproic acid, such as divalproex sodium, may inhibit hepatic metabolism of tricyclic antidepressants (TCAs).

Effect
Levels and adverse effects of TCAs may increase.

Nursing considerations
- Use these drugs together cautiously.
- If the patient is stable on valproic acid, start TCA at reduced dosage, and adjust upward slowly to address symptoms and serum level.
- If the patient is stable on a TCA, monitor serum level and patient status closely when starting or stopping valproic acid.
- Explain to the patient the signs and symptoms to watch for.
- Other TCAs may interact with valproic acid. If you suspect an interaction, consult the prescriber or pharmacist.

---

docetaxel ◀▶ ketoconazole
Taxotere   Nizoral

Risk rating: 1
Severity: Major   **Onset: Delayed**   **Likelihood: Suspected**

Cause
Ketoconazole inhibits CYP3A4 metabolism of docetaxel.

Effect
Docetaxel level, effects, and risk of toxicity may increase.

Nursing considerations
- Avoid using these drugs together if possible.
- If the patient must take both, the dose of docetaxel may need to be decreased.
- Monitor the patient's white blood cell count.
- Notify the prescriber immediately if the patient has a fever, sore throat, red or inflamed areas, or other signs of infection.

---

dofetilide ◀▶ azole antifungals
Tikosyn   itraconazole, ketoconazole

Risk rating: 1
Severity: Major   **Onset: Delayed**   **Likelihood: Suspected**

Cause
Dofetilide renal elimination may be inhibited.

Effect
Dofetilide level and risk of ventricular arrhythmias, including torsades de pointes, may increase.

Nursing considerations
▶ **ALERT** Use of dofetilide with itraconazole or ketoconazole is contraindicated.
■ Monitor ECG for excessive prolongation of QTc interval or development of ventricular arrhythmias.
■ Consult the prescriber about alternative anti-infective therapy.
■ Urge the patient to tell the prescriber about increased adverse effects.
■ Other azole antifungals may interact with dofetilide. If you suspect an interaction, consult the prescriber or pharmacist.

---

dofetilide ▶◀ cimetidine
Tikosyn   Tagamet

Risk rating: 1
Severity: Major   **Onset: Delayed**   **Likelihood: Suspected**

Cause
Dofetilide renal elimination may be inhibited.

Effect
Dofetilide level and risk of ventricular arrhythmias, including torsades de pointes, may increase.

Nursing considerations
▶ **ALERT** Use of dofetilide with cimetidine is contraindicated.
■ Monitor ECG for excessive prolongation of QTc interval and development of ventricular arrhythmias.
■ Omeprazole, ranitidine, and aluminum and magnesium antacids don't affect dofetilide elimination. Ask the prescriber or pharmacist about them as alternatives to cimetidine.
■ During dofetilide therapy, monitor renal function and QTc interval every 3 months.

---

dofetilide ▶◀ hydrochlorothiazide
Tikosyn   Microzide

Risk rating: 1
Severity: Major   **Onset: Delayed**   **Likelihood: Suspected**

Cause
Use of a thiazide diuretic increases potassium excretion.

Effect
Hypokalemia increases the risk of ventricular arrhythmias, including torsades de pointes.

Nursing considerations
⚠ **ALERT** Use of dofetilide with a thiazide diuretic is contraindicated.
■ Monitor ECG for excessive prolongation of the QTc interval and development of ventricular arrhythmias.
■ A similar interaction is likely with loop diuretics.
■ Dofetilide clearance is decreased when used with a thiazide diuretic.

---

dofetilide ━━━━━▶◀━━━━━ macrolide antibiotics
Tikosyn

azithromycin, clarithromycin, erythromycin, telithromycin

Risk rating: 1
Severity: Major   **Onset: Delayed**   **Likelihood: Suspected**

Cause
An additive increase in the QT interval is seen when administering macrolide antibiotics and antiarrhythmic agents.

Effect
The risk of life-threatening cardiac arrhythmias, including torsades de pointes, is increased.

Nursing considerations
⚠ **ALERT** Monitor patient for prolonged QT interval and torsades de pointes.
■ This interaction appears to be dose-related.
■ Instruct the patient to let the prescriber know if he experiences dizziness, palpitations, or light-headedness.
■ The QT interval returns to normal within 3 days of stopping the medications.

---

dofetilide ━━━━━▶◀━━━━━ megestrol
Tikosyn

Megace

Risk rating: 1
Severity: Major   **Onset: Delayed**   **Likelihood: Suspected**

Cause
Dofetilide renal elimination may be inhibited.

Effect
Dofetilide level and the risk of ventricular arrhythmias, including torsades de pointes, increase.

Nursing considerations
⚠ **ALERT** Use of dofetilide with megestrol is contraindicated.

- Monitor ECG for excessive prolongation of QTc interval and development of ventricular arrhythmias.
- During dofetilide therapy, monitor renal function and QTc interval every 3 months.
- Watch for prolonged diarrhea, sweating, and vomiting, and alert the prescriber. Electrolyte imbalance may increase risk of arrhythmias.
- Urge the patient to tell the prescriber about increased adverse effects.

---

dofetilide ▶◀ **prochlorperazine**

Tikosyn   Compazine

Risk rating: 1
Severity: Major   **Onset: Rapid**   **Likelihood: Suspected**

Cause
Dofetilide renal elimination may be inhibited.

Effect
Dofetilide level and risk of ventricular arrhythmias, including torsades de pointes, increase.

Nursing considerations
◼ ALERT Use of dofetilide with prochlorperazine is contraindicated.
- Monitor ECG for excessive prolongation of QTc interval and development of ventricular arrhythmias.
- During dofetilide therapy, monitor renal function and QTc interval every 3 months.
- Consult the prescriber or pharmacist for alternative to prochlorperazine to control nausea and vomiting or symptoms of psychosis.

---

dofetilide ▶◀ **trimethoprim, trimethoprim-sulfamethoxazole**

Tikosyn   Proloprim, Septra

Risk rating: 1
Severity: Major   **Onset: Delayed**   **Likelihood: Suspected**

Cause
Dofetilide renal elimination may be inhibited.

Effect
Dofetilide level and risk of ventricular arrhythmias, including torsades de pointes, increase.

Nursing considerations
⚠ **ALERT** Use of dofetilide with trimethoprim or trimethoprim-sulfamethoxazole is contraindicated.
- Monitor ECG for excessive prolongation of QTc interval and development of ventricular arrhythmias.
- During dofetilide therapy, monitor renal function and QTc interval every 3 months.
- Watch for prolonged diarrhea, sweating, and vomiting, and alert the prescriber. Electrolyte imbalance may increase risk of arrhythmias.
- Consult the prescriber or pharmacist about substituting an alternative anti-infective.

---

dofetilide ━━━━◄► verapamil
Tikosyn   Calan

Risk rating: 1
Severity: Major   **Onset: Delayed**   **Likelihood: Suspected**

Cause
Verapamil may increase dofetilide absorption.

Effect
Dofetilide level and risk of ventricular arrhythmias, including torsades de pointes, increase.

Nursing considerations
⚠ **ALERT** Use of dofetilide with verapamil is contraindicated.
- Monitor ECG for excessive prolongation of QTc interval and development of ventricular arrhythmias.
- During dofetilide therapy, monitor renal function and QTc interval every 3 months.

---

dofetilide ━━━━◄► ziprasidone
Tikosyn   Geodon

Risk rating: 1
Severity: Major   **Onset: Delayed**   **Likelihood: Suspected**

Cause
Each of these drugs may lengthen the QTc interval; joint use may have additive effects.

Effect
Risk of ventricular arrhythmias, including torsades de pointes, increases.

Nursing considerations
⚠ ALERT Use of dofetilide with ziprasidone is contraindicated.
■ Monitor ECG for excessive prolongation of QTc interval and development of ventricular arrhythmias.
■ During dofetilide therapy, monitor renal function and QTc interval every 3 months.
■ If the patient takes dofetilide, consult the prescriber or pharmacist about antipsychotics other than ziprasidone.
■ Urge the patient to tell the prescriber about increased adverse effects.

---

dolasetron ▸◂ ziprasidone
Anzemet   Geodon

Risk rating: 1
Severity: Major   **Onset: Delayed**   **Likelihood: Suspected**

Cause
Possible additive prolongation of the QTc interval.

Effect
Risk of life-threatening arrhythmias, including torsades de pointes, increases.

Nursing considerations
⚠ ALERT Use of dolasetron with ziprasidone is contraindicated.
■ Ask the patient if he or anyone in his family has a history of prolonged QT intervals or arrhythmias.
■ Monitor the patient for other risk factors for torsades de pointes, including bradycardia, hypokalemia, and hypomagnesemia.
■ Measure the QTc interval at baseline and throughout therapy.
■ Monitor the patient for bradycardia.

---

dopamine ▸◂ MAO inhibitors
phenelzine, tranylcypromine

Risk rating: 1
Severity: Major   **Onset: Rapid**   **Likelihood: Established**

Cause
Norepinephrine accumulates with MAO inhibition and is released by indirect and mixed-acting sympathomimetics such as dopamine.

Effect
The pressor response at receptor sites increases, increasing the risk of severe headache, hypertension, high fever, and hypertensive crisis.

Nursing considerations
- Avoid giving dopamine with an MAO inhibitor.
- Direct-acting sympathomimetics interact minimally.
- **ALERT** Warn the patient that OTC medicines, such as decongestants, may cause this interaction.
- Phentolamine can be administered to block epinephrine- and norepinephrine-induced vasoconstriction and reduce blood pressure.

dopamine ━━━━▶◀━━━━ phenytoin
Dilantin

Risk rating: 1
Severity: Major   **Onset: Rapid**   **Likelihood: Suspected**

Cause
Hypotension may result from phenytoin-induced myocardial depression and dopamine-related depletion of catecholamines.

Effect
Profound, life-threatening hypotension may occur.

Nursing considerations
- Use together with extreme caution and frequent blood pressure monitoring.
- **ALERT** Life-threatening hypotension can occur in a few minutes of co-administration. Cardiac arrest and death may occur.
- Stop phenytoin infusion at the first sign of hypotension.
- It isn't known if phenytoin reacts similarly to sympathomimetics other than dopamine. Approach this combination with the same level of caution.

doxazosin ━━━━▶◀━━━━ tadalafil
Cardura   Cialis

Risk rating: 1
Severity: Major   **Onset: Rapid**   **Likelihood: Suspected**

Cause
The cause of the interaction is unknown.

Effect
The hypotensive effects of alpha$_1$-adrenergic blockers may be increased.

Nursing considerations

⚠ ALERT Administering tadalafil and an alpha$_1$-adrenergic blocker together is contraindicated.

■ If the patient has taken tadalafil and an alpha$_1$-adrenergic blocker, carefully monitor his blood pressure and cardiac output.

■ Alert the prescriber that the patient is taking tadalafil and an alpha$_1$-adrenergic blocker together and their use is contraindicated.

■ Make sure the patient has readily available I.V. access so fluids can be administered, if needed, for hypotension.

---

doxazosin ▬▬▬►◄ vardenafil
Cardura   Levitra

Risk rating: 2
Severity: Moderate   **Onset: Rapid**   **Likelihood: Suspected**

Cause
Vardenafil causes an additive pharmacological action.

Effect
The risk of hypotension may be increased.

Nursing considerations

⚠ ALERT Administering vardenafil and an alpha$_1$-adrenergic blocker together is contraindicated.

■ If the patient has taken vardenafil and an alpha$_1$-adrenergic blocker, carefully monitor his blood pressure and cardiac output.

■ Alert the prescriber that the patient is taking vardenafil and an alpha$_1$-adrenergic blocker together and their use is contraindicated.

■ Make sure the patient has readily available I.V. access so fluids can be administered, if needed for hypotension.

---

doxepin ▬▬▬►◄ carbamazepine
Sinequan   Carbatrol, Epitol, Equetro, Tegretol

Risk rating: 2
Severity: Moderate   **Onset: Delayed**   **Likelihood: Probable**

Cause
Tricyclic antidepressants (TCAs), such as doxepin, may compete with carbamazepine for hepatic metabolism. Carbamazepine may induce hepatic TCA metabolism.

Effect
Carbamazepine level and risk of toxicity may increase. TCA level and effects may decrease.

Nursing considerations
- Other TCAs may interact with carbamazepine. If you suspect a drug interaction, consult the prescriber or pharmacist.
- Monitor carbamazepine level; therapeutic range is 4 to 12 mcg/ml.
- Watch for evidence of carbamazepine toxicity, including dizziness, ataxia, respiratory depression, tachycardia, arrhythmias, blood pressure changes, impaired consciousness, abnormal reflexes, nystagmus, seizures, nausea, vomiting, and urine retention.

doxepin ▶◀ cimetidine
Sinequan   Tagamet

Risk rating: 2
Severity: Moderate   **Onset: Rapid**   **Likelihood: Probable**

Cause
Cimetidine may interfere with metabolism of tricyclic antidepressants (TCAs) such as doxepin.

Effect
TCA level and bioavailability increase.

Nursing considerations
- When starting or stopping cimetidine, monitor TCA level and adjust dosage as needed.
- If needed, consult the prescriber about possible change from cimetidine to ranitidine.
- Urge the patient and family to watch for, and report, any increased anticholinergic effects, dizziness, drowsiness, and psychosis.

doxepin ▶◀ fluoxetine
Sinequan   Prozac, Sarafem

Risk rating: 2
Severity: Moderate   **Onset: Delayed**   **Likelihood: Probable**

Cause
Fluoxetine may inhibit hepatic metabolism of tricyclic antidepressants (TCAs) such as doxepin.

Effect
Serum TCA level and toxicity may increase.

Nursing considerations
■ Monitor serum TCA level and watch closely for evidence of toxicity, such as increased anticholinergic effects, delirium, dizziness, drowsiness, and psychosis.
■ Report evidence of increased TCA level or toxicity; dosage may need to be decreased.
■ If the patient already takes fluoxetine, and starts on doxepin, the dose may need to be decreased by up to 75% to avoid this interaction.
■ Other TCAs may interact with fluoxetine. If you suspect an interaction, consult the prescriber or pharmacist.

doxycycline ▶◀ amoxicillin
Vibramycin   Amoxil

Risk rating: 1
Severity: Major   **Onset: Delayed**   **Likelihood: Suspected**

Cause
Tetracyclines such as doxycycline may disrupt bactericidal activity of penicillins such as amoxicillin.

Effect
Penicillin efficacy may be reduced.

Nursing considerations
■ If possible, avoid giving tetracyclines with penicillins.
■ Monitor the patient closely for lack of penicillin effect.

doxycycline ▶◀ carbamazepine
Vibramycin   Carbatrol, Epitol, Equetro,
                                    Tegretol

Risk rating: 2
Severity: Moderate   **Onset: Delayed**   **Likelihood: Probable**

Cause
Carbamazepine may increase hepatic metabolism of doxycycline.

Effect
Doxycycline level and therapeutic effects may decrease.

Nursing considerations
■ Dose of doxycycline may need to be increased during carbamazepine administration.

- Monitor patient for resolving infection. If the infection doesn't resolve, discuss the interaction with the prescriber.
- If possible, consider the use of another tetracycline; the interaction isn't seen in other tetracyclines.

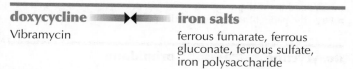

doxycycline   ▶◀   iron salts
Vibramycin

ferrous fumarate, ferrous gluconate, ferrous sulfate, iron polysaccharide

Risk rating: 2
Severity: Moderate   Onset: Delayed   Likelihood: Probable

Cause
Doxycycline and other tetracyclines form insoluble chelates with iron salts, which may reduce absorption of both substances.

Effect
Tetracycline and iron salt levels and effects may decrease.

Nursing considerations
◧ ALERT Avoid giving tetracyclines with iron salts if possible.
- If they must be given together, separate doses by 3 to 4 hours.
- If you suspect an interaction, consult the prescriber or pharmacist; an enteric-coated or sustained-release iron salt may reduce this interaction.
- Monitor the patient for expected response to tetracycline.
- Assess for evidence of iron deficiency, including fatigue, dyspnea, tachycardia, palpitations, dizziness, and orthostatic hypotension.

doxycycline   ▶◀   phenytoin
Vibramycin

Dilantin

Risk rating: 2
Severity: Moderate   Onset: Delayed   Likelihood: Probable

Cause
Phenytoin induces doxycycline metabolism, and doxycycline may be displaced from plasma proteins.

Effect
Doxycycline elimination may increase and effects may decrease.

Nursing considerations
- Hydantoins other than phenytoin may interact with doxycycline. If you suspect an interaction, consult the prescriber or pharmacist.

- If the patient takes phenytoin, watch for expected doxycycline effects.
- Doxycycline dose may need to be doubled to maintain therapeutic level; consult the prescriber for dosage increase.
- Consult the prescriber or pharmacist about using a tetracycline that doesn't interact with phenytoin.
- Urge the patient to tell the prescriber if he isn't improving.

---

doxycycline ▶◀ primidone
Vibramycin   Mysoline

Risk rating: 2
Severity: Moderate   Onset: Delayed   Likelihood: Suspected

Cause
Barbiturates such as primidone may increase hepatic metabolism of doxycycline, a tetracycline.

Effect
Doxycycline level and effects may decrease.

Nursing considerations
- Monitor the patient for expected doxycycline effects.
- Doxycycline dose may need to be increased.
- Effects of barbiturates on doxycycline may persists for weeks after the barbiturate is stopped.
- Consult the prescriber or pharmacist about using a tetracycline that doesn't interact with barbiturates, such as demeclocycline or tetracycline.
- Urge the patient to tell the prescriber if he isn't improving with doxycycline.

---

doxycycline ▶◀ rifampin
Vibramycin   Rifadin, Rimactane

Risk rating: 2
Severity: Moderate   Onset: Delayed   Likelihood: Suspected

Cause
Rifampin may increase hepatic metabolism of doxycycline.

Effect
Doxycycline level and effects may decrease.

Nursing considerations
- Monitor the patient for expected doxycycline effects.
- Doxycycline dose may need to be increased.
- Consult the prescriber or pharmacist about using a tetracycline such as streptomycin that doesn't interact with rifampin.
- Urge the patient to tell the prescriber if he isn't improving with doxycycline.

---

droperidol ◣◢ ziprasidone
Vibramycin   Geodon

Risk rating: 1
Severity: Major   **Onset: Delayed**   **Likelihood: Suspected**

Cause
Possible additive prolongation of the QT interval.

Effect
The risk of life-threatening arrhythmias, including torsades de pointes, increases.

Nursing considerations
◤ **ALERT** Use of ziprasidone with droperidol is contraindicated.
- Ask the patient if he or anyone in his family has a history of prolonged QT interval or arrhythmias.
- Monitor the patient for other risk factors for torsades de pointes, including bradycardia, hypokalemia, and hypomagnesemia.
- Monitor the patient for bradycardia.
- Measure the QTc interval at baseline and throughout therapy.

---

duloxetine ◣◢ MAO inhibitors
Cymbalta   isocarboxazid, phenelzine, selegine, tranylcypromine

Risk rating: 1
Severity: Major   **Onset: Rapid**   **Likelihood: Probable**

Cause
Serotonin may accumulate rapidly in the CNS.

Effect
The risk of serotonin syndrome increases.

Nursing considerations
◤ **ALERT** Don't use these drugs together.

- Allow 2 weeks after stopping duloxetine before giving an MAO inhibitor.
- Allow 2 weeks after stopping an MAO inhibitor before giving an SSRI such as duloxetine.
- Describe the traits of serotonin syndrome, including confusion, restlessness, incoordination, muscle tremors and rigidity, fever, and sweating.
- Explain that serotonin-induced symptoms can be fatal if not treated immediately.

duloxetine ▶◀ thioridazine
Cymbalta

Risk rating: 1
Severity: Major   **Onset: Delayed**   **Likelihood: Suspected**

Cause
Inhibition of thioridazine metabolism.

Effect
Thioridazine levels and risk of life-threatening arrhythmias and sudden death increases.

Nursing considerations
⚠ **ALERT** Don't use these drugs together.
- Thioridazine has the risk of increasing the QT interval, causing serious ventricular arrhythmias and sudden death.
- Because of the seriousness of the interaction, this interaction is based on pharmacodynamics, not actual patient studies.

edrophonium ▶◀ succinylcholine
Tensilon   Anectine, Quelicin

Risk rating: 2
Severity: Moderate   **Onset: Rapid**   **Likelihood: Probable**

Cause
Anticholinesterases, such as edrophonium, inhibit plasma cholinesterase, which delays the breakdown of succinylcholine. Also, increased levels of acetylcholine may increase the neuromuscular blockade.

Effect
The combination prolongs the neuromuscular blockade.

Nursing considerations
- Use this combination with caution.
- This interaction is more likely in patients receiving succinylcholine by continuous infusion.

⚠ ALERT Provide respiratory support and mechanical ventilation if needed.

---

efavirenz ▶◀ benzodiazepines
Sustiva

alprazolam, midazolam, triazolam

Risk rating: 2
Severity: Moderate　　　**Onset: Rapid**　　　**Likelihood: Suspected**

Cause
Nonnucleoside reverse-transcriptase inhibitors, such as efavirenz, may inhibit CYP3A4 metabolism of certain benzodiazepines.

Effect
Sedative effects of benzodiazepines may be increased or prolonged.

Nursing considerations
⚠ ALERT Don't combine benzodiazepines with efavirenz.
- Explain the risk of oversedation and respiratory depression.
- Urge the patient to report any suspected interaction promptly.
- Other benzodiazepines and nonnucleoside reverse-transcriptase inhibitors may interact. If you suspect an interaction, consult the prescriber or pharmacist.

---

efavirenz ▶◀ ergot derivatives
Sustiva

dihydroergotamine, ergotamine

Risk rating: 1
Severity: Major　　　**Onset: Delayed**　　　**Likelihood: Suspected**

Cause
Nonnucleoside reverse-transcriptase inhibitors, such as efavirenz, may decrease CYP3A4 metabolism of ergot derivatives.

Effect
The risk of ergot-induced peripheral vasospasm and ischemia increases.

Nursing considerations
⚠ ALERT Use of ergot derivatives with efavirenz is contraindicated.

- Monitor the patient for peripheral ischemia: pain in limb muscles while exercising and later at rest; numbness and tingling of fingers and toes; cool, pale, or cyanotic limbs; red or violet blisters on hands or feet; and gangrene.
- Ergot toxicity also may cause nausea, vomiting, lassitude, impaired mental function, delirium, severe dyspnea, hypotension, hypertension, rapid or weak pulse, unconsciousness, limb spasms, seizures, and shock.
- Give a vasodilator for vasospasm and diazepam for seizures as needed.
- Other nonnucleoside reverse-transcriptase inhibitors, such as nevirapine, may interact with ergot derivatives. If you suspect an interaction, consult the prescriber or pharmacist.

---

efavirenz ◀▶ methadone

Sustiva   Methadose

Risk rating: 2
Severity: Moderate   Onset: Delayed   Likelihood: Probable

Cause
Increased CYP3A4 hepatic metabolism of methadone.

Effect
Action of methadone may be reduced, resulting in opiate withdrawal symptoms.

Nursing considerations
- When starting a patient on an nonnucleoside reverse-transcriptase inhibitor, such as efavirenz, carefully monitor the patient's clinical response to methadone.
- Be prepared to increase methadone dose.
- Monitor the patient for methadone overdose when efavirenz therapy is stopped.
- Monitor the patient for dilated pupils, diarrhea, abdominal pain, sweating, agitation, nausea, and vomiting.
- Instruct the patient not to change the dose of his medications before consulting with the prescriber or pharmacist.

efavirenz ■■■■■►◄ protease inhibitors
Sustiva

atazanavir, fosamprenavir,
indinavir, lopinavir/ritonavir,
nelfinavir, ritonavir

Risk rating: 2
Severity: Moderate   **Onset: Delayed**   **Likelihood: Suspected**

Cause
This combination increases CYP3A4 metabolism of protease inhibitors.

Effect
Protease inhibitor plasma levels and efficacy may be reduced.

Nursing considerations
■ Monitor the patient's protease inhibitor levels and clinical response
when starting or stopping an nonnucleoside reverse-transcriptase inhibitor such as efavirenz.
■ Adjust protease inhibitor dosage as needed.
■ Tell the patient not to alter his HIV regimen without consulting his
prescriber.

efavirenz ■■■■■►◄ voriconazole
Sustiva

Vfend

Risk rating: 1
Severity: Major   **Onset: Delayed**   **Likelihood: Suspected**

Cause
This combination increases CYP3A4 metabolism of voriconazole.
Voriconazole may inhibit the CYP3A4 metabolism of efavirenz.

Effect
Voriconazole plasma levels and efficacy may be reduced. Efavirenz
levels and adverse effects may be increased.

Nursing considerations
◤ **ALERT** Use of voriconazole with efavirenz is contraindicated.
■ This interaction is based on pharmacodynamics. Due to the serious-
ness of this interaction, it hasn't been studied in humans.

eletriptan ➤◀ azole antifungals
Relpax   fluconazole, itraconazole,
                           ketoconazole

Risk rating: 2
Severity: Moderate   Onset: Delayed   Likelihood: Suspected

Cause
Azole antifungals inhibit CYP3A4 metabolism of certain 5-HT$_1$ receptor agonists such as eletriptan.

Effect
Selective 5-HT$_1$ receptor agonist level and adverse effects increase.

Nursing considerations
◪ **ALERT** Don't give eletriptan within 72 hours or almotriptan within 7 days of itraconazole or ketoconazole.
■ Adverse effects of selective 5-HT$_1$ receptor agonists include coronary artery vasospasm, dizziness, nausea, paresthesia, and somnolence.

eletriptan ➤◀ dihydroergotamine
Relpax   D.H.E. 45

Risk rating: 1
Severity: Major   Onset: Rapid   Likelihood: Suspected

Cause
Combined use may have additive effects.

Effect
The risk of vasospastic effects increases.

Nursing considerations
◪ **ALERT** Use of these drugs or any two selective 5-HT$_1$ receptor agonists within 24 hours of each other is contraindicated.
■ Combined use may cause severe vasospastic effects, including sustained coronary artery vasospasm that triggers an MI.
■ Warn the patient not to mix migraine drugs within 24 hours of each other and to call his prescriber if a drug isn't effective.

enalapril ◄► aspirin

Vasotec

Bayer, Ecotrin

Risk rating: 2
Severity: Moderate **Onset: Rapid** **Likelihood: Suspected**

Cause
Salicylates inhibit synthesis of prostaglandins, which enalapril, an ACE inhibitor, needs to lower blood pressure.

Effect
ACE inhibitor's hypotensive effect decreases.

Nursing considerations
- This interaction is more likely in people with hypertension, coronary artery disease, and possibly heart failure.
- Monitor the patient's blood pressure carefully.
- The dose of aspirin may need to be decreased to less than 100 mg/day.
- If an interaction occurs, the patient may need to be placed on a nonaspirin antiplatelet agent or an angiotensin-receptor blocker.

enalapril ◄► glyburide

Vasotec

Diabeta, Micronase

Risk rating: 2
Severity: Moderate **Onset: Rapid** **Likelihood: Probable**

Cause
ACE inhibitors such as enalapril increase insulin sensitivity.

Effect
Risk of hypoglycemia increases.

Nursing considerations
- Start ACE inhibitor therapy carefully, monitoring the patient for hypoglycemia.
- Describe signs and symptoms of hypoglycemia, including diaphoresis, fatigue, headache, hunger, irritability, malaise, nervousness, rapid heart rate, tension, and trembling.
- Instruct the patient to eat a small carbohydrate snack or meal if hypoglycemia develops, preferably after checking blood glucose level.

enalapril ▰▰▰►◄▰▰▰ indomethacin
Vasotec   Indocin

Risk rating: 2
Severity: Moderate   Onset: Rapid   Likelihood: Probable

Cause
Indomethacin inhibits synthesis of prostaglandins, which enalapril, an ACE inhibitor, needs to lower blood pressure.

Effect
ACE inhibitor's hypotensive effect decreases.

Nursing considerations
◪ **ALERT** Monitor blood pressure closely. Severe hypertension may persist until indomethacin is stopped.
■ If indomethacin can't be avoided, the patient may need a different antihypertensive.
■ Remind the patient that hypertension commonly causes no physical symptoms but sometimes may cause headache and dizziness.
■ Other ACE inhibitors may interact with indomethacin. If you suspect an interaction, consult the prescriber or pharmacist.

enalapril ▰▰▰►◄▰▰▰ lithium
Vasotec   Eskalith

Risk rating: 2
Severity: Moderate   Onset: Delayed   Likelihood: Suspected

Cause
The mechanism of this interaction is unknown.

Effect
Lithium level may be elevated and neurotoxicity may occur.

Nursing considerations
■ If the patient takes lithium, consider an antihypertensive other than an ACE inhibitor.
■ Monitor lithium level. Steady state lithium level should be 0.6 to 1.2 mEq/L.
■ Adjust lithium dose as needed.
■ Watch for evidence of lithium toxicity, such as diarrhea, vomiting, dehydration, drowsiness, muscle weakness, tremor, fever, and ataxia.
■ Use with added caution in elderly patients and those with heart failure, renal insufficiency, or volume depletion. Dehydration may increase the effects of this interaction.

enalapril ━━━━▶◀ potassium-sparing diuretics

Vasotec

amiloride, spironolactone

Risk rating: 1
Severity: Major   **Onset: Delayed**   **Likelihood: Probable**

Cause
The mechanism of this interaction is unknown.

Effect
Serum potassium level may increase.

Nursing considerations
■ Use cautiously in patients at high risk for hyperkalemia, especially those with renal impairment.
■ Monitor BUN, creatinine, and serum potassium levels as needed.
■ ACE inhibitors other than enalapril may interact with potassium-sparing diuretics. If you suspect an interaction, consult the prescriber or pharmacist.
■ Urge the patient to report an irregular heartbeat, a slow pulse, weakness, and other evidence of hyperkalemia immediately.

enflurane ━━━━▶◀ nondepolarizing muscle relaxants

Ethrane

atracurium, pancuronium, vecuronium

Risk rating: 1
Severity: Major   **Onset: Rapid**   **Likelihood: Established**

Cause
These drugs potentiate pharmacologic actions.

Effect
The actions of nondepolarizing muscle relaxants are potentiated.

Nursing considerations
■ Closely monitor respiratory function.
■ The dose of both the inhalation anesthetic and nondepolarizing muscle relaxant may need to be adjusted.
■ Provide ventilatory support as needed.
■ The interaction is dose-dependant.
■ If the patient is receiving a nondepolarizing muscle relaxant continuously, the maintenance dose may need to be decreased 25% to 30%.

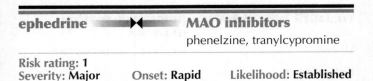

ephedrine ▶◀ MAO inhibitors
phenelzine, tranylcypromine

Risk rating: 1
Severity: Major   **Onset: Rapid**   **Likelihood: Established**

Cause
Norepinephrine accumulates with MAO inhibition and is released by indirect and mixed-acting sympathomimetics such as ephedrine.

Effect
The pressor response at receptor sites increases, elevating the risk of severe headache, hypertension, high fever, and hypertensive crisis.

Nursing considerations
■ Avoid giving indirect or mixed-acting sympathomimetics with an MAO inhibitor.
■ If drugs are given together, phentolamine can block epinephrine- and norepinephrine-induced vasoconstriction and reduce blood pressure.
■ Direct-acting sympathomimetics interact minimally.
◄ **ALERT** Warn the patient that OTC medicines such as decongestants may cause this interaction.

ephedrine ▶◀ reserpine
Serpalan

Risk rating: 2
Severity: Moderate   **Onset: Rapid**   **Likelihood: Suspected**

Cause
Receptor sensitivity to sympathomimetics, such as ephedrine, is increased.

Effect
The pressor response of ephedrine may increase, resulting in hypertension. The pressor response may be decreased.

Nursing considerations
■ Monitor the patient's blood pressure closely.
■ The dose of ephedrine may need to be increased or decreased, depending on the patient's clinical response.

epinephrine ━━━▶◀━━━ beta-adrenergic blockers

Adrenalin   nadolol, propranolol

Risk rating: 1
Severity: Major   **Onset: Rapid**   **Likelihood: Established**

Cause
Alpha-receptor effects of epinephrine supersede the effects of non-selective beta-adrenergic blockers, increasing vascular resistance.

Effect
Marked hypertensive effects are followed by reflex bradycardia.

Nursing considerations
◼ **ALERT** Three days before planned use of epinephrine, stop the beta-adrenergic blocker. Better yet, avoid using epinephrine if possible.
◼ If drugs must be used together, monitor blood pressure and pulse closely. If interaction occurs, give I.V. chlorpromazine, hydralazine, aminophylline, or atropine if needed.
◼ Explain the risks of interaction. Caution the patient to carry medical identification at all times.
◼ Other beta-adrenergic blockers may interact with epinephrine. If you suspect an interaction, consult the prescriber or pharmacist.

epinephrine ━━━▶◀━━━ tricyclic antidepressants

Adrenalin   amitriptyline, desipramine, imipramine, nortriptyline, protriptyline

Risk rating: 2
Severity: Moderate   **Onset: Rapid**   **Likelihood: Established**

Cause
Tricyclic antidepressants (TCAs) increase the effects of direct-acting sympathomimetics such as epinephrine.

Effect
When sympathomimetic effects increase, the risk of hypertension and arrhythmias increases.

Nursing considerations
◼ If possible, avoid using these drugs together.
◼ Watch the patient closely for hypertension and heart rhythm changes; they may warrant reduction of sympathomimetic dosage.

■ Other TCAs and sympathomimetics may interact. If you suspect an interaction, consult the prescriber or pharmacist.

---

eplerenone ━━━▶◀━━━ azole antifungals

Inspra   itraconazole, ketoconazole

Risk rating: 1
Severity: Major　　　**Onset: Delayed**　　　**Likelihood: Suspected**

Cause
Azole antifungals inhibit eplerenone metabolism.

Effect
Eplerenone level rises, causing hyperkalemia and increasing the risk of life-threatening arrhythmias.

Nursing considerations
⚡ **ALERT** Use of azole antifungals with eplerenone is contraindicated.
■ Potent CYP3A4 inhibitors increase the eplerenone level and the risk of hyperkalemia-induced arrhythmias—some fatal.
■ Monitor the patient's serum potassium level.
■ Tell the patient to report nausea, irregular heartbeat, or slowed pulse to the prescriber.

---

eplerenone ━━━▶◀━━━ clarithromycin

Inspra   Biaxin

Risk rating: 1
Severity: Major　　　**Onset: Delayed**　　　**Likelihood: Suspected**

Cause
Macrolide antibiotics such as clarithromycin inhibit the CYP3A4 metabolism of eplerenone.

Effect
Eplerenone level increases, which may increase risk of hyperkalemia and serious arrhythmias.

Nursing considerations
⚡ **ALERT** Administration of clarithromycin and eplerenone is contraindicated.
■ The basis for this interaction is the risk of hyperkalemia from eplerenone therapy.
■ The interaction is based on pharmacodynamics, not actual patient studies.

eplerenone ◀▶ nefazodone

Inspra

Risk rating: 1
Severity: Major   **Onset: Delayed**   **Likelihood: Suspected**

Cause
Nefazodone inhibits the CYP3A4 metabolism of eplerenone.

Effect
Eplerenone level increases, which may increase risk of hyperkalemia and serious arrhythmias.

Nursing considerations
◼ **ALERT** Administration of nefazodone and eplerenone is contraindicated.
◾ The risk of hyperkalemia from eplerenone therapy is the basis for this interaction.
◾ The interaction is based on pharmacodynamics, not actual patient studies.

eplerenone ◀▶ potassium-sparing diuretics

Inspra

amiloride, spironolactone, triamterene

Risk rating: 1
Severity: Major   **Onset: Delayed**   **Likelihood: Suspected**

Cause
Potassium-sparing diuretics decrease renal elimination of potassium ions.

Effect
Serum potassium levels increase.

Nursing considerations
◼ **ALERT** Taking eplerenone and potassium-sparing diuretics together is contraindicated.
◾ If the patient is taking eplerenone and a potassium-sparing diuretic together, notify the prescriber that this combination is contraindicated.
◾ Monitor the patient for signs of hyperkalemia, such as muscle weakness and cardiac arrhythmias.
◾ Monitor serum potassium levels closely.
◾ Urge the patient to report an irregular heart beat, a slow pulse, weakness, and other evidence of hyperkalemia immediately.

eplerenone ▶◀ protease inhibitors
Inspra   nelfinavir, ritonavir

Risk rating: 1
Severity: Major   **Onset: Delayed**   **Likelihood: Suspected**

Cause
Protease inhibitors hinder eplerenone metabolism.

Effect
Eplerenone level rises, causing hyperkalemia and increasing the risk of life-threatening arrhythmias.

Nursing considerations
⚠ **ALERT** Use of nelfinavir or ritonavir with eplerenone is contraindicated.
■ Potent CYP3A4 inhibitors increase the eplerenone level and the risk of hyperkalemia-induced arrhythmias—some fatal.
■ Monitor the patient's serum potassium level.
■ Tell the patient to report nausea, irregular heartbeat, or slowed pulse to the prescriber.

ergonovine ▶◀ azole antifungals
Ergotrate   itraconazole, ketoconazole, voriconazole

Risk rating: 1
Severity: Major   **Onset: Delayed**   **Likelihood: Suspected**

Cause
Azole antifungals may inhibit CYP3A4 metabolism of ergot derivatives.

Effect
Risk of ergot toxicity may be increased.

Nursing considerations
⚠ **ALERT** Use of these drugs together is contraindicated.
■ Signs of ergot toxicity include peripheral vasospasm and ischemia.
■ Caution the patient to avoid ergot derivatives (for migraine, for example) while taking azole antifungals; consult the prescriber about alternative therapies.

ergonovine ▬▬▶◀▬▬ protease inhibitors
Ergotrate

amprenavir, atazanavir,
darunavir, indinavir, lopinavir-
ritonavir, nelfinavir, ritonavir,
saquinavir

Risk rating: 1
Severity: Major   **Onset: Delayed**   **Likelihood: Probable**

Cause
Protease inhibitors may interfere with CYP3A4 metabolism of ergot
derivatives such as ergonovine.

Effect
Risk of ergot-induced peripheral vasospasm and ischemia may increase.

Nursing considerations
◼ **ALERT** Use of ergot derivatives with protease inhibitors is contraindicated.
◼ Monitor the patient for evidence of peripheral ischemia, including
pain in limb muscles while exercising and later at rest; numbness and
tingling of fingers and toes; cool, pale, or cyanotic limbs; red or violet
blisters on hands or feet; and gangrene.
◼ Sodium nitroprusside may be given for ergot-induced vasospasm.
◼ If the patient takes a protease inhibitor, consult the prescriber or
pharmacist about alternative treatments for migraine pain.
◼ Urge the patient to tell the prescriber about increased adverse effects.

ergotamine ▬▬▶◀▬▬ azole antifungals
Ergomar

itraconazole, voriconazole

Risk rating: 1
Severity: Major   **Onset: Delayed**   **Likelihood: Suspected**

Cause
Azole antifungals inhibit CYP3A4 metabolism of ergot derivatives
such as ergotamine.

Effect
Risk of ergot toxicity may increase.

Nursing considerations
◼ **ALERT** Use of these drugs together is contraindicated.

■ Signs of ergot toxicity include peripheral vasospasm and ischemia.
■ Caution against use of ergot derivatives (for migraine, for example) while taking azole antifungals; consult the prescriber about alternatives.

ergotamine ▶◀ macrolide antibiotics

Ergomar

clarithromycin, erythromycin, telithromycin

Risk rating: 1
Severity: Major   **Onset: Rapid**   **Likelihood: Probable**

Cause
Macrolide antibiotics interfere with hepatic metabolism of ergot derivatives such as ergotamine.

Effect
Symptoms of acute ergotism, mainly peripheral ischemia, may develop.

Nursing considerations
■ Monitor the patient for evidence of peripheral ischemia, including pain in limb muscles while exercising and later at rest; numbness and tingling of fingers and toes; cool, pale, or cyanotic limbs; red or violet blisters on hands or feet; and gangrene.
■ Dosage of ergot derivative may need to be decreased, or both drugs may need to be stopped.
■ Consider a different anti-infective drug that's less likely to interact with ergot derivatives.
◪ ALERT Sodium nitroprusside may be given for macrolide-ergot–induced vasospasm.
■ Explain evidence of ergot-induced peripheral ischemia. Urge the patient to report it promptly to his prescriber.

ergotamine ▶◀ non-nucleoside reverse-transcriptase inhibitors

Ergomar

delavirdine, efavirenz

Risk rating: 1
Severity: Major   **Onset: Delayed**   **Likelihood: Suspected**

Cause
Nonnucleoside reverse-transcriptase inhibitors may decrease CYP3A4 metabolism of ergot derivatives such as ergotamine.

Effect
Risk of ergot-induced peripheral vasospasm and ischemia may increase.

Nursing considerations
⚠ ALERT Use of ergot derivatives with delavirdine or efavirenz is contraindicated.

■ Monitor the patient for evidence of peripheral ischemia: pain in limb muscles while exercising and later at rest; numbness and tingling of fingers and toes; cool, pale, or cyanotic limbs; red or violet blisters on hands or feet; and gangrene.

■ Ergot toxicity also may cause nausea, vomiting, lassitude, impaired mental function, delirium, severe dyspnea, hypotension, hypertension, rapid or weak pulse, unconsciousness, limb spasm, seizures, and shock.

■ Give a vasodilator for vasospasm and diazepam for seizures as needed.

■ Other nonnucleoside reverse-transcriptase inhibitors, such as nevirapine, may interact with ergot derivatives. If you suspect an interaction, consult the prescriber or pharmacist.

---

ergotamine ➤◀ propranolol
Ergomar   Inderal

Risk rating: 2
Severity: Moderate   **Onset: Delayed**   **Likelihood: Suspected**

Cause
Vasoconstriction and blockade of peripheral beta$_2$-receptors allow unopposed ergot action.

Effect
The vasoconstrictive effects of ergot derivatives, such as ergotamine, increase.

Nursing considerations
■ Watch for peripheral ischemia, cold limbs, and possible gangrene.
■ If needed, stop propranolol and adjust ergot derivative.
■ Other ergot derivatives may interact with beta-adrenergic blockers. If you suspect an interaction, consult the prescriber or pharmacist.

ergotamine ➤◄ protease inhibitors

Ergomar

amprenavir, atazanavir, darunavir, indinavir, lopinavir-ritonavir, nelfinavir, ritonavir, saquinavir

Risk rating: 1
Severity: Major   **Onset: Delayed**   **Likelihood: Probable**

Cause
Protease inhibitors may interfere with CYP3A4 metabolism of ergot derivatives such as ergotamine.

Effect
Risk of ergot-induced peripheral vasospasm and ischemia may increase.

Nursing considerations
◆ **ALERT** Use of ergotamine with protease inhibitors is contraindicated.
■ Watch for evidence of peripheral ischemia: pain in limb muscles while exercising and later at rest; numbness and tingling of fingers and toes; cool, pale, or cyanotic limbs; red or violet blisters on hands or feet; and gangrene.
■ Sodium nitroprusside may be given for ergot-induced vasospasm.
■ If the patient takes a protease inhibitor, consult the prescriber or pharmacist about alternative treatments for migraine pain.
■ Urge the patient to tell the prescriber about increased adverse effects.

ergotamine ➤◄ selective 5-HT$_1$ receptor agonists

Ergomar

eletriptan, frovatriptan, naratriptan, rizatriptan, sumatriptan, zolmitriptan

Risk rating: 1
Severity: Major   **Onset: Rapid**   **Likelihood: Suspected**

Cause
Combined use may have additive effects.

Effect
The risk of vasospastic effects increases.

Nursing considerations
🔰 **ALERT** Use of these drugs or any two selective 5-HT$_1$ receptor agonists within 24 hours of each other is contraindicated.
■ Combined use may cause severe vasospastic effects, including a sustained coronary artery vasospasm that triggers an MI.
■ Warn the patient not to mix migraine headache drugs within 24 hours of each other, but to call his prescriber if a drug isn't effective.

---

erlotinib ▶◀ rifamycins
Tarceva   rifabutin, rifampin, rifapentine

Risk rating: 2
Severity: Moderate   **Onset: Delayed**   **Likelihood: Suspected**

Cause
Rifamycins induce CYP3A4 metabolism of erlotinib.

Effect
Erlotinib level and effects may be reduced.

Nursing considerations
■ If possible, consider using another class of drug besides rifamycins if the patient is taking erlotinib.
■ If the patient must take a rifamycin and erlotinib, the dose of erlotinib may need to be increased to greater than 150 mg.

---

erythromycin ▶◀ amiodarone
E-mycin, Eryc   Cordarone, Pacerone

Risk rating: 1
Severity: Major   **Onset: Delayed**   **Likelihood: Suspected**

Cause
An additive increase in the QT interval is seen when administering antiarrhythmic agents and macrolide antibiotics such as erythromycin.

Effect
The risk of life-threatening cardiac arrhythmias, including torsades de pointes, is increased.

Nursing considerations
🔰 **ALERT** Monitor the patient for prolonged QT interval and torsades de pointes.

■ This interaction may be more likely with telithromycin; avoid administering with antiarrhythmics.
■ This interaction appears to be dose-related.
■ Instruct the patient to let the prescriber know if he experiences dizziness, palpitations, or light-headedness.
■ The QT interval returns to normal within 3 days of stopping the medications.

---

erythromycin ➤◀ benzodiazepines
E-mycin, Eryc   alprazolam, diazepam,
                                 midazolam, triazolam

Risk rating: 2
Severity: Moderate   **Onset: Rapid**   **Likelihood: Suspected**

Cause
Macrolide antibiotics such as erythromycin may decrease metabolism of certain benzodiazepines.

Effect
Sedative effects of benzodiazepines may be increased or prolonged.

Nursing considerations
■ Talk with the prescriber about decreasing benzodiazepine dosage during antibiotic therapy.
■ Lorazepam, oxazepam, and temazepam probably don't interact with macrolide antibiotics; substitution may be possible.
■ Urge the patient to report oversedation promptly.

---

erythromycin ➤◀ bromocriptine
E-mycin, Eryc   Parlodel

Risk rating: 2
Severity: Moderate   **Onset: Delayed**   **Likelihood: Suspected**

Cause
Erythromycin inhibits hepatic metabolism, resulting in increased bioavailability.

Effect
The therapeutic and toxic effects of bromocriptine may increase.

Nursing considerations
■ Monitor the patient for increased response to bromocriptine, and adjust the dose accordingly.
■ Monitor the patient for dizziness and orthostatic hypotension.

- The most common increased adverse effect is vomiting.
- Give bromocriptine with food to minimize adverse effects.

---

erythromycin ━━▶◀━━ buspirone
E-mycin, Eryc   BuSpar

Risk rating: 2
Severity: Moderate   Onset: Delayed   Likelihood: Suspected

Cause
Macrolide antibiotics such as erythromycin may inhibit CYP3A4 metabolism of buspirone.

Effect
Buspirone level and adverse effects may increase.

Nursing considerations
◪ **ALERT** Use of other macrolide antibiotics (such as azithromycin or dirithromycin) should be considered because they probably don't interact with buspirone. Consult the prescriber or pharmacist.
- During buspirone therapy, monitor the patient closely if a macrolide antibiotic is started or stopped or its dosage is changed.
- If the patient takes a macrolide antibiotic, the starting buspirone dose should be conservative.
- Monitor the patient for signs of buspirone toxicity, including increased CNS effects (such as dizziness, drowsiness, and headache), vomiting, and diarrhea.
- Adjust buspirone dose as needed.

---

erythromycin ━━▶◀━━ carbamazepine
E-mycin, Eryc   Carbatrol, Epitol, Equetro, Tegretol

Risk rating: 1
Severity: Major   Onset: Rapid   Likelihood: Established

Cause
CYP3A4 metabolism of carbamazepine is inhibited, decreasing carbamazepine clearance.

Effect
Carbamazepine level and toxicity may increase.

Nursing considerations
◪ **ALERT** If possible, avoid use together.

■ Consult the prescriber or pharmacist about an alternative macrolide antibiotic (such as azithromycin) or an alternative anti-infective drug unlikely to interact with carbamazepine.
■ If using a macrolide antibiotic, monitor carbamazepine level; the therapeutic range is 4 to 12 mcg/ml.
■ Monitor the patient for evidence of carbamazepine toxicity, including dizziness, ataxia, respiratory depression, tachycardia, arrhythmias, blood pressure changes, impaired consciousness, abnormal reflexes, nystagmus, seizures, nausea, vomiting, and urine retention.
■ Carbamazepine dosage may need adjustment.

erythromycin ━━▶◀━━ cilostazol
E-mycin, Eryc   Pletal

Risk rating: 1
Severity: Major   **Onset: Delayed**   **Likelihood: Suspected**

Cause
Certain macrolide antibiotics such as erythromycin inhibit CYP3A4 metabolism of cilostazol.

Effect
Cilostazol effects, including adverse effects, may increase.

Nursing considerations
■ Cilostazol dose may need to be decreased during combined therapy; consider cilostazol 50 mg b.i.d.
■ Watch for evidence of cilostazol toxicity, including severe headache, diarrhea, hypotension, tachycardia, and arrhythmias.
■ Urge the patient to tell the prescriber about all drugs and supplements he takes and about any increase in adverse effects.
■ Other macrolide antibiotics may interact with cilostazol. If you suspect a drug interaction, consult the prescriber or pharmacist.

erythromycin ━━▶◀━━ colchicine
E-mycin, Eryc

Risk rating: 1
Severity: Major   **Onset: Delayed**   **Likelihood: Suspected**

Cause
Metabolism of colchicine is inhibited.

Effect
Colchicine levels and risk of toxicity increase.

Nursing considerations
- Monitor the serum levels of colchicine.
- If using a macrolide antibiotic and colchicine together, it may be necessary to decrease the dose of colchicine.
- Monitor the patient for fever, diarrhea, abdominal pain, myalgia, convulsions, and hair loss.
- Patients with hepatic or renal impairment are more at risk for toxicity.

---

erythromycin ▶◀ cyclosporine
E-mycin, Eryc   Gengraf, Neoral, Sandimmune

Risk rating: 2
Severity: Moderate   **Onset: Delayed**   **Likelihood: Established**

Cause
Macrolide antibiotics, such as erythromycin, interfere with cyclosporine metabolism. The rate and extent of absorption may increase, and the volume of distribution may decrease.

Effect
Elevated cyclosporine levels and increased risk of toxicity may occur.

Nursing considerations
▶ ALERT Monitor the patient carefully for nephrotoxicity or neurotoxicity.
- Closely monitor BUN and serum creatinine levels.
- The dose of cyclosporine may need to be decreased.
- Of all the macrolide antibiotics, azithromycin appears to interact the least with cyclosporine.

---

erythromycin ▶◀ digoxin
E-mycin, Eryc   Lanoxin

Risk rating: 1
Severity: Major   **Onset: Delayed**   **Likelihood: Established**

Cause
Macrolide antibiotics, such as erythromycin, may alter GI flora and increase digoxin absorption.

Effect
Digoxin level and risk of toxicity may increase.

Nursing considerations
- Monitor digoxin level. Therapeutic range is 0.8 to 2 ng/ml.

■ Watch for evidence of digoxin toxicity: arrhythmias (bradycardia, AV blocks, and ventricular ectopy), lethargy, drowsiness, confusion, hallucinations, headaches, syncope, visual disturbances, nausea, anorexia, vomiting, and diarrhea.

■ Digoxin dosage may need reduction.

⚠ ALERT Erythromycin doesn't affect the serum level of digoxin given I.V. Capsule form of digoxin may increase digoxin availability and decrease risk of interaction.

■ Other macrolide antibiotics may interact with digoxin. If you suspect an interaction, consult the prescriber or pharmacist.

---

erythromycin ➡◀ ergot derivatives
E-mycin, Eryc   dihydroergotamine, ergotamine

Risk rating: 1
Severity: Major   **Onset: Rapid**   **Likelihood: Probable**

Cause
Macrolide antibiotics such as erythromycin interfere with hepatic metabolism of ergotamine.

Effect
Symptoms of acute ergotism, primarily peripheral ischemia, may develop.

Nursing considerations
■ Watch for evidence of peripheral ischemia, including cool, pale, or cyanotic limbs; pain in limb muscles while exercising and later at rest; numbness and tingling of fingers and toes; red or violet blisters on hands or feet; and gangrene.

■ Dosage of ergot derivative may need to be decreased, or both drugs may need to be stopped.

■ Consider a different anti-infective that's less likely to interact with ergot derivatives.

■ Sodium nitroprusside may be given for macrolide-ergot–induced vasospasm.

■ Make sure the patient is aware of the signs and symptoms of ergot-induced peripheral ischemia. Tell him to report them promptly to the prescriber.

erythromycin 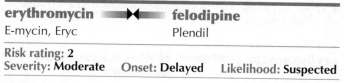 felodipine
E-mycin, Eryc   Plendil

Risk rating: 2
Severity: Moderate   **Onset: Delayed**   **Likelihood: Suspected**

Cause
Erythromycin inhibits the metabolism of felodipine.

Effect
Felodipine level, effects, and risk of adverse effects may increase.

Nursing considerations
- Monitor the patient's response to felodipine when erythromycin therapy is started, altered, or stopped.
- Watch for increased felodipine effects: prolonged hypotension, bradycardia, palpitation, flushing, headache, dizziness, and edema.
- Urge the patient to tell the prescriber about increased adverse effects.
- If an interaction is suspected, notify the prescriber or pharmacist; the dose may need to be altered.

erythromycin 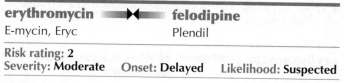 food, grapefruit juice
E-mycin, Eryc

Risk rating: 1
Severity: Major   **Onset: Delayed**   **Likelihood: Suspected**

Cause
Food may decrease GI absorption of erythromycin stearate and certain erythromycin base forms. Grapefruit may inhibit metabolism of erythromycin and other macrolide antibiotics.

Effect
With food, efficacy of certain macrolide antibiotics may decrease. With grapefruit, macrolide level and adverse effects may increase.

Nursing considerations
- Give erythromycin stearate and non–enteric-coated erythromycin base tablets 2 hours before or after a meal.
- Enteric-coated tablets aren't affected by food and may be taken without regard to meals.
- Give erythromycin estolate, erythromycin ethylsuccinate, and enteric-coated tablets of erythromycin base with food to decrease GI adverse effects.

■ Advise the patient to take a macrolide antibiotic with a beverage other than grapefruit juice.

---

erythromycin ▬▬►◄▬▬	HMG-CoA reductase inhibitors
E-mycin, Eryc	atorvastatin, lovastatin, simvastatin

Risk rating: 1
Severity: Major   **Onset: Delayed**   **Likelihood: Probable**

Cause
CYP3A4 metabolism of certain HMG-CoA reductase inhibitors may be decreased.

Effect
HMG-CoA reductase inhibitor level and risk of severe myopathy or rhabdomyolysis may increase.

Nursing considerations
⚡ **ALERT** If these drugs are given with a macrolide antibiotic, such as erythromycin, watch for evidence of rhabdomyolysis, especially 5 to 21 days after macrolide is started. Evidence may include fatigue; muscle aches and weakness; joint pain; dark, red, or cola-colored urine; weight gain; seizures; and greatly increased serum CK level.
■ Fluvastatin and pravastatin are metabolized by other enzymes and may be better choices when used with a macrolide antibiotic.
■ Urge the patient to report muscle pain, tenderness, or weakness.

---

erythromycin ▬▬►◄▬▬	methylprednisolone
E-mycin, Eryc	Medrol

Risk rating: 2
Severity: Moderate   **Onset: Delayed**   **Likelihood: Established**

Cause
The mechanism of this interaction is unclear.

Effect
Methylprednisolone effects, including toxic effects, may increase.

Nursing considerations
■ This interaction may be used for therapeutic benefit because it may be possible to reduce methylprednisolone dosage.
■ Monitor the patient for adverse or toxic effects, such as euphoria, insomnia, peptic ulceration, and cushingoid effects.

erythromycin ▰▰▰◀▶▰▰▰ pimozide
E-mycin, Eryc   Orap

Risk rating: 1
Severity: Major   **Onset: Delayed**   **Likelihood: Probable**

Cause
Macrolide antibiotics such as erythromycin may inhibit CYP3A4 metabolism of pimozide.

Effect
The risk of life-threatening arrythmias, including torsades de pointes, may increase.

Nursing considerations
◼ **ALERT** Combined use of these drugs is contraindicated.
◼ Arrhythmias are related to prolonged QT interval, a known risk of pimozide.
◼ **ALERT** People with normal baseline ECG and no history of arrhythmias have died from pimozide blood levels 2.5 times the upper limit of normal from this interaction.

erythromycin ▰▰▰◀▶▰▰▰ quinolones
E-mycin, Eryc   gatifloxacin, levofloxacin,
                                       moxifloxacin

Risk rating: 1
Severity: Major   **Onset: Delayed**   **Likelihood: Suspected**

Cause
The mechanism of this interaction is unknown.

Effect
The risk of life-threatening arrhythmias, including torsades de pointes, increases.

Nursing considerations
◼ Avoid use of levofloxacin with erythromycin because doing so may prolong the QT interval.
◼ Use cautiously with gatifloxacin and moxifloxacin.
◼ Monitor ECG for prolonged QTc interval and arrhythmias.
◼ Tell the patient to report palpitations, dizziness, shortness of breath, and chest pain.
◼ Macrolides other than erythromycin may interact with quinolones. If you suspect an interaction, consult the prescriber or pharmacist.

■ Monitor serum electrolyte levels; electrolyte disturbances increase the risk of ventricular arrhythmias.

---

erythromycin ▰▰▶◀▰▰ tacrolimus
E-mycin, Eryc   Prograf

Risk rating: 2
Severity: Moderate   Onset: Delayed   Likelihood: Suspected

Cause
Certain macrolide antibiotics such as erythromycin inhibit CYP3A4 metablism of tacrolimus.

Effect
Tacrolimus level and risk of toxicity may increase.

Nursing considerations
■ If possible, use a different class of antibiotic.
■ Monitor tacrolimus level and renal function test results. Expected trough level of tacrolimus is 6 to 10mcg/L.
■ Tacrolimus may need to be stopped temporarily because reduced dosages may not prevent renal changes.
■ Other macrolide antibiotics may have the same interaction.

---

erythromycin ▰▰▶◀▰▰ theophyllines
E-mycin, Eryc   aminophylline, theophylline

Risk rating: 2
Severity: Moderate   Onset: Delayed   Likelihood: Established

Cause
Certain macrolide antibiotics such as erythromycin inhibit theophylline metabolism. Theophyllines increase renal clearance and decrease availability of oral erythromycin.

Effect
Theophylline level and risk of toxicity may increase. Erythromycin level may decrease.

Nursing considerations
■ When starting or stopping a macrolide antibiotic, monitor theophylline level. Therapeutic range is 10 to 20 mcg/ml for adults and 5 to 15 mcg/ml for children.
■ If the patient takes a theophylline, watch for decreased erythromycin efficacy; tell the prescriber promptly.

■ Consult the prescriber about the possibility of using another antibiotic.

■ Watch for evidence of toxicity: tachycardia, anorexia, nausea, vomiting, diarrhea, seizures, restlessness, irritability, and headache.

■ Describe the adverse effects of theophylline and signs of toxicity, and tell the patient to report them immediately to the prescriber.

erythromycin ▶◀ verapamil

E-mycin, Eryc　　　　　　　Calan

Risk rating: 1
Severity: Major **Onset: Delayed** **Likelihood: Probable**

Cause
Certain macrolides such as erythromycin inhibit CYP3A4 metabolism of verapamil. Verapamil increases erythromycin absorption and decreases erythromycin metabolism.

Effect
Risk of cardiotoxicity increased.

Nursing considerations
■ Closely monitor cardiac function in patients taking this combination of drugs.

■ Evidence of cardiotoxcity, if present, will appear within 2 days to 1 week.

■ Monitor the patient for dizziness, shortness of breath, weakness, profound hypotension, bradycardia, QTc prolongation, and complete atrioventricular heart block.

■ Consult the prescriber about the possibilty of using another antibiotic class.

■ Tell the patient to report palpitations, dizziness, shortness of breath, unexplained weakness, and chest pain.

erythromycin ▶◀ vinblastine

E-mycin, Eryc　　　　　　　Velban

Risk rating: 1
Severity: Major **Onset: Delayed** **Likelihood: Suspected**

Cause
Erythromycin inhibits metabolism of vinblastine.

Effect
Risk of vinblastine toxicity increases.

Nursing considerations
■ If possible, avoid this drug combination.
■ If erythromycin and vinblastine must be given together, keep the dose of vinblastine conservative.
■ Watch for evidence of toxicity, such as constipation, myalgia, hypertension, hyponatremia, and neutropenia.
■ If both drugs are taken together, and erythromycin is stopped because of the resulting adverse reactions, the patient's myalgia and neutropenia may resolve completely or decrease. Be aware, however, that both can recur after symptoms seemingly resolve.
■ Explain adverse reactions of vinblastine to the patient. Tell the patient to report them to the prescriber.

---

erythromycin ➤◀ **warfarin**
E-mycin, Eryc   Coumadin

Risk rating: 1
Severity: Major   **Onset: Delayed**   **Likelihood: Probable**

Cause
Combining both reduces warfarin clearance.

Effect
Anticoagulant effects and risk of bleeding increase.

Nursing considerations
■ Monitor PT and INR closely when a patient who's taking warfarin starts—or stops—taking a macrolide antibiotic such as erythromycin. The PT may be prolonged within a few days.
■ Warfarin dose adjustment may need to continue for several days after the patient stops antibiotic therapy. Now that the antibiotic is no longer present to intefere with warfarin clearance, warfarin levels will decrease.
■ Treat excessive anticoagulation with vitamin K.
■ Tell the patient to report unusual bruising or bleeding.
■ Remind the patient that warfarin interacts with many drugs and that he should report any change in drug regimen.
■ Advise the patient to keep all follow-up medical appointments for proper monitoring and dosage adjustments.

esomeprazole ━━▶◀━━ clarithromycin
Nexium   Biaxin

Risk rating: 2
Severity: Moderate   **Onset: Delayed**   **Likelihood: Suspected**

Cause
Clarithromycin inhibits the CYP3A metabolism of certain proton pump inhibitors such as esomeprazole.

Effect
Proton pump inhibitor levels and risk of adverse effects increase.

Nursing considerations
- Monitor the patient for adverse reactions.
- Watch the patient for headache, abdominal pain, constipation, diarrhea, dry mouth, nausea, and vomiting.
- Teach the patient about adverse reactions to watch for; tell him to notify the prescriber if adverse reactions increase.
- Administration of clarithromycin with other proton pump inhibitors may not cause this interaction.

esomeprazole ━━▶◀━━ protease inhibitors
Nexium   atazanavir, indinavir,
                             saquinavir

Risk rating: 1
Severity: Major   **Onset: Delayed**   **Likelihood: Suspected**

Cause
GI absorption of protease inhibitors may be decreased.

Effect
Antiviral activity of protease inhibitors may be reduced.

Nursing considerations
- Use of protease inhibitors and proton pump inhibitors isn't recommended.
- Monitor the patient for a decrease in antiviral activity.
- Adjust the dose of the protease inhibitor as needed.

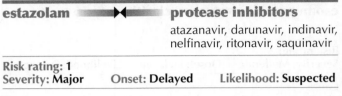

estazolam ━━━━►◄━━ **protease inhibitors**
atazanavir, darunavir, indinavir, nelfinavir, ritonavir, saquinavir

Risk rating: 1
Severity: Major   **Onset: Delayed**   **Likelihood: Suspected**

Cause
Protease inhibitors may inhibit CYP3A4 metabolism of certain benzodiazepines such as estazolam.

Effect
Sedative effects may be increased and prolonged.

Nursing considerations
⚠ **ALERT** Don't combine estazolam with protease inhibitors.
■ If the patient takes any benzodiazepine–protease inhibitor combination, notify the prescriber. Interaction could involve others in the class.
■ Watch for evidence of oversedation and respiratory depression.
■ Teach the patient and his family about the risks of combining these drugs.

estrogens ━━━━►◄━━ **bosentan**
ethinyl estradiol   Tracleer

Risk rating: 1
Severity: Major   **Onset: Delayed**   **Likelihood: Suspected**

Cause
Bosentan may increase CYP3A4 metabolism of estrogens.

Effect
Estrogen level and efficacy may be reduced.

Nursing considerations
■ Inform the patient of the increased risk of oral contraceptive failure when combined with taking bosentan.
■ The patient should consider an alternative nonhormonal contraceptive or an additional method of contraception while taking bosentan.
■ Watch for menstrual disturbances, such as spotting, intermenstrual bleeding, or amenorrhea.
■ Estrogen dose may need to be increased; consult the prescriber.

estrogens ◄►◄ corticosteroids

conjugated estrogens,
esterified estrogens,
estradiol, estrone,
estropipate, ethinyl
estradiol

prednisone, prednisolone

Risk rating: 2
Severity: Moderate   **Onset: Delayed**   **Likelihood: Suspected**

Cause
Estrogens may inhibit hepatic metabolism of corticosteroids.

Effect
Therapeutic and toxic corticosteroid effects may increase.

Nursing considerations
- Assess the effect of corticosteroids when given with estrogens.
- Watch for evidence of corticosteroid toxicity: nervousness, sleepiness, depression, psychosis, weakness, decreased hearing, lower leg edema, skin disorders, hypertension, muscle weakness, and seizures.
- If a problem is noted, decrease corticosteroid dosage.
- Estrogen may continue to affect corticosteroid therapy for an unknown length of time after estrogen is stopped.
- Other corticosteroids may interact with estrogens. If you suspect an interaction, consult the prescriber or the pharmacist.
- Tell the patient to report increased adverse effects.

estrogens ◄►◄ modafinil

ethinyl estradiol

Provigil

Risk rating: 2
Severity: Moderate   **Onset: Delayed**   **Likelihood: Suspected**

Cause
Modafinil induces gastrointestinal and hepatic metabolism of estrogens.

Effect
Estrogen level and efficacy may be reduced.

Nursing considerations
- Inform the patient that taking modafinil increases the risk that oral contraceptives may fail to prevent pregnancy.

■ The patient should consider using a nonhormonal contraceptive instead, or—if she wants to stay on a hormonal contraceptive—adding another contraceptive method while taking modafinil.

■ Caution the patient to watch for, and report, menstrual disturbances, such as spotting, intermenstrual bleeding, or amenorrhea.

■ Estrogen dose may need to be adjusted; consult the prescriber.

estrogens ◄►► phenytoin

conjugated estrogens   Dilantin

Risk rating: 2
Severity: Moderate   Onset: Delayed   Likelihood: Suspected

Cause
Phenytoin may induce hepatic metabolism of estrogens. Estrogens may increase water retention, worsen seizures, and alter phenytoin protein-binding.

Effect
Risk of spotting, breakthrough bleeding, and pregnancy increases. Seizure control may decrease.

Nursing considerations
◤ **ALERT** Advise the patient that breakthrough bleeding, spotting, and amenorrhea are signs of contraceptive failure.

■ Estrogen dose may need to be altered so the patient can obtain cycle control.

■ Seizures may worsen in patients who take hormonal contraceptives.

■ Watch for increased seizure activity when estrogen therapy starts.

■ Hydantoins other than phenytoin may interact with estrogens. If you suspect an interaction, consult the prescriber or the pharmacist.

■ If the patient takes phenytoin, suggest a nonhormonal contraceptive.

estrogens ◄►► rifampin

estradiol, ethinyl estradiol   Rifadin, Rimactane

Risk rating: 2
Severity: Moderate   Onset: Delayed   Likelihood: Suspected

Cause
Rifampin induces hepatic metabolism of estrogens.

Effect
Estrogen level and efficacy may be reduced.

Nursing considerations

■ Watch for menstrual disturbances, such as spotting, intermenstrual bleeding, or amenorrhea.
■ Explain that contraception may fail during combined therapy.
■ Estrogen dose may need to be increased; consult the prescriber.
■ If the patient takes rifampin, suggest a nonhormonal contraceptive.
■ Urge the patient to take the full course of rifampin exactly as prescribed to minimize risk of continued infection.

---

estrogens ▶◀ topiramate

ethinyl estradiol   Topamax

Risk rating: 2
Severity: Moderate   **Onset: Delayed**   **Likelihood: Suspected**

Cause
Topiramate may increase estrogen metabolism.

Effect
Estrogen efficacy may decrease.

Nursing considerations
■ Watch for worsening vasomotor symptoms: hot flashes, diaphoresis, headache, nausea, palpitations, dizziness, and a skin-crawling feeling.
■ Estrogen replacement or hormonal contraceptive dosage may need to be increased; consult the prescriber or pharmacist.
■ Tell the patient that topiramate may decrease estrogen efficacy.
■ Urge the patient to report loss of effect—such as spotting, breakthrough bleeding, and amenorrhea—or increased adverse effects.
■ If the patient takes topiramate, suggest a nonhormonal contraceptive.

---

ethacrynic acid ▶◀ aminoglycosides

Edecrin   gentamicin, streptomycin, tobramycin

Risk rating: 1
Severity: Major   **Onset: Rapid**   **Likelihood: Suspected**

Cause
The mechanism of the interaction is unknown.

Effect
Synergistic ototoxicity increases the risk of hearing loss, possibly permanently.

Nursing considerations
◨ **ALERT** Patients with renal insufficiency are at increased risk for ototoxicity.
■ Perform baseline and periodic hearing function tests.
■ Other aminoglycosides may interact with loop diuretics such as ethacrynic acid. If you suspect an interaction, consult the prescriber or pharmacist.
■ Tell the patient to immediately report ringing or roaring in the ears, muffled sounds, or any noticeable changes in hearing.
■ Advise family members to stay alert for evidence of hearing loss.

---

ethacrynic acid ➠◀ cisplatin
Edecrin   Platinol

Risk rating: 2
Severity: Moderate   **Onset: Rapid**   **Likelihood: Suspected**

Cause
The mechanism of this interaction is unknown.

Effect
Interaction may cause additive ototoxicity.

Nursing considerations
■ Combined, these drugs may cause ototoxicity that's much more severe than that caused by either drug alone; the combination may possibly result in permanent damage.
■ Avoid giving a loop diuretic such as ethacrynic acid with cisplatin.
■ Advise the patient to obtain hearing tests to detect early hearing loss.
■ Tell the patient to report ringing in the ears, change in balance, or muffled sounds. Also, ask family members to watch for changes.

---

ethacrynic acid ➠◀ digoxin
Edecrin   Lanoxin

Risk rating: 1
Severity: Major   **Onset: Delayed**   **Likelihood: Probable**

Cause
Urinary excretion of potassium and magnesium is increased.

Effect
Electrolyte disturbances may predispose the patient to digitalis-induced arrhythmias.

Nursing considerations
- Monitor serum potassium and magensium levels; decreased levels may predispose the patient to arrhythmias.
- Carefully monitor the patient's ECG while receiving digoxin and a loop diuretic such as ethacrynic acid.
- If the patient develops hypomagnesemia or hypokalemia, be prepared to administer supplements.
- Monitor the patient for increased serum sodium.
- Changing the patient from a loop diuretic to a potassium-sparing diuretic will minimize the risk of arrhythmias.
- This interaction appears to be dose related.

ethacrynic acid ▶◀ lithium
Edecrin   Eskalith

Risk rating: 2
Severity: Moderate   Onset: Delayed   Likelihood: Suspected

Cause
The cause of this interaction is unknown.

Effect
Lithium level, effects, and risk of toxicity may increase.

Nursing considerations
- Monitor lithium level. Steady state lithium level should be 0.6 to 1.2 mEq/L.
- Adjust lithium dose as needed.
- Monitor the patient for evidence of lithium toxicity, such as diarrhea, vomitong, dehydration, drowsiness, muscle weakness, tremor, fever, and ataxia.

ethosuximide ▶◀ primidone
Zarontin   Mysoline

Risk rating: 2
Severity: Moderate   Onset: Delayed   Likelihood: Suspected

Cause
The cause of this interaction is unknown.

Effect
Primodone levels and pharmacologic effects may be reduced.

Nursing considerations
- Monitor serum primodone levels.

- Adjustments to ethosuximide dosage may neccesitate a change in primodone.
- Monitor the patient for increased seizure activity.
- Therapeutic level of primidone is 5 to 12 mcg/ml.

etoposide ━━━◄ cyclosporine
VePesid   Gengraf, Neoral, Sandimmune

Risk rating: 2
Severity: Moderate   Onset: Delayed   Likelihood: Established

Cause
Etoposide clearance may be decreased and metabolism inhibited by cyclosporine.

Effect
Etoposide level and risk of toxicity may increase.

Nursing considerations
- Monitor the patient for evidence of etoposide toxicity, including myelosuppression, nausea, vomiting, and diarrhea.
- Monitor CBC for evidence of leukopenia and thrombocytopenia.
- Adjust etoposide dosage as needed.

etoposide ━━━◄ warfarin
VePesid   Coumadin

Risk rating: 2
Severity: Moderate   Onset: Delayed   Likelihood: Suspected

Cause
Warafin metabolism, clotting factor synthesis, and possibly protein displacement may be inhibited.

Effect
Anticoagulant effects increase.

Nursing considerations
- Monitor the patient PT and INR closely during and after chemo-therapy.
- Tell the patient to report any unusual bruising or bleeding.
- Remind the patient that warafin interacts with many drugs and that he should report any change in drug regimen.

ezetimibe ▬▶◀▬ cyclosporine

Zetia   Gengraf, Neoral, Sandimmune

Risk rating: 2
Severity: Moderate   Onset: Delayed   Likelihood: Suspected

Cause
The cause of this interaction is unknown.

Effect
Exposure to cyclosporine and ezetimibe may be increased, which consequently increases the therapeutic and adverse effects of both drugs.

Nursing considerations
- Monitor cyclosporine level.
- Adjust the dose of cyclosporine as needed.
- Carefully monitor cyclosporine level when starting, stopping, or adjusting ezetimibe therapy.
- Monitor the patient for adverse effects including shakiness, headache, tremor, hypertension, and fatigue.
- Monitor serum cholesterol and lipid levels to assess the patient's response to therapy.

felbamate ▬▶◀▬ carbamazepine

Felbatol   Carbatrol, Epitol, Equetro,
                               Tegretol

Risk rating: 2
Severity: Moderate   Onset: Delayed   Likelihood: Suspected

Cause
The mechanism of this interaction is unknown. Carbamazepine metabolism may increase, or conversion of carbamazepine metabolites may decrease. Also, felbamate metabolism may increase.

Effect
Carbamazepine and felbamate levels and effects may decrease.

Nursing considerations
- **⚠ ALERT** Monitor the patient for loss of seizure control.
- Monitor carbamazepine level; therapeutic range is 4 to 12 mcg/ml.
- Dosage may need adjustment when felbamate starts.
- Urge the patient to tell the prescribers about all drugs and supplements he takes.

felbamate ━━━▶◀━━━ phenytoin
Felbatol   Dilantin

Risk rating: 2
Severity: Moderate   Onset: Delayed   Likelihood: Probable

Cause
The mechanism of this interaction is unknown. Possibly felbamate inhibits metabolism of phenytoin. Phenytoin may increase the metabolism of felbamate.

Effect
Phenytoin levels, pharmacologic effects, and risk of toxicity may increase. Felbamate levels may decrease.

Nursing considerations
- Monitor the patient for changes in seizure control.
- If felbmate is added, consider reducing phenytoin dosage by 20%.
- Monitor phenytoin level; therapeutic range is 10 to 20 mcg/ml.
- Monitor the patient for signs of phenytoin toxicity, including drowsiness, nausea, vomiting, nystagmus, ataxia, dysarthria, tremor, slurred speech, hypotension, arrhythmias, respiratory depression, and coma.
- Toxic effects can occur at therapuetic level. Adjust the measured level for hypoalbuminemia or renal impairment, which can increase free drug level.

felbamate ━━━▶◀━━━ valproic acid
Felbatol   Depakene

Risk rating: 2
Severity: Moderate   Onset: Delayed   Likelihood: Probable

Cause
Felbamate inhibits metabolism of valproic acid.

Effect
Valproic acid level and risk of toxicity may increase.

Nursing considerations
- Monitor serum valproic acid level when the patient starts or stops felbamate, or takes an adjusted dose. Valproic acid dosage may need adjustment.
- If the patient takes valproic acid, start felbamate slowly, if possible.
- If felbamate must start quickly, valproic acid dosage may need to be reduced. Watch the patient closely.
- Watch for valproic acid toxicity, sedation, nausea, vomiting, pancreatitis, hemorrhage, emotional changes, and serious rash.

■ Teach the patient to watch for signs and symptoms of valproic toxicity, and to report them to the prescriber.

felodipine ◄►◄ carbamazepine
Plendil

Carbatrol, Epitol, Equetro, Tegretol

Risk rating: 2
Severity: Moderate   Onset: Delayed   Likelihood: Suspected

Cause
Felodipine metabolism may increase and availability decrease.

Effect
Felodipine effects may decrease.

Nursing considerations
■ Watch for loss of blood pressure control if the patient is started on carbamazepine.
■ Felodipine dose may need to be increased.
■ Watch for evidence of felodipine toxicity (peripheral vasodilation, hypotension, bradycardia, and palpitations) if the patient stops taking carbamazepine.
■ Advise the patient to tell the prescriber about all drugs and supplements he takes and about any increase in adverse effects.
■ Urge the patient to have blood pressure monitored if he starts on carbamazepine. Remind the patient that hypertension may cause no symptoms.

felodipine ◄►◄ erythromycin
Plendil

E-mycin, Eryc

Risk rating: 2
Severity: Moderate   Onset: Delayed   Likelihood: Suspected

Cause
Erythromycin inhibits the metabolism of felodipine.

Effect
Felodipine level, effects, and risk of adverse effects may increase.

Nursing considerations
■ Monitor the patient's response to felodipine when he starts or stops erythromycin therapy, or alters it in anyway, including changing the dose.

■ Wach for increased felodipine effects: prolonged hypotension, bradycardia, palpitation, flushing, headache, dizziness, and edema.
■ Urge the patient to tell the prescriber about increased adverse effects.
■ If an interaction is suspected, notify the prescriber or pharmacist. The dose may need to be altered.

---

felodipine ▶◀ grapefruit juice
Plendil

Risk rating: 2
Severity: Moderate   **Onset: Rapid**   **Likelihood: Probable**

Cause
Felodipine metabolism may be decreased by grapefruit juice.

Effect
Felodipine level, effects, and risk of adverse effects may increase.

Nursing considerations
⚡ **ALERT** Avoid giving felodipine with grapefruit juice.
■ Watch for increased felodipine effects: prolonged hypotension, bradycardia, palpitations, flushing, headache, dizziness, and edema.
■ Urge the patient to take felodipine with a beverage other than grapefruit juice.
■ Urge the patient to tell the prescriber about increased adverse effects.

---

felodipine ▶◀ itraconazole
Plendil   Sporanox

Risk rating: 2
Severity: Moderate   **Onset: Delayed**   **Likelihood: Suspected**

Cause
Itraconazole may inhibit felodipine CYP3A4 metabolism.

Effect
Felodipine level and adverse effects may increase.

Nursing considerations
■ Felodipine dose may need to be adjusted.
■ Closely monitor patients age 65 and older and patients with liver impairment. Both are at increased risk for elevated felodipine levels.
■ Monitor the patient for adverse felodipine effects, including increased peripheral edema, hypotension, and tachycardia.

■ Azole antifungals other than itraconazole may interact with felodipine. If you suspect an interaction, consult the prescriber or pharmacist.

■ Urge the patient to tell the prescriber about increased adverse effects.

felodipine ➤◄ phenytoin
Plendil   Dilantin

Risk rating: 2
Severity: Moderate   Onset: Delayed   Likelihood: Suspected

Cause
Phenytoin may increase felodipine metabolism and decrease its availability.

Effect
Felodipine effects may decrease.

Nursing considerations
■ Felodipine dose may need to be increased.
■ Watch for loss of blood pressure control in a patient who's taking felodipine and starts phenytoin.
■ Watch for evidence of felodipine toxicity (peripheral vasodilation, hypotension, bradycardia, and palpitations) if the patient stops phenytoin.
■ Urge the patient to have blood pressure monitored if phenytoin therapy starts. Remind the patient that hypertension may cause no symptoms.
■ Urge the patient to tell the prescriber about increased adverse effects.

fenofibrate ➤◄ HMG-CoA reductase inhibitors
Tricor   atorvastatin, lovastatin,
                                 pravastatin, rosuvastatin,
                                 simvastatin

Risk rating: 1
Severity: Major   Onset: Delayed   Likelihood: Suspected

Cause
The mechanism of interaction is unknown.

Effect
Severe myopathy or rhabdomyolysis may occur.

Nursing considerations
■ Avoid this combination.
■ If the patient has severe hyperlipidemia, combined therapy may be an option, but only with careful monitoring.
■ **ALERT** Assess the patient for evidence of rhabdomyolysis, including fatigue, muscle aches and weakness; joint pain; dark, red, or cola-colored urine; weight gain; seizures; and greatly increased serum CK level.
■ Watch for evidence of acute renal failure, including decreased urine output, elevated BUN and creatinine levels, edema, dyspnea, tachycardia, distended jugular veins, nausea, vomiting, poor appetite, weakness, fatigue, confusion, and agitation.
■ Urge the patient to report unexplained muscle pain, tenderness, or weakness to the prescriber.

---

fenofibrate ➤◄ warfarin
Coumadin

Risk rating: 1		
Severity: **Major**	Onset: **Delayed**	Likelihood: **Established**

Cause
Coagulation factor synthesis may be altered.

Effect
Hypoprothrombinemic effects of warfarin may increase.

Nursing considerations
■ Avoid use together if possible. If unavoidable, INR should be checked often.
■ **ALERT** Plasma warfarin level isn't affected by this interaction, but INR will increase. Hemorrhage and death may occur.
■ Tell the patient to report unusual bruising or bleeding.
■ Remind the patient that warfarin interacts with many drugs and that he should report any change in drug regimen.
■ Advise the patient to keep all follow-up medical appointments for proper monitoring and dosage adjustments

fentanyl ▶◀ amiodarone
Sublimaze   Cordarone, Pacerone

Risk rating: 1
Severity: Major   **Onset: Rapid**   **Likelihood: Suspected**

Cause
The mechanism of this interaction is unknown.

Effect
Risk of profound bradycardia, sinus arrest, and hypotension increases.

Nursing considerations
◄ **ALERT** Bradycardia caused by this interaction usually doesn't respond to atropine.
■ It isn't known if these effects are related to fentanyl anesthesia or anesthesia in general; use fentanyl and amiodarone cautiously together.
■ Monitor hemodynamic function.
■ Keep inotropic, chronotropic, and pressor support available.

fentanyl ▶◀ azole antifungals
Sublimaze   fluconazole, voriconazole

Risk rating: 1
Severity: Major   **Onset: Rapid**   **Likelihood: Suspected**

Cause
Azole antifungals inhibit CYP3A4 metabolism of fentanyl.

Effect
Fentanyl pharmacologic and adverse effects may increase.

Nursing considerations
◄ **ALERT** Carefully monitor the patient for increased effects of opioid analgesics, including respiratory depression, decreased LOC, and bradycardia.
■ Alert the prescriber about the risk of interaction between the opioid analgesic and the azole antifungal and discuss a possible decrease in opioid dosage.
■ Keep naloxone available to treat respiratory depression.
■ Monitor the patient's pain level and administer pain medication as needed to keep him comfortable, taking care not to prevent significant adverse effects.

fentanyl ━━━━▶◀ protease inhibitors
Sublimaze   atazanavir, ritonavir, saquinavir

Risk rating: 2
Severity: Moderate   **Onset: Delayed**   **Likelihood: Suspected**

Cause
Metabolism of fentanyl in the GI tract and liver may be inhibited.

Effect
Fentanyl level may increase and half-life lengthen.

Nursing considerations
◣ **ALERT** If the patient takes a protease inhibitor, watch closely for respiratory depression if fentanyl is added.
■ Because fentanyl half-life is prolonged, monitoring period should be extended, even after fentanyl is stopped.
■ Keep naloxone available to treat respiratory depression.
■ If fentanyl is continuously infused, dosage should be decreased.

fentanyl ━━━━▶◀ rifampin
Sublimaze   Rifadin, Rimactane

Risk rating: 2
Severity: Moderate   **Onset: Rapid**   **Likelihood: Suspected**

Cause
Rifampin may induce CYP3A4 metabolism of fentanyl

Effect
Fentanyl level and pharmacologic effects may decrease.

Nursing considerations
■ Monitor the patient's response when rifampin is started or discontinued. Be prepared to adjust fentanyl dosage as needed.
■ Explain that taking these drugs together may decrease therapuetic effects of fentanyl.
■ Monitor for adequate pain relief.

---

fexofenadine ▸◂ itraconazole
Allegra   Sporanox

Risk rating: 3
Severity: Minor   **Onset: Rapid**   **Likelihood: Suspected**

Cause
Itraconazole may increase absorption of fexofenadine.

Effect
Fexofenadine levels and pharmacologic and adverse effects may increase.

Nursing considerations
■ Monitor the patient for fexofenadine adverse reactions: drowsiness, headache, fatigue, nausea, dyspepsia, and dysmenorrhea.
■ Watch for expected clinical effects, including relief of seasonal allergic rhinitis or relief of chronic urticaria.
■ In patients with impaired renal function, maximum daily dosage recommendations of fexofenadine are 60 mg for adults and 30 mg for children.

---

flecainide ▸◂ amiodarone
Tambocor   Cordarone

Risk rating: 2
Severity: Moderate   **Onset: Delayed**   **Likelihood: Suspected**

Cause
Amiodarone decreases the metabolism of flecainide.

Effect
Flecainide plasma levels may be increased.

Nursing considerations
◤ **ALERT** Monitor the patient for prolonged QRS interval when giving both drugs together.
■ Decreasing flecainide dosage by 33% to 50% is recommended when the patient is also receiving amiodarone.
■ The full extent of the interaction may not be seen for up to 2 weeks.
■ Patients with heart failure may be at greater risk.

flecainide ━━━▶◀━━━ ritonavir
Tambocor   Norvir

Risk rating: 1
Severity: Major   **Onset: Delayed**   **Likelihood: Suspected**

Cause
Ritonavir may inhibit CYP2D6 metabolism of flecainide.

Effect
Flecainide level and risk of toxicity may increase.

Nursing considerations
▨ **ALERT** Ritonavir is contraindicated in patients taking flecainide.
■ Monitor serum flecainide level; therapeutic range is 0.2 to 1 mcg/ml.
■ Watch for flecainide toxicity: slowed or irregular pulse, palpitations, shortness of breath, hypotension, and new or worsened heart failure.
■ Monitor ECG for conduction disturbances (prolonged PR, QRS, and QT intervals), new or worsened arrhythmias, ventricular tachycardia, ventricular fibrillation, tachycardia, bradycardia, second- or third-degree AV block, and sinus arrest.

fluconazole ━━━▶◀━━━ benzodiazepines
Diflucan   alprazolam, chlordiazepoxide,
                                      midazolam, quazepam,
                                      triazolam

Risk rating: 2
Severity: Moderate   **Onset: Delayed**   **Likelihood: Established**

Cause
Azole antifungals such as fluconazole decrease CYP3A4 metabolism of certain benzodiazepines.

Effect
Benzodiazepine effects are increased and prolonged, which may cause CNS depression and psychomotor impairment.

Nursing considerations
■ If the patient takes fluconazole, talk with the prescriber about giving a lower benzodiazepine dose or a drug not metabolized by CYP3A4, such as temazepam or lorazepam.
■ Caution that the effects of this interaction may last several days after stopping the azole antifungal.
■ Explain the risk of sedation; tell the patient to report it promptly.

■ Explain alternative methods of inducing sleep or relieving anxiety during antifungal therapy.
■ Various azole antifungal–benzodiazepine combinations may interact. If you suspect an interaction, consult the prescriber or pharmacist.

fluconazole ━━━━▶◀━━━ carbamazepine
Diflucan   Carbatrol, Epitol, Equetro, Tegretol

Risk rating: 2
Severity: Moderate   **Onset: Delayed**   **Likelihood: Suspected**

Cause
Azole antifungals such as fluconazole may inhibit CYP3A4 metabolism of carbamazepine.

Effect
Carbamazepine effects, including adverse effects, may increase.

Nursing considerations
■ Monitor the patient's response when fluconazole is started or stopped.
■ Monitor carbamazepine level; therapeutic range is 4 to 12 mcg/ml.
🔰 **ALERT** Watch for signs of anorexia or subtle appetite changes, which may indicate an excessive carbamazepine level.
■ Monitor the patient for signs of carbamazepine toxicity, including dizziness, ataxia, respiratory depression, tachycardia, arrhythmias, blood pressure changes, impaired consciousness, abnormal reflexes, nystagmus, seizures, nausea, vomiting, and urine retention.
■ Other azole antifungals may interact with carbamazepine. If you suspect an interaction, consult the prescriber or pharmacist.

fluconazole ━━━━▶◀━━━ cyclophosphamide
Diflucan   Cytoxan

Risk rating: 2
Severity: Moderate   **Onset: Delayed**   **Likelihood: Suspected**

Cause
Fluconazole may inhibit cyclophosphamide hepatic metabolism.

Effect
Cyclophosphamide adverse effects may increase.

Nursing considerations

■ Closely monitor the patient for cyclophosphamide adverse effects during coadministration of fluconazole.
■ Watch for evidence of cyclophosphamide adverse effects including: cardiotoxcity, nausea, vomiting, cystitis, leukopenia, thrombocytopenia, hepatotoxcity, and pulmonary fibrosis.
■ Monitor CBC and renal and liver function tests.
■ Advise the patient to watch for signs of infection (fever, sore throat, fatigue) and bleeding (easy bruising, nosebleeds, bleeding gums, tarry stools).

---

fluconazole ➤◀ cyclosporine

Diflucan   Gengraf, Neoral, Sandimmune

Risk rating: 2
Severity: Moderate   **Onset: Delayed**   **Likelihood: Established**

Cause
Azole antifungals such as fluconazole decrease cyclosporine metabolism.

Effect
Cyclosporine level and toxicity may increase.

Nursing considerations
■ Cyclosporine level may increase 1 to 3 days after starting an azole antifungal and persist for more than 1 week after stopping it.
■ Monitor cyclosporine level.
■ Adjust cyclosporine dosage to maintain therapeutic level.
■ Cyclosporine dose may need to be decreased by 68% to 97%.
■ Monitor the patient for hepatotoxicity and nephrotoxicity.

---

fluconazole ➤◀ HMG-CoA reductase inhibitors

Diflucan   atorvastatin, fluvastatin, lovastatin, pravastatin, rosuvastatin, simvastatin

Risk rating: 1
Severity: Major   **Onset: Rapid**   **Likelihood: Probable**

Cause
Azole antifungals such as fluconazole may inhibit hepatic metabolism of HMG-CoA reductase inhibitors.

Effect
HMG-CoA reductase inhibitor level and adverse effects may increase.

Nursing considerations
- If possible, avoid the combination.
- HMG-CoA reductase inhibitor dosage may need to be decreased.
- Monitor serum cholesterol and lipid levels.

⚠ ALERT Assess the patient for evidence of rhabdomyolysis: fatigue; muscle aches and weakness; joint pain; dark, red, or cola-colored urine; weight gain; seizures; and greatly increased serum CK level.

- Pravastatin is least affected by this interaction and may be preferable for use with an azole antifungal, if needed.

---

fluconazole ➤◀ losartan
Diflucan   Cozaar

Risk rating: 3
Severity: Minor   **Onset: Delayed**   **Likelihood: Suspected**

Cause
Fluconazole inhibits the metabolism of losartan.

Effect
Losartan antihypertensive and adverse effects may increase.

Nursing considerations
- Closely monitor blood pressure response to losartan when fluconazole therapy is started, stopped, or doseage is adjusted.
- Observe the patient for adverse effects of losartan including hypotension, dizziness, chest pain, nausea, myalgia, cough, and angioedema.
- Monitor renal function including creatinine and BUN levels.

---

fluconazole ➤◀ NSAIDs
Diflucan   flurbiprofen, ibuprofen

Risk rating: 2
Severity: Moderate   **Onset: Delayed**   **Likelihood: Suspected**

Cause
Fluconazole inhibits metabolism of NSAIDs.

Effect
NSAID levels, pharmacologic effects, and adverse reactions increase.

Nursing considerations
■ Observe the patient for any increase in NSAID adverse reactions and adjust NSAID dose as needed.
■ Monitor for NSAID adverse reactions including: dizziness, fluid retention, tinnitus, abdominal pain, heartburn, acute renal failure, leukopenia, prolonged bleeding time, and thrombocytopenia.
■ Tell the patient to watch for and report signs and symptoms of GI bleeding, including blood in vomit, urine, or stool; coffee ground vomit; and black tarry stools.
■ Maximum daily NSAID dose should not exceed 1200 mg for adults.

---

fluconazole ▬▶◀▬ opioid analgesics
Diflucan   alfentanil, fentanyl

Risk rating: 1
Severity: Major   **Onset: Rapid**   **Likelihood: Suspected**

Cause
Azole antifungals such as fluconazole inhibit CYP3A4 metabolism of opioid analgesics.

Effect
Opioid pharmacologic and adverse effects may increase.

Nursing considerations
◪ ALERT Carefully monitor the patient for increased effects of opioid analgesics, including respiratory depression, decreased LOC, and bradycardia.
■ Alert the prescriber of the risk of interaction between the opioid analgesic and the azole antifungal and discuss a possible decrease in opioid dosage.
■ Keep naloxone available to treat respiratory depression.
■ Monitor the patient's pain level and administer pain medication as needed to keep him comfortable, but without significant adverse effects.

---

fluconazole ▬▶◀▬ phenytoin
Diflucan   Dilantin

Risk rating: 2
Severity: Moderate   **Onset: Delayed**   **Likelihood: Probable**

Cause
Fluconazole may inhibit hepatic meatabolism of phenytoin.

Effect

Phenytoin levels, pharmacologic, and risk of toxicity may increase.

Nursing considerations

- Monitor phenytoin levels and patient response if fluconazole therapy is started or stopped. Therapeutic range for phenytion is 10 to 20 mcg/ml.
- Phenytoin dose may need to be adjusted when fluconazole therapy is started or stopped.
- Toxic effects can occur at therapeutic levels. Adjust the measured level for patients who have hypoalbuminemia or renal impairment, which can increase the free drug level.
- Monitor the patient for signs and symptons of phenytoin toxicity, including drowsiness, nausea, vomiting, nystagmus, ataxia, dysarthria, tremor, slurred speech, hypotension, arryhythmias, respiratory depression, and coma.

---

fluconazole ━━▶◀━━ protease inhibitors

Diflucan   amprenavir, indinavir,
                                  ritonavir, saquinavir

Risk rating: 2
Severity: Moderate   **Onset: Delayed**   **Likelihood: Suspected**

Cause

Azole antifungals such as fluconazole may inhibit metabolism of protease inhibitors.

Effect

Protease inhibitor level may increase.

Nursing considerations

- Protease inhibitor dosage may need to be decreased.
- Watch for increased protease inhibitor effects: hyperglycemia, onset of diabetes, rash, GI complaints, and altered liver function tests.
- Advise the patient to report increased hunger or thirst, frequent urination, fatigue, and dry, itchy skin.
- Tell the patient not to change dosage or stop either drug without consulting the prescriber.

fluconazole ➤◀ rifamycins

Diflucan   rifabutin, rifampin

Risk rating: 2
Severity: Moderate   Onset: Delayed   Likelihood: Suspected

Cause
Rifamycins may decrease level of azole antifungals such as fluconazole.

Effect
Infection may recur.

Nursing considerations
■ Tell the prescriber about combined use; an alternative may be available.
■ If drugs must be taken together and the antifungal appears ineffective, antifungal dosage may need to be increased.
■ Teach the patient to recognize evidence of infection and to contact the prescriber promptly if it recurs.

fluconazole ➤◀ selective 5-HT1 receptor agonists

Diflucan   almotriptan, eletriptan

Risk rating: 2
Severity: Moderate   Onset: Delayed   Likelihood: Suspected

Cause
Azole antifungals such as fluconazole inhibit CYP3A4 metabolism of 5-HT_1 receptor agonists.

Effect
Selective 5-HT_1 receptor agonist level and adverse effects increase.

Nursing considerations
⚡ **ALERT** Don't give selective 5-HT_1 receptor agonists within 72 hours of azole antifungals.
■ Adverse effects of selective 5-HT_1 receptor agonists include coronary artery vasospasm, dizziness, nausea, paresthesia, and somnolence.
■ Other azole antifungals may have the same interaction.

fluconazole ━━━━►◄━━━━ sulfonylureas
Diflucan   glimepiride, tolbutamide

Risk rating: 2
Severity: Moderate   Onset: Delayed   Likelihood: Suspected

Cause
Fluconazole inhibits metabolism of sulfonylureas.

Effect
Hypoglycemic effects increase.

Nursing considerations
■ Monitor blood glucose levels.
■ Watch for evidence of hypoglycemia: tingling of lips and tongue, nausea, vomiting, epigastric pain, lethargy, confusion, agitation, tachycardia, diaphoresis, tremor, seizures, and coma.
■ Other sulfonylureas may interact with fluconazole. If you suspect an interaction, consult the prescriber or pharmacist.
■ If the patient takes a sulfonylurea, consult the prescriber about a different antifungal.
■ Urge the patient to monitor blood glucose level at home and to report increased episodes of hypoglycemia.

fluconazole ━━━━►◄━━━━ tacrolimus
Diflucan   Prograf

Risk rating: 2
Severity: Moderate   Onset: Delayed   Likelihood: Probable

Cause
Fluconazole inhibits tacrolimus metabolism in the liver and GI tract.

Effect
Tacrolimus level and risk of adverse effects may increase.

Nursing considerations
■ Monitor renal function and mental status closely.
■ Check tacrolimus level often. Normal trough level is 6 to 10 mcg/L.
■ Tacrolimus dosage may need to be decreased when the patient takes fluconazole.
■ Signs of toxicity often occur within 3 days of combined use.
◼ **ALERT** Watch for renal failure, nephrotoxicity, hyperkalemia, hyperglycemia, delirium, and other changes in mental status.

fluconazole ━━━━▶◀━━━━ tricyclic antidepressants
Diflucan   amitriptyline, imipramine,
                                  nortriptyline

Risk rating: 2
Severity: Moderate   **Onset: Delayed**   **Likelihood: Suspected**

Cause
Azole antifungals such as fluconazole may inhibit metabolism of tricyclic antidepressants (TCAs).

Effect
Serum TCA level and risk of toxicity may increase.

Nursing considerations
■ When starting or stopping an azole antifungal, monitor serum TCA level and adjust dosage as needed.
■ After starting fluconazole, check sitting and standing blood pressure for changes.
■ If the patient takes a TCA and an azole antifungal, assess symptoms and behavior for evidence of adverse reactions, such as increased drowsiness, dizziness, confusion, heart rate or rhythm changes, and urine retention.

fluconazole ━━━━▶◀━━━━ warfarin
Diflucan   Coumadin

Risk rating: 1
Severity: Major   **Onset: Delayed**   **Likelihood: Established**

Cause
Warfarin metabolism is inhibited.

Effect
Anticoagulant effects may increase.

Nursing considerations
■ Monitor PT and INR at least every 2 days.
■ Patients with renal insufficiency may be at greater risk.
■ Although all azole antifungals, including fluconazole, interact with warfarin, some interactions may be more significant than others.
■ Watch for evidence of bleeding.
■ Tell the patient to report unusual bruising or bleeding.
■ Remind the patient that warfarin interacts with many drugs, so he should report any change in drug regimen.

fluconazole ━━━▶◀━━━ zolpidem
Diflucan   Ambien

Risk rating: 2
Severity: Moderate   **Onset: Delayed**   **Likelihood: Suspected**

Cause
Fluconazole inhibits CYP3A4 metabolism of zolpidem.

Effect
Zolpidem levels and therapeutic effects may increase.

Nursing considerations
■ If the patient is taking fluconazole and zolpidem, monitor the patient's response. Zolpidem dosage may need to be decreased.
■ Teach the patient how to recognize the signs and symptoms that zolpidem levels are too high. Signs and symptoms include headache, daytime drowsiness, hangover, lethargy, lightheadedness, palpitations, abdominal pain, nausea, myalgia, and back or chest pain.
■ Caution the patient to avoid activities that require mental alertness or physical coordination during therapy.

fludrocortisone ━━━▶◀━━━ phenytoin
Florinef   Dilantin

Risk rating: 2
Severity: Moderate   **Onset: Delayed**   **Likelihood: Established**

Cause
Phenytoin induces liver enzymes, which stimulate metabolism of corticosteroids such as fludrocortisone.

Effect
Corticosteroid effects may decrease.

Nursing considerations
■ Avoid giving phenytoin with corticosteroids if possible.
■ Monitor the patient for decreased fludrocortisone effects. Also monitor phenytoin level, and adjust dosage of either drug as needed.
■ Corticosteroid effects may decrease within days of starting phenytoin and may stay at those levels for 3 weeks after the patient stops taking phenytoin.
■ Dosage of one—or both—drugs may need to be increased.

fludrocortisone ➤◀ rifampin
Florinef   Rifadin, Rimactane

Risk rating: 1
Severity: Major   **Onset: Delayed**   **Likelihood: Established**

Cause
Rifampin increases hepatic metabolism of corticosteroids such as fludrocortisone.

Effect
Corticosteroid effects may be decreased.

Nursing considerations
- If possible, avoid giving rifampin with corticosteroids such as fludrocortisone.
- Monitor the patient for decreased fludrocortisone effects, including loss of control over the disease.
- Watch closely for symptom control after increasing rifampin dose. The rifampin may need to be stopped so that fludrocortisone can do its work without interference, and help the patient regain control of the disease.
- Corticosteroid effects may decrease within days of starting rifampin and may stay at those levels for 2 to 3 weeks after the patient stops taking rifampin.
- Fludrocortisone dose may need to be doubled after adding rifampin to the patient's drug regimen.

fluorouracil ➤◀ warfarin
Adrucil, Carac,   Coumadin
Efudex

Risk rating: 1
Severity: Major   **Onset: Delayed**   **Likelihood: Suspected**

Cause
Warfarin metabolism, clotting factor synthesis, and possibly protein displacement may be inhibited.

Effect
Anticoagulant effects increase.

Nursing considerations
- Monitor PT and INR closely during and after chemotherapy.
- Tell the patient to report unusual bruising or bleeding.

■ Remind the patient that warfarin interacts with many drugs, so he should report any change in drug regimen to the prescriber or pharmacist.

---

fluoxetine ▬▬▶◀▬▬ carbamazepine
Prozac   Tegretol

Risk rating: 2
Severity: Moderate   Onset: Delayed   Likelihood: Suspected

Cause
The mechanism of this interaction is unknown. Fluoxetine may inhibit carbamazepine metabolism.

Effect
Carbamazepine level and risk of toxicity may increase.

Nursing considerations
■ Monitor carbamazepine level; therapeutic range is 4 to 12 mcg/ml.
⚠ ALERT Watch for signs of anorexia or subtle appetite changes, which may indicate an excessive carbamazepine level.
■ Monitor the patient for evidence of carbamazepine toxicity, including dizziness, ataxia, respiratory depression, tachycardia, arrhythmias, blood pressure changes, impaired consciousness, abnormal reflexes, nystagmus, seizures, nausea, vomiting, and urine retention.
■ Carbamazepine dosage may need adjustment if patient starts or stops taking fluoxetine.
■ If the patient starts fluoxetine during stabilized carbamazepine therapy, advise the patient to report nausea, vomiting, dizziness, visual disturbances, difficulty balancing, tremors, or any new adverse effects.
■ SSRIs other than fluoxetine may interact with carbamazepine. If you suspect a drug interaction, consult the prescriber or pharmacist.

---

fluoxetine ▬▬▶◀▬▬ clozapine
Prozac   Clozaril

Risk rating: 1
Severity: Major   Onset: Delayed   Likelihood: Established

Cause
SSRIs such as fluoxetine inhibit hepatic metabolism of clozapine.

Effect
Clozapine level and risk of toxicity increase.

Nursing considerations
- Not all SSRIs share this interaction. If you suspect an interaction, consult the prescriber or pharmacist.
- Monitor serum clozapine level.
- Assess the patient for increased adverse effects or toxicity, including agranulocytosis, ECG changes, and seizures.
- Adjust clozapine dose as needed when adding or withdrawing an SSRI to the patient's drug regimen.

---

fluoxetine ➤◀ cyclosporine
Prozac   Gengraf, Neoral, Sandimmune

Risk rating: 2
Severity: Moderate   Onset: Delayed   Likelihood: Suspected

Cause
SSRIs such as fluoxetine inhibit cyclosporine metabolism.

Effect
Cyclosporine level and risk of toxicity may increase.

Nursing considerations
- Consider use of citalopram as an alternative to fluoxetine because this interaction probably won't occur.
- Monitor cyclosporine level when adding or stopping fluoxetine.
- Adjust cyclosporine dose as needed.

---

fluoxetine ➤◀ cyproheptadine
Prozac   Periactin

Risk rating: 2
Severity: Moderate   Onset: Rapid   Likelihood: Suspected

Cause
Because cyproheptadine is a serotonin antagonist, the interaction is thought to occur at the receptor level.

Effect
Pharmacologic effects of SSRIs decrease.

Nursing considerations
- Monitor the clinical response to SSRIs such as fluoxetine.
- If loss of antidepressant efficacy occurs, discuss discontinuing cyproheptadine.

■ Depressive symptoms may resolve within 5 days of discontinuing this combination.

---

fluoxetine ━━━▶◀━━━ linezolid

Prozac   Zyvox

Risk rating: 1
Severity: Major   **Onset: Delayed**   **Likelihood: Suspected**

Cause
Serotonin may accumulate rapidly in the CNS.

Effect
The risk of serotonin syndrome increases.

Nursing considerations
⚠ **ALERT** Don't use these drugs together.
■ Allow 2 weeks after stopping linezoid before starting the patient on fluoxetine.
■ Allow 2 weeks after stopping an an SSRI such as fluoxetine and starting the patient on linezoid.
■ Make the patient aware of the signs and symptoms of serotonin syndrome, which include confusion, restlessness, uncoordination, muscle tremors and rigidity, fever, and sweating.
■ Explain that serotonin syndrome can be fatal if not treated immediately.

---

fluoxetine ━━━▶◀━━━ MAO inhibitors

Prozac, Sarafem   isocarboxazid, phenelzine,
                                selegiline, tranylcypromine

Risk rating: 1
Severity: Major   **Onset: Rapid**   **Likelihood: Probable**

Cause
Serotonin may accumulate rapidly in the CNS.

Effect
Risk of serotonin syndrome increases.

Nursing considerations
⚠ **ALERT** Don't use these drugs together.
■ Allow 5 weeks after stopping fluoxetine before starting the patient on an MAO inhibitor. Allow 2 weeks after stopping an MAO inhibitor before starting the patient on an SSRI such as fluoxetine.

■ The selective MAO type-B inhibitor selegiline has been given with fluoxetine, paroxetine, or sertraline—without negative effects—to patients with Parkinson's disease.

■ Make the patient aware of the signs and symptoms of serotonin syndrome, including CNS irritability, motor weakness, shivering, myoclonus, and altered consciousness.

■ Urge the patient to promptly report these and other adverse effects to the prescriber.

---

fluoxetine ▶◀ olanzapine

Prozac, Sarafem   Zyprexa, Symbyax

Risk rating: 3
Severity: Minor   **Onset: Delayed**   **Likelihood: Suspected**

Cause
Fluoxetine inhibits CYP2D6 metabolism of olanzapine.

Effect
Olanzapine levels may be increased.

Nursing considerations
■ Use together cautiously. Adjust olanzapine dose if an interaction is suspected.

■ Observe the patient's response to olanzapine when starting, stopping, or adjusting the dose.

■ Monitor olanzapine levels.

■ No significant adverse effects were reported due to this interaction.

---

fluoxetine ▶◀ phenothiazines

Prozac, Sarafem   chlorpromazine, thioridazine

Risk rating: 1
Severity: Major   **Onset: Delayed**   **Likelihood: Suspected**

Cause
Fluoxetine inhibits the metabolism of phenothiazines such as chlorpromazine.

Effect
Chlorpromazine levels and risk of life-threatening arrhythmias such as torsades de pointes may increase.

Nursing considerations
■ Closely monitor the ECG and QTc interval when administering chlorpromazine and fluoxetine together.

■ The risk of arrhythmias increases if the patient takes any other drugs that increase the QTc interval.
■ Ask the patient if he or any member of his family has a history of prologned QTc interval.

fluoxetine ▸◂ phenytoin
Prozac, Sarafem   Dilantin

Risk rating: 2
Severity: Moderate   Onset: Delayed   Likelihood: Suspected

Cause
Fluoxetine may inhibit phenytoin metabolism.

Effect
Serum phenytoin level, effects, and risk of toxicity may increase.

Nursing considerations
■ Monitor serum phenytoin level. Therapeutic range for phenytoin is 10 to 20 mcg/ml.
■ Phenytoin dosage may need adjustment.
■ Watch for evidence of phenytoin toxicity: drowsiness, nausea, vomiting, nystagmus, ataxia, dysarthria, tremor, slurred speech, hypotension, arrhythmias, respiratory depression, and coma.
■ Urge the patient to tell the prescriber about increased adverse effects.

fluoxetine ▸◂ propafenone
Prozac, Sarafem   Rythmol

Risk rating: 2
Severity: Moderate   Onset: Delayed   Likelihood: Suspected

Cause
Certain SSRIs such as fluoxetine may inhibit CYP2D6 metabolism of propafenone.

Effect
Propafenone level and risk of adverse effects may increase.

Nursing considerations
■ Monitor cardiac function closely.
■ Tell the patient to promptly report dizziness, drowsiness, ataxia, tremor, palpitations, chest pain, edema, dyspnea, and other new symptoms.
■ Citalopram doesn't inhibit CYP2D6 and may be a safer choice.

fluoxetine ➤◀ risperidone

Prozac, Sarafem   Risperdal

Risk rating: 1
Severity: Major   **Onset: Rapid**   **Likelihood: Suspected**

Cause
SSRIs such as fluoxetine may inhibit CYP2D6 metabolism of risperidone.

Effect
Risperidone level, risk of adverse reactions, and rapid accumulation of serotonin in the CNS may increase.

Nursing considerations
- Monitor the patient carefully if SSRI therapy starts or stops or if the dosage changes during risperidone therapy.
- Assess the patient for CNS irritability, increased muscle tone, muyscle twitching or jerking, and changes in level of consciousness.
- Advise the patient not to alter the dose of either drug without the advice of his prescriber.
- Average doses of fluoxetine may cause this interaction.

fluoxetine ➤◀ ritonavir

Prozac, Sarafem   Norvir

Risk rating: 2
Severity: Moderate   **Onset: Delayed**   **Likelihood: Suspected**

Cause
Fluoxetine and ritonavir may inhibit the CYP2D6 metabolism of each other.

Effect
The level of ritionavir may be increased. Risk of serotonin syndrome increases.

Nursing considerations
- If serotonin syndrome occurs, immediately stop fluoxetine.
- The increase level of ritonavir from this interaction doesn't increase the risk of adverse effects.
- Ritonavir may increase level of fluoxetine, causing cardiac and neurologic events such as syncope, vasodilation, anxiety, depression, dizziness, and seizures.
- Watch carefully for serotonin syndrome; it requires immediate attention.

- Describe the traits of serotonin syndrome: CNS irritability, motor weakness, shivering, muscle twitching, and altered consciousness.
- Explain that serotonin syndrome can be fatal if not treated immediately.

---

fluoxetine ▶◀ sibutramine
Prozac, Sarafem　　　　　Meridia

Risk rating: 1
Severity: Major　　　**Onset: Rapid**　　　**Likelihood: Suspected**

Cause
Serotonin may accumulate rapidly in the CNS.

Effect
Risk of serotonin syndrome increases.

Nursing considerations
◪ **ALERT** If possible, don't give these drugs together.
- Watch carefully for adverse effects; they need immediate attention.
- Describe traits of serotonin syndrome: CNS irritability, motor weakness, shivering, muscle twitching, and altered consciousness.
- Explain that serotonin syndrome can be fatal if not treated immediately.

---

fluoxetine ▶◀ sumatriptan
Prozac, Sarafem　　　　　Imitrex

Risk rating: 1
Severity: Major　　　**Onset: Rapid**　　　**Likelihood: Suspected**

Cause
Serotonin may accumulate rapidly in the CNS.

Effect
Risk of serotonin syndrome increases.

Nursing considerations
◪ **ALERT** If possible, avoid combined use of these drugs.
- Start with lowest dosages possible, and assess the patient closely.
- Stop sumatriptan at the first sign of interaction, and start an antiserotonergic.
- In some patients, migraine frequency may increase and antimigraine drug efficacy may decrease when an SSRI such as fluoxetine is started.

■ Describe traits of serotonin syndrome: CNS irritability, motor weakness, shivering, muscle twitching, and altered consciousness.
■ Explain that serotonin syndrome can be fatal if not treated immediately.

---

fluoxetine ▶◀ sympathomimetics

Prozac, Sarafem

amphetamine,
dextroamphetamine,
phentermine

Risk rating: 2
Severity: Moderate   **Onset: Rapid**   **Likelihood: Suspected**

Cause
The mechanism of this interaction is unknown.

Effect
Sympathomimetic effects and risk of serotonin syndrome increase.

Nursing considerations
■ Watch closely for increased CNS effects, such as anxiety, jitteriness, agitation, and restlessness.
■ Mild serotonin-like symptoms may develop, including anxiety, dizziness, restlessness, nausea, and vomiting.
■ Explain to the patient the risk posed by the interaction and why it's necessary to avoid sympathomimetics.
■ Make the patient aware of the signs and symptoms of serotonin syndrome: CNS irritability, motor weakness, shivering, myoclonus, and altered consciousness.

---

fluoxetine ▶◀ tricyclic antidepressants

Prozac, Sarafem

amitriptyline, desipramine,
doxepin, imipramine,
nortriptyline, protriptyline

Risk rating: 2
Severity: Moderate   **Onset: Rapid**   **Likelihood: Established**

Cause
Fluoxetine may inhibit hepatic metabolism of tricyclic antidepressants (TCAs).

Effect
Serum TCA level and toxicity may increase.

Nursing considerations

- Monitor serum TCA level and watch closely for evidence of toxicity, such as increased anticholinergic effects, delirium, dizziness, drowsiness, and psychosis.
- Report evidence of increased TCA level or toxicity; dosage may need to be decreased.
- If TCA starts when the patient already takes fluoxetine, TCA dosage may need to be decreased by up to 75% to avoid interaction.
- Inhibitory effects of fluoxetine may take several weeks to dissipate after drug is stopped.
- Other TCAs may interact with fluoxetine. If you suspect an interaction, consult the prescriber or pharmacist.

---

fluoxetine ◄►► tramadol

Prozac, Sarafem   Ultram, Ultracet

Risk rating: 1

Severity: Major   **Onset: Delayed**   **Likelihood: Suspected**

Cause
Additive serotonergic effects may occur.

Effect
Serotonin syndrome may occur.

Nursing considerations

- Watch closely for increased CNS effects, such as anxiety, jitteriness, agitation, and restlessness.
- If serotonin syndrome occurs, have patient stop the fluoxetine and obtain immediate medical attention.
- Make the patient aware of the signs and symptoms of serotonin syndrome: CNS irritability, motor weakness, shivering, myoclonus, and altered consciousness.
- Urge the patient to promptly report adverse effects.

---

fluphenazine ◄►► alcohol

Prolixin

Risk rating: 2

Severity: Moderate   **Onset: Rapid**   **Likelihood: Probable**

Cause
These substances may produce CNS depression by working on different sites in the brain. Also, alcohol may lower resistance to neurotoxic effects of phenothiazines such as fluphenazine.

Effect
CNS depression may increase.

Nursing considerations
■ Watch for extrapyramidal reactions, such as dystonic reactions and acute akathisia or restlessness.
■ If the patient takes a phenothiazine, warn that alcohol may worsen CNS depression and impair psychomotor skills.
■ Discourage alcohol consumption during phenothiazine therapy.

---

flurazepam ━━━▶◀━━━ **cimetidine**
Dalmane   Tagamet

Risk rating: 3		
Severity: **Minor**	Onset: **Rapid**	Likelihood: **Probable**

Cause
Hepatic metabolism of flurazepam may be decreased.

Effect
Serum levels of flurazepam may be increased, causing increased sedation.

Nursing considerations
◪ ALERT Carefully monitor the patient for increased sedation after taking cimetidine and flurazepam.
■ Warn the patient about the risk of increased sedation when taking cimetidine and flurazepam together.
■ If the patient has increased sedation, discuss the possibility of decreasing the dose of flurazepam with the prescriber.
■ Monitor serum benzodiazepine levels while the patient is taking cimetidine and flurazepam together.
◪ ALERT Elderly patients are at a higher risk for increased levels of sedation.

---

flurazepam ━━━▶◀━━━ **omeprazole**
Dalmane   Prilosec

Risk rating: 3		
Severity: **Minor**	Onset: **Delayed**	Likelihood: **Suspected**

Cause
Metabolism of benzodiazepines such as flurazepam may be decreased.

Effect
Half-life of flurazepam may be increased, leading to increased levels. Sedation or ataxia may be enhanced.

Nursing considerations
- Monitor the patient for increased sedation or CNS impairment.
- Consult the prescriber about reducing diazepam dosage.
- Other benzodiazepines may not have this interaction.

---

flurazepam ◄► **protease inhibitors**
Dalmane   atazanavir, darunavir, indinavir, nelfinavir, ritonavir, saquinavir

Risk rating: 1
Severity: Major   **Onset: Delayed**   **Likelihood: Suspected**

Cause
Protease inhibitors may inhibit CYP3A4 metabolism of certain benzodiazepines such as flurazepam.

Effect
Sedative effects may be increased and prolonged.

Nursing considerations
⚠ ALERT Don't combine flurazepam with protease inhibitors.
- If the patient takes any benzodiazepine-protease inhibitor combination, notify the prescriber. Interaction could involve related drugs.
- Watch for oversedation and respiratory depression.
- Teach the patient and his family about risks of taking these drugs together.

---

fluticasone ◄► **azole antifungals**
Flovent   itraconazole, ketoconazole

Risk rating: 2
Severity: Moderate   **Onset: Delayed**   **Likelihood: Suspected**

Cause
Inhibition of CYP3A4 metabolism of fluticasone and decrease in elimination.

Effect
Corticosteroid effects and toxicity may be increased.

Nursing considerations
- Monitor the patient for increased adverse effects of fluticasone and adjust dose as needed.
- Monitor the patient taking a corticosteroid and an azole antifungal for Cushing syndrome.
- Watch the patient closely for infection, edema, and increased serum glucose level.
- Caution the patient not to abruptly stop fluticasone; the drug dose should gradually be tapered to prevent withdrawal symptoms.

---

fluvastatin ━━━▶◀━━━ **azole antifungals**
Lescol   fluconazole, itraconazole, ketoconazole

Risk rating: 1
Severity: Major   **Onset: Rapid**   **Likelihood: Probable**

Cause
Azole antifungals may inhibit hepatic metabolism of HMG-CoA reductase inhibitors such as fluvastatin.

Effect
Fluvastatin level and adverse effects may increase.

Nursing considerations
- If possible, avoid this combination.
- Fluvastatin dosage may need to be decreased.
- Monitor serum cholesterol and lipid levels.
- ◪ ALERT Assess the patient for evidence of rhabdomyolysis, including fatigue; muscle aches and weakness; joint pain; dark, red, or cola-colored urine; weight gain; seizures; and greatly increased CK level.
- Pravastatin is the HMG-CoA reductase inhibitor least affected by this interaction and may be preferable to use with an azole antifungal.

---

fluvastatin ━━━▶◀━━━ **cholestyramine**
Lescol   Locholest, Prevalite, Questran

Risk rating: 4
Severity: Moderate   **Onset: Delayed**   **Likelihood: Possible**

Cause
GI absorption of HMG-CoA reductase inhibitor may decrease.

Effect
HMG-CoA reductase inhibitor and pharmacologic effects may decrease.

Nursing considerations
⚠ **ALERT** Separate doses of HMG-CoA reductase inhibitor and cholestyramine, a bile acid sequestrant, by at least 4 hours.
■ If possible, give cholestyramine before meals and the HMG-CoA reductase inhibitor in the evening.
■ Monitor serum cholesterol and lipid levels to assess patient's response to therapy.
■ Help the patient develop a daily plan to ensure proper intervals between drug doses.

---

fluvastatin ▶◀ warfarin
Lescol   Coumadin

Risk rating: 2
Severity: Moderate   **Onset: Delayed**   **Likelihood: Probable**

Cause
Hepatic metabolism of warfarin may be inhibited.

Effect
Anticoagulant effects may increase.

Nursing considerations
■ Monitor PT and INR closely when starting or stopping fluvastatin.
■ Atorvastatin and pravastatin, other HMG-CoA reductase inhibitors, don't appear to have this interaction with warfarin and may be better treatment options.
■ Tell the patient to report unusual bruising or bleeding.
■ Remind the patient that warfarin interacts with many drugs and that he should report any change in drug regimen.
■ Advise the patient to keep all follow-up medical appointments for proper monitoring and dosage adjustments.

---

fluvoxamine ▶◀ buspirone
Luvox   BuSpar

Risk rating: 3
Severity: Minor   **Onset: Delayed**   **Likelihood: Suspected**

Cause
CYP3A4 metabolism of buspirone may be inhibited by fluvoxamine.

Effect
Buspirone level may increase.

Nursing considerations
■ Monitor the patient's clinical response to buspirone while taking fluvoxamine.
■ The dose of buspirone may need to be adjusted.

---

fluvoxamine ▶◀ **clozapine**

Luvox   Clozaril

Risk rating: 1
Severity: Major   **Onset: Delayed**   **Likelihood: Established**

Cause
SSRIs such as fluvoxamine inhibit hepatic metabolism of clozapine.

Effect
Clozapine level and risk of toxicity increase.

Nursing considerations
■ Not all SSRIs share this interaction. If you suspect an interaction, consult the prescriber or pharmacist.
■ Monitor serum clozapine level.
■ Assess the patient for increased adverse effects or toxicity, including agranulocytosis, ECG changes, and seizures.
■ Observe the patient's clinical response when adjusting clozapine dose or when adding or withdrawing an SSRI.

---

fluvoxamine ▶◀ **cyclosporine**

Luvox   Gengraf, Neoral, Sandimmune

Risk rating: 2
Severity: Moderate   **Onset: Delayed**   **Likelihood: Suspected**

Cause
SSRIs inhibit cyclosporine metabolism.

Effect
Cyclosporine level and risk of toxicity may increase.

Nursing considerations
■ Consider use of citalopram as an alternative to fluvoxamine because this interaction probably won't occur.
■ Monitor cyclosporine level when adding or stopping fluvoxamine.
■ Adjust cyclosporine dose as needed.

fluvoxamine ━━━▶◀━━━ phenytoin
Luvox   Dilantin

Risk rating: 2
Severity: Moderate   **Onset: Delayed**   **Likelihood: Suspected**

Cause
Fluvoxamine may inhibit CYP2C9 and CYP2C19 metabolism of
phenytoin.

Effect
Phenytoin level, pharmacologic, and risk of toxic effects may increase.

Nursing considerations
■ Monitor serum phenytoin level. Therapeutic range for phenytoin is
10 to 20 mcg/ml.
■ Phenytoin dosage may need adjustment.
■ When fluvoxamine starts, watch for phenytoin toxicity: drowsiness,
nausea, vomiting, nystagmus, ataxia, dysarthria, tremor, slurred
speech, hypotension, arrhythmias, respiratory depression, and coma.
■ When fluvoxamine stops, watch for loss of anticonvulsant effect and
increased seizure activity.

fluvoxamine ━━━▶◀━━━ sibutramine
Luvox   Meridia

Risk rating: 1
Severity: Major   **Onset: Rapid**   **Likelihood: Suspected**

Cause
Serotonin may accumulate rapidly in the CNS.

Effect
Risk of serotonin syndrome increases.

Nursing considerations
◪ **ALERT** If possible, don't give these drugs together.
■ Watch carefully for adverse effects; they need immediate attention.
■ Teach the patient to recognize signs and symptoms of serotonin syn-
drome: CNS irritability, motor weakness, shivering, muscle twitching,
and altered consciousness.
■ Explain that serotonin syndrome can be fatal if not treated immedi-
ately.

fluvoxamine ━━▶◀━━ tacrine
Luvox   Cognex

Risk rating: 2
Severity: Moderate   Onset: Delayed   Likelihood: Suspected

Cause
Fluvoxamine may inhibit CYP1A2 metabolism of tacrine.

Effect
Tacrine level, effects, and adverse effects may increase.

Nursing considerations
- Avoid this combination if possible.
- If combined use can't be avoided, watch for tacrine toxicity: nausea, vomiting, salivation, sweating, bradycardia, hypotension, and seizures.
- **⚡ ALERT** Watch for progressive muscle weakness (a symptom of tacrine toxicity), which can be fatal if respiratory muscles are involved.
- Monitor liver function tests. Urge the patient to report signs of hepatotoxicity: abdominal pain, loss of appetite, fatigue, yellow skin or eye discoloration, and dark urine.
- Consult the prescriber or pharmacist; SSRIs such as fluoxetine that aren't metabolized by CYP1A2 metabolism may be safer alternatives.

fluvoxamine ━━▶◀━━ theophylline
Luvox   Theo-dur, Theolair

Risk rating: 2
Severity: Moderate   Onset: Delayed   Likelihood: Suspected

Cause
Fluvoxamine inhibits hepatic CYP1A2 metabolism of theophylline.

Effect
Theophylline level and risk of toxicity may increase.

Nursing considerations
- When adding fluvoxamine to the regimen, monitor theophylline level closely. Therapeutic range is 10 to 20 mcg/ml for adults and 5 to 15 mcg/ml for children.
- If a patient who takes fluvoxamine starts theophylline, theophylline dosage may be reduced by 33%.
- Watch for evidence of toxicity: tachycardia, anorexia, nausea, vomiting, diarrhea, seizures, restlessness, irritability, and headache.

■ Describe adverse effects of theophylline and signs of toxicity, and tell the patient to report them immediately.

fluvoxamine ▸◂ thioridazine
Luvox

Risk rating: 1
Severity: Major   **Onset: Delayed**   **Likelihood: Suspected**

Cause
Fluvoxamine may inhibit metabolism of thioridazine.

Effect
Risk of life-threatening arrhythmias and other adverse effects may increase.

Nursing considerations
◩ ALERT Use of these drugs together is contraindicated.
■ Life-threatening torsades de pointes may result.
■ This interaction continues for more than 2 weeks after fluvoxamine is stopped.
■ Other possible adverse effects include tardive dyskinesia, neuroleptic malignant syndrome, constipation, orthostatic hypotension, and urine retention.

fluvoxamine ▸◂ tricyclic antidepressants
Luvox   amitriptyline, clomipramine, imipramine, trimipramine

Risk rating: 2
Severity: Moderate   **Onset: Delayed**   **Likelihood: Probable**

Cause
Fluvoxamine may inhibit oxidative metabolism of tricyclic antidepressants (TCAs) via CYP2D6 pathway.

Effect
TCA level and risk of toxicity increase.

Nursing considerations
■ If combined use can't be avoided, TCA dosage may be decreased.
■ When starting or stopping fluvoxamine, monitor serum TCA level.
■ Report evidence of toxicity or increased TCA level.
■ Inhibitory effects of fluvoxamine may take up to 2 weeks to dissipate after drug is stopped.
■ Using the TCA, desipramine, may avoid this interaction.

■ Urge the patient and his family to watch for and report increased anticholinergic effects, such as confusion, blurred vision, constipation, dry mouth and dizziness, along with drowsiness and psychosis.

---

folic acid ━━━━━━▸◂━━━━━ phenytoin
Folvite   Dilantin

Risk rating: 2
Severity: Moderate   Onset: Delayed   Likelihood: Suspected

Cause
The mechanism of this interaction is unknown but probably involves altered metabolic process.

Effect
Phenytoin level and effects may decrease.

Nursing considerations
■ Monitor phenytoin level. Therapeutic range for phenytoin is 10 to 20 mcg/ml.
■ Phenytoin dosage may need adjustment.
■ If folic acid is started during phenytoin therapy, watch for loss of anticonvulsant effect and increased seizure activity.
■ If folic acid is stopped during phenytoin therapy, watch for evidence of phenytoin toxicity: drowsiness, nausea, vomiting, nystagmus, ataxia, dysarthria, tremor, slurred speech, hypotension, arrhythmias, respiratory depression, and coma.
■ Urge the patient to tell the prescriber about increased adverse effects.

---

fosamprenavir ━━━━▸◂━━━ non-nucleoside reverse transcriptase inhibitors
Lexiva   efavirenz, nevirapine

Risk rating: 2
Severity: Moderate   Onset: Delayed   Likelihood: Suspected

Cause
Increased CYP3A4 metabolism of protease inhibitors such as fosamprenavir.

Effect
Protease inhibitor plasma levels and efficacy may be reduced.

Nursing considerations
- Monitor protease inhibitor levels and clinical response when the patient starts or stops a non-nucleoside reverse transcriptase inhibitor such as efavirenz.
- Adjust protease inhibitor dosage as needed.
- Tell the patient not to alter HIV regimen without consulting the prescriber.

---

fosamprenavir ►◄ pimozide
Lexiva   Orap

Risk rating: 1
Severity: Major   **Onset: Delayed**   **Likelihood: Suspected**

Cause
Protease inhibitors such as fosamprenavir may inhibit CYP3A4 metabolism of pimozide.

Effect
Risk of life-threatening arrhythmias may increase.

Nursing considerations
- **ALERT** Combined use of these drugs is contraindicated.
- Arrhythmias are related to prolonged QT interval, a known risk of pimozide.
- Interaction warning is based on pharmokinetics of these drugs, not actual patient studies.

---

foscarnet ►◄ cyclosporine
Foscavir   Gengraf, Neoral, Sandimmune

Risk rating: 1
Severity: Major   **Onset: Delayed**   **Likelihood: Suspected**

Cause
Synergistic drug effects may cause nephrotoxicity.

Effect
Risk of renal failure may be increased.

Nursing considerations
- Base foscarnet dosage on the patient's renal function.
- Expect cyclosporine level to stay within normal limits.
- Monitor renal function carefully.
- If nephrotoxicity occurs, foscarnet may need to be stopped.
- Nephrotoxicity should resolve once foscarnet is stopped.

fosphenytoin ━━▶◀━━ chloramphenicol
Cerebyx   Chloromycetin

Risk rating: 2
Severity: Moderate   **Onset: Delayed**   **Likelihood: Suspected**

Cause
Fosphenytoin metabolism is altered.

Effect
 Fosphenytoin level and increased toxicty may occur. Chloramphenicol concentration may change.

Nursing considerations
- Monitor drug levels closely. Dosage may need to be adjusted.
- The therapeutic range for phenytoin is 10 to 20 mcg/ml.
- Toxic effects of fosphenytoin can occur at therapeutic level. Adjust the measured level for hypoalbuminia or renal impairment.
- Signs and symptoms of phenytoin toxicity include nystagmus, slurred speech, ataxia, blurred or double vision, confusion, drowsiness, and lethargy.
- This interaction may occur with other hydantoins.

frovatriptan ━━▶◀━━ ergot derivatives
Frova   dihydroergotamine, ergotamine

Risk rating: 1
Severity: Major   **Onset: Rapid**   **Likelihood: Suspected**

Cause
Combined use may have additive effects.

Effect
Risk of vasospastic effects increases.

Nursing considerations
 ⚑ **ALERT** Use of these drugs or any two selective 5-HT$_1$ receptor agonists within 24 hours of each other is contraindicated.
- Combined use may cause severe vasospastic effects, including sustained coronary artery vasospasm that triggers MI.
- Warn the patient not to mix migraine headache drugs within 24 hours of each other, but to call the prescriber if a drug isn't effective.

furosemide ▶◀ aminoglycosides
Lasix

gentamicin, streptomycin, tobramycin

Risk rating: 1
Severity: Major   **Onset: Rapid**   **Likelihood: Suspected**

Cause
The mechanism of this interaction is unknown.

Effect
Synergistic ototoxicity may cause hearing loss of varying degrees, possibly permanent.

Nursing considerations
⚠ **ALERT** Patients with renal insufficiency are at increased risk for ototoxicity.
■ Perform baseline and periodic hearing function tests.
■ Other aminoglycosides may interact with loop diuretics such as furosemide. If you suspect an interaction, consult the prescriber or pharmacist.
■ Tell the patient to immediately report ringing or roaring in the ears, muffled sounds, or any noticeable changes in hearing.
■ Advise family members to stay alert for evidence of hearing loss.

furosemide ▶◀ captopril
Lasix

Capoten

Risk rating: 3
Severity: Minor   **Onset: Delayed**   **Likelihood: Suspected**

Cause
Inhibition of angiotensin II production by captopril.

Effect
The effects of loop diuretics such as furosemide may be decreased.

Nursing considerations
■ Monitor fluid status and body weight in a patient taking furosemide when captopril therapy is started, stopped, or the dosage is adjusted.
■ Weigh the patient daily.
■ Monitor the patient for expected furosemide effects: reduction in peripheral edema, resolution of pulmonary edema, or decreased blood pressure in hypertensive patients.

furosemide ◄►► cholestyramine

Lasix   Locholest, Prevalite, Questran

Risk rating: 2
Severity: Moderate   **Onset: Rapid**   **Likelihood: Suspected**

Cause
Cholestyramine may bind to furosemide, inhibiting furosemide absorption.

Effect
Furosemide effects may decrease.

Nursing considerations
■ Cholestyramine should be taken at least 2 hours after furosemide.
■ Monitor the patient for expected furosemide effects, including reduction in peripheral edema, resolution of pulmonary edema, and decreased blood pressure in hypertensive patients.
■ If furosemide is needed, consult the prescriber or pharmacist about alternative cholesterol-lowering therapy.
■ Bile acid sequestrants other than cholestyramine may interact with furosemide. If you suspect a drug interaction, consult the prescriber or pharmacist.

furosemide ◄►► cisplatin

Lasix   Platinol

Risk rating: 2
Severity: Moderate   **Onset: Rapid**   **Likelihood: Suspected**

Cause
The mechanism of this interaction is unknown.

Effect
Additive ototoxicity may be much more severe than that of either drug used alone, causing permanent hearing loss.

Nursing considerations
■ If possible, avoid giving loop diuretics such as furosemide with cisplatin.
■ Obtain hearing tests to detect early hearing loss.
■ Tell the patient to report ringing in the ears, change in balance, or muffled sounds. Also, ask family members to watch for changes.

furosemide ◄► colestipol
Lasix   Colestid

Risk rating: 2
Severity: Moderate   **Onset: Rapid**   **Likelihood: Suspected**

Cause
Colestipol may bind to furosemide, inhibiting furosemide absorption.

Effect
Furosemide effects may decrease.

Nursing considerations
- Separate doses; colestipol should be taken at least 2 hours after furosemide.
- Monitor the patient for expected furosemide effects, including reduction in peripheral edema, resolution of pulmonary edema, and decreased blood pressure in hypertensive patients.
- Monitor urine output and blood pressure to assess diuretic effect.
- If furosemide must be used, consult the prescriber or pharmacist about alternative cholesterol-lowering therapy.
- Help the patient develop a daily plan to ensure proper intervals between drug doses.
- Bile acid sequestrants other than colestipol may interact with furosemide. If you suspect an interaction, consult the prescriber or pharmacist.

furosemide ◄► digoxin
Lasix   Lanoxin

Risk rating: 1
Severity: Major   **Onset: Delayed**   **Likelihood: Probable**

Cause
Urinary excretion of potassium and magnesium is increased.

Effect
Electrolyte disturbances may predispose the patient to digitalis-induced arrhythmias.

Nursing considerations
- Monitor serum potassium and magensium levels; decreased levels may predispose the patient to arrhythmias.
- Carefully monitor the patient's ECG while receiving digoxin and a loop diuretic such as furosemide.
- If the patient develops hypomagnesimia or hypokalemia, be prepared to administer supplements.

- Monitor the patient for increased serum sodium.
- Changing the patient from a loop-diuretic to a potassium-sparing diuretic will minimize the risk of arrhythmias.
- This interaction appears to be dose related.

---

furosemide ━━━▶◀━━━ lithium

Lasix   Eskalith

Risk rating: 2
Severity: Moderate   Onset: Delayed   Likelihood: Suspected

Cause
The mechanism of this interaction is unknown.

Effect
Increased lithium levels and risk of toxicity may occur.

Nursing considerations
- Monitor serum lithium levels. Steady state lithium level should be 0.6 to 1.2 mEq/L.
- Adjust lithium dose as needed.
- Monitor the patient for evidence of lithium toxicity, such as diarrhea, vomiting, dehydration, drowsiness, muscle weakness, tremor, fever, and ataxia.
- Despite this interaction, lithium and loop diuretics may be used together safely, with close monitoring of the lithium level.

---

furosemide ━━━▶◀━━━ phenytoin

Lasix   Dilantin

Risk rating: 3
Severity: Minor   Onset: Delayed   Likelihood: Suspected

Cause
Reduced oral absorption of furosemide may occur.

Effect
Phenytoin may reduce furosemide effects.

Nursing considerations
- Patients taking phenytoin, may need to have an increase in furosemide dose.
- Monitor diuretic response.
- Monitor the patient for expected furosemide effects: reduction in peripheral edema, resolution of pulmonary edema, or decreased blood pressure in hypertensive patients.

furosemide ━━━━▶◀━━━━ thiazide diuretics
Lasix   hydrochlorothiazide,
                                   metolazone

Risk rating: 2
Severity: Moderate   **Onset: Rapid**   **Likelihood: Probable**

Cause
The mechanism of this interaction is likely a renal tubular mechanism.

Effect
Because these drugs work synergistically, they may cause profound diuresis and serious electrolyte abnormalities.

Nursing considerations
- This combination may be used for therapeutic benefit.
- Expect increased sodium, potassium, and chloride excretion and greater diuresis during combined therapy.
- Monitor the patient for dehydration and electrolyte abnormalities.

ganciclovir ━━━━▶◀━━━━ zidovudine
Cytovene   AZT, Retrovir

Risk rating: 1
Severity: Major   **Onset: Delayed**   **Likelihood: Probable**

Cause
The mechanism of interaction is unknown.

Effect
Combining ganciclovir with zidovudine increases the risk of severe hematologic toxicities, including anemia, neutropenia, and leukopenia.

Nursing considerations
- Use together should be avoided. Foscarnet may be an adequate substitute for ganciclovir.
- Monitor CBC with differential.
- Use together may warrant reduction of ganciclovir dosage.
- Explain that adverse hematologic effects may not appear for 3 to 5 weeks. Tell the patient to report symptoms of infection, such as fever, sore throat, and unexplained tiredness.

gatifloxacin ━━━▶◀━━━ antiarrhythmics

Tequin

amiodarone, bretylium,
disopyramide, procainamide,
quinidine, sotalol

Risk rating: 1
Severity: Major   **Onset: Delayed**   **Likelihood: Suspected**

Cause
The mechanism of this interaction is unknown.

Effect
Risk of life-threatening arrhythmias, including torsades de pointes,
increases when certain quinolones such as gatifloxacin are combined
with antiarrhythmics.

Nursing considerations
- Avoid giving class IA or class III antiarrhythmics with gatifloxacin.
- Quinolones that aren't metabolized by CYP3A4 isoenzymes or that
don't prolong the QT interval may be given with antiarrhythmics.
- Monitor ECG for prolonged QTc interval.
- Tell the patient to report a rapid heartbeat, shortness of breath,
dizziness, fainting, and chest pain.

gatifloxacin ━━━▶◀━━━ erythromycin

Tequin

E-mycin, Eryc

Risk rating: 1
Severity: Major   **Onset: Delayed**   **Likelihood: Suspected**

Cause
The mechanism of this interaction is unknown.

Effect
Risk of life-threatening arrhythmias, including torsades de pointes,
increases when certain quinolones such as gatifloxacin are combined
with erythromycin.

Nursing considerations
- Use gatifloxacin cautiously with erythromycin.
- Monitor the QTc interval closely.
- Tell the patient to report palpitations, dizziness, shortness of breath,
and chest pain.

gatifloxacin ▰▰▰▰►◄ imipramine
Tequin   Tofranil

Risk rating: 1
Severity: Major **Onset: Delayed**   **Likelihood: Suspected**

Cause
The mechanism of this interaction is unknown.

Effect
Life-threatening arrhythmias, including torsades de pointes, may increase when certain quinolones such as gatifloxacin are combined with tricyclic antidepressants (TCAs) such as imipramine.

Nursing considerations
- Use gatifloxacin cautiously with TCAs such as imipramine.
- If possible, use other quinolone antibiotics that don't prolong the QTc interval or aren't metabolized by the CYP3A4 isoenzyme.

gatifloxacin ▰▰▰▰►◄ ziprasidone
Tequin   Geodon

Risk rating: 1
Severity: Major   **Onset: Delayed**   **Likelihood: Suspected**

Cause
The mechanism of this interaction is unknown.

Effect
Risk of life-threatening arrhythmias, including torsades de pointes, increases.

Nursing considerations
⚠ **ALERT** Use of ziprasidone with a quinolone such as gatifloxacin is contraindicated.
- Monitor the patient for other risk factors for torsades de pointes, including bradycardia, hypokalemia, and hypomagnesemia.
- Ask the patient if he or anyone in his family has a history of prolonged QT intervals or arrhythmias.
- Monitor the patient for bradycardia.
- Measure the QTc interval at baseline and throughout therapy.

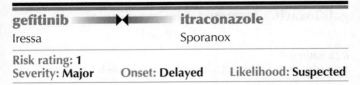

gefitinib ▶◀ itraconazole
Iressa   Sporanox

Risk rating: 1
Severity: Major   **Onset: Delayed**   **Likelihood: Suspected**

Cause
Azole antifungals such as itraconazole may inhibit metabolism (CYP3A4) of gefitinib.

Effect
Gefitinib levels and risk of adverse reactions may be increased.

Nursing considerations
■ If the patient receives gefitinib, observe for adverse reactions if itraconazole is added to the treatment.
■ Encourage the patient to report signs and symptoms of adverse reactions including: eye problems such as pain, redness, or vision changes; diarrhea, vomiting, or loss of appetite; rash or itching; weakness; weight loss; and liver damage.
⚠ **ALERT** The FDA has limited the use of gefitinib to certain patient populations. New clinical trials are being developed to determine future benefits of this drug.

gefitinib ▶◀ rifampin
Iressa   Rifadin, Rimactane

Risk rating: 2
Severity: Moderate   **Onset: Delayed**   **Likelihood: Suspected**

Cause
Rifamycins such as rifampin may increase the metabolism of gefitinib.

Effect
Gefitinib levels and efficacy may may be reduced.

Nursing considerations
■ Monitor clinical response to gefitinib when starting or stopping rifampin therapy.
■ Adjust the gefitinib dose as needed.
■ Encourage the patient to report signs and symptoms of adverse reactions including: eye problems such as pain, redness, or vision changes; diarrhea, vomiting, or loss of appetite; rash or itching; weakness; weight loss; and liver damage.

ALERT The FDA has limited the use of gefitinib to certain patient populations. New clinical trials are being developed to determine future benefits of this drug.

---

gefitinib 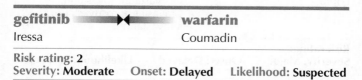 warfarin
Iressa   Coumadin

Risk rating: 2
Severity: Moderate   Onset: Delayed   Likelihood: Suspected

Cause
The mechanism of this interaction is unknown.

Effect
Anticoagulant effects and risk of bleeding may increase.

Nursing considerations
- Monitor coagulation values closely when starting or stopping gefitinib.
- Adjust the wafarin dose as needed.
- Tell the patient to report unusual bruising or bleeding.
- Remind the patient that warfarin interacts with many other drugs, and tell the patient to report any change in drug regimen.

ALERT The FDA has limited the use of gefitinib to certain patient populations. New clinical trials are being developed to determine future benefits of this drug.

---

gemcitabine 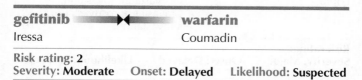 warfarin
Gemzar   Coumadin

Risk rating: 1
Severity: Major   Onset: Delayed   Likelihood: Suspected

Cause
Warfarin metabolism, clotting factor synthesis, and possibly protein displacement may be inhibited.

Effect
Anticoagulant effects increase.

Nursing considerations
- Monitor PT and INR closely during and after chemotherapy.
- Tell the patient to report unusual bruising or bleeding.
- Remind the patient that warfarin interacts with many drugs, and tell the patient to report any change in drug regimen.

gemfibrozil ━━━▶◀━━━ HMG-CoA reductase inhibitors

Lopid

atorvastatin, lovastatin, pravastatin, rosuvastatin, simvastatin

Risk rating: 1
Severity: Major   **Onset: Delayed**   **Likelihood: Suspected**

Cause
The mechanism of this interaction is unknown.

Effect
Severe myopathy or rhabdomyolysis may occur.

Nursing considerations
⚡ **ALERT** Avoid use together.
■ If the patient has severe hyperlipidemia, combined therapy may be an option, but only with careful monitoring.
■ Assess the patient for evidence of rhabdomyolysis: fatigue; muscle aches and weakness; joint pain; dark, red, or cola-colored urine; weight gain; seizures; and greatly increased CK level.
■ Watch for evidence of acute renal failure: decreased urine output, elevated BUN and creatinine levels, edema, dyspnea, tachycardia, distended jugular veins, nausea, vomiting, poor appetite, weakness, fatigue, confusion, and agitation.
■ Urge the patient to report muscle pain, tenderness, or weakness.

gemfibrozil ━━━▶◀━━━ warfarin

Lopid

Coumadin

Risk rating: 1
Severity: Major   **Onset: Delayed**   **Likelihood: Established**

Cause
Coagulation factor synthesis may be altered.

Effect
Hypoprothrombinemic effects of warfarin may increase.

Nursing considerations
■ Avoid use together if possible. If unavoidable, INR should be checked often.
⚡ **ALERT** Plasma warfarin level isn't affected by this interaction, but INR will increase. Hemorrhage and death may occur.
■ Tell the patient to report unusual bruising or bleeding.

■ Remind the patient that warfarin interacts with many drugs, and tell the patient to report any change in drug regimen.
■ Advise the patient to keep all follow-up medical appointments for proper monitoring and dosage adjustments.

gentamicin ▶◀ cephalosporins
Garamycin   ceftazidime, cephalothin

Risk rating: 2
Severity: Moderate   Onset: Delayed   Likelihood: Suspected

Cause
The mechanism of this interaction is unknown.

Effect
Bactericidal activity may increase against some organisms, but risk of nephrotoxicity may also increase.

Nursing considerations
⚠ **ALERT** Check peak and trough gentamicin level after third dose. For peak level, draw blood 30 minutes after I.V. or 60 minutes after I.M. dose. For trough level, draw blood just before a dose.
■ Assess BUN and creatinine levels.
■ Monitor urine output, and check urine for increased protein, cell, or cast levels.
■ If renal insufficiency develops, notify the prescriber. Dosage may need to be reduced, or drug may need to be stopped.
■ Aminoglycosides other than gentamicin may interact with cephalosporins. If you suspect an interaction, consult the prescriber or pharmacist.

gentamicin ▶◀ indomethacin
Garamycin   Indocin

Risk rating: 2
Severity: Moderate   Onset: Delayed   Likelihood: Suspected

Cause
Indomethacin and other NSAIDs may reduce glomerular filtration rate (GFR), causing aminoglycosides to accumulate.

Effect
Aminoglycoside level in premature infants may increase.

Nursing considerations
■ Before administering NSAIDs, adjust the dose of gentamicin.

⚡ **ALERT** Check peak and trough gentamicin levels after third dose. For peak level, draw blood 30 minutes after I.V. or 60 minutes after I.M. dose. For trough level, draw blood just before a dose.
- Monitor the patient's renal function.
- Although only indomethacin is known to interact with aminoglycosides such as gentamicin, other NSAIDs probably do as well. If you suspect an interaction, consult the prescriber or pharmacist.
- Other drugs cleared by GFR may have a similar interaction.

---

gentamicin ▰▰▰◄▮ loop diuretics
Garamycin   ethacrynic acid, furosemide

Risk rating: 1
Severity: Major   **Onset: Rapid**   **Likelihood: Suspected**

Cause
The mechanism of this interaction is unknown.

Effect
Synergistic ototoxicity may cause hearing loss of varying degrees, possibly permanent.

Nursing considerations
⚡ **ALERT** Patients with renal insufficiency are at increased risk for ototoxicity.
- Perform baseline and periodic hearing function tests.
- Aminoglycosides other than gentamicin may interact with loop diuretics. If you suspect an interaction, consult the prescriber or pharmacist.
- Tell the patient to immediately report ringing or roaring in the ears, muffled sounds, or any noticeable changes in hearing.
- Advise family members to stay alert for evidence of hearing loss.

---

gentamicin ▰▰▰◄▮ nondepolarizing muscle relaxants
Garamycin   atracurium, pancuronium, rocuronium

Risk rating: 1
Severity: Major   **Onset: Rapid**   **Likelihood: Probable**

Cause
These drugs may be synergistic.

Effect
The effects of nondepolarizing muscle relaxants may increase.

Nursing considerations
■ Give these drugs together only when needed.
■ The nondepolarizing muscle relaxant dose may need adjustment based on neuromuscular response.
■ Monitor the patient for prolonged respiratory depression.
■ Provide ventilatory support as needed.

gentamicin ■■■■▶◀ penicillins

Garamycin

ampicillin, penicillin G, piperacillin, ticarcillin

Risk rating: 2
Severity: Moderate   Onset: Delayed   Likelihood: Probable

Cause
The mechanism of this interaction is unknown.

Effect
Penicillins may inactivate certain aminoglycosides such as gentamicin decreasing their therapeutic effects.

Nursing considerations
◪ **ALERT** Check peak and trough aminoglycoside levels after third dose. For peak level, draw blood 30 minutes after I.V. or 60 minutes after I.M. dose. For trough level, draw blood just before a dose.
■ Penicillin affects gentamicin more than amikacin and netilmicin.
■ Monitor the patient's renal function.
■ Other aminoglycosides may interact with penicillins. If you suspect an interaction, consult the prescriber or pharmacist.

glimepiride ■■■■▶◀ fluconazole

Amaryl

Diflucan

Risk rating: 2
Severity: Moderate   Onset: Delayed   Likelihood: Suspected

Cause
Fluconazole may inhibit CYP2C9 metabolism of certain sulfonylureas such as glimepiride.

Effect
Hypoglycemic effect may increase.

Nursing considerations
- Monitor blood glucose level.
- Watch for evidence of hypoglycemia: tingling of lips and tongue, nausea, vomiting, epigastric pain, lethargy, confusion, agitation, tachycardia, diaphoresis, tremor, seizures, and coma.
- Other sulfonylureas may interact with fluconazole. If you suspect an interaction, consult the prescriber or pharmacist.
- If the patient takes a sulfonylurea, consult the prescriber about a different antifungal.
- Urge the patient to monitor blood glucose level at home and to report any increase in episodes of hypoglycemia.

---

glimepride ◄► rifampin
Amaryl   Rifadin, Rimactane

Risk rating: 2
Severity: Moderate   Onset: Delayed   Likelihood: Probable

Cause
Rifampin may increase hepatic metabolism of certain sulfonylureas such as glimepride.

Effect
The risk of hyperglycemia increases.

Nursing considerations
- Use these drugs together cautiously.
- Monitor the patient's blood glucose level regularly; consult the prescriber about adjustments to either drug to maintain stable glucose level.
- Teach the patient to use a self-monitoring glucose meter and to report significant changes to the prescriber.
- Tell the patient to stay alert for increased fatigue, thirst, eating, or urination and possible blurred vision or dry skin and mucous membranes as evidence of high blood glucose level.

---

glipizide ◄► alcohol
Glucotrol

Risk rating: 2
Severity: Moderate   Onset: Rapid   Likelihood: Established

Cause
Chronic alcohol use may delay absorption and elimination of sulfonylureas such as glipizide.

Effect
Risk of hypoglycemia increases.

Nursing considerations
■ Describe consequences of a disulfiram-like reaction: flushing and possible burning of the face and neck, headache, nausea, and tachycardia. Explain that a reaction typically occurs within 20 minutes of alcohol intake and lasts for 1 to 2 hours.
■ Tell the patient who takes an oral antidiabetic to avoid ingesting more alcohol than an occasional single drink.
■ Naloxone may be used to antagonize a disulfiram-like reaction.
■ Urge the patient to have regular follow-up blood tests to monitor diabetic status and decrease episodes of hyperglycemia and hypoglycemia.
■ Other sulfonylureas may interact with alcohol.

---

glyburide ▶◀ alcohol
DiaBeta, Micronase

Risk rating: 2
Severity: Moderate   **Onset: Rapid**   **Likelihood: Established**

Cause
Alcohol use inhibits gluconeogenesis.

Effect
The risk of hypoglycemia increases.

Nursing considerations
■ Tell the patient who takes an oral antidiabetic to avoid alcohol in general, and to limit any alcohol to an occasional single drink.
■ Urge the patient to have regular follow-up blood tests to monitor diabetes and decrease episodes of hyperglycemia and hypoglycemia.
■ Sulfonylureas other than glyburide also interact with alcohol.

---

glyburide ▶◀ aspirin
DiaBeta, Micronase   Ecotrin, Bayer

Risk rating: 2
Severity: Moderate   **Onset: Delayed**   **Likelihood: Probable**

Cause
Salicylates such as aspirin reduce blood glucose level and prompt insulin secretion.

Effect
The hypoglycemic effects of glyburide and other sulfonylureas increase.

Nursing considerations
■ Monitor the patient for hypoglycemia.
■ Consult the prescriber and the patient about possibly replacing aspirin with acetaminophen or an NSAID.
■ Acquaint the patient with signs and symptoms of hypoglycemia, including diaphoresis, fatigue, headache, hunger, irritability, malaise, nervousness, rapid heart rate, tension, and trembling.
■ Instruct the patient to eat a small carbohydrate snack or meal if hypoglycemia develops, preferably after checking blood glucose level.

glyburide ■■■■■►◄■■■■ bosentan
DiaBeta, Micronase   Tracleer

Risk rating: 1
Severity: Major   **Onset: Delayed**   **Likelihood: Suspected**

Cause
Bosentan increases the CYP3A4 and CYP2C9 metabolism of glyburide.

Effect
Plasma levels of bosentan and glyburide may be decreased. Liver enzymes may increase, resulting in serious liver injury.

Nursing considerations
◘ ALERT Administration of bosentan and glyburide together is contraindicated.
■ Discuss the use of another hypoglycemic agent with the prescriber.
■ Monitor the patient's liver enzymes and report any increase to the prescriber.
■ Monitor the patient for signs of liver damage, including icterius, jaundice, dark urine, and confusion.

glyburide ■■■■■►◄■■■■ enalapril
DiaBeta, Micronase   Vasotec

Risk rating: 2
Severity: Moderate   **Onset: Rapid**   **Likelihood: Suspected**

Cause
ACE inhibitors such as enalapril increase insulin sensitivity.

Effect
Risk of hypoglycemia increases.

Nursing considerations
■ Start enalapril therapy carefully, monitoring the patient for hypoglycemia.
■ Describe signs and symptoms of hypoglycemia, including diaphoresis, fatigue, headache, hunger, irritability, malaise, nervousness, rapid heart rate, tension, and trembling.
■ Instruct the patient to eat a small carbohydrate snack or meal if hypoglcemia develops, prefereably after checking his blood glucose level.

---

glyburide ▬▬▬►◄ rifampin
DiaBeta, Micronase   Rifadin, Rimactane

Risk rating: 2
Severity: Moderate   **Onset: Delayed**   **Likelihood: Probable**

Cause
Rifampin may increase hepatic metabolism of certain sulfonylureas such as glyburide.

Effect
Risk of hyperglycemia increases.

Nursing considerations
■ Use these drugs together cautiously.
■ Monitor the patient's blood glucose level regularly; consult the prescriber about adjustments to either drug to maintain a stable glucose level.
■ Tell the patient to be alert for evidence of high blood glucose level: increased fatigue, thirst, eating, or urination and possible blurred vision or dry skin and mucous membranes.

---

griseofulvin ▬▬▬►◄ hormonal contraceptives
Grisactin

Risk rating: 2
Severity: Moderate   **Onset: Delayed**   **Likelihood: Suspected**

Cause
Griseofulvin may induce hepatic metabolism of contraceptives.

Effect
Patient may experience a decrease in the efficacy of hormonal contraceptives.

Nursing considerations
■ Advise the patient to use alternative or additional nonhormonal contraceptive methods during griseofulvin therapy.
■ Instruct the patient to use barrier contraception.
■ Warn the patient about the risk of breakthrough bleeding and pregnancy.

---

griseofulvin ━━▶◀━━ **primidone**
Grisactin   Mysoline

Risk rating: 2
Severity: Moderate   Onset: Delayed   Likelihood: Suspected

Cause
Primidone may decrease griseofulvin absorption, and increase hepatic metabolism.

Effect
Griseofulvin levels decrease.

Nursing considerations
■ Separate drug administration times.
■ Give primidone in divided doses.
■ Griseofulvin dose may need to be increased.
■ Consider stopping either drug; alternative therapy may be needed.

---

griseofulvin ━━▶◀━━ **warfarin**
Grisactin   Coumadin

Risk rating: 2
Severity: Moderate   Onset: Delayed   Likelihood: Suspected

Cause
The mechanism of this interaction is unknown.

Effect
Anticoagulant effects decrease.

Nursing considerations
■ Monitor the patient for inadequate response to warfarin.

■ If the patient's INR is stabilized while taking griseofulvin, monitor closely when griseofulvin stops. The warfarin dose may need to be reduced to prevent serious bleeding.
■ Urge the patient to keep all follow-up medical appointments for monitoring and dosage adjustments. Monitoring may take several weeks.
■ Tell the patient to report unusual bruising or bleeding.
■ Remind the patient that warfarin interacts with many drugs, and tell the patient to report any change in drug regimen.

haloperidol ▶◀ anticholinergics
Haldol

benztropine, procyclidine, trihexyphenidyl

Risk rating: 2
Severity: Moderate   Onset: Delayed   Likelihood: Suspected

Cause
The mechanism of this interaction is unknown. It may involve central cholinergic pathways rather than a true pharmacokinetic interaction.

Effect
Effects may vary and include decreased haloperidol level, worsened schizophrenic symptoms, and development of tardive dyskinesia.

Nursing considerations
⚠ **ALERT** If the patient takes haloperidol, avoid anticholinergics if possible.
■ Watch for signs of worsening schizophrenia, including delusions, hallucinations, disorganized speech or behavior, inappropriate affect, and abnormal psychomotor activity.
■ Watch for development of tardive dyskinesia—involuntary abnormal repetitive movements, including lip smacking, cheek puffing, chewing motions, tongue thrusting, finger flicking, and trunk twisting.
■ Consult the prescriber if adverse effects occur; anticholinergic drug may need to be stopped, or haloperidol dosage may need adjustment.
■ Other anticholinergics may interact with haloperidol. If you suspect an interaction, consult the prescriber or pharmacist.

haloperidol ━━━▶◀ carbamazepine
Haldol
Carbatrol, Epitol, Equetro, Tegretol

Risk rating: 2
Severity: Moderate   Onset: Delayed   Likelihood: Suspected

Cause
Carbamazepine may increase haloperidol hepatic metabolism; haloperidol may inhibit carbamazepine metabolism.

Effect
Haloperidol effects may decrease. Therapeutic and adverse effects of carbamazepine may increase.

Nursing considerations
- Assess the patient for loss of haloperidol effects: psychomotor agitation, obsessive-compulsive rituals, withdrawn behavior, auditory hallucinations, delusions, and delirium.
- Monitor haloperidol level (therapeutic range, 5 to 20 nanograms/ml) and carbamazepine level (therapeutic range, 4 to 12 mcg/ml).
- **⚠ ALERT** Watch for signs of anorexia or subtle appetite changes, which may indicate excessive carbamazepine level.
- Watch for evidence of carbamazepine toxicity, including dizziness, ataxia, respiratory depression, tachycardia, arrhythmias, blood pressure changes, impaired consciousness, abnormal reflexes, nystagmus, seizures, nausea, vomiting, and urine retention.
- If adverse effects occur, consult the prescriber; the dosages of one or both drugs may need adjustment.

haloperidol ━━━▶◀ itraconazole
Haldol
Sporanox

Risk rating: 2
Severity: Moderate   Onset: Delayed   Likelihood: Suspected

Cause
Itraconazole inhibits CYP3A4 metabolism of haloperidol.

Effect
Haloperidol levels and risk of adverse reactions increase.

Nursing considerations
- Observe the patient's clinical response to haloperidol when itraconazole is started or stopped. Adjust the dose as needed.
- Monitor haloperidol level (therapeutic range, 5 to 20 nanograms/ml).

- Monitor for adverse reactions including: neurologic toxicity (altered mental status, rigidity, hyperpyrexia, weakness, lethargy, stupor, fever, severe extrapyrmidal symptoms, and dystonia).
- Advise the patient to tell the prescriber about increased adverse effects.

haloperidol ━━━▶◀━━━ lithium
Haldol   Eskalith

Risk rating: 1
Severity: Major   **Onset: Delayed**   **Likelihood: Suspected**

Cause
The exact mechanism of this interaction is unknown.

Effect
The patient may have an altered level of consciousness, encephalopathy, extrapyramidal effects, fever, leukocytosis, and increased enzyme levels.

Nursing considerations
⚠ **ALERT** Monitor the patient closely, especially the first 3 weeks.
- Watch for early evidence of neurologic toxicity, such as altered mental status, rigidity, or hyperpyrexia; treatment should be stopped promptly if such signs appear.
- Evidence of more severe neurologic toxicity includes weakness, lethargy, tremulousness, confusion, stupor, fever, severe extrapyramidal symptoms, and dystonias. Some patients may have permanent brain damage.
- Check lab studies for leukocytosis, elevated serum enzyme levels, and increased BUN level. Therapeutic lithium level is 0.6 to 1.2 mEq/L; therapeutic haloperidol level is 5 to 20 nanograms/ml.
- If an interaction occurs, alert the prescriber. One or both drugs may need to be stopped. Give supportive treatment for symptoms.

haloperidol ━━━▶◀━━━ rifampin
Haldol   Rifadin, Rimactane

Risk rating: 2
Severity: Moderate   **Onset: Delayed**   **Likelihood: Suspected**

Cause
Haloperidol metabolism may increase.

Effect
Haloperidol level and effects may decrease.

Nursing considerations
■ Watch for expected haloperidol effects if the patient starts or stops rifampin, a rifamycin.
■ Monitor haloperidol level (therapeutic range, 5 to 20 nanograms/ml).
■ Watch for loss of haloperidol effects: psychomotor agitation, obsessive-compulsive rituals, withdrawn behavior, auditory hallucinations, delusions, and delirium.
■ Consult prescriber if haloperidol effects decline; haloperidol dosage may need adjustment.
■ Advise patient to tell prescriber about increased adverse effects.

---

heparin ◢◤ alteplase
Activase, tPA

Risk rating: 1
Severity: Major   **Onset: Rapid**   **Likelihood: Suspected**

Cause
The combined effect of this interaction may be greater than the sum of each individual effect.

Effect
Risk of serious bleeding is increased.

Nursing considerations
◥ **ALERT** Use of heparin with alteplase is contraindicated.
◥ **ALERT** Use of alteplase in patients with acute ischemic stroke is contraindicated if the patient has a bleeding diathesis, has used heparin within 48 hours before onset of stroke, or has an elevated APTT. This poses an increased risk of bleeding that may cause disability or death.

---

heparin ◢◤ aspirin
Bayer

Risk rating: 2
Severity: Moderate   **Onset: Rapid**   **Likelihood: Probable**

Cause
Aspirin may inhibit platelet aggregation and cause bleeding; this effect may be additive to heparin anticoagulation.

Effect
Risk of bleeding increases.

Nursing considerations
- Monitor coagulation studies.
- Assess patient for signs of bleeding: bleeding gums, bruises on arms or legs, petechiae, epistaxis, melena, hematuria, or hematemesis.
- Advise patient to report signs of bleeding or bruising immediately.
- Provide treatment for symptoms as needed.
- Urge patient to tell prescriber about increased adverse effects.

hydralazine ►◄ beta-adrenergic blockers
Apresoline   metoprolol, propranolol

Risk rating: 2
Severity: Moderate   **Onset: Rapid**   **Likelihood: Probable**

Cause
Hydralazine may cause transient increase in visceral blood flow and decreased first-pass hepatic metabolism of some oral beta-adrenergic blockers.

Effect
The effects of both drugs may increase.

Nursing considerations
- Monitor blood pressure regularly; dosage of both drugs may need adjustment based on the patient's response.
- With propranolol, interaction involves only oral, immediate-release form and not extended-release or I.V. drug.
- Other beta-adrenergic blockers may interact with hydralazine. If you suspect an interaction, consult the prescriber or pharmacist.
- Explain that both drugs can affect blood pressure. Urge the patient to report evidence of hypotension, such as light-headedness or dizziness when changing positions.

hydrochlorothiazide ►◄ dofetilide
Microzide   Tikosyn

Risk rating: 1
Severity: Major   **Onset: Delayed**   **Likelihood: Suspected**

Cause
Use of a thiazide diuretic increases potassium excretion.

Effect
Hypokalemia increases risk of ventricular arrhythmias, including torsades de pointes.

Nursing considerations
ALERT Use of dofetilide with a thiazide diuretic is contraindicated.
- Monitor ECG for excessive prolongation of the QTc interval and development of ventricular arrhythmias.
- A similar interaction is likely with loop diuretics.
- Dofetilide clearance is decreased when taken with a thiazide diuretic.

hydrochlorothiazide ▸◂ lithium
Microzide   Eskalith

Risk rating: 2
Severity: Moderate   Onset: Delayed   Likelihood: Established

Cause
Thiazide diuretics such as hydrochlorothiazide may decrease lithium clearance.

Effect
Lithium level, effects, and risk of toxicity may increase.

Nursing considerations
- Despite this interaction, lithium and thiazide diuretics may be used together safely, with close monitoring of lithium level.
- Reduction in lithium clearance may depend on thiazide dose.
- Monitor lithium level, and adjust dose as needed.
- Monitor the patient for evidence of lithium toxicity, such as diarrhea, vomiting, dehydration, drowsiness, muscle weakness, tremor, fever, and ataxia.

hydrochlorothiazide ▸◂ loop diuretics
Microzide   bumetanide, furosemide

Risk rating: 2
Severity: Moderate   Onset: Rapid   Likelihood: Probable

Cause
The mechanism of this interaction is unclear.

Effect
Because these drugs work synergistically, they may cause profound diuresis and serious electrolyte abnormalities.

Nursing considerations
- These drugs may be used together for therapeutic benefit.
- Expect increased sodium, potassium, and chloride excretion and greater diuresis during combined therapy.

- Monitor the patient for dehydration and electrolyte abnormalities.
- Carefully adjust drugs, using small or intermittent doses.

hydrochlorothiazide ►◄ sulfonylureas
Microzide   chlorpropamide, tolbutamide

Risk rating: 2
Severity: Moderate   **Onset: Delayed**   **Likelihood: Probable**

Cause
Thiazide diuretics such as hydrochlorothiazide may decrease insulin secretion and tissue sensitivity, and may increase potassium loss.

Effect
Risk of hyperglycemia and hyponatremia may increase.

Nursing considerations
- Use these drugs together cautiously.
- Check the patient's blood glucose level regularly, and consult the prescriber about adjustments to either drug to maintain stable glucose level.
- This interaction may occur several days to many months after dual therapy starts but is readily reversible when the diuretic stops.
- Describe signs and symptoms of hypoglycemia, including diaphoresis, fatigue, headache, hunger, irritability, malaise, nervousness, rapid heart rate, tension, and trembling.
- Instruct the patient to eat a small carbohydrate snack or meal if hypoglycemia develops, preferably after checking blood glucose level.

hydrocortisone ►◄ anticholinergics
Cortef   neostigmine, pyridostigmine

Risk rating: 1
Severity: Major   **Onset: Delayed**   **Likelihood: Probable**

Cause
In myasthenia gravis, corticosteroids such as hydrocortisone antagonize anticholinesterases by an unknown mechanism.

Effect
The patient may develop severe muscular depression refractory to the cholinesterase inhibitor.

Nursing considerations
- Corticosteroids such as hydrocortisone may have long-term benefits in myasthenia gravis.

■ Combined therapy may be attempted under strict supervision.

■ In myasthenia gravis, monitor the patient for severe muscle deterioration.

ALERT Be prepared to provide respiratory support and mechanical ventilation if needed.

■ Consult the prescriber or pharmacist about safe hydrocortisone delivery to maximize improvement in muscle strength.

hydrocortisone ➡◄ barbiturates
Cortef   pentobarbital, primidone

Risk rating: 2
Severity: Moderate   Onset: Delayed   Likelihood: Established

Cause
Barbiturates induce liver enzymes, which stimulate metabolism of corticosteroids such as hydrocortisone.

Effect
Corticosteroid effects may decrease.

Nursing considerations
■ Avoid giving barbiturates with corticosteroids if possible.

■ If the patient takes hydrocortisone, watch for aggravation of symptoms when he starts or stops a barbiturate.

■ Hydrocortisone dosage may need to be increased.

hydrocortisone ➡◄ bile acid sequestrants
Cortef   cholestyramine, colestipol

Risk rating: 2
Severity: Moderate   Onset: Delayed   Likelihood: Suspected

Cause
Bile acid sequestrants disrupt GI absorption of hydrocortisone.

Effect
Hydrocortisone effects may decrease.

Nursing considerations
■ If the patient needs hydrocortisone, consider a different cholesterol-lowering drug.

■ If drugs must be taken together, giving them at separate times may help improve hydrocortisone absorption, although that hasn't been proven.

■ Check for expected hydrocortisone effects.

- If needed, consult the prescriber about increasing hydrocortisone dosage to achieve desired effect.
- Help the patient develop a plan to ensure proper dosage intervals.

hydrocortisone ➤◀ phenytoin
Cortef   Dilantin

Risk rating: 2
Severity: Moderate   Onset: Delayed   Likelihood: Established

Cause
Hydantoins such as phenytoin induce liver enzymes, which stimulate metabolism of corticosteroids such as hydrocortisone.

Effect
Corticosteroid effects may decrease.

Nursing considerations
- Avoid giving phenytoin with corticosteroids if possible.
- If drugs must be given together, monitor the patient for decreased hydrocortisone effects. Also monitor phenytoin level, and adjust dosage of either drug as needed.

hydrocortisone ➤◀ rifampin
Cortef   Rifadin, Rimactane

Risk rating: 1
Severity: Major   Onset: Delayed   Likelihood: Established

Cause
Rifampin increases hepatic metabolism of corticosteroids such as hydrocortisone.

Effect
Corticosteroid effects may decrease.

Nursing considerations
- If possible, avoid giving rifamycins with corticosteroids.
- Monitor the patient for decreased corticosteroid effects, including loss of disease control.
- Watch closely for symptom control after increasing rifampin dose. The drug may need to be stopped so the patient can regain control of disease.
- Hydrocortisone effects may decrease within days of starting rifampin and may stay at reduced for 2 to 3 weeks after the patient stops taking it.

- Hydrocortisone dose may need to be doubled after adding rifampin.

---

hydrocortisone ➤◀ salicylates
Cortef

aspirin, choline salicylate,
sodium salicylate

Risk rating: 2
Severity: Moderate   Onset: Delayed   Likelihood: Probable

Cause
Hydrocortisone and other corticosteroids stimulate hepatic metabolism of salicylates and may increase renal excretion.

Effect
Salicylate level and effects decrease.

Nursing considerations
- If the patient takes a salicylate and hydrocortisone, monitor salicylate efficacy and level; dosage may need adjustment.
- **⚡ ALERT** Giving a salicylate while tapering hydrocortisone may result in salicylate toxicity.
- Watch for evidence of salicylate toxicity, including diaphoresis, nausea, vomiting, tinnitus, hyperventilation, and CNS depression.
- Patients with renal impairment may be at greater risk.

---

ibuprofen ➤◀ beta-adrenergic blockers
Advil, Motrin

atenolol, pindolol,
propranolol

Risk rating: 2
Severity: Moderate   Onset: Delayed   Likelihood: Probable

Cause
Ibuprofen and other NSAIDs may inhibit renal prostaglandin synthesis, allowing pressor systems to be unopposed.

Effect
Beta-adrenergic blocker may not be able to lower blood pressure.

Nursing considerations
- Avoid using these drugs together if possible.
- Monitor blood pressure and related signs and symptoms of hypertension closely.
- Consult the prescriber about ways to minimize interaction, such as adjusting beta-adrenergic blocker dosage or switching to sulindac as the NSAID.

■ Explain the risks of using these drugs together, and teach the patient how to monitor his blood pressure.
■ Other NSAIDs may interact with beta-adrenergic blockers. If you suspect an interaction, consult the prescriber or pharmacist.

---

imatinib ▸◂ levothyroxine
Gleevec   Synthroid

Risk rating: 2
Severity: Moderate   Onset: Delayed   Likelihood: Suspected

Cause
Imatinib may increase levothyroxine's hepatic clearance.

Effect
Thyroid-stimulating hormone (TSH) levels may be increased. Symptoms of hypothyroidism may occur.

Nursing considerations
■ Monitor thyroid function during coadminstration of imatinib.
■ Levothyroxine dosage may need adjusting when starting or stopping imatinib treatment.
■ Monitor for signs and symptoms of hypothyroidism, by monitoring TSH, T_3, and T_4 levels. Therapeutic range for TSH is 0.2 to 5.4 microunits/ml; for T_3, 80 to 200 nanograms/dl; and for T_4, 5.4 to 11.5 mcg/dl.
■ Watch for evidence of hypothyroidism: weakness, fatigue, weight gain, coarse dry hair, rough skin, cold intolerance, muscle aches, constipation, depression, irritability, and memory loss. Urge the patient to report such symptoms to the prescriber.

---

imatinib ▸◂ rifampin
Gleevec   Rifadin, Rimactane

Risk rating: 2
Severity: Moderate   Onset: Delayed   Likelihood: Suspected

Cause
Rifampin increases CYP3A4 metabolism of imatinib.

Effect
Imatinib levels and therapeutic effect decrease.

Nursing considerations
■ Monitor the patient's clinical response when rifampin therapy is started or stopped.

- Consider alternative rifamycin therapy.
- Use these drugs together cautiously.

imipenem and cilastatin ⧓ cyclosporine

Primaxin — Gengraf, Neoral, Sandimmune

Risk rating: 2
Severity: Moderate **Onset: Rapid** **Likelihood: Suspected**

Cause
Additive or synergistic toxicity may occur.

Effect
Adverse CNS effects of both drugs may increase.

Nursing considerations
- Monitor the patient for adverse CNS effects, including confusion, agitation, and tremors.
- Decreasing cyclosporine dose may decrease risk of adverse effects.
- Consider giving an alternative antibiotic if an interaction is suspected.
- Adverse effects should improve after stopping imipenem and cilastatin.

imipenem and cilastatin ⧓ valproic acid

Primaxin — Depakote

Risk rating: 2
Severity: Moderate **Onset: Delayed** **Likelihood: Suspected**

Cause
The mechanism of this interaction is unknown.

Effect
Valproic acid plasma levels may be decreased.

Nursing considerations
- Monitor the patient's valproic acid levels and observe the patient for seizure activity when starting a carbapenem antibiotic, such as imipenem and cilastatin.
- Consider giving an alternative antibiotic if an interaction is suspected.

■ If imipenem and cilastatin is stopped, you may have to decrease the dose of valproic acid.

---

imipramine ━━━━▶◀━━━━ azole antifungals
Tofranil   fluconazole, ketoconazole

Risk rating: 2
Severity: Moderate   Onset: Delayed   Likelihood: Suspected

Cause
Azole antifungals may inhibit metabolism of imipramine, a tricyclic antidepressant (TCA), by varying CYP pathways.

Effect
Serum TCA level and risk of toxicity may increase.

Nursing considerations
■ When starting or stopping an azole antifungal, monitor serum TCA level and adjust dosage as needed.
■ After starting an azole antifungal, check sitting and standing blood pressure for changes.
■ Assess symptoms and behavior for adverse reactions, such as increased drowsiness, dizziness, confusion, heart rate or rhythm changes, and urine retention.

---

imipramine ━━━━▶◀━━━━ carbamazepine
Tofranil   Carbatrol, Epitol, Equetro, Tegretol

Risk rating: 2
Severity: Moderate   Onset: Delayed   Likelihood: Probable

Cause
Tricyclic antidepressants (TCAs) such as imipramine may compete with carbamazepine for hepatic metabolism. Carbamazepine may induce hepatic metabolism of imipramine.

Effect
Carbamazepine levels, pharmacologic, and toxic effects may be elevated. Imipramine levels may be decreased.

Nursing considerations
■ Imipramine and other TCAs may interact with carbamazepine. If you suspect a drug interaction, consult the prescriber or pharmacist.
■ Monitor carbamazepine level; therapeutic range is 4 to 12 mcg/ml.

■ Watch for evidence of carbamazepine toxicity, including dizziness, ataxia, respiratory depression, tachycardia, arrhythmias, blood pressure changes, impaired consciousness, abnormal reflexes, nystagmus, seizures, nausea, vomiting, and urine retention.

imipramine ▶◀ chlorpromazine
Tofranil   Thorazine

Risk rating: 3
Severity: Minor   **Onset: Delayed**   **Likelihood: Probable**

Cause
Taking these two drugs together fosters competitive inhibition of imipramine metabolism.

Effect
This leads to increased levels of impramine.

Nursing considerations
■ Monitor the patient's clinical response to imipramine and decrease the dose if needed.
■ No toxic effects were noted from this interaction.

imipramine ▶◀ cimetidine
Tofranil   Tagamet

Risk rating: 2
Severity: Moderate   **Onset: Rapid**   **Likelihood: Probable**

Cause
Cimetidine may interfere with metabolism of tricyclic antidepressants (TCAs) such as imipramine.

Effect
TCA level and bioavailability increase.

Nursing considerations
■ Monitor serum imipramine level and adjust dosage as prescribed.
■ If needed, consult the prescriber about possible changes from cimetidine to ranitidine.
■ Urge the patient and his family to watch for and report increased anticholinergic effects, dizziness, drowsiness, and psychosis.

imipramine ━━━▶◀━━━ clonidine
Tofranil   Catapres

Risk rating: 1
Severity: Major   **Onset: Rapid**   **Likelihood: Probable**

Cause
Tricyclic antidepressants such as imipramine inhibit alpha$_2$-adrenergic receptors, which clonidine stimulates for blood pressure control.

Effect
Clonidine's efficacy in reducing blood pressure decreases.

Nursing considerations
- Life-threatening increases in blood pressure may occur.
- The intensity of this effect depends on the dosage of both drugs.
- ⚠ ALERT Tell the prescriber that the patient takes imipramine.
- Tell the patient to keep an up-to-date list of all drugs he takes, so the prescriber can avoid possible interactions.
- Other types of antidepressants can be used as an alternative treatment without this potential interaction.

imipramine ━━━▶◀━━━ fluoxetine
Tofranil   Prozac, Sarafem

Risk rating: 2
Severity: Moderate   **Onset: Delayed**   **Likelihood: Probable**

Cause
Fluoxetine may inhibit hepatic metabolism of tricyclic antidepressants (TCAs) such as imipramine.

Effect
TCA level and risk of toxicity may increase.

Nursing considerations
- Monitor serum TCA level and watch closely for evidence of toxicity, such as increased anticholinergic effects, delirium, dizziness, drowsiness, and psychosis.
- Report evidence of increased TCA level or toxicity; dosage may need to be decreased.
- If TCA starts when the patient already takes fluoxetine, TCA dosage may need to be decreased by up to 75% to avoid interaction.
- Other TCAs may interact with fluoxetine. If you suspect an interaction, consult the prescriber or pharmacist.

imipramine ━━━━━▶◀━━━━ fluvoxamine
Tofranil   Luvox

Risk rating: 2
Severity: Moderate   Onset: Delayed   Likelihood: Probable

Cause
Fluvoxamine may inhibit oxidative metabolism of tricyclic antidepressants (TCAs) such as imipramine via CYP2D6 pathway.

Effect
TCA level and risk of toxicity increase.

Nursing considerations
- If combined use can't be avoided, TCA dosage may need to be decreased.
- When starting or stopping fluvoxamine, monitor serum TCA level.
- Report evidence of toxicity or increased TCA level.
- Inhibitory effects of fluvoxamine may take up to 2 weeks to dissipate after drug is stopped.
- Using the TCA, desipramine, may avoid this interaction.
- Urge the patient and his family to watch for and report increased anticholinergic effects, dizziness, drowsiness, and psychosis.

imipramine ━━━━━▶◀━━━━ MAO inhibitors
Tofranil   isocarboxazid, phenelzine,
                                  tranylcypromine

Risk rating: 1
Severity: Major   Onset: Rapid   Likelihood: Suspected

Cause
The mechanism of this interaction is unknown.

Effect
The risk of hyperpyretic crisis, seizures, and death increases.

Nursing considerations
- ◤ **ALERT** Don't give a tricyclic antidepressant (TCA) such as imipramine with or within 2 weeks of an MAO inhibitor.
- Imipramine and clomipramine may be more likely than other TCAs to interact with MAO inhibitors.
- Watch for adverse effects, including confusion, hyperexcitability, rigidity, seizures, increased temperature, increased pulse, increased respiration, sweating, mydriasis, flushing, headache, coma, and DIC.

imipramine ◄► paroxetine
Tofranil   Paxil

Risk rating: 2
Severity: Moderate   **Onset: Delayed**   **Likelihood: Suspected**

Cause
Paroxetine may decrease imipramine metabolism in some people and increase it in others.

Effect
Therapeutic and toxic effects of certain tricyclic antidepressants (TCAs) such as imipramine may increase.

Nursing considerations
- When starting or stopping paroxetine, monitor TCA level and adjust dosage as needed.
- Assess symptoms and behavior for evidence of adverse reactions, such as increased drowsiness, dizziness, confusion, heart rate or rhythm changes, and urine retention.
- Watch closely for evidence of serotonin syndrome, such as delirium, bizarre movements, and tachycardia. Alert the prescriber if they occur; TCA may need to be stopped.
- Symptoms of serotonin syndrome may resolve within 24 hours of stopping a TCA and starting a short course of cyproheptadine.

---

imipramine ◄► quinolones
Tofranil   gatifloxacin, levofloxacin,
                                          moxifloxacin

Risk rating: 1
Severity: Major   **Onset: Delayed**   **Likelihood: Suspected**

Cause
The mechanism of this interaction is unknown.

Effect
Life-threatening arrhythmias, including torsades de pointes, may increase when certain tricyclic antidepressants (TCAs) such as imipramine are used with certain quinolones.

Nursing considerations
- **⚠ ALERT** Avoid giving levofloxacin with a TCA.
- Use gatifloxacin and moxifloxacin cautiously with TCAs.
- If possible, use other quinolone antibiotics that don't prolong the QTc interval or aren't metabolized by the CYP3A4 isoenzyme.

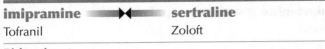

imipramine ━━━▶◀━━━ sertraline
Tofranil   Zoloft

Risk rating: 2
Severity: Moderate   **Onset: Delayed**   **Likelihood: Suspected**

Cause
Hepatic metabolism of imipramine, a tricyclic antidepressant (TCA), may be inhibited.

Effect
Therapeutic and toxic effects of certain TCAs may increase.

Nursing considerations
- If possible, avoid this drug combination.
- Watch for evidence of TCA toxicity and serotonin syndrome.
- Signs of serotonin syndrome include delirium, bizarre movements, and tachycardia.
- Monitor TCA level when starting or stopping sertraline.
- If abnormalities occur, decrease TCA dosage or stop drug.

imipramine ━━━━▶◀━━━ sympathomimetics
Tofranil   epinephrine, norepinephrine
                         phenylephrine

Risk rating: 2
Severity: Moderate   **Onset: Rapid**   **Likelihood: Established**

Cause
Tricyclic antidepressants (TCAs) such as imipramine increase the effects of direct-acting sympathomimetics and decrease the effects of indirect-acting sympathomimetics.

Effect
When sympathomimetic effects increase, the risk of hypertension and arrhythmias increases. When sympathomimetic effects decrease, blood pressure control decreases.

Nursing considerations
- If possible, avoid using these drugs together.
- Watch the patient closely for hypertension and heart rhythm changes; they may warrant reduced sympathomimetic dosage.
- If the patient takes a mixed-acting sympathomimetic, watch for negative effects; dosage may need to be altered.
- Other TCAs and sympathomimetics may interact. If you suspect an interaction, consult the prescriber or pharmacist.

imipramine ━━━━▶◀━━━━ terbinafine
Tofranil   Lamisil

Risk rating: 2
Severity: **Moderate**   Onset: **Delayed**   Likelihood: **Suspected**

Cause
Hepatic metabolism of a tricyclic antidepressant (TCA) such as imipramine may be inhibited.

Effect
Therapeutic and toxic effects of certain TCAs may increase.

Nursing considerations
■ Check for toxic TCA level; report an abnormal level to the prescriber.
■ TCA dosage may be decreased while the patient takes terbinafine.
■ Adverse effects or toxicity may include vertigo, fatigue, loss of appetite, ataxia, muscle twitching, and trouble swallowing. Acquaint the patient with these signs and symptoms.
■ Terbinafine's inhibitory effects may take several weeks to dissipate after the patient stops taking the drug.

indinavir ━━━━▶◀━━━━ aldesleukin
Crixivan   Proleukin

Risk rating: 2
Severity: **Moderate**   Onset: **Delayed**   Likelihood: **Suspected**

Cause
Aldesleukin causes the formation of interleukin-6, an enzyme which inhibits the metabolism of indinavir.

Effect
The plasma concentrations of indinavir may be elevated, along with an increased risk of toxicity.

Nursing considerations
■ Aldesleukin taken with protease inhibitors other than indinavir may cause a similar interaction.
■ Monitor the patient and be prepared for adjustments in the dose of indinavir when aldesleukin therapy is initiated or stopped.
■ Instruct the patient to notify the prescriber if he develops signs and symptoms of indinavir toxicity, including hematuria, flank pain, nausea, and vomiting.

indinavir ◀▶ amiodarone

Crixivan   Cordarone, Pacerone

Risk rating: 1
Severity: Major   **Onset: Delayed**   **Likelihood: Suspected**

Cause
Protease inhibitors such as indinavir inhibit the CYP3A4 metabolism of amiodarone.

Effect
Amiodarone level increases, increasing the risk of toxicity.

Nursing considerations
◼ **ALERT** Other protease inhibitors are contraindicated for use with amiodarone because of large increase in amiodarone level.
◼ Increased amiodarone level may prolong the QT interval and cause life-threatening arrhythmias.
◼ Monitor ECG and QTc interval closely during combined therapy.
◼ Tell the patient to immediately report slowed pulse or fainting.

indinavir ◀▶ azole antifungals

Crixivan   fluconazole, itraconazole,
                                  ketoconazole

Risk rating: 2
Severity: Moderate   **Onset: Delayed**   **Likelihood: Suspected**

Cause
Azole antifungals may inhibit metabolism of protease inhibitors such as indinavir.

Effect
Indinavir level may increase.

Nursing considerations
◼ Indinavir dosage may be decreased when therapy starts.
◼ Monitor the patient for increased protease inhibitor effects, including hyperglycemia, onset of diabetes, rash, GI complaints, and altered liver function tests.
◼ Advise the patient to report increased hunger or thirst, frequent urination, fatigue, and dry, itchy skin.
◼ Tell the patient not to change dosage or stop either drug without consulting the prescriber.

indinavir ◄► benzodiazepines

Crixivan

alprazolam, clorazaepate, estazolam, flurazepam, triazolam, midazolam, diazepam

Risk rating: 2
Severity: Moderate   Onset: Delayed   Likelihood: Suspected

Cause
Protease inhibitors such as indinavir may inhibit CYP3A4 metabolism of certain benzodiazepines.

Effect
Sedative effects may be increased and prolonged, leading to severe respiratory depression.

Nursing considerations
⚠ **ALERT** Don't combine these benzodiazepines with protease inhibitors such as indinavir.
■ If the patient takes any benzodiazepine–protease inhibitor combination, notify the prescriber. Interaction could involve other drugs in the class.
■ Watch for evidence of oversedation and respiratory depression.
■ Teach the patient and his family about the risks of combining these drugs.

indinavir ◄► carbamazepine

Crixivan

Tegretol

Risk rating: 2
Severity: Moderate   Onset: Rapid   Likelihood: Suspected

Cause
Indinaviir may inhibit hepatic metabolism (CYP3A4) of carbamazepine. Carbamazepine may induce metabolism (CYP3A4) of indinavir.

Effect
Carbamazepine levels and risk of toxicity may increase. Indinavir levels may decrease.

Nursing considerations
■ Closely monitor carbamazepine levels when starting, stopping, or changing the dose of indinavir.

■ Observe the patient's clinical response to indinavir therapy. Adjust the dose as needed.
◤ ALERT If indinavir level decreases, antiretroviral treatment therapy may fail.
■ Monitor carbamazepine level; therapeutic range is 4 to 12 mcg/ml.
◤ ALERT Watch for signs of anorexia or subtle appetite changes, which may indicate excessive carbamazepine level.
■ Monitor the patient for evidence of carbamazepine toxicity, including dizziness, ataxia, respiratory depression, tachycardia, arrhythmias, blood pressure changes, impaired consciousness, abnormal reflexes, nystagmus, seizures, nausea, vomiting, and urine retention.

indinavir ◄►◄ conivaptan
Crixivan   Vaprisol

Risk rating: 1
Severity: Major   **Onset: Delayed**   **Likelihood: Suspected**

Cause
Indinavir may inhibt metabolism (CYP3A4) of conivaptan.

Effect
Conivaptan plasma levels and risk of adverse reactions may be increased.

Nursing considerations
◤ ALERT Coadministration of conivaptan and indinavir is contraindicated.
■ The consequences of increased conivaptan levels are unknown.

indinavir ◄►◄ delavirdine
Crixivan   Rescriptor

Risk rating: 2
Severity: Moderate   **Onset: Delayed**   **Likelihood: Probable**

Cause
Indinavir may have decreased metabolism (CYP3A4) and post absorptive clearance.

Effect
Indinavir plasma levels, pharmacologic effects and adverse reactions may be increased.

Nursing considerations
- Closely monitor the patient and adjust therapy as needed.
- Monitor the patient for indinavir adverse reactions, including hyperglycemia, onset of diabetes, rash, GI complaints, and altered liver function tests.
- Advise the patient to report increased hunger or thirst, frequent urination, fatigue, and dry, itchy skin.
- Tell the patient not to change dosage or stop either drug without consulting the prescriber.

---

indinavir ▶◀ didanosine
Crixivan   Videx

Risk rating: 2
Severity: Moderate   **Onset: Rapid**   **Likelihood: Suspected**

Cause
Indinavir absorption may be decreased by buffers in didanosine.

Effect
Indinavir effects may decrease.

Nursing considerations
⚠ **ALERT** Give indinavir and didanosine at least 1 hour apart on an empty stomach.
- Watch for expected therapeutic effects of indinavir, including improvement in HIV symptoms.
- Monitor lab values for an increased CD4+ T-cell count and a decreased HIV-1 RNA level.
- Help the patient develop a plan to ensure proper dosage intervals.

---

indinavir ▶◀ ergot derivatives
Crixivan   dihydroergotamine,
                            ergonovine, ergotamine,
                            methylergonovine

Risk rating: 1
Severity: Major   **Onset: Delayed**   **Likelihood: Probable**

Cause
Protease inhibitors such as indinavir may interfere with CYP3A4 metabolism of ergot derivatives.

Effect
Risk of ergot-induced peripheral vasospasm and ischemia may increase.

Nursing considerations
ALERT Use of ergot derivatives with protease inhibitors is contraindicated.

■ Monitor the patient for evidence of peripheral ischemia: pain in limb muscles while exercising and later at rest; numbness and tingling of fingers and toes; cool, pale, or cyanotic limbs; red or violet blisters on hands or feet; and gangrene.

■ Sodium nitroprusside may be used to treat ergot-induced vasospasm.

■ If the patient takes a protease inhibitor, consult the prescriber or pharmacist about alternative treatments for migraine pain.

■ Urge the patient to tell the prescriber about increased adverse effects.

---

indinavir ▶◀ grapefruit juice
Crixivan

Risk rating: 3
Severity: Minor   **Onset: Rapid**   **Likelihood: Suspected**

Cause
Grapefruit juice may delay absorption of indinavir because of increase in gastric pH.

Effect
Indinavir peak plasma levels may be delayed.

Nursing considerations
ALERT Instruct the patient to avoid chronic ingestion of grapefruit with indinavir. A single dose of indinavir taken with grapefruit juice or grapefruit products has no effects.

■ Teach the patient to separate ingestion of grapefruit juice and grapefruit products as much as possible from indinavir.

■ Additional studies are needed to determine the effects of chronic ingestion of grapefruit juice on the pharmacokinetics of indinavir.

indinavir ■■■■■►◄ non-nucleoside reverse transcriptase inhibitors

Crixivan

efavirenz, nevirapine

Risk rating: 2
Severity: Moderate   Onset: Delayed   Likelihood: Suspected

Cause
Non-nucleoside reverse transcriptase (NNRT) inhibiters may increase hepatic metabolism of protease inhibitors such as indinavir.

Effect
Protease inhibitor level and effects decrease.

Nursing considerations
■ When an NNRT inhibitor is started or stopped, monitor indinavir level closely.
■ Indiniavir dosage may need adjustment.
■ Monitor CD4+ and T-cell counts, and tell the prescriber if they decrease.
■ Urge the patient to report opportunistic infections.
■ Tell the patient not to change an HIV regimen without consulting the prescriber.

indinavir ■■■■■►◄ pimozide

Crixivan

Orap

Risk rating: 1
Severity: Major   Onset: Delayed   Likelihood: Suspected

Cause
Protease inhibitors such as indinavir may inhibit CYP3A4 metabolism of pimozide.

Effect
Risk of life-threatening arrhythmias may increase.

Nursing considerations
◾ **ALERT** Combined use of these drugs is contraindicated.
■ Arrhythmias are related to prolonged QT interval, a known risk of pimozide.
■ Interaction warning is based on pharmacokinetics of these drugs, not actual patient studies.

indinavir ━━━━▶◀ proton pump inhibitors
Crixivan

esomeprazole, lansoprazole, omeprazole, pantoprazole, rabeprazole

Risk rating: 1
Severity: Major   **Onset: Delayed**   **Likelihood: Suspected**

Cause
GI absorption of protease inhibitors, including indinavir, may be decreased.

Effect
Antiviral activity of indinavir may be reduced.

Nursing considerations
- Use of indinavir and proton pump inhibitors is not recommended.
- Monitor the patient for a decrease in antiviral activity.
- Adjust the dose of the protease inhibitor as needed.

indinavir ━━━━▶◀ rifamycins
Crixivan

rifabutin, rifampin, rifapentine

Risk rating: 2
Severity: Moderate   **Onset: Delayed**   **Likelihood: Probable**

Cause
Indinavir decreases CYP3A4 metabolism of rifamycins, while rifamycins increase the metabolism of indinavir.

Effect
Antiviral activity of indinavir may be reduced. The rifamycin levels and risk of toxicity increase.

Nursing considerations
- Decrease rifamycin dose to half the standard dose when administering together.
- Use of these drugs together isn't recommended.
- Adjust the dose of the protease inhibitor such as indinavir as needed.
- Monitor CD4+ and T-cell counts; tell the prescriber if they decrease.
- Tell the patient not to change an HIV regimen without consulting the prescriber.
- Monitor the patient for increased rifamycin adverse effects, such as abdominal pain, anorexia, nausea, vomiting, diarrhea, and rash.

indinavir ◄► ritonavir
Crixivan   Norvir

Risk rating: 2
Severity: Moderate   **Onset: Delayed**   **Likelihood: Probable**

Cause
Ritonavir may decrease CYP3A4 metabolism and clearance of indinavir.

Effect
Indinavir level, effects, and risk of adverse effects may increase.

Nursing considerations
◪ ALERT Both drugs may need dosage adjustment.
■ Watch for increased indinavir adverse effects, including nausea, vomiting, diarrhea, and adverse renal effects.
■ Monitor the patient for nephrolithiasis; the patient may experience flank pain and hematuria.
■ Advise the patient to drink at least six 8-oz glasses of fluid (1.5 L) daily.
■ Help the patient develop a plan to ensure proper dosage intervals.

indinavir ◄► sildenafil
Crixivan   Viagra

Risk rating: 1
Severity: Major   **Onset: Rapid**   **Likelihood: Suspected**

Cause
Hepatic metabolism of the phosphodiesterase-5 (PDE-5) inhibitor such as sildenafil is inhibited.

Effect
PDE-5 inhibitor level may increase, possibly leading to fatal hypotension.

Nursing considerations
◪ ALERT Warn the patient about potentially fatal low blood pressure if these drugs are taken together. Tell the patient to take sildenafil exactly as prescribed.
■ Dosage of sildenafil may be reduced and interval extended.
■ Tell the patient to notify the prescriber if he has dizziness, fainting, or chest pain.

indinavir ===►◄=== St. John's wort
Crixivan

Risk rating: 1
Severity: Major   **Onset: Delayed**   **Likelihood: Suspected**

Cause
Hepatic metabolism of protease inhibitors such as indinavir may increase.

Effect
Protease inhibitor level and effects may decrease.

Nursing considerations
- If the patient starts or stops taking St. John's wort, monitor protease inhibitor level closely.
- Monitor CD4+ and T-cell counts; tell the prescriber if they decrease.
- Urge the patient to report opportunistic infections.
- Tell the patient not to change an HIV drug regimen without consulting the prescriber.
- Urge the patient to tell the prescribers about all drugs, supplements, and alternative therapies he uses.

indinavir ===►◄=== tacrolimus
Crixivan   Prograf

Risk rating: 2
Severity: Moderate   **Onset: Delayed**   **Likelihood: Suspected**

Cause
Hepatic metabolism of tacrolimus is inhibited.

Effect
Tacrolimus level and risk of toxicity may increase.

Nursing considerations
- Monitor renal function and mental status closely.
- Check tacrolimus level often. Normal trough level is 6 to 10 mcg/ml.
- Tacrolimus dosage may need to be decreased when the patient takes a protease inhibitor such as indinavir.
- Other protease inhibitors may have this same interaction.
- Watch for renal failure, nephrotoxicity, hyperkalemia, hyperglycemia, delirium, and other changes in mental status.

indomethacin ➤◀ ACE inhibitors
Indocin   captopril, enalapril

Risk rating: 2
Severity: Moderate   **Onset: Rapid**   **Likelihood: Probable**

Cause
Indomethacin inhibits synthesis of prostaglandins, which ACE inhibitors need to lower blood pressure.

Effect
ACE inhibitor's hypotensive effect will decrease.

Nursing considerations
■ **ALERT** Monitor blood pressure closely. Severe hypertension may persist until indomethacin is stopped.
■ If indomethacin can't be avoided, the patient may need a different antihypertensive.
■ Other ACE inhibitors may interact with indomethacin. If you suspect an interaction, consult the prescriber or pharmacist.
■ Remind the patient that hypertension commonly causes no physical symptoms but sometimes may cause headache and dizziness.

indomethacin ➤◀ aminoglycosides
Indocin   amikacin, gentamicin

Risk rating: 2
Severity: Moderate   **Onset: Delayed**   **Likelihood: Suspected**

Cause
Indomethacin and other NSAIDs may reduce glomerular filtration rate (GFR), causing aminoglycosides to accumulate.

Effect
Aminoglycoside level in premature infants may increase.

Nursing considerations
■ Before starting an NSAID, reduce aminoglycoside dose.
■ **ALERT** Check peak and trough aminoglycoside levels after third dose. For peak level, draw blood 30 minutes after I.V. or 60 minutes after I.M. dose. For trough level, draw blood just before a dose.
■ Monitor the patient's renal function.
■ Although only indomethacin is known to interact with aminoglycosides, other NSAIDs probably do as well. If you suspect an interaction, consult the prescriber or pharmacist.
■ Other drugs cleared by GFR may have a similar interaction.

indomethacin ◄►► aspirin
Indocin   Bayer, Ecotrin

Risk rating: 1
Severity: Major   **Onset: Delayed**   **Likelihood: Suspected**

Cause
Increased metabolism and displaced protein binding of NSAIDs such as indomethacin may occur.

Effect
The pharmacologic effects of indomethacin may be decreased. The cardioprotective effect of low-dose, uncoated aspirin may be decreased. These drugs are also gastric irritants.

Nursing considerations
- If possible, use analgesics that don't interfere with the platelet effect for pain control such as acetaminophen in place of NSAIDs.
- If possible, administer indomethacin 8 hours before or 30 minutes after immediate-release aspirin.
- Monitor the patient for signs of bleeding, including bleeding gums, bruises on arms or legs, petechiae, epistaxis, melena, hematuria, and hematemesis.
- Instruct the patient to notify the prescriber if he notices increased bleeding or bruising.
- NSAIDs used occasionally for pain relief don't interact with aspirin; only regular, long-term use may cause a problem.

---

indomethacin ◄►► digoxin
Indocin   Lanoxin

Risk rating: 2
Severity: Moderate   **Onset: Delayed**   **Likelihood: Suspected**

Cause
Indomethacin may reduce renal digoxin elimination.

Effect
Digoxin level, effects, and adverse effects may increase.

Nursing considerations
- Interaction may not occur in patients with normal renal function.
- **⚠ ALERT** Digoxin dose may need to be reduced by 50% when indomethacin is started in these patients.
- Monitor digoxin level. Therapeutic range is 0.8 to 2 nanograms/ml.
- Monitor renal function tests and urine output.

■ Monitor the patient for evidence of digoxin toxicity: arrhythmias (bradycardia and AV blocks, more common in children; ventricular ectopy, more common in adults), lethargy, drowsiness, confusion, hallucinations, headaches, syncope, visual disturbances, nausea, vomiting, diarrhea, and anorexia.

indomethacin ▶◀ losartan
Indocin   Cozaar

Risk rating: 2
Severity: Moderate   **Onset: Delayed**   **Likelihood: Suspected**

Cause
The mechanism of this interaction is unknown.

Effect
Hypotensive effect of losartan may be reduced.

Nursing considerations
■ Other antihypertensives may not share this interaction.
■ Monitor blood pressure closely.
■ If you suspect an interaction, notify the prescriber. Indomethacin may need to be stopped or a different antihypertensive considered.

insulin ▶◀ alcohol

Risk rating: 1
Severity: Major   **Onset: Rapid**   **Likelihood: Probable**

Cause
Alcohol enhances insulin release in response to glucose and inhibits gluconeogenesis (glucose formation).

Effect
Glucose-lowering effect of insulin may be potentiated.

Nursing considerations
■ Monitor the patient for evidence of hypoglycemia: tachycardia, palpitations, anxiety, diaphoresis, nausea, hunger, dizziness, restlessness, headache, confusion, tremors, and speech and motor dysfunction.
■ Teach the patient to avoid alcohol because it lowers the glucose level.
■ Advise the patient to monitor glucose level carefully if consuming alcohol.

⚠ **ALERT** If a patient taking insulin plans to consume alcohol, advise him to drink in moderation and with food.
- Make sure the patient and family can recognize hypoglycemia and respond appropriately.

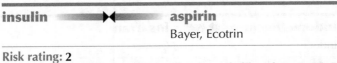

insulin ◀▶ **aspirin**
Bayer, Ecotrin

Risk rating: 2
Severity: Moderate   Onset: Delayed   Likelihood: Probable

Cause
Basal insulin level is increased; salicylates such as aspirin enhance release of insulin in response to glucose.

Effect
Glucose-lowering effect of insulin may be potentiated.

Nursing considerations
- Monitor glucose level closely if a patient who takes insulin starts a salicylate.
- Watch for evidence of hypoglycemia: tachycardia, palpitations, anxiety, diaphoresis, nausea, hunger, dizziness, restlessness, headache, confusion, tremors, and speech and motor dysfunction.
- Consult the prescriber if the patient experiences hypoglycemia; insulin dosage may need to be decreased.
- Treat hypoglycemia as needed, such as with fast-acting oral carbohydrates, parenteral glucagon, or I.V. $D_{50}W$ bolus.
- Urge the patient to tell the prescriber about increased adverse effects.
- Make sure the patient and family can recognize hypoglycemia and respond appropriately.

insulin ◀▶ **beta-adrenergic blockers, nonselective**
pindolol, propranolol, timolol

Risk rating: 2
Severity: Moderate   Onset: Rapid   Likelihood: Established

Cause
Beta-adrenergic blockers lessen the sympathetic-mediated response to hypoglycemia.

Effect
Hypoglycemia may be prolonged and hypoglycemic symptoms masked.

Nursing considerations
- Nonselective beta-adrenergic blockers should be used cautiously in patients with diabetes; if possible, use a selective beta-adrenergic blocker or one with intrinsic sympathomimetic activity, such as acebutolol, atenolol, and metoprolol.
- Watch for evidence of hypoglycemia: tachycardia, palpitations, anxiety, diaphoresis, nausea, hunger, dizziness, restlessness, headache, confusion, tremors, and speech and motor dysfunction.

⚠ ALERT Hypoglycemic symptoms such as tachycardia may be lessened or absent in patients taking a nonselective beta-adrenergic blocker; other symptoms, such as dizziness and diaphoresis, will still be present.

- Monitor glucose level closely when beta-adrenergic blocker starts or dosage changes.
- Consult the prescriber if the patient continues to experience hypoglycemia; insulin dosage may need to be decreased.
- Make sure the patient and family can recognize hypoglycemia and respond appropriately.

---

insulin ━━━━▶◀ **MAO inhibitors**

isocarboxazid, phenelzine, tranylcypromine

Risk rating: 2
Severity: Moderate   **Onset: Delayed**   **Likelihood: Established**

Cause
MAO inhibitors stimulate insulin secretion and inhibit gluconeogenesis (glucose formation).

Effect
Hypoglycemic response to insulin may be increased and prolonged.

Nursing considerations
- Monitor glucose level closely if MAO inhibitor starts or dosage changes.
- The extent of MAO inhibitor effect on glucose level may not be known for several weeks.
- Watch for evidence of hypoglycemia: tachycardia, palpitations, anxiety, diaphoresis, nausea, hunger, dizziness, restlessness, headache, confusion, tremors, and speech and motor dysfunction.
- Consult the prescriber if the patient experiences hypoglycemia; insulin dosage may need to be decreased.

- Treat hypoglycemia as needed, such as with fast-acting oral carbohydrates, parenteral glucagon, or I.V. $D_{50}W$ bolus.
- Make sure the patient and family can recognize hypoglycemia and respond appropriately.

irbesartan ➤◄ spironolactone
Avapro   Aldactone

Risk rating: 1
Severity: Major   **Onset: Delayed**   **Likelihood: Suspected**

Cause
Angiotensin II receptor antagonists such as irbesartan and potassium-sparing diuretics such as spironolactone each may increase serum potassium level.

Effect
Risk of hyperkalemia may increase, especially in high-risk patients.

Nursing considerations
- High-risk patients include elderly people and those with renal impairment, type 2 diabetes, or decreased renal perfusion; monitor these patients closely.
- Check serum potassium, BUN, and creatinine levels regularly. If they increase, notify the prescriber.
- Advise the patient to immediately report an irregular heartbeat, slow pulse, weakness, or other evidence of hyperkalemia.
- Give the patient a list of foods high in potassium; stress the need to eat them only in moderate amounts.

irinotecan ➤◄ St. John's wort
Camptosar

Risk rating: 2
Severity: Moderate   **Onset: Delayed**   **Likelihood: Suspected**

Cause
The exact mechanism of this interaction is unknown. CYP3A4 hepatic metabolism of irinotecan may be altered by St. John's wort.

Effect
Irinotecan level and effects may decrease.

Nursing considerations
- Those who take irinotecan shouldn't take St. John's wort.

■ If the patient stops St. John's wort during irinotecan therapy, watch for severe diarrhea, nausea, vomiting, electrolyte disturbances, and hematologic toxicities.
■ Urge the patient to tell the prescriber about all supplements he takes.

iron salts ■■■■►◄ chloramphenicol
ferrous fumarate,
ferrous gluconate,
ferrous sulfate,
iron dextran

Chloromycetin

Risk rating: 2
Severity: Moderate   Onset: Delayed   Likelihood: Suspected

Cause
Chloramphenicol causes bone marrow toxicity, which leads to decreased iron clearance and erythropoiesis.

Effect
Iron levels may increase.

Nursing considerations
■ If the patient shows signs of bone marrow suppression, use an alternative antimicrobial agent, if possible.
■ Carefully monitor iron stores, and adjust the iron dosage as needed.
■ Serum iron levels may begin to increase within 5 to 7 days of beginning chloramphenicol.
■ Assess the patient for evidence of iron deficiency, including fatigue, dyspnea, tachycardia, palpitations, dizzziness, and orthostatic hypotension.

iron salts ■■■■►◄ levodopa
ferrous fumarate,
ferrous gluconate,
ferrous sulfate,
iron dextran

Risk rating: 2
Severity: Moderate   Onset: Delayed   Likelihood: Probable

Cause
Levodopa may form chelates with iron salts, which decreases levodopa absorption and serum level.

Effect
Levodopa effects may decrease.

Nursing considerations
- Separate doses as much as possible.
- If these drugs are used together, watch for recurring or worsening Parkinson's symptoms: increased tremors, muscle rigidity, bradykinesia (slowing of voluntary movement), shuffling gait, loss of facial expression, speech disturbances, and drooling.
- Notify the prescriber about loss of symptom control.
- Help the patient or caregiver develop a plan to ensure proper dosage intervals.
- Warn the patient or caregiver not to change levodopa dosage without consulting the prescriber.

---

iron salts ➤◄ **levothyroxine**

ferrous fumarate,   Synthroid
ferrous gluconate,
ferrous sulfate,
iron polysaccharide

Risk rating: 2
Severity: Moderate   Onset: Delayed   Likelihood: Suspected

Cause
Levothyroxine absorption may decrease, probably because it forms a complex with iron salt.

Effect
Levothyroxine effects may decrease, resulting in hypothyroidism.

Nursing considerations
- **ALERT** Separate levothyroxine and iron salts as much as possible.
- Monitor TSH, T_3, and T_4 levels. Therapeutic range for TSH is 0.2 to 5.4 microunits/ml; for T_3, 80 to 200 nanograms/dl; and for T_4, 5.4 to 11.5 mcg/dl.
- Levothyroxine dosage may need adjustment.
- Watch for evidence of hypothyroidism: weakness, fatigue, weight gain, coarse dry hair, rough skin, muscle aches, constipation, depression, irritability, and memory loss.
- Explain that levothyroxine dosage may need adjustment.
- Urge the patient to tell the prescriber about evidence of hypothyroidism, such as fatigue, weight gain, cold intolerance, and constipation.

iron salts ▶◀ mycophenolate mofetil

ferrous fumarate,
ferrous gluconate,
ferrous sulfate,
iron polysaccharide

CellCept

Risk rating: 2
Severity: Moderate   **Onset: Rapid**   **Likelihood: Suspected**

Cause
Mycophenolate mofetil absorption may decrease because the drug may form a complex with iron salt in the GI tract.

Effect
Mycophenolate mofetil level and effects may decrease.

Nursing considerations
◖ ALERT Avoid combining iron salts with mycophenolate mofetil.
▪ If you must give both, separate doses as much as possible.
▪ Watch for evidence of rejection or decreased drug effect.
▪ Tell the patient to report signs of organ rejection: reduced urine output after kidney transplant or shortness of breath after heart transplant.
▪ Help the patient develop a plan to ensure proper dosage intervals.

iron salts ▶◀ quinolones

ferrous fumarate,
ferrous gluconate,
ferrous sulfate,
iron polysaccharide

ciprofloxacin, moxifloxacin,
norfloxacin, ofloxacin

Risk rating: 2
Severity: Moderate   **Onset: Rapid**   **Likelihood: Probable**

Cause
Formation of an iron-quinolone complex decreases GI absorption of the quinolone.

Effect
Quinolone effects decrease.

Nursing considerations
▪ Monitor the patient for quinolone efficacy.
▪ Tell the patient to separate quinolone dose from iron by at least 2 hours.
▪ Other quinolones may interact with iron.
▪ Help the patient develop a plan to ensure proper dosage intervals.

iron salts ▰▰▰◀▶▰▰▰ tetracyclines, oral

ferrous fumarate,
ferrous gluconate,
ferrous sulfate,
iron polysaccharide

doxycycline, minocycline,
tetracycline

Risk rating: 2
Severity: Moderate   Onset: Delayed   Likelihood: Probable

Cause
Tetracyclines form insoluble chelates with iron salts, which may reduce absorption of both substances.

Effect
Tetracycline and iron salt levels and effects may decrease.

Nursing considerations
◨ **ALERT** If possible, avoid giving tetracyclines with iron salts.
▪ If they must be given together, separate doses by 3 to 4 hours.
▪ If you suspect an interaction, consult the prescriber or pharmacist; an enteric-coated or sustained-release iron salt may reduce the effects of the interaction.
▪ Monitor the patient for expected therapeutic response to tetracycline.
▪ Assess the patient for evidence of iron deficiency, including fatigue, dyspnea, tachycardia, palpitations, dizziness, and orthostatic hypotension.

isocarboxazid ▰▰▰◀▶▰▰▰ atomoxetine

Marplan

Strattera

Risk rating: 1
Severity: Major   Onset: Rapid   Likelihood: Suspected

Cause
Level of monoamine in the brain may change.

Effect
Possible risk increases for serious or fatal reaction resembling neuroleptic malignant syndrome.

Nursing considerations
◨ **ALERT** Use of atomoxetine and an MAO inhibitor such as isocarboxazid concurrently or within 2 weeks of each other is contraindicated.

■ Before starting atomoxetine, ask the patient when he last took an MAO inhibitor. Before starting an MAO inhibitor, ask the patient when he last took atomoxetine.
■ Monitor the patient for hyperthermia, rapid changes in vital signs, rigidity, muscle twitching, and mental status changes.

isocarboxazid ▬▬◄▬▬ bupropion
Marplan   Wellbutrin, Zyban

Risk rating: 1
Severity: Major   Onset: Delayed   Likelihood: Suspected

Cause
The cause of this interaction is unknown.

Effect
Risk of acute bupropion toxicity is increased.

Nursing considerations
◲ ALERT Administration of bupropion and MAO inhibitors such as isocarboxazid together is contraindicated.
■ Allow at least 14 days between discontinuining an MAO inhibitor and starting buproprion.
■ Interaction warning is based on animal trials, not actual patient studies.

isocarboxazid ▬▬◄▬▬ carbamazepine
Marplan   Carbatrol, Epitol, Equetro, Tegretol

Risk rating: 1
Severity: Major   Onset: Delayed   Likelihood: Suspected

Cause
The mechanism of this interaction is unknown.

Effect
Risk of severe adverse effects, including hyperpyrexia, hyperexcitability, muscle rigidity, and seizures, may increase.

Nursing considerations
◲ ALERT Use of carbamazepine with an MAO inhibitor such as isocarboxazid is contraindicated.
◲ ALERT Carbamazepine is structurally related to tricyclic antidepressants, which may cause hypertensive crisis, seizures, and death when given with MAO inhibitors.

■ MAO inhibitor should be stopped at least 14 days before carba-mazepine starts.
■ Urge the patient to tell the prescriber about all drugs and supple-ments he takes and about any increase in adverse effects.

---

isocarboxazid ━━▶◀━━ dextromethorphan
Marplan   Robitussin DM

Risk rating: 1
Severity: Major   **Onset: Rapid**   **Likelihood: Suspected**

Cause
MAO inhibitor such as isocarboxazid may decrease serotonin metabolism. Dextromethorphan may decrease synaptic reuptake of serotonin.

Effect
Risk of serotonin syndrome increases.

Nursing considerations
■ If possible, avoid giving these drugs together.
◪ **ALERT** Combined use may cause hyperpyrexia, abnormal muscle movement, hypotension, coma, and death.
■ If the patient takes an MAO inhibitor, caution against taking OTC cough and cold medicines that contain dextromethorphan.

---

isocarboxazid ━━▶◀━━ insulin
Marplan

Risk rating: 2
Severity: Moderate   **Onset: Delayed**   **Likelihood: Established**

Cause
MAO inhibitors such as isocaroxazid stimulate insulin secretion and inhibit gluconeogenesis (glucose formation).

Effect
Hypoglycemic response to insulin may be increased and prolonged.

Nursing considerations
■ Monitor glucose level closely if MAO inhibitor starts or dosage changes.
■ The extent of MAO inhibitor effect on glucose level may not be known for several weeks.

■ Watch for evidence of hypoglycemia: tachycardia, palpitations, anxiety, diaphoresis, nausea, hunger, dizziness, restlessness, headache, confusion, tremors, and speech and motor dysfunction.
■ Consult the prescriber if the patient experiences hypoglycemia; insulin dosage may need to be decreased.
■ Treat hypoglycemia as needed, such as with fast-acting oral carbohydrates, parenteral glucagon, or I.V. $D_{50}W$ bolus.
■ Make sure the patient and family can recognize hypoglycemia and respond appropriately.

isocarboxazid ━━▶◀━━	selective 5-HT$_1$ receptor agonists
Marplan	rizatriptan, sumatriptan, zolmitriptan

Risk rating: 1
Severity: Major   **Onset: Rapid**   **Likelihood: Suspected**

Cause
MAO inhibitors, subtype-A, such as isocarboxazid may inhibit metabolism of selective 5-HT$_1$ receptor agonists.

Effect
Serum level and the risk of cardiac toxicity from certain selective 5-HT$_1$ receptor agonists may increase.

Nursing considerations
◤ **ALERT** Use of certain selective 5-HT$_1$ receptor agonists with or within 2 weeks of stopping an MAO inhibitor is contraindicated.
■ If these drugs must be used together, naratriptan is less likely to interact with an MAO inhibitor.
■ Cardiac toxicity may include coronary artery vasospasm and transient myocardial ischemia.

isocarboxazid ━━▶◀━━	serotonin reuptake inhibitors
Marplan	citalopram, duloxetine, fluoxetine, sertraline, venlafaxine

Risk rating: 1
Severity: Major   **Onset: Rapid**   **Likelihood: Suspected**

Cause
Serotonin may accumulate rapidly in the CNS.

Effect
Risk of serotonin syndrome increases.

Nursing considerations
⚠ ALERT Don't use these drugs together.
▪ Allow 1 week after stopping venlafaxine (2 weeks after stopping citalopram or sertraline; 5 weeks after stopping fluoxetine) before giving an MAO inhibitor such as isocarboxazid.
▪ Allow 2 weeks after stopping an MAO inhibitor before giving a serotonin reuptake inhibitor.
▪ The selective MAO type-B inhibitor selegiline has been given with fluoxetine, paroxetine, or sertraline to patients with Parkinson's disease without negative effects.
▪ Make the patient aware of the traits of serotonin syndrome, which include CNS irritability, motor weakness, shivering, myoclonus, and altered consciousness.
▪ Urge the patient to promptly report adverse effects to the prescriber.

---

isocarboxazid ▬◄▬ tricyclic antidepressants
Marplan   amitriptyline, clomipramine,
                             desipramine, imipramine

Risk rating: 1
Severity: Major   **Onset: Rapid**   **Likelihood: Suspected**

Cause
The mechanism of this interaction is unknown.

Effect
Risk of hyperpyretic crisis, seizures, and death increase.

Nursing considerations
⚠ ALERT Don't give a tricyclic antidepressant with or within 2 weeks of an MAO inhibitor such as isocarboxazid.
▪ Imipramine and clomipramine may be more likely to interact with MAO inhibitors.
▪ Watch for adverse effects, including confusion, hyperexcitability, rigidity, seizures, increased temperature, increased pulse, increased respiration, sweating, mydriasis, flushing, headache, coma, and DIC.

isoflurane ◄►◄ labetalol
Forane   Trandate

Risk rating: 2
Severity: Moderate   **Onset: Rapid**   **Likelihood: Probable**

Cause
Additive myocardial depressant effects.

Effect
Excessive hypotension may result.

Nursing considerations
- Use these drugs together cautiously.
- Closely monitor blood pressure.
- The degree and duration of this interaction appears to be dose-dependent.
- This interaction may be used to induce deliberate hypotension for some surgical procedures.

isoflurane ◄►◄ nondepolarizing muscle relaxants
Forane   atracurium, pancuronium, vecuronium

Risk rating: 1
Severity: Major   **Onset: Rapid**   **Likelihood: Established**

Cause
These drugs potentiate pharmacologic actions.

Effect
The actions of nondepolarizing muscle relaxants are potentiated.

Nursing considerations
- Closely monitor respiratory function.
- The dose of both isoflurane and the nondepolarizing muscle relaxant may need to be adjusted.
- Provide ventilatory support as needed.
- The interaction is dose-dependent.
- If the the patient is receiving a nondepolarizing muscle relaxant continuously, the maintenance dose may need to be decreased 25% to 30%.

isoniazid ━━━▶◀━━━ carbamazepine
Nydrazid   Carbatrol, Epitol, Equetro,
                                    Tegretol

Risk rating: 2
Severity: Moderate   Onset: Delayed   Likelihood: Suspected

Cause
Isoniazid may inhibit carbamazepine metabolism. Carbamazepine
may increase isoniazid hepatotoxicity.

Effect
Risk of carbamazepine toxicity and isoniazid hepatotoxicity increase.

Nursing considerations
- Monitor carbamazepine level; therapeutic range is 4 to 12 mcg/ml.
- Watch for evidence of carbamazepine toxicity: dizziness, ataxia, respiratory depression, tachycardia, arrhythmias, blood pressure changes, impaired consciousness, abnormal reflexes, nystagmus, seizures, nausea, vomiting, and urine retention.
- Carbamazepine dosage may need adjustment.
- Monitor liver function tests. If hepatotoxicity develops, consult the prescriber about stopping isoniazid.
- Advise the patient to report signs of hepatotoxicity: abdominal pain, appetite loss, fatigue, yellow skin or eye discoloration, and dark urine.

isoniazid ━━━▶◀━━━ chlorzoxazone
Nydrazid   Parafon Forte DSC

Risk rating: 2
Severity: Moderate   Onset: Delayed   Likelihood: Suspected

Cause
Isoniazid inhibits the CYP2E1 hepatic metabolism of chlorzoxazone.

Effect
Chlorzoxazone levels and therapeutic and adverse effects may increase.

Nursing considerations
- Monitor the patient for increased CNS adverse effects including dizziness, drowsiness, headache, and light-headedness.
- Signs of more severe toxicity include nausea, vomiting, diarrhea, loss of muscle tone, decreased or absent deep tendon reflexes, respiratory depression, and hypotension.

■ Advise the patient to avoid hazardous activities that require alertness or physical coordination until CNS depressant effects are determined.
■ Chlorzoxazone dose may need to be reduced during combined therapy.

---

isoniazid ━━━▶◀━━━ phenytoin
Nydrazid   Dilantin

Risk rating: 2
Severity: Moderate   Onset: Delayed   Likelihood: Established

Cause
Hepatic microsomal enzyme metabolism of phenytoin is inhibited.

Effect
Phenytoin level, effects, and risk of toxicity increase.

Nursing considerations
■ Monitor phenytoin level closely. Dosage may need to be adjusted. Therapeutic range for phenytoin is 10 to 20 mcg/ml.
■ Toxic effects can occur at therapeutic levels. Adjust the measured level for hypoalbuminemia or renal impairment, which can increase free drug level.
■ Signs and symptoms of phenytoin toxicity include nystagmus, slurred speech, ataxia, blurred or double vision, confusion, drowsiness, and lethargy.
■ If the patient's phenytoin level has been stabilized with isoniazid and isoniazid stops, watch for loss of seizure control.
■ Hydantoins other than phenytoin may have a similar interaction.

---

isoniazid ━━━▶◀━━━ rifampin
Nydrazid   Rifadin, Rimactane

Risk rating: 1
Severity: Major   Onset: Delayed   Likelihood: Probable

Cause
Rifampin may alter isoniazid metabolism.

Effect
Risk of hepatotoxicity increases over either drug given alone.

Nursing considerations
■ Monitor liver function tests in patients taking both drugs.

■ Consult the prescriber about increased liver enzyme levels; one or both drugs may need to be stopped.
■ Monitor the patient's liver enzymes and condition even after one or both drugs are stopped because of possible severity of reaction.
■ Advise the patient to report signs of hepatotoxicity: abdominal pain, appetite loss, fatigue, yellow skin or eye discoloration, and dark urine.

isosorbide dinitrate ▶◀ dihydroergotamine
Isordil   D.H.E. 45

Risk rating: 2
Severity: Moderate   **Onset: Rapid**   **Likelihood: Suspected**

Cause
Metabolism of dihydroergotamine decreases, increasing its availability, which antagonizes coronary vasodilation caused by nitrates such as isosorbide dinitrate.

Effect
Increased dihydroergotamine availability may increase systolic blood pressure and decrease the antianginal effects of the nitrate.

Nursing considerations
■ Use these drugs together cautiously in patients with angina.
■ I.V. dihydroergotamine may antagonize coronary vasodilation.
■ Watch for evidence of ergotism, such as peripheral ischemia, paresthesia, headache, nausea, and vomiting.
■ Teach the patient to immediately report signs of peripheral ischemia, such as numbness or tingling in fingers and toes or red blisters on hands or feet. Dihydroergotamine dosage may need to be decreased.

isosorbide dinitrate, ▶◀ phosphodiesterase-5 isosorbide inhibitors mononitrate
Imdur, Isordil   sildenafil, tadalafil, vardenafil

Risk rating: 1
Severity: Major   **Onset: Rapid**   **Likelihood: Suspected**

Cause
Phosphodiesterase-5 inhibitors potentiate hypotensive effects of nitrates, such as isosorbide.

Effect
Risk of severe hypotension increases.

Nursing considerations
⚠ ALERT Combined use of nitrates and erectile dysfunction (ED) drugs may be fatal and is contraindicated.
- Carefully screen the patient for ED drug use before giving a nitrate.
- Even during an emergency, before giving a nitrate, find out if a patient with chest pain has taken an ED drug during the previous 2 hours.
- Monitor the patient for orthostatic hypotension, dizziness, sweating, and headache.

---

itraconazole ▶◀ alfuzosin
Sporanox   Uroxatral

Risk rating: 2
Severity: Moderate   Onset: Delayed   Likelihood: Suspected

Cause
Azole antifungals such as itraconazole may inhibit the metabolism of alfuzosin.

Effect
The pharmacologic and adverse effects of alfuzosin may be increased.

Nursing considerations
ALERT
Avoid giving alfuzosin and azole antifungals together.
- Notify the the prescriber that the patient is taking an azole antifungal and alfuzosin together, which is contraindicated.
- Monitor the patient for development of adverse effects of alfuzosin, including dizziness, abdominal pain, nausea, and fatigue.

---

itraconazole ▶◀ aripiprazole
Sporanox   Abilify

Risk rating: 2
Severity: Moderate   Onset: Delayed   Likelihood: Suspected

Cause
Azole antifungals such as itraconazole may inhibit CYP3A4 metabolism of aripiprazole.

Effect
Plasma concentrations of aripiprazole may be increased, increasing pharmacologic and adverse effects.

Nursing considerations
- When azole antifungals are administered with aripiprazole, reduce the dose of aripiprazole by 50%.
- The dose of aripiprazole will need to be increased when itraconazole is discontinued.
- Instruct the the patient to notify the prescriber of increased adverse effects, such as anxiety, insomnia, nausea and vomiting, and flu-like symptoms.

itraconazole ➤◄	benzodiazepines
Sporanox	alprazolam, chlordiazepoxide, midazolam, quazepam, triazolam

Risk rating: 2
Severity: Moderate   Onset: Delayed   Likelihood: Established

Cause
Azole antifungals such as itraconazole decrease CYP3A4 metabolism of certain benzodiazepines.

Effect
Benzodiazepine effects are increased and prolonged, which may cause CNS depression and psychomotor impairment.

Nursing considerations
⚠ **ALERT** Use of alprazolam or triazolam with itraconazole is contraindicated.
- Caution that the effects of this interaction may last several days after stopping the azole antifungal.
- Explain that taking these drugs together may increase sedative effects; tell the patient to report such effects promptly.
- Explain alternative methods of inducing sleep or relieving anxiety during antifungal therapy.
- Various azole antifungal–benzodiazepine combinations may interact. If you suspect an interaction, consult the prescriber or pharmacist.

itraconazole ━━━▶◀━━━ buspirone
Sporanox   BuSpar

Risk rating: 2
Severity: Moderate   **Onset: Delayed**   **Likelihood: Probable**

Cause
Azole antifungals such as itraconazole may inhibit the CYP3A4 isoen-zyme responsible for buspirone metabolism.

Effect
Plasma buspirone level may increase.

Nursing considerations
■ If the patient is taking buspirone, monitor him closley when an azole antifungal is started or stopped or its dosage is changed.
■ If the patient is taking itraconazole, initial buspirone dose should be conservative.
■ Monitor the patient for signs of buspirone toxicity, including in-creased CNS effects (such as dizziness, drowsiness, and headache), vomiting, and diarrhea.
■ Urge the patient to tell prescribers about all drugs and supplements he takes and about any increase in adverse effects.

itraconazole ━━━▶◀━━━ busulfan
Sporanox   Myleran

Risk rating: 2
Severity: Moderate   **Onset: Delayed**   **Likelihood: Suspected**

Cause
The mechanism of the interaction is unknown.

Effect
Itraconazole may increase plasma busulfan levels, increasing the risk of toxicity.

Nursing considerations
■ Monitor the patient taking busulfan and itraconazole for increased toxicity.
■ If a patient taking busulfan is started on itraconazole, the dose of busulfan may need to be decreased.
■ Monitor the patient for persistent cough, labored breathing, throm-bocytopenia, and signs of infection.
■ Tell the patient to call the prescriber if he notices increased bleed-ing or bruising, jaundice, or fever, sore throat, or fatigue.

■ Fluconazole may be used as a safe alternative instead of itraconazole.

---

itraconazole ▬▶◀▬ conivaptan
Sporanox   Vaprisol

Risk rating: 1
Severity: Major   **Onset: Delayed**   **Likelihood: Suspected**

Cause
Azole antifungals such as itraconazole may inhibit the CYP3A4 metabolism of conivaptan.

Effect
Conivaptan levels and risk of adverse reactions may increase.

Nursing considerations
⚡ **ALERT** Use of conivaptan and azole antifungals together is contraindicated.
■ The basis for this interaction is pharmacodynamics, not actual patient studies.

---

itraconazole ▬▶◀▬ corticosteroids
Sporanox   budesonide, dexamethasone,
                            fluticasone, methylpredniso-
                            lone, prednisolone/prednisone

Risk rating: 2
Severity: Moderate   **Onset: Delayed**   **Likelihood: Suspected**

Cause
Itraconazole inhibits CYP3A4 metabolism of corticosteroid and decreases elimination.

Effect
Corticosteroid effects and toxicity may be increased.

Nursing considerations
■ Monitor the patient for increased adverse effects to corticosteroids, and adjust dose as needed.
■ Monitor the patient taking corticosteroid and itraconazole for Cushing syndrome.
■ Carefully monitor the patient for infection, edema, and increased serum glucose level.
■ Instruct the patient not to abruptly stop the corticosteroid; it should gradually be tapered to prevent withdrawal symptoms.

itraconazole ▶◀ cyclophosphamide
Sporanox   Cytoxan

Risk rating: 2
Severity: Moderate   **Onset: Delayed**   **Likelihood: Suspected**

Cause
Inhibition of cyclophosphamide hepatic metabolism is suspected.

Effect
Cyclophosphamide exposure and its metabolites may be increased, increasing the risk of adverse effects.

Nursing considerations
- Monitor the patient for increased adverse effects.
- Monitor liver and renal function tests.
- Watch the patient for hemorrhagic cystitis, infection, cardiotoxicity, and anemia.
- Teach the patient the adverse effects of cyclophosphamide, and instuct him to call the prescriber immediately if seen.

itraconazole ▶◀ cyclosporine
Sporanox   Gengraf, Neoral, Sandimmune

Risk rating: 2
Severity: Moderate   **Onset: Delayed**   **Likelihood: Established**

Cause
Azole antifungals such as itraconazole decrease cyclosporine metabolism.

Effect
Cyclosporine level and toxicity may increase.

Nursing considerations
- Cyclosporine level may increase 1 to 3 days after starting an azole antifungal and persist for more than 1 week after stopping it.
- Monitor cyclosporine level.
- Adjust cyclosporine dosage to maintain therapeutic level.
- Cyclosporine dose may need to be decreased by 68% to 97%.
- Monitor the patient for hepatotoxicity and nephrotoxicity.

itraconazole ➤◀ didanosine
Sporanox   Videx

Risk rating: 2
Severity: Moderate   **Onset: Rapid**   **Likelihood: Suspected**

Cause
Inert ingredients in chewable didanosine tablets decrease absorption of azole antifungals such as itraconazole.

Effect
Efficacy of azole antifungal may decrease.

Nursing considerations
■ To minimize interaction, instruct the patient to take antifungal drug 2 hours before didanosine.
■ Monitor the patient for lack of response to antifungal drug.
■ Help the patient develop a plan to ensure proper dosage intervals.
■ Other azole antifungals may interact with didanosine. If you suspect an interaction, consult the prescriber or pharmacist.

itraconazole ➤◀ digoxin
Sporanox   Lanoxin

Risk rating: 2
Severity: Moderate   **Onset: Delayed**   **Likelihood: Established**

Cause
Renal clearance of digoxin may decrease and absorption increase.

Effect
Digoxin level, effects, and adverse effects may increase.

Nursing considerations
■ Monitor digoxin level. Therapeutic range is 0.8 to 2 nanogram/ml.
■ Watch for evidence of digoxin toxicity: arrhythmias (such as brady-cardia, AV blocks, and ventricular ectopy), lethargy, drowsiness, confusion, hallucinations, headaches, syncope, visual disturbances, nausea, anorexia, vomiting, and diarrhea.
■ Digoxin dosage may need reduction.
■ Azole antifungals other than itraconazole may also interact with digoxin. If you suspect an interaction, consult the prescriber or pharmacist.

itraconazole ➤◀ dofetilide
Sporanox   Tikosyn

Risk rating: 1
Severity: Major   **Onset: Delayed**   **Likelihood: Suspected**

Cause
Dofetilide renal elimination may be inhibited.

Effect
Dofetilide level and risk of ventricular arrhythmias, including torsades de pointes, may increase.

Nursing considerations
◼ **ALERT** Use of dofetilide with itraconazole is contraindicated.
■ Monitor ECG for excessive prolongation of QTc interval or development of ventricular arrhythmias.
■ Consult the prescriber about alternative anti-infective therapy.
■ Urge the patient to tell the prescriber about increased adverse effects.
■ Azole antifungals other than itraconazole may interact with dofetilide. If you suspect an interaction, consult the prescriber or pharmacist.

itraconazole ➤◀ eplerenone
Sporanox   Inspra

Risk rating: 1
Severity: Major   **Onset: Delayed**   **Likelihood: Suspected**

Cause
Azole antifungals, such as itraconazole, inhibit eplerenone metabolism.

Effect
Eplerenone level rises, causing hyperkalemia and increasing the risk of life-threatening arrhythmias.

Nursing considerations
◼ **ALERT** Use of azole antifungals with eplerenone is contraindicated.
■ Potent CYP3A4 inhibitors increase the eplerenone level and the risk of hyperkalemia-induced arrhythmias—some fatal.
■ Monitor the patient's serum potassium level.
■ Tell the patient to report nausea, irregular heartbeat, or slowed pulse to the prescriber.

itraconazole ━━━►◄━━━ ergot derivatives
Sporanox   dihydroergotamine, ergotamine

Risk rating: 1
Severity: Major   **Onset: Delayed**   **Likelihood: Suspected**

Cause
Itraconazole may inhibit CYP3A4 metabolism of ergot derivatives.

Effect
Risk of ergot toxicity may be increased.

Nursing considerations
◼ **ALERT** Use of these drugs together is contraindicated.
■ Signs of ergot toxicity include peripheral vasospasm and ischemia.
■ Caution the patient to avoid ergot derivatives (for migraine, for example) while taking itraconazole; consult the prescriber about alternative therapies.

itraconazole ━━━►◄━━━ felodipine
Sporanox   Plendil

Risk rating: 2
Severity: Moderate   **Onset: Delayed**   **Likelihood: Suspected**

Cause
Itraconazole may inhibit felodipine CYP3A4 metabolism.

Effect
Felodipine level and adverse effects may increase.

Nursing considerations
■ Felodipine dose may need to be adjusted.
■ Closely monitor patients age 65 and older and patients with liver impairment; they're at increased risk for elevated felodipine level.
■ Monitor the patient for adverse felodipine effects, including increased peripheral edema, hypotension, and tachycardia.
■ Azole antifungals other than itraconazole may interact with felodipine. If you suspect an interaction, consult the prescriber or pharmacist.
■ Urge the patient to tell the prescriber about increased adverse effects.

itraconazole ➤◀ fexofenadine

Sporanox   Allegra

Risk rating: 3
Severity: Minor   **Onset: Rapid**   **Likelihood: Suspected**

Cause
Itraconazole may increase absorption of fexofenadine.

Effect
Fexofenadine levels and pharmacologic and adverse effects may increase.

Nursing considerations
- Monitor for fexofenadine adverse reactions: drowsiness, headache, fatigue, nausea, dyspepsia, and dysmenorrhea.
- Watch for expected clinical effects, including relief of seasonal allergic rhinitis or relief of chronic urticaria.
- In patients with impaired renal function, maximum daily dosage recommendations are 60 mg for adults and 30 mg for children.

itraconazole ➤◀ food

Sporanox   cola, food, grapefruit juice, orange juice

Risk rating: 2
Severity: Moderate   **Onset: Rapid**   **Likelihood: Suspected**

Cause
Cola and food may increase itraconazole absorption. Grapefruit juice may decrease it. The exact mechanism of the interaction with orange juice is unknown.

Effect
Itraconazole level may increase (cola, food) or decrease (grapefruit juice, orange juice), with the latter resulting in decreased itraconazole effects.

Nursing considerations
- Advise the patient to take itraconazole capsules after meals.
- **ALERT** Itraconazole oral solution should be taken without food for maximum absorption.
- Advise the patient to avoid taking itraconazole with grapefruit products, orange juice, or cola.

itraconazole 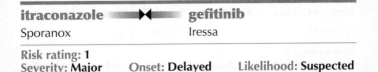 gefitinib
Sporanox   Iressa

Risk rating: 1
Severity: Major   **Onset: Delayed**   **Likelihood: Suspected**

Cause
Azole antifungals such as itraconazole may inhibit CYP3A4 metabolism of gefitinib.

Effect
Gefitinib levels and risk of adverse reactions may be increased.

Nursing considerations
■ If the patient receives gefitinib, observe for adverse reactions if itraconazole is added to the treatment.
■ Encourage the patient to report signs and symptoms of adverse reactions, including eye problems such as pain, redness, or vision changes; diarrhea, vomiting, loss of appetite, or weight loss; rash or itching; weakness; and liver damage.
◪ ALERT The FDA has limited the use of gefitinib to certain patient populations. New clinical trials are being developed to determine future benefits of this drug.

itraconazole 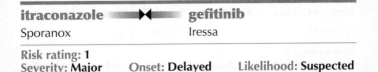 H2 antagonists
Sporanox   cimetidine, ranitidine

Risk rating: 2
Severity: Moderate   **Onset: Delayed**   **Likelihood: Suspected**

Cause
Azole antifungal availability may decrease because elevated gastric pH may reduce tablet dissolution.

Effect
Azole antifungal effects may decrease.

Nursing considerations
■ If possible, don't adminsiter itraconazole with an H2 antagonist.
■ If combined use is needed, give 680 mg of glutamic acid hydrochloride 15 mintues before itraconazole.
■ Watch for expected antifungal effects.
■ Explain that other drugs that increase gastric pH such as antacids also may decrease azole antifungal absorption.

itraconazole ━━━▶◀ haloperidol
Sporanox   Haldol

Risk rating: 2
Severity: Moderate   **Onset: Delayed**   **Likelihood: Suspected**

Cause
Itraconazole inhibits CYP3A4 metabolism of haloperidol.

Effect
Haloperidol levels and risk of adverse reactions increases.

Nursing considerations
■ Observe the patient's clinical response to haloperidol when itraconazole is started or stopped. Adjust the dose as needed.
■ Monitor haloperidol level (therapeutic range, 5 to 20 nanograms/ml).
■ Monitor for adverse reactions, which include neurologic toxicity, altered mental status, rigidity, hyperpyrexia, weakness, lethargy, stupor,
fever, severe extrapyrmidal symptoms, and dystonia.
■ Advise the patient to tell the prescriber about increased adverse effects.

itraconazole ━━━▶◀ HMG-CoA reductase inhibitors
Sporanox   atorvastatin, fluvastatin,
                                  lovastatin, pravastatin,
                                  rosuvastatin, simvastatin

Risk rating: 1
Severity: Major   **Onset: Rapid**   **Likelihood: Probable**

Cause
Azole antifungals such as itraconazole may inhibit hepatic metabolism of HMG-CoA reductase inhibitors.

Effect
HMG-CoA reductase inhibitor level and adverse effects may increase.

Nursing considerations
■ If possible, avoid use together.
■ HMG-CoA reductase inhibitor dosage may need to be decreased.
■ Monitor serum cholesterol and lipid levels.
◖ **ALERT** Assess the patient for evidence of rhabdomyolysis, includ-
ing fatigue; muscle aches and weakness; joint pain; dark, red, or cola-

colored urine; weight gain; seizures; and greatly increased serum CK level.
■ Pravastatin is the HMG-CoA reductase inhibitor least affected by this interaction and may be preferable for use with an azole antifungal, if needed.

itraconazole ▶◀ omeprazole
Sporanox   Prilosec

Risk rating: 2
Severity: Moderate   Onset: Rapid   Likelihood: Suspected

Cause
Proton pump inhibitors such as omeprazole increase gastric pH, which may impair dissolution of azole antifungals, such as itraconazole.

Effect
Efficacy of azole antifungals may decrease.

Nursing considerations
■ Notify the prescriber if the patient takes both drugs; an alternative may be available.
■ If no alternative is possible, suggest taking the azole antifungal with an acidic beverage such as cola.
■ Monitor the patient for lack of response to the antifungal drug.
■ If the patient can't tolerate acidic beverages and the antifungal therapy appears to be ineffective, antifungal dosage may need to be increased.
■ Other drugs that increase gastric pH may interact with azole antifungals. If you suspect an interaction, consult the prescriber or pharmacist.

itraconazole ▶◀ phenytoin
Sporanox   Dilantin

Risk rating: 2
Severity: Moderate   Onset: Delayed   Likelihood: Suspected

Cause
Metabolism of itraconazole increases, and phenytoin metabolism is inhibited.

Effect
Efficacy of itraconazole may decrease. Phenytoin effects increase.

Nursing considerations
- Avoid use of these drugs together.
- More research is being done on this interaction.
- Monitor the patient for lack of response to the antifungal drug.
- Monitor phenytoin level closely. Dosage may need to be adjusted. Therapeutic range for phenytoin is 10 to 20 mcg/ml.
- Signs and symptoms of phenytoin toxicity include nystagmus, slurred speech, ataxia, blurred or double vision, confusion, drowsiness, and lethargy.

---

itraconazole ◄►► phosphodiesterase-5 inhibitors
Sporanox   sildenafil, tadalafil, vardenafil

Risk rating: 2
Severity: Moderate   **Onset: Delayed**   **Likelihood: Suspected**

Cause
Azole antifungals such as itraconazole inhibit CYP3A4 metabolism of PDE-5 inhibitors.

Effect
PDE-5 inhibitor levels, pharmacologic effects, and risk of adverse effects may increase.

Nursing considerations
- Dosage of PDE-5 inhibitor may need to be decreased.
- Administer these drugs together cautiously.
- Instruct the patient to take PDE-5 exactly as instructed.
- Warn the patient of adverse effects, including prolonged, painful erection.

---

itraconazole ◄►► pimozide
Sporanox   Orap

Risk rating: 1
Severity: Major   **Onset: Delayed**   **Likelihood: Suspected**

Cause
Azole antifungals such as itraconazole may inhibit CYP3A4 metabolism of pimozide.

Effect
Risk of life-threatening arrhythmias may increase.

Nursing considerations
⚠ ALERT Combined use of these drugs is contraindicated.
■ Arrhythmias are related to prolonged QT interval, a known risk of pimozide.
■ Interaction warning is based on pharmokinetics of these drugs, not actual patient studies.

---

itraconazole ━━━━◄► protease inhibitors
Sporanox

amprenavir, indinavir, ritonavir, saquinavir

Risk rating: 2
Severity: Moderate   **Onset: Delayed**   **Likelihood: Suspected**

Cause
Azole antifungals such as itraconazole may inhibit metabolism of protease inhibitors.

Effect
Protease inhibitor level may increase.

Nursing considerations
■ Protease inhibitor dosage may be decreased when therapy starts.
■ Watch for increased protease inhibitor effects: hyperglycemia, onset of diabetes, rash, GI complaints, and altered liver function tests.
■ Advise the patient to report increased hunger or thirst, frequent urination, fatigue, and dry, itchy skin.
■ Tell the patient not to alter regimen without consulting the prescriber.

---

itraconazole ━━━━◄► quinidine
Sporanox

Risk rating: 1
Severity: Major   **Onset: Delayed**   **Likelihood: Probable**

Cause
Azole antifungals such as itraconazole may inhibit metabolism and excretion of quinidine.

Effect
Quinidine level and risk of adverse effects, including serious cardiovascular events, increases.

Nursing considerations
⚠ ALERT Combined use of these drugs is contraindicated.

- Monitor quinidine level closely; dose may need to be reduced.
- Therapeutic range of quinidine is 2 to 6 mcg/ml. More specific assays have levels of less than 1 mcg/ml.
- Carefully monitor the QT interval, and notify the prescriber if interval increases.

itraconazole ━━▶◀━ rifamycins

Sporanox   rifabutin, rifampin

Risk rating: 2
Severity: Moderate   **Onset: Delayed**   **Likelihood: Suspected**

Cause
Rifamycins may decrease the level of an azole antifungal such as itraconazole.

Effect
Infection may recur.

Nursing considerations
- Notify the prescriber if the patient takes both drugs; an alternative may be available.
- If drugs must be taken together and the antifungal appears ineffective, antifungal dosage may need to be increased.
- Teach the patient to recognize signs and symptoms of his infection and to contact the prescriber promptly if they occur.

itraconazole ━━▶◀━ selective 5-HT$_1$ receptor agonists

Sporanox   almotriptan, eletriptan

Risk rating: 2
Severity: Moderate   **Onset: Delayed**   **Likelihood: Suspected**

Cause
Azole antifungals, such as itraconazole, inhibit CYP3A4 metabolism of certain 5-HT$_1$ receptor agonists.

Effect
Serum level and adverse effects of the selective 5-HT$_1$ receptor agonist may increase.

Nursing considerations
⚡ ALERT Don't give eletriptan within 72 hours or almotriptan within 7 days of itraconazole.

■ Adverse effects of selective 5-HT$_1$ receptor agonists may include coronary artery vasospasm, dizziness, nausea, paresthesia, and somnolence.

itraconazole ➤◀ sirolimus
Sporanox   Rapamune

Risk rating: 2
Severity: Moderate   Onset: Delayed   Likelihood: Probable

Cause
Azole antifungals such as itraconazole inhibit CYP3A4, which is needed for sirolimus metabolism.

Effect
Sirolimus level, effects, and risk of adverse effects may increase.

Nursing considerations
■ Monitor trough level of sirolimus in whole blood when starting or stopping an azole antifungal. Therapeutic level varies depending on which other drugs the patient receives such as cyclosporine, for example.
■ Watch for signs of sirolimus toxicity, such as anemia, leukopenia, thrombocytopenia, hypokalemia, hyperlipemia, fever, interstitial lung disease, and diarrhea.
■ Other CYP3A4 inhibitors may interact with sirolimus. If you suspect an interaction, consult the prescriber or pharmacist.
■ Urge the patient to promptly report new onset of fever higher than 100°F (38° C), fatigue, shortness of breath, easy bruising, gum bleeding, muscle twitches, palpitations, or chest discomfort or pain.

itraconazole ➤◀ tacrolimus
Sporanox   Prograf

Risk rating: 2
Severity: Moderate   Onset: Delayed   Likelihood: Probable

Cause
Itraconazole inhibits tacrolimus metabolism in the liver and GI tract.

Effect
Tacrolimus level and risk of adverse effects may increase.

Nursing considerations
■ Monitor renal function and mental status closely.
■ Check tacrolimus level often. Normal trough level is 6 to 10 mcg/L.

- Tacrolimus dosage may need to be decreased when the patient takes itraconaozle.
- Signs of toxicity often occur within 3 days of combined use.
- **ALERT** Watch for renal failure, nephrotoxicity, hyperkalemia, hyperglycemia, delirium, and other changes in mental status.

---

itraconazole ▶◀ vincristine
Sporanox   Oncovin

Risk rating: 1
Severity: Major   **Onset: Delayed**   **Likelihood: Probable**

Cause
Azole antifungals such as itraconazole inhibit CYP3A4, which is needed for vinca alkaloid metabolism.

Effect
Risk of vinca alkaloid toxicity increases.

Nursing considerations
- If possible, avoid giving these drugs together.
- **ALERT** The risk of serious toxicity is increased with itraconazole.
- If use together is unavoidable, watch for evidence of toxicity, such as constipation, myalgia, hypertension, hyponatremia, and neutropenia.
- Explain adverse vinca alkaloid effects and the need to report them promptly.
- Stop azole antifungal as soon as possible.

---

itraconazole ▶◀ warfarin
Sporanox   Coumadin

Risk rating: 1
Severity: Major   **Onset: Delayed**   **Likelihood: Established**

Cause
Warfarin metabolism is inhibited.

Effect
Anticoagulant effects may increase.

Nursing considerations
- Monitor PT and INR at least every 2 days.
- Patients with renal insufficiency may be at greater risk.
- Although all azole antifungals interact with warfarin, some interactions may be more significant than others.
- Watch for evidence of bleeding.

■ Tell the patient to report unusual bruising or bleeding.
■ Remind the patient that warfarin interacts with many drugs, and tell the patient to report any change in drug regimen.

itraconazole ▶◀ zolpidem
Sporanox   Ambien

Risk rating: 2
Severity: Moderate   Onset: Delayed   Likelihood: Suspected

Cause
Itraconazole inhibits CYP3A4 metabolism of zolpidem.

Effect
Zolpidem levels and therapeutic effects may increase.

Nursing considerations
■ If itraconazole and zolpidem are coadministered, monitor the patient's response. Zolpidem dosage may need to be decreased.
■ Instruct the patient on signs and symptoms of increased effects of zolpidem, including headache, daytime drowsiness, hangover, lethargy, light-headedness, palpitations, abdominal pain, nausea, myalgia, and back or chest pain.
■ Caution the patient to avoid performing activities that require mental alertness or physical coordination during therapy.

ketamine ▶◀ atracurium
Ketalar

Risk rating: 2
Severity: Moderate   Onset: Rapid   Likelihood: Probable

Cause
Increased acetylcholine release and decreased postsynaptic membrane sensitivity is suspected.

Effect
The actions of nondepolarizing muscle relaxants, including atracurium, are enhanced, leading to profound and severe respiratory depression.

Nursing considerations
■ Use these drugs together cautiously.
■ The nondepolarizing muscle relaxant dosage may need adjustment.
■ Provide ventilatory support as needed.
■ The recovery time from atracurium may also be increased.

ketoconazole ━━▶◀━━ alfuzosin
Nizoral   Uroxatral

Risk rating: 2
Severity: Moderate   Onset: Delayed   Likelihood: Suspected

Cause
Azole antifungals such as ketoconazole may inhibit the metabolism of alfuzosin.

Effect
The pharmacologic and adverse effects of alfuzosin may be increased.

Nursing considerations
◪ **ALERT** Avoid giving alfuzosin and azole antifungals together.
■ Notifty the prescriber that the patient is taking an azole antifungal and alfuzosin together, which is contraindicated.
■ Monitor the patient for the development of adverse effects from alfuzosin, which include dizziness, abdominal pain, nausea, and fatigue.

ketoconazole ━━▶◀━━ aripiprazole
Nizoral   Abilify

Risk rating: 2
Severity: Moderate   Onset: Delayed   Likelihood: Suspected

Cause
Azole antifungals such as ketoconazole may inhibit CYP3A4 metabolism of aripiprazole.

Effect
Plasma concentrations of aripiprazole may be increased, increasing pharmacologic and adverse effects.

Nursing considerations
■ When azole antifungals are administered with aripiprazole, reduce the dose of aripiprazole by 50%.
■ The dose of aripiprazole will need to be increased when ketoconazole is discontinued.
■ Instruct the patient to notify the prescriber of increased adverse effects, such as anxiety, insomnia, nausea and vomiting, and flu-like symptoms.

ketoconazole ■■■▶◀■■■ benzodiazepines

Nizoral

alprazolam, chlordiazepoxide, midazolam, quazepam, triazolam

Risk rating: 2
Severity: Moderate   Onset: Delayed   Likelihood: Established

Cause
Azole antifungals such as ketoconazole decrease CYP3A4 metabolism of certain benzodiazepines.

Effect
Benzodiazepine effects are increased and prolonged, which may cause CNS depression and psychomotor impairment.

Nursing considerations
◤ **ALERT** Use of alprazolam or triazolam with ketoconazole is contra-indicated.
■ Caution that the effects of this interaction may last several days after stopping the azole antifungal.
■ Explain that taking these drugs together may increase sedative effects; tell the patient to report such effects promptly.
■ Explain alternative methods of inducing sleep or relieving anxiety during antifungal therapy.
■ Various azole antifungal–benzodiazepine combinations may interact. If you suspect an interaction, consult the prescriber or pharmacist.

ketoconazole ■■■▶◀■■■ bosentan

Nizoral

Tracleer

Risk rating: 2
Severity: Moderate   Onset: Delayed   Likelihood: Suspected

Cause
Azole antifungals such as ketoconazole inhibit CYP3A4 metabolism of bosentan.

Effect
Plasma concentration of bosentan may be increased, increasing pharmacologic and adverse effects.

Nursing considerations
■ Closely monitor clinical response to bosentan when starting or stopping ketoconazole.

- Observe the patient for an increase in adverse effects to bosentan.
- An increased number of patients receiving both drugs complained of a headache.
- Monitor the patient for increased shortness of breath, edema, and heart failure.

---

ketoconazole ◄ carbamazepine
Nizoral

Carbatrol, Epitol, Equetro, Tegretol

Risk rating: 2
Severity: Moderate   Onset: Delayed   Likelihood: Suspected

Cause
Azole antifungals such as ketoconazole may inhibit CYP3A4 metabolism of carbamazepine.

Effect
Carbamazepine effects, including adverse effects, may increase.

Nursing considerations
- Monitor the patient's response when an azole antifungal is started or stopped.
- Monitor carbamazepine level; therapeutic range is 4 to 12 mcg/ml.
- **ALERT** Watch for signs of anorexia or subtle appetite changes, which may indicate an excessive carbamazepine level.
- Monitor the patient for signs of carbamazepine toxicity, including dizziness, ataxia, respiratory depression, tachycardia, arrhythmias, blood pressure changes, impaired consciousness, abnormal reflexes, nystagmus, seizures, nausea, vomiting, and urine retention.
- Other azole antifungals may interact with carbamazepine. If you suspect an interaction, consult the prescriber or pharmacist.

---

ketoconazole ◄ conivaptan
Nizoral

Vaprisol

Risk rating: 1
Severity: Major   Onset: Delayed   Likelihood: Suspected

Cause
Azole antifungals such as ketoconazole may inhibit the CYP3A4 metabolism of conivaptan.

Effect
Conivaptan levels and risk of adverse reactions may increase.

Nursing considerations
ALERT Use of conivaptan and azole antifungals together is contra-indicated.
■ The basis for this interaction is pharmacodynamics, not actual patient studies.

ketoconazole ▶◀ corticosteroids

Nizoral

budesonide, dexamethasone, fluticasone, methylpredniso-lone, prednisolone/prednisone

Risk rating: 2
Severity: Moderate   Onset: Delayed   Likelihood: Suspected

Cause
Inhibition of CYP3A4 metabolism of corticosteroid and decrease in elimination.

Effect
Corticosteroid effects and toxicity may be increased.

Nursing considerations
■ Monitor the patient for increased adverse effects to corticosteroids, and adjust dose as needed.
■ Monitor the patient taking corticosteroid and ketoconazole for Cushing syndrome.
■ Carefully monitor the patient for infection, edema, and increased serum glucose level.
■ Instruct the patient not to abruptly stop the corticosteroid; it should gradually be tapered to prevent withdrawal symptoms.

ketoconazole ▶◀ cyclosporine

Nizoral

Gengraf, Neoral, Sandimmune

Risk rating: 2
Severity: Moderate   Onset: Delayed   Likelihood: Established

Cause
Azole antifungals such as ketoconazole decrease cyclosporine metabolism.

Effect
Cyclosporine level and toxicity may increase.

Nursing considerations
■ Cyclosporine level may increase 1 to 3 days after starting an azole antifungal and persist for more than 1 week after stopping it.
■ Monitor cyclosporine level.
■ Adjust cyclosporine dosage to maintain therapeutic level.
■ Cyclosporine dose may need to be decreased by 68% to 97%.
■ Monitor the patient for hepatotoxicity and nephrotoxicity.

ketoconazole ▬▶◀▬ didanosine
Nizoral   Videx

Risk rating: 2
Severity: Moderate   **Onset: Rapid**   **Likelihood: Suspected**

Cause
Inert ingredients in chewable didanosine tablets decrease absorption of azole antifungals such as ketoconazole.

Effect
Efficacy of azole antifungals may decrease.

Nursing considerations
■ To minimize interaction, instruct the patient to take the antifungal drug 2 hours before didanosine.
■ Monitor the patient for lack of response to the antifungal drug.
■ Other azole antifungals may interact with didanosine. If you suspect an interaction, consult the prescriber or pharmacist.
■ Help the patient develop a plan to ensure proper dosage intervals.

ketoconazole ▬▶◀▬ docetaxel
Nizoral   Taxotere

Risk rating: 1
Severity: Major   **Onset: Delayed**   **Likelihood: Suspected**

Cause
Ketoconazole inhibits CYP3A4 metabolism of docetaxel.

Effect
Docetaxol level, effects, and risk of toxicity may increase.

Nursing considerations
■ If possible, avoid using these drugs together.
■ If the patient must take both drugs, the dose of docetaxel may need to be decreased.
■ Monitor the patient's WBC count.

■ Notify the prescriber immediately if the patient has a fever, sore throat, red or inflamed areas, or other signs of infection.

ketoconazole ➤◀ dofetilide
Nizoral   Tikosyn

Risk rating: 1
Severity: Major   **Onset: Delayed**   **Likelihood: Suspected**

Cause
Dofetilide renal elimination may be inhibited.

Effect
Dofetilide level and risk of ventricular arrhythmias, including torsades de pointes, may increase.

Nursing considerations
◼ **ALERT** Use of dofetilide with ketoconazole is contraindicated.
■ Monitor ECG for excessive prolongation of QTc interval or development of ventricular arrhythmias.
■ Consult the prescriber about alternative anti-infective therapy.
■ Urge the patient to tell the prescriber about increased adverse effects.
■ Azole antifungals other than ketoconazole may interact with dofetilide. If you suspect an interaction, consult the prescriber or pharmacist.

ketoconazole ➤◀ eplerenone
Nizoral   Inspra

Risk rating: 1
Severity: Major   **Onset: Delayed**   **Likelihood: Suspected**

Cause
Azole antifungals such as ketoconazole inhibit eplerenone metabolism.

Effect
Eplerenone level rises, causing hyperkalemia and increasing the risk of life-threatening arrhythmias.

Nursing considerations
◼ **ALERT** Use of azole antifungals with eplerenone is contraindicated.
■ Potent CYP3A4 inhibitors increase the eplerenone level and the risk of hyperkalemia-induced arrhythmias—some fatal.

- Monitor the patient's serum potassium level.
- Tell the patient to report nausea, irregular heartbeat, or slowed pulse to the prescriber.

---

ketoconazole ➤◄ H₂ antagonists

Nizoral

cimetidine, ranitidine

Risk rating: 2
Severity: Moderate   **Onset: Delayed**   **Likelihood: Suspected**

Cause
Ketoconazole availability may decrease because elevated gastric pH may reduce tablet dissolution.

Effect
Ketoconazole effects may decrease.

Nursing considerations
- If possible, don't give ketoconazole, an azole antifungal, with an H₂ antagonist.
- If combined use is needed, give 680 mg of glutamic acid hydrochloride 15 minutes before ketoconazole.
- Watch for expected antifungal effects.
- Explain that other drugs that increase gastric pH such as antacids also may decrease ketoconazole absorption.

---

ketoconazole ➤◄ HMG-CoA reductase inhibitors

Nizoral

atorvastatin, fluvastatin, lovastatin, pravastatin, rosuvastatin, simvastatin

Risk rating: 1
Severity: Major   **Onset: Rapid**   **Likelihood: Probable**

Cause
Azole antifungals such as ketoconazole may inhibit hepatic metabolism of HMG-CoA reductase inhibitors.

Effect
HMG-CoA reductase inhibitor level and adverse effects may increase.

Nursing considerations
- If possible, avoid use together.

■ If drugs must be taken together, HMG-CoA reductase inhibitor dosage may need to be decreased.

■ Monitor serum cholesterol and lipid levels.

⚠ ALERT Assess the patient for evidence of rhabdomyolysis: fatigue; muscle aches and weakness; joint pain; dark, red, or cola-colored urine; weight gain; seizures; and greatly increased CK level.

■ Pravastatin is the HMG-CoA reductase inhibitor least affected by this interaction and may be best for use with an azole antifungal.

ketoconazole ━━▶◀━━ omeprazole
Nizoral   Prilosec

Risk rating: 2
Severity: Moderate   **Onset: Rapid**   **Likelihood: Suspected**

Cause
Proton pump inhibitors such as omeprazole increase gastric pH, which may impair dissolution of azole antifungals such as ketoconazole.

Effect
Azole antifungal efficacy may decrease.

Nursing considerations
■ Tell the prescriber if the patient takes both drugs; an alternative may be available.

■ If no alternative is possible, suggest taking the azole antifungal with an acidic beverage such as cola.

■ Monitor the patient for lack of response to the antifungal.

■ If the patient can't tolerate acidic beverages and antifungal therapy appears to be ineffective, the antifungal dosage may need to be increased.

■ Other drugs that increase gastric pH may interact with azole antifungals. If you suspect an interaction, consult the prescriber or pharmacist.

ketoconazole ━━▶◀━━ nisoldipine
Nizoral   Sular

Risk rating: 2
Severity: Moderate   **Onset: Delayed**   **Likelihood: Suspected**

Cause
Azole antifungals such as ketoconazole inhibit CYP3A4, which is needed for nisoldipine metabolism.

Effect

Nisoldipine level, effects, and risk of adverse effects may increase.

Nursing considerations

■ Tell the prescriber if the patient takes both drugs; an alternative may be available.

■ If drugs must be taken together, watch for orthostatic hypotension, which stems from increased nisoldipine effect.

■ Tell the patient to report adverse nisoldipine effects, including chest pain, dizziness, headache, weight gain, nausea, palpitations, and peripheral edema.

---

ketoconazole ▶◀ phosphodiesterase-5 inhibitors

Nizoral   sildenafil, tadalafil, vardenafil

Risk rating: 2

Severity: Moderate   Onset: Delayed   Likelihood: Suspected

Cause

Azole antifungals such as ketoconazole inhibit CYP3A4 metabolism of PDE-5 inhibitors.

Effect

PDE-5 inhibitor levels, pharmacologic, and risk of adverse effects may increase.

Nursing considerations

■ Dosage of PDE-5 inhibitor may need to be decreased.

■ Administer these drugs together cautiously.

■ Instruct the patient to take PDE-5 exactly as instructed.

■ Warn the patient of adverse effects, including prolonged, painful erection.

---

ketoconazole ▶◀ pimozide

Nizoral   Orap

Risk rating: 1

Severity: Major   Onset: Delayed   Likelihood: Suspected

Cause

Azole antifungals such as ketoconazole may inhibit CYP3A4 metabolism of pimozide.

Effect

Risk of life-threatening arrhythmias may increase.

Nursing considerations
◨ **ALERT** Combined use of these drugs is contraindicated.
■ Arrhythmias are related to prolonged QT interval, a known risk of pimozide.
■ Interaction warning is based on pharmacokinetics of these drugs, not actual patient studies.

---

ketoconazole ━━━▶◀━━━ protease inhibitors
Nizoral   amprenavir, indinavir, ritonavir, saquinavir

Risk rating: 2
Severity: Moderate   **Onset: Delayed**   **Likelihood: Suspected**

Cause
Azole antifungals such as ketoconazole may inhibit metabolism of protease inhibitors.

Effect
Protease inhibitor level may increase.

Nursing considerations
■ Protease inhibitor dosage may be decreased when therapy starts.
■ Monitor the patient for increased protease inhibitor effects, including hyperglycemia, onset of diabetes, rash, GI complaints, and altered liver function tests.
■ Advise the patient to report increased hunger or thirst, frequent urination, fatigue, and dry, itchy skin.
■ Tell the patient not to change dosage or stop either drug without consulting the prescriber.

---

ketoconazole ━━━▶◀━━━ quinine derivatives
Nizoral   quinidine, quinine

Risk rating: 2
Severity: Moderate   **Onset: Delayed**   **Likelihood: Suspected**

Cause
Hepatic CYP3A4 metabolism of quinine derivatives is inhibited.

Effect
Quinine derivative level may increase, resulting in toxicity.

Nursing considerations
■ When starting or stopping ketoconazole, monitor quinidine level.

- Therapeutic range of quinidine is 2 to 6 mcg/ml. More specific assays have levels of less than 1 mcg/ml.
- Monitor ECG for conduction disturbances, prolonged QTc interval, and increased ventricular ectopy.
- Urge the patient to report palpitations, chest pain, dizziness, and shortness of breath.

ketoconazole ➤◀ rifamycins
Nizoral   rifabutin, rifampin, rifapentine

Risk rating: 2
Severity: Moderate   **Onset: Delayed**   **Likelihood: Suspected**

Cause
Rifamycins may decrease level of ketoconazole, an azole antifungal. Also, ketoconazole may decease rifampin level.

Effect
Infection may recur.

Nursing considerations
- Tell the prescriber if the patient takes both drugs; an alternative may be available.
- If ketoconazole and a rifamycin must be taken together, separate doses by 12 hours.
- If drugs must be taken together and the antifungal appears ineffective, antifungal dosage may need to be increased.
- Teach the patient to recognize signs and symptoms of infection and to contact the prescriber promptly if they occur.

ketoconazole ➤◀ selective 5-HT$_1$ receptor agonists
Nizoral   almotriptan, eletriptan

Risk rating: 2
Severity: Moderate   **Onset: Delayed**   **Likelihood: Suspected**

Cause
Azole antifungals such as ketoconazole inhibit CYP3A4 metabolism of certain 5-HT$_1$ receptor agonists.

Effect
Serum level and adverse effects of the selective 5-HT$_1$ receptor agonist may increase.

Nursing considerations
⚠ ALERT Don't give eletriptan within 72 hours or almotriptan within 7 days of ketoconazole.

■ Adverse effects of selective 5-HT$_1$ receptor agonists may include coronary artery vasospasm, dizziness, nausea, paresthesia, and somnolence.

---

ketoconazole ➤◄ sirolimus
Nizoral   Rapamune

Risk rating: 2
Severity: Moderate   Onset: Delayed   Likelihood: Probable

Cause
Azole antifungals such as ketoconazole inhibit CYP3A4, which is needed for sirolimus metabolism.

Effect
Sirolimus level, effects, and risk of toxicity may increase.

Nursing considerations
■ Monitor trough level of sirolimus in whole blood when starting or stopping an azole antifungal. Therapeutic level varies depending on which other drugs the patient receives—cyclosporine, for example.
■ Watch for signs of sirolimus toxicity, such as anemia, leukopenia, thrombocytopenia, hypokalemia, hyperlipemia, fever, interstitial lung disease, and diarrhea.
■ Other CYP3A4 inhibitors may interact with sirolimus. If you suspect an interaction, consult the prescriber or pharmacist.
■ Urge the patient to promptly report new onset of fever higher than 100° F (38° C), fatigue, shortness of breath, easy bruising, gum bleeding, muscle twitches, palpitations, or chest discomfort or pain.

---

ketoconazole ➤◄ tacrolimus
Nizoral   Prograf

Risk rating: 2
Severity: Moderate   Onset: Delayed   Likelihood: Probable

Cause
Ketoconazole inhibits tacrolimus metabolism in the liver and GI tract.

Effect
Tacrolimus level and risk of adverse effects may increase.

Nursing considerations
⚠ ALERT
Watch for renal failure, nephrotoxicity, hyperkalemia, hyperglycemia, delirium, and other changes in mental status.
- Monitor renal function and mental status closely.
- Check tacrolimus level often. Normal trough level is 6 to 10 mcg/L.
- Tacrolimus dosage may need to be decreased when the patient takes ketoconazole.
- Signs of toxicity often occur within 3 days of combined use.

---

ketoconazole ▶◀ TCAs
Nizoral

amitriptyline, imipramine, nortriptyline

Risk rating: 2
Severity: Moderate   Onset: Delayed   Likelihood: Suspected

Cause
Azole antifungals such as ketoconazole may inhibit metabolism of tricyclic antidepressants (TCAs).

Effect
Serum TCA level and risk of toxicity may increase.

Nursing considerations
- When starting or stopping an azole antifungal, monitor serum TCA level, and adjust dosage as needed.
- After starting ketoconazole, check sitting and standing blood pressure for changes.
- If the patient takes a TCA and an azole antifungal, assess symptoms and behavior for evidence of adverse reactions, such as increased drowsiness, dizziness, confusion, heart rate or rhythm changes, and urine retention.

---

ketoconazole ▶◀ tolterodine
Nizoral

Detrol

Risk rating: 2
Severity: Moderate   Onset: Delayed   Likelihood: Suspected

Cause
Azole antifungals such as ketoconazole inhibit CYP3A4, which is needed for tolterodine metabolism.

Effect
Tolterodine level, effects, and risk of toxicity may increase.

Nursing considerations
■ Tell the prescriber if the patient takes both drugs; an alternative may be available.
■ Watch for evidence of tolterodine overdose, such as dry mouth, urine retention, constipation, dizziness, and headache.
■ Other CYP3A4 inhibitors may interact with tolterodine. If you suspect an interaction, consult the prescriber or pharmacist.
■ Explain adverse tolterodine effects and need to report them promptly.

---

ketoconazole ■■■■▶◀■■■■ warfarin
Nizoral   Coumadin

Risk rating: 1
Severity: Major   **Onset: Delayed**   **Likelihood: Established**

Cause
Warfarin metabolism is inhibited.

Effect
Anticoagulant effects may increase.

Nursing considerations
■ Monitor PT and INR at least every 2 days.
■ Patients with renal insufficiency may be at greater risk.
■ Although all azole antifungals interact with warfarin, some interactions may be more significant than others.
■ Watch for evidence of bleeding.
■ Tell the patient to report unusual bruising or bleeding.
■ Remind the patient that warfarin interacts with many drugs and that he should report any change in drug regimen.

---

ketoconazole ■■■■▶◀■■■■ zolpidem
Nizoral   Ambien

Risk rating: 2
Severity: Moderate   **Onset: Delayed**   **Likelihood: Suspected**

Cause
Ketoconazole inhibits CYP3A4 metabolism of zolpidem.

Effect
Zolpidem levels and therapeutic effects may increase.

Nursing considerations
■ If coadministration of ketoconazole and zolpidem is given, monitor the patient's response. Zolpidem dosage may need to be decreased.
■ Instruct the patient on signs and symptoms of increased effects of zolpidem, including headache, daytime drowsiness, hangover, lethargy, light-headedness, palpitations, abdominal pain, nausea, myalgia, and back or chest pain.
■ Caution the patient to avoid performing activities that require mental alertness or physical coordination during therapy

---

ketorolac ━━━▶◀━━━ aspirin
Toradol   Bayer, Ecotrin

Risk rating: 1
Severity: Major   **Onset: Delayed**   **Likelihood: Suspected**

Cause
Aspirin may displace ketorolac from protein-binding sites, increasing unbound ketorolac level.

Effect
Risk of serious ketorolac-related adverse effects increases.

Nursing considerations
◣ **ALERT** Ketorolac is contraindicated in patients taking aspirin or other NSAIDs.
■ If drugs are inadvertently taken together, watch for adverse effects, such as GI bleeding, neurotoxicity, renal failure, blood dyscrasias, and hepatotoxicity.
■ Ketorolac therapy isn't meant to exceed 5 days.
■ Urge the patient to tell the prescriber and pharmacist about all drugs (prescribed and OTC), and any supplements he takes.

L-tryptophan ━━━▶◀━━━ MAO inhibitors
                                     phenelzine, tranylcypromine

Risk rating: 1
Severity: Major   **Onset: Rapid**   **Likelihood: Suspected**

Cause
Giving these drugs together may cause additive serotonergic effects.

Effect
The risk of serotonin syndrome increases.

Nursing considerations
⚠ ALERT Combined use of these drugs is contraindicated.
- They may cause CNS irritability, motor weakness, shivering, muscle twitching, and altered consciousness.

---

labetalol ➤◄ isoflurane
Trandate   Forane

Risk rating: 2
Severity: Moderate   Onset: Rapid   Likelihood: Probable

Cause
Additive myocardial depressant effects may occur.

Effect
Excessive hypotension may result.

Nursing considerations
- Use these drugs together cautiously.
- Closely monitor blood pressure.
- The degree and duration of this interaction appears to be dose-dependent.
- This interaction may be used to induce deliberate hypotension for some surgical procedures.

---

lamotrigine ➤◄ carbamazepine
Lamictal   Carbatrol, Epitol, Equetro, Tegretol

Risk rating: 2
Severity: Moderate   Onset: Delayed   Likelihood: Suspected

Cause
Lamotrigine metabolism may increase. Carbamazepine metabolite levels may increase.

Effect
Lamotrigine effects may decrease. Risk of carbamazepine toxicity may increase.

Nursing considerations
- Watch for expected lamotrigine effects when starting therapy in a patient taking carbamazepine.
- Lamotrigine dosage may need adjustment when the patient starts, changes, or stops carbamazepine therapy.

- Monitor carbamazepine level when adding lamotrigine; carbamazepine therapeutic range is 4 to 12 mcg/ml.
- Watch for evidence of carbamazepine toxicity: dizziness, ataxia, respiratory depression, tachycardia, arrhythmias, blood pressure changes, impaired consciousness, abnormal reflexes, nystagmus, seizures, nausea, vomiting, and urine retention.
- Carbamazepine dosage may need reduction.

lamotrigine ▶◀ hormonal contraceptives
Lamictal

Risk rating: 2
Severity: Moderate   Onset: Delayed   Likelihood: Probable

Cause
Hormonal contraceptives increase lamotrigine metabolism.

Effect
Lamotrigine effects may decrease.

Nursing considerations
- Watch for expected lamotrigine effects after starting therapy in a patient taking hormonal contraceptives.
- Lamotrigine dosage may need to be adjusted when the patient starts, changes, or stops hormonal contraceptive therapy.

lamotrigine ▶◀ valproic acid
Lamictal   divalproex sodium, valproate
                        sodium, valproic acid

Risk rating: 2
Severity: Moderate   Onset: Delayed   Likelihood: Probable

Cause
Valproic acid may inhibit lamotrigine metabolism.

Effect
Both drugs may have increased effects.

Nursing considerations
- Observe the patient closely for Stevens-Johnson rash, disabling tremor, and other signs of toxicity when starting the second anticonvulsant.
- Monitor serum valproic acid and lamotrigine levels, and report increasing level of either drug.

■ Explain that combined use may improve seizure control; instruct the patient to be alert for adverse effects and toxicity.
■ Lamotrigine level decreases readily when valproic acid is stopped.

---

lansoprazole ▰▰▰◄► clarithromycin
Prevacid   Biaxin

Risk rating: 2
Severity: Moderate   **Onset: Delayed**   **Likelihood: Suspected**

Cause
Clarithromycin inhibits the CYP3A metabolism of certain proton pump inhibitors such as lansoprazole.

Effect
Proton pump inhibitor levels and risk of adverse effects increase.

Nursing considerations
■ Monitor the patient for adverse reactions.
■ Watch the patient for headache, abdominal pain, constipation, diarrhea, dry mouth, nausea, and vomiting.
■ Teach the patient about adverse reactions to watch for, and tell the patient to notify the prescriber if adverse reactions increase.
■ Administration of clarithromycin with other proton pump inhibitors may not cause this interaction.

---

lansoprazole ▰▰▰◄► protease inhibitors
Prevacid   atazanavir, indinavir, saquinavir

Risk rating: 2
Severity: Moderate   **Onset: Delayed**   **Likelihood: Suspected**

Cause
GI absorption of protease inhibitors may be decreased.

Effect
Antiviral activity of protease inhibitors may be reduced.

Nursing considerations
■ Use of protease inhibitors with proton pump inhibitors such as lansoprazole is not recommended.
■ Monitor the patient for a decrease in antiviral activity.
■ Adjust the dose of the protease inhibitor as needed.

levodopa ◀▶ iron salts

Larodopa

ferrous fumarate, ferrous
gluconate, ferrous sulfate,
iron polysaccharide

Risk rating: 1
Severity: Major   **Onset: Delayed**   **Likelihood: Suspected**

Cause
Levodopa may form chelates with iron salts, which decreases levodopa absorption and serum level.

Effect
Levodopa effects may decrease.

Nursing considerations
- Separate doses as much as possible.
- Watch for loss of levodopa effects if iron salts are added to a stable regimen. Evidence of recurring or worsening Parkinson's symptoms may include increased tremors, muscle rigidity, bradykinesia (slowing of voluntary movement), shuffling gait, loss of facial expression, speech disturbances, and drooling.
- Notify the prescriber about loss of symptom control.
- Warn the patient or caregiver not to change levodopa dosage without consulting the prescriber.
- Help the patient develop a plan to ensure proper dosage intervals.

levodopa ◀▶ phenytoin

Larodopa

Dilantin

Risk rating: 2
Severity: Moderate   **Onset: Delayed**   **Likelihood: Suspected**

Cause
The exact mechanism of this interaction is unknown.

Effect
Levodopa effects may decrease.

Nursing considerations
- Avoid this combination, if possible.
- If these drugs are used together, watch for recurring or worsening Parkinson's symptoms: increased tremors, muscle rigidity, bradykinesia (slowing of voluntary movement), shuffling gait, loss of facial expression, speech disturbances, and drooling.

- In patients treated for chronic manganese poisoning, watch for recurring or worsening symptoms of manganese toxicity: muscle weakness, difficulty walking, tremors, salivation, and psychological disturbances, such as irritability, aggressiveness, and hallucinations.
- If you suspect a drug interaction, consult the prescriber or pharmacist; an alternative therapy may need to be considered.
- Warn the patient or caregiver not to change levodopa dosage without consulting the prescriber.

---

levodopa ━━━━▶◀━━━ MAO inhibitors
Larodopa   phenelzine, tranylcypromine

Risk rating: 1
Severity: Major   **Onset: Rapid**   **Likelihood: Established**

Cause
Peripheral metabolism of levodopa-derived dopamine is inhibited, increasing level at dopamine receptors.

Effect
Risk of hypertensive reaction increases.

Nursing considerations
- If possible, avoid giving these drugs together.
- Interaction occurs within 1 hour and appears to be dose-related.
- Monitor the patient for flushing, light-headedness, and palpitations.
- Selegiline doesn't cause hypertensive reaction and may be used instead of other MAO inhibitors in patients taking levodopa.

---

levodopa ━━━━▶◀━━━ pyridoxine (vitamin B₆)
Larodopa   Aminoxin

Risk rating: 2
Severity: Moderate   **Onset: Rapid**   **Likelihood: Established**

Cause
Pyridoxine increases peripheral metabolism of levodopa, decreasing the level available for penetration into the CNS.

Effect
Pyridoxine reduces levodopa efficacy in Parkinson's disease.

Nursing considerations
- Avoid combined use of pyridoxine and levodopa in patients taking levodopa alone.

- Watch for recurring or worsening Parkinson's symptoms: increased tremors, muscle rigidity, bradykinesia (slowing of voluntary movement), shuffling gait, loss of facial expression, speech disturbances, and drooling.
- Advise the patient and caregivers that multivitamins, fortified cereals, and certain OTC drugs may contain pyridoxine.
- The effect of pyridoxine is minimal or negligible in patients taking levodopa-carbidopa combination products.

levofloxacin ▶◀ amiodarone
Levaquin   Cordarone, Pacerone

Risk rating: 1
Severity: Major   **Onset: Delayed**   **Likelihood: Suspected**

Cause
The mechanism of this interaction is unknown.

Effect
Risk of life-threatening arrhythmias, including torsades de pointes, increases.

Nursing considerations
⚠ ALERT Use of some quinolones such as levofloxacin with an antiarrhythmic such as amiodarone is contraindicated.
- Quinolones that aren't metabolized by CYP3A4 isoenzymes or that don't prolong the QT interval may be given with antiarrhythmics.
- Avoid giving class IA or class III antiarrhythmics with levofloxacin.
- Tell the patient to report a rapid heart rate, shortness of breath, dizziness, fainting, and chest pain.

levofloxacin ▶◀ antiarrhythmics
Levaquin   amiodarone, bretylium,
                                  disopyramide, procainamide,
                                  quinidine, sotalol

Risk rating: 1
Severity: Major   **Onset: Delayed**   **Likelihood: Suspected**

Cause
The mechanism of this interaction is unknown.

Effect
Risk of life-threatening arrhythmias, including torsades de pointes, increases.

Nursing considerations
- Avoid giving class IA or class III antiarrhythmics with the quinolone levofloxacin.
- Monitor the ECG for prolonged QTc interval.
- Tell the patient to report a rapid heartbeat, shortness of breath, dizziness, fainting, and chest pain.
- Quinolones that aren't metabolized by CYP3A4 isoenzymes or that don't prolong the QT interval may be given with antiarrhythmics.

levofloxacin ▶◀ erythromycin
Levaquin   E-Mycin, Eryc

Risk rating: 1
Severity: Major   **Onset: Delayed**   **Likelihood: Suspected**

Cause
The mechanism of this interaction is unknown.

Effect
Risk of life-threatening arrhythmias, including torsades de pointes, increases.

Nursing considerations
- Avoid use of levofloxacin with erythromycin because doing so may prolong the QT interval.
- Monitor the QTc interval closely.
- Tell the patient to report palpitations, dizziness, shortness of breath, and chest pain.

levofloxacin ▶◀ imipramine
Levaquin   Tofranil

Risk rating: 1
Severity: Major   **Onset: Delayed**   **Likelihood: Suspected**

Cause
The mechanism of this interaction is unknown.

Effect
Life-threatening arrhythmias, including torsades de pointes, may increase when certain of these drugs are used together.

Nursing considerations
◼ ALERT Avoid giving the quinolone, levofloxacin, with a tricyclic antidepressant.

■ If possible, use other quinolone antibiotics that don't prolong the QTc interval or aren't metabolized by the CYP3A4 isoenzyme.

---

levofloxacin ➤◀ warfarin
Levaquin   Coumadin

Risk rating: 2
Severity: Moderate   Onset: Delayed   Likelihood: Suspected

Cause
The mechanism of the interaction is unknown.

Effect
Anticoagulant effects may increase.

Nursing considerations
■ Monitor PT and INR closely.
■ Tell the patient to report unusual bleeding or bruising.
■ Remind the patient that warfarin interacts with many drugs and that he should report any change in drug regimen.

---

levofloxacin ➤◀ ziprasidone
Levaquin   Geodon

Risk rating: 1
Severity: Major   Onset: Delayed   Likelihood: Suspected

Cause
The mechanism of this interaction is unknown.

Effect
Risk of life-threatening arrhythmias, including torsades de pointes, increases.

Nursing considerations
◪ **ALERT** Use of ziprasidone with a quinolone such as levofloxacin is contraindicated.
■ Monitor the patient for other risk factors for torsades de pointes, including bradycardia, hypokalemia, and hypomagnesemia.
■ Ask the patient if he or anyone in his family has a history of prolonged QT interval or arrhythmias.
■ Monitor the patient for bradycardia.
■ Measure the QTc interval at baseline and throughout therapy.

levothyroxine ➤◀ cholestyramine

Levoxyl, Synthroid   Locholest, Prevalite, Questran

Risk rating: 2
Severity: Moderate   Onset: Delayed   Likelihood: Suspected

Cause
Cholestyramine may prevent GI absorption of thyroid hormones, such as levothyroxine.

Effect
Effects of exogenous thyroid hormone may be lost, and hypothyroidism may recur.

Nursing considerations
■ Separate doses by 6 hours.
■ Monitor the patient for evidence of hypothyroidism, including weakness, fatigue, weight gain, coarse dry hair and skin, cold intolerance, muscle aches, constipation, depression, irritability, and memory loss.
■ Monitor thyroid function tests during combined therapy (TSH, 0.2 to 5.4 microunits/ml; T_3, 80 to 200 nanograms/dl; and T_4, 5.4 to 11.5 mcg/dl).
■ Other thyroid hormones may interact with cholestyramine. If you suspect a drug interaction, consult the prescriber or pharmacist.

levothyroxine ➤◀ digoxin

Levoxyl, Synthroid   Lanoxin

Risk rating: 2
Severity: Moderate   Onset: Delayed   Likelihood: Established

Cause
Digoxin level may decrease in hyperthyroidism or when a hypothyroid patient becomes euthyroid.

Effect
Digoxin effects may decrease.

Nursing considerations
■ Monitor digoxin level. Therapeutic range is 0.8 to 2 nanograms/ml.
■ Watch for expected digoxin effects: decreased heart rate, arrhythmia conversion, maintenance of converted rhythm, and improvement of heart failure symptoms.
■ Monitor thyroid function tests (TSH, 0.2 to 5.4 microunits/ml; T_3, 80 to 200 nanograms/dl; and T_4, 5.4 to 11.5 mcg/dl).

■ If a hypothyroid patient becomes euthyroid, digoxin dosage may need to be increased.

■ If the patient is euthyroid and already taking a thyroid hormone when starting on digoxin, no special precautions are needed.

---

levothyroxine ■■■▶◀ food
Levoxyl, Synthroid   grapefruit juice

Risk rating: 3
Severity: Minor   **Onset: Delayed**   **Likelihood: Suspected**

Cause
Grapefruit juice interferes with the intestinal absorption of levothyroxine.

Effect
Absorption of levothyroxine is delayed.

Nursing considerations
■ No adverse effects are noted from this interaction.
■ Monitor thyroid function tests (TSH, 0.2 to 5.4 microunits/ml; T_3, 80 to 200 nanograms/dl; and T_4, 5.4 to 11.5 mcg/dl).
■ This interaction is not thought to be clinically important.

---

levothyroxine ■■■▶◀ imatinib
Levoxyl, Synthroid   Gleevec

Risk rating: 2
Severity: Moderate   **Onset: Delayed**   **Likelihood: Suspected**

Cause
Imatinib may increase levothyroxine's hepatic clearance.

Effect
TSH levels may be increased. Symptoms of hypothyroidism may occur.

Nursing considerations
■ Monitor thyroid function during coadministration of imatinib.
■ Levothyroxine dosage may need adjusting when starting or stopping imatinib treatment.
■ Monitor for signs and symptoms of hypothyroidism, including TSH, T_3, and T_4 levels. Therapeutic range for TSH is 0.2 to 5.4 microunits/ml; T_3, 80 to 200 nanograms/dl; and T_4, 5.4 to 11.5 mcg/dl.
■ Watch for evidence of hypothyroidism: weakness, fatigue, weight gain, coarse dry hair, rough skin, cold intolerance, muscle aches, con-

stipation, depression, irritability, and memory loss. Urge the patient to report such symptoms to the prescriber.

---

levothyroxine ━━▶◀━━ iron salts

Levoxyl, Synthroid

ferrous fumarate, ferrous gluconate, ferrous sulfate, iron polysaccharide

Risk rating: 2
Severity: Moderate   Onset: Delayed   Likelihood: Suspected

Cause
Levothyroxine absorption may be decreased, probably because it forms a complex with iron salt.

Effect
Levothyroxine effects may decrease, resulting in hypothyroidism.

Nursing considerations
■ **ALERT** Separate levothyroxine from iron salts as much as possible.
■ Monitor TSH, T_3, and T_4 levels. Therapeutic range for TSH is 0.2 to 5.4 microunits/ml; T_3, 80 to 200 nanograms/dl; and T_4, 5.4 to 11.5 mcg/dl.
■ Levothyroxine dosage may need adjustment.
■ Watch for evidence of hypothyroidism: weakness, fatigue, weight gain, coarse dry hair, rough skin, cold intolerance, muscle aches, constipation, depression, irritability, and memory loss. Urge the patient to report such symptoms to the prescriber.

---

levothyroxine ━━▶◀━━ theophyllines

Levoxyl, Synthroid

aminophylline, theophylline

Risk rating: 2
Severity: Moderate   Onset: Delayed   Likelihood: Suspected

Cause
Thyroxine level is directly related to theophylline level. Patients who are hyperthyroid or hypothyroid may have varying interactions.

Effect
In hypothyroidism, theophylline metabolism decreases, and serum level—and risk of toxicity—increase.

Nursing considerations
■ Monitor theophylline level and dosage carefully; adjust dosage as needed to avoid theophylline toxicity.

■ Normal therapeutic range is 10 to 20 mcg/ml for adults and 5 to 15 mcg/ml for children.
■ Watch for increased adverse effects of theophylline, such as tachycardia, anorexia, nausea, vomiting, diarrhea, seizures, restlessness, irritability, and headache.
■ Once a patient becomes euthyroid, theophylline clearance returns to normal.
■ Explain common side effects of theophylline and signs of toxicity, and tell the patient to report them immediately to the prescriber.

---

levothyroxine ▶◀ warfarin

Levoxyl, Synthroid   Coumadin

Risk rating: 1
Severity: Major   **Onset: Delayed**   **Likelihood: Probable**

Cause
Thyroid hormones increase the breakdown of vitamin K–dependent clotting factors.

Effect
Anticoagulant effects and risk of bleeding may increase.

Nursing considerations
■ Monitor coagulation values carefully.
■ A lower warfarin dose may be needed.
■ If the patient's anticoagulant values are stabilized during combined therapy and the thyroid hormones are stopped, the warfarin dose may need to be increased.
■ Tell the patient to report unusual bruising or bleeding.
■ Remind the patient that warfarin interacts with many drugs and that he should report any change in drug regimen.

---

lidocaine ▶◀ beta-adrenergic blockers

Xylocaine   atenolol, metoprolol, nadolol, pindolol, propranolol

Risk rating: 2
Severity: Moderate   **Onset: Rapid**   **Likelihood: Established**

Cause
Beta-adrenergic blockers reduce hepatic metabolism of lidocaine.

Effect
Lidocaine level and risk of toxicity may increase.

Nursing considerations
- Check for normal therapeutic level of lidocaine: 2 to 5 mcg/ml.
- Assess the patient for evidence of lidocaine toxicity, including dizziness, somnolence, confusion, paresthesias, and seizures.
- Slow the I.V. bolus rate to decrease the risk of high peak level and toxic reaction.
- Explain the warning signs of toxicity to the patient and family, and tell them to contact the prescriber if they have concerns.

---

lidocaine ➤◄ cimetidine
Xylocaine   Tagamet

Risk rating: 2
Severity: Moderate   **Onset: Rapid**   **Likelihood: Established**

Cause
Hepatic metabolism of lidocaine may decrease.

Effect
Risk of lidocaine toxicity increases.

Nursing considerations
- Ask the prescriber or pharmacist about an H_2-receptor antagonist other than cimetidine, such as ranitidine or famotidine, that may be safer in combination. Monitor lidocaine level; therapeutic range is 1.5 to 6 mcg/ml.
- Assess the patient for evidence of lidocaine toxicity: dizziness, somnolence, confusion, tremors, paresthesias, seizures, hypotension, arrhythmias, respiratory depression, and coma.
- Adjust lidocaine dosage as ordered.
- Other H_2-receptor antagonists may interact with lidocaine. If you suspect an interaction, consult the prescriber or pharmacist.

---

lidocaine ➤◄ succinylcholine
Xylocaine

Risk rating: 2
Severity: Moderate   **Onset: Rapid**   **Likelihood: Suspected**

Cause
The mechanism of this interaction is unknown.

Effect
Neuromuscular blockade may increase.

Nursing considerations
- Monitor respiratory function closely.
- Prolonged respiratory depression may occur; provide ventilatory support as needed.
- There is no evidence that suggests a change in therapy is indicated.

---

linezolid ▶◀	serotonin reuptake inhibitors
Zyvox	citalopram, fluoxetine, paroxetine, sertraline, venlafaxine

Risk rating: 1
Severity: **Major**   Onset: **Delayed**   Likelihood: **Suspected**

Cause
Serotonin may accumulate rapidly in the CNS.

Effect
The risk of serotonin syndrome increases.

Nursing considerations
 ☒ ALERT Don't use these drugs together.
- Allow 2 weeks after stopping linezoid and administering a serotonin reuptake inhibitor.
- Allow 2 weeks after stopping an SSRI and administering linezoid.
- Describe the traits of serotonin syndrome, including confusion, restlessness, incoordination, muscle tremors and rigidity, fever, and sweating.
- Explain that serotonin-induced symptoms can be fatal if not treated immediately.

---

liothyronine ▶◀	digoxin
Cytomel	Lanoxin

Risk rating: 2
Severity: **Moderate**   Onset: **Delayed**   Likelihood: **Established**

Cause
Digoxin level may decrease in hyperthyroidism or when a hypothyroid patient becomes euthyroid.

Effect
Digoxin effects may decrease.

Nursing considerations
■ Monitor digoxin level. Therapeutic range is 0.8 to 2 nanograms/ml.
■ Watch for expected digoxin effects: decreased heart rate, arrhythmia conversion, maintenance of converted rhythm, and improvement of heart failure symptoms.
■ Monitor thyroid function tests (TSH, 0.2 to 5.4 microunits/ml; T_3, 80 to 200 nanograms/dl; and T_4, 5.4 to 11.5 mcg/dl).
■ If a hypothyroid patient becomes euthyroid, digoxin dosage may need to be increased.
■ If the patient is euthyroid and taking a thyroid hormone such as liothyronine when starting on digoxin, no special precautions are needed.

---

liothyronine ▶◀ warfarin
Cytomel   Coumadin

Risk rating: 1
Severity: Major   **Onset: Delayed**   **Likelihood: Probable**

Cause
Thyroid hormones such as liothyronine increase the breakdown of vitamin K–dependent clotting factors.

Effect
Anticoagulant effects and risk of bleeding may increase.

Nursing considerations
■ Monitor coagulation values carefully.
■ A lower warfarin dose may be needed.
■ If the patient's anticoagulant values are stabilized during combined therapy and the thyroid hormones are stopped, the warfarin dose may need to be increased.
■ Tell the patient to report unusual bruising or bleeding.
■ Remind the patient that warfarin interacts with many drugs and that he should report any change in drug regimen.

---

lisinopril ▶◀ aspirin
Prinivil, Zestril   Bayer, Ecotrin

Risk rating: 2
Severity: Moderate   **Onset: Rapid**   **Likelihood: Suspected**

Cause
Salicylates such as aspirin inhibit synthesis of prostaglandins, which ACE inhibitors such as lisinopril need to lower blood pressure.

Effect
The ACE inhibitor's hypotensive effect will be reduced.

Nursing considerations
■ This interaction is more likely in people with hypertension, coronary artery disease, or possibly heart failure.
■ Aspirin, at doses less than 100 mg daily, is less likely to interact with ACE inhibitors.

---

lisinopril ◄►◄ **lithium**

Prinivil, Zestril   Eskalith

Risk rating: 2
Severity: Moderate   Onset: Delayed   Likelihood: Suspected

Cause
The mechanism of this interaction is unknown.

Effect
Lithium level may be elevated, and neurotoxicity may occur.

Nursing considerations
■ If the patient takes lithium, consider an antihypertensive other than an ACE inhibitor.
■ Monitor lithium level. Steady state lithium level should be 0.6 to 1.2 mEq/L.
■ Adjust lithium dose as needed.
■ Watch for evidence of lithium toxicity, such as diarrhea, vomiting, dehydration, drowsiness, muscle weakness, tremor, fever, and ataxia.
■ Use with added caution in elderly patients and those with heart failure, renal insufficiency, or volume depletion. Dehydration may increase the effects of this interaction.

---

lisinopril ◄►◄ **potassium-sparing diuretics**

Prinivil, Zestril   amiloride, spironolactone

Risk rating: 1
Severity: Major   Onset: Delayed   Likelihood: Probable

Cause
The mechanism of this interaction is unknown.

Effect
Serum potassium level may increase.

Nursing considerations
■ Use cautiously in patients at high risk for hyperkalemia, especially those with renal impairment.
■ Monitor BUN, creatinine, and serum potassium levels as needed.
■ ACE inhibitors other than lisinopril may interact with potassium-sparing diuretics. If you suspect an interaction, consult the prescriber or pharmacist.
■ Urge the patient to immediately report an irregular heartbeat, a slow pulse, weakness, and other evidence of hyperkalemia.

---

lithium ▶◀	ACE inhibitors
Eskalith	enalapril, lisinopril

Risk rating: 2
Severity: Moderate   **Onset: Delayed**   **Likelihood: Suspected**

Cause
The mechanism for this interaction is unknown.

Effect
Lithium level may be elevated, and neurotoxicity may occur.

Nursing considerations
■ If the patient takes lithium, consider an antihypertensive other than an ACE inhibitor.
■ Monitor lithium level. Steady state lithium level should be 0.6 to 1.2mEq/L.
■ Adjust the lithium dose as needed.
■ Watch for evidence of lithium toxicity, such as diarrhea, vomiting, dehydration, drowsiness, muscle weakness, tremor, fever, and ataxia.
■ Use with added caution in elderly patients and those with heart failure, renal insufficiency, or volume depletion. Dehydration may increase the effects of this interaction.

---

lithium ▶◀	angiotensin II receptor antagonists
Eskalith	candesartan, losartan, valsartan

Risk rating: 2
Severity: Moderate   **Onset: Delayed**   **Likelihood: Suspected**

Cause
Angiotensin II receptor antagonists may decrease lithium excretion.

Effect
Lithium level, effects, and risk of toxicity may increase.

Nursing considerations
■ If the patient takes lithium, consider an antihypertensive other than an angiotensin II receptor antagonist.
■ Monitor lithium level. Steady state lithium level should be 0.6 to 1.2 mEq/L.
■ Adjust lithium dose as needed.
■ Monitor the patient for evidence of lithium toxicity, such as diarrhea, vomiting, dehydration, drowsiness, muscle weakness, tremor, fever, and ataxia.

lithium ◄►◄ carbamazepine
Eskalith   Carbatrol, Epitol, Equetro, Tegretol

Risk rating: 2
Severity: Moderate   Onset: Delayed   Likelihood: Suspected

Cause
The mechanism of this interaction is unknown.

Effect
Risk of adverse CNS effects—including lethargy, muscle weakness, ataxia, tremor, and hyperreflexia—increases.

Nursing considerations
■ Combining lithium and carbamazepine may help in treating bipolar disorder.
■ This combination may be justified if the benefits outweigh the risks; some patients can tolerate it without adverse effects.

lithium ◄►◄ haloperidol
Eskalith   Haldol

Risk rating: 1
Severity: Major   Onset: Delayed   Likelihood: Suspected

Cause
The exact mechanism of this interaction is unknown.

Effect
Patients may have altered level of consciousness, encephalopathy, extrapyramidal effects, fever, leukocytosis, and increased enzyme levels.

Nursing considerations

▌◧ **ALERT** Monitor the patient closely, especially during the first
3 weeks.
■ Watch for early evidence of neurologic toxicity, such as altered mental status, rigidity, or hyperpyrexia; treatment should be stopped
promptly if such signs appear.
■ Evidence of more severe neurologic toxicity includes weakness,
lethargy, tremulousness, confusion, stupor, fever, severe extrapyramidal symptoms, and dystonias. Some patients may have permanent
brain damage.
■ Check lab studies for leukocytosis, elevated serum enzyme levels,
and increased BUN. Therapeutic lithium level is 0.6 to 1.2 mEq/ L;
therapeutic haloperidol level is 5 to 20 nanograms/ml.
■ If an interaction occurs, alert the prescriber. One or both drugs may
need to be stopped. Give supportive treatment for symptoms.

---

lithium ━━━━▶◀━━━ loop diuretics

Eskalith

bumetanide, ethacrynic acid,
furosemide

Risk rating: 2
Severity: Moderate   Onset: Delayed   Likelihood: Suspected

Cause
The mechanism of this interaction is unknown.

Effect
Increased lithium levels and risk of toxicity may occur.

Nursing considerations
■ Monitor serum lithium levels. Steady state lithium level should be
0.6 to 1.2 mEq/L.
■ Adjust lithium dose as needed.
■ Monitor the patient for evidence of lithium toxicity, such as diarrhea, vomiting, dehydration, drowsiness, muscle weakness, tremor,
fever, and ataxia.
■ Despite this interaction, lithium and loop diuretics may be used together safely, with close monitoring of lithium level.

lithium ◄► NSAIDs

Eskalith

celecoxib, diclofenac, ibuprofen, indomethacin, ketorolac, meloxicam, naproxen, piroxicam, sulindac

Risk rating: 2
Severity: Moderate   Onset: Delayed   Likelihood: Suspected

Cause
Lithium elimination may decrease because NSAIDs interfere with prostaglandin production in the kidneys.

Effect
Lithium level, effects, and risk of toxicity may increase.

Nursing considerations
■ Monitor lithium level. Steady state lithium level should be 0.6 to 1.2 mEq/L.
■ Adjust lithium dose as needed.
■ Monitor the patient for evidence of lithium toxicity, such as diarrhea, vomiting, dehydration, drowsiness, muscle weakness, tremor, fever, and ataxia.
■ Expect lithium level to return to pretreatment value within 7 days of stopping the NSAID.

lithium ◄► sibutramine

Eskalith

Meridia

Risk rating: 1
Severity: Major   Onset: Rapid   Likelihood: Suspected

Cause
The serotonergic effects of these drugs may be additive.

Effect
A serotonin syndrome, including CNS irritability, motor weakness, shivering, myoclonus, and altered consciousness, may occur.

Nursing considerations
■ Avoid using these drugs together.
■ Monitor the patient for adverse effects.
⚠ **ALERT** If signs and symptoms of serotonin syndrome occur, provide immediate treatment.
■ This interaction is rare, but it may be fatal.

lithium ━━━▶◀━━━ thiazide diuretics

Eskalith

chlorothiazide, chlorthalidone, hydrochlorothiazide, methyclothiazide

Risk rating: 2
Severity: Moderate   **Onset: Delayed**   **Likelihood: Established**

Cause
Thiazide diuretics may decrease lithium clearance.

Effect
Lithium level, effects, and risk of toxicity may increase.

Nursing considerations
■ Despite this interaction, lithium and thiazide diuretics may be used together safely, with close monitoring of lithium level.
■ Reduction in lithium clearance may depend on thiazide dose.
■ Monitor lithium level, and adjust dose as needed.
■ Monitor the patient for evidence of lithium toxicity, such as diarrhea, vomiting, dehydration, drowsiness, muscle weakness, tremor, fever, and ataxia.

lomefloxacin ━━━▶◀━━━ sucralfate

Maxaquin

Carafate

Risk rating: 2
Severity: Moderate   **Onset: Rapid**   **Likelihood: Probable**

Cause
Sucralfate decreases GI absorption of quinolones such as lomefloxacin.

Effect
Quinolone effects decrease.

Nursing considerations
■ Don't use together. If that can't be avoided, give sucralfate at least 6 hours after the quinolone.
■ Monitor the patient for resolving infection.
■ Help the patient develop a plan to ensure proper dosage intervals.

loperamide ▶◀ ritonavir
Imodium   Norvir

Risk rating: 3
Severity: Minor   **Onset: Delayed**   **Likelihood: Suspected**

Cause
Ritonavir inhibits CYP3A4 metabolism of loperamide.

Effect
Loperamide levels may increase.

Nursing considerations
- The pharmacodynamics of loperamide aren't affected.
- The dose of loperamide may be decreased.
- No special precautions are needed for patients taking these drugs.

lopinavir-ritonavir ▶◀ carbamazepine
Kaletra   Tegretol

Risk rating: 2
Severity: Moderate   **Onset: Rapid**   **Likelihood: Suspected**

Cause
Lopinavir-ritonavir may inhibit CYP3A4 hepatic metabolism of carbamazepine, boosting serum levels. Carbamazepine, a powerful CYP34A enzyme inducer, may induce lopinavir-ritonavir metabolism.

Effect
Carbamazepine levels and risk of toxicity may increase. Lopinavir-ritonavir levels may decrease.

Nursing considerations
- Closely monitor carbamazepine levels when starting, stopping, or changing the dose of lopinavir-ritonavir.
- Observe the patient's clinical response to lopinavir-ritonavir therapy. Adjust the dose as needed.
- If lopinavir-ritonavir level decreases, antiretroviral treatment therapy may fail.
- Monitor carbamazepine level; therapeutic range is 4 to 12 mcg/ml.
- **⚡ ALERT** Watch for signs of anorexia or subtle appetite changes, which may indicate excessive carbamazepine level.
- Monitor the patient for evidence of carbamazepine toxicity, including dizziness, ataxia, respiratory depression, tachycardia, arrhythmias, blood pressure changes, impaired consciousness, abnormal reflexes, nystagmus, seizures, nausea, vomiting, and urine retention.

lopinavir-ritonavir ➡◀ ergot derivatives

Kaletra   dihydroergotamine,
                                 ergonovine, ergotamine,
                                 methylergonovine

Risk rating: 1
Severity: Major   **Onset: Delayed**   **Likelihood: Probable**

Cause
Protease inhibitors such as lopinavir-ritonavir may interfere with
CYP3A4 metabolism of ergot derivatives.

Effect
Risk of ergot-induced peripheral vasospasm and ischemia may increase.

Nursing considerations
◪ **ALERT** Use of ergot derivatives with protease inhibitors is contraindicated.
■ Monitor the patient for evidence of peripheral ischemia: pain in
limb muscles while exercising and later at rest; numbness and tingling
of fingers and toes; cool, pale, or cyanotic limbs; red or violet blisters
on hands or feet; and gangrene.
■ Sodium nitroprusside may be used to treat ergot-induced vasospasm.
■ If the patient takes a protease inhibitor, consult the prescriber or
pharmacist about alternative treatments for migraine pain.
■ Urge the patient to tell the prescriber about increased adverse effects.

lopinavir-ritonavir ➡◀ methadone

Kaletra

Risk rating: 2
Severity: Moderate   **Onset: Delayed**   **Likelihood: Suspected**

Cause
Protease inhibitors such as lopinavir-ritonavir may increase metabolism of methadone.

Effect
Pharmacologic effects of methadone may decrease. Patients on maintenance methadone treatment may experience opiate withdrawal
symptoms.

Nursing considerations
- Methadone dosage may need adjustment.
- If protease inhibitor therapy starts while the patient is taking methadone, watch for signs of opioid withdrawal.
- If protease inhibitor is stopped, methadone dosage may need to be decreased.
- Urge the patient to tell the prescriber about loss of methadone effect.

lopinavir-ritonavir ➥◀ nonnucleoside reverse transcriptase inhibitors
Kaletra   efavirenz, nevirapine

Risk rating: 2
Severity: Moderate   Onset: Delayed   Likelihood: Suspected

Cause
Nevirapine may increase hepatic metabolism of protease inhibitors, such as lopinavir-ritonavir.

Effect
Protease inhibitor level and effects decrease.

Nursing considerations
- If nevirapine is started or stopped, monitor protease inhibitor level.
- Protease inhibitor dosage may need adjustment.
- Monitor CD4+ and T-cell counts; tell the prescriber if they decrease.
- Urge the patient to report opportunistic infections.
- Tell the patient not to change an HIV regimen without consulting the prescriber.

lopinavir-ritonavir ➥◀ pimozide
Kaletra   Orap

Risk rating: 1
Severity: Major   Onset: Delayed   Likelihood: Suspected

Cause
Protease inhibitors such as lopinavir-ritonavir may inhibit CYP3A4 metabolism of pimozide.

Effect
Risk of life-threatening arrhythmias may increase.

Nursing considerations
🔌 **ALERT** Combined use of these drugs is contraindicated.

■ Arrhythmias are related to prolonged QT interval, a known risk of pimozide.
■ Interaction warning is based on pharmacokinetics of these drugs, not actual patient studies.

lopinavir-ritonavir ▰▸◀▰ tacrolimus
Kaletra   Prograf

Risk rating: 2
Severity: Moderate   **Onset: Delayed**   **Likelihood: Suspected**

Cause
Hepatic metabolism of tacrolimus is inhibited.

Effect
Tacrolimus level and risk of toxicity may increase.

Nursing considerations
■ Monitor renal function and mental status closely.
■ Check tacrolimus level often. Normal trough level is 6 to 10 mcg/ml.
■ Tacrolimus dosage may need to be decreased when the patient takes a protease inhibitor such as lopinavir-ritonavir.
■ Other protease inhibitors may have this same interaction.
◣ALERT Watch for renal failure, nephrotoxicity, hyperkalemia, hyperglycemia, delirium, and other changes in mental status.

lorazepam ▰▰▰▸◀▰▰▰ alcohol
Ativan

Risk rating: 2
Severity: Moderate   **Onset: Rapid**   **Likelihood: Established**

Cause
Alcohol inhibits hepatic enzymes, which decreases clearance and increases peak levels of benzodiazepines such as lorazepam.

Effect
Combining a benzodiazepine and alcohol may have additive or synergistic effects.

Nursing considerations
■ Before benzodiazepine therapy starts, assess the patient thoroughly for a history or evidence of alcohol use.
■ Advise the patient not to consume alcohol while taking a benzodiazepine.

■ Watch for additive CNS effects, which may suggest benzodiazepine overdose.

---

losartan ▶◀	fluconazole
Cozaar	Diflucan

Risk rating: 3
Severity: Minor   **Onset: Delayed**   **Likelihood: Suspected**

Cause
Fluconazole inhibits the metabolism of losartan.

Effect
Losartan antihypertensive and adverse effects may increase.

Nursing considerations
■ Closely monitor blood pressure response to losartan if the patient starts or stops fluconazole therapy, or the dosage is adjusted.
■ Observe the patient for adverse effects of losartan, which include hypotension, dizziness, chest pain, nausea, myalgia, cough, and angioedema.
■ Monitor renal function, including creatinine and BUN levels.

---

losartan ▶◀	indomethacin
Cozaar	Indocin

Risk rating: 2
Severity: Moderate   **Onset: Delayed**   **Likelihood: Suspected**

Cause
The mechanism of this interaction is unknown.

Effect
Hypotensive effect of losartan may decrease.

Nursing considerations
■ Antihypertensives other than losartan may not share this interaction.
■ Monitor blood pressure closely.
■ If you suspect an interaction, notify the prescriber. Indomethacin may need to be stopped or a different antihypertensive considered.

losartan ▶◀ lithium

Cozaar   Eskalith

Risk rating: 2
Severity: Moderate   Onset: Delayed   Likelihood: Suspected

Cause
Angiotensin II receptor antagonists may decrease lithium excretion.

Effect
Lithium level, effects, and risk of toxicity may increase.

Nursing considerations
■ If the patient takes lithium, consider an antihypertensive other than an angiotensin II receptor antagonist.
■ Monitor lithium level. Steady state lithium level should be 0.6 to 1.2 mEq/L.
■ Adjust lithium dose as needed.
■ Monitor the patient for evidence of lithium toxicity, such as diarrhea, vomiting, dehydration, drowsiness, muscle weakness, tremor, fever, and ataxia.

losartan ▶◀ spironolactone

Cozaar

Risk rating: 1
Severity: Major   Onset: Delayed   Likelihood: Suspected

Cause
Both angiotensin II receptor antagonists such as losartan and potassium-sparing diuretics such as spironolactone may increase the serum potassium level.

Effect
Risk of hyperkalemia may increase, especially among high-risk patients.

Nursing considerations
■ High-risk patients include elderly people and those with renal impairment, type 2 diabetes, or decreased renal perfusion. Monitor these patients closely.
■ Check serum potassium, BUN, and creatinine levels regularly. If they increase, notify the prescriber.
■ Advise the patient to immediately report an irregular heartbeat, slow pulse, weakness, or other evidence of hyperkalemia.

■ Give the patient a list of foods high in potassium; stress the need to eat them only in moderate amounts.

---

lovastatin ━━━━▶◀━━━━ azole antifungals

Mevacor   fluconazole, itraconazole, ketoconazole

Risk rating: 1
Severity: Major   **Onset: Rapid**   **Likelihood: Probable**

Cause
Azole antifungals may inhibit hepatic metabolism of HMG-CoA reductase inhibitors such as lovastatin.

Effect
Lovastatin level and adverse effects may increase.

Nursing considerations
■ If possible, avoid use together.
■ Lovastatin dosage may need to be decreased.
■ Monitor serum cholesterol and lipid levels.
■ **ALERT** Assess the patient for evidence of rhabdomyolysis, including fatigue; muscle aches and weakness; joint pain; dark, red, or cola-colored urine; weight gain; seizures; and greatly increased CK level.
■ Pravastatin is the HMG-CoA reductase inhibitor least affected by this interaction and may be preferred for use with an azole antifungal.

---

lovastatin ━━━━▶◀━━━━ cyclosporine

Mevacor   Neoral

Risk rating: 1
Severity: Major   **Onset: Delayed**   **Likelihood: Probable**

Cause
The metabolism of certain HMG-CoA reductase inhibitors such as lovastatin may decrease.

Effect
Plasma levels and adverse effects of HMG-CoA reductase inhibitors may increase.

Nursing considerations
■ If possible, avoid use together.
■ HMG-CoA reductase inhibitor dosage may need to be decreased.
■ Monitor serum cholesterol and lipid levels to assess the patient's response to therapy.

⚡ **ALERT** Assess the patient for evidence of rhabdomyolysis, including fatigue; muscle aches and weakness; joint pain; dark, red, or cola-colored urine; weight gain; seizures; and greatly increased CK level.
- Urge the patient to report muscle pain, tenderness, or weakness.

---

lovastatin ➤◄ diltiazem
Mevacor   Cardizem

Risk rating: 2
Severity: Moderate   Onset: Delayed   Likelihood: Probable

Cause
CYP3A4 metabolism of certain HMG-CoA reductase inhibitors such as lovastatin may be inhibited.

Effect
HMG-CoA reductase inhibitor level may increase, raising the risk of toxicity, including myositis and rhabdomyolysis.

Nursing considerations
- If possible, avoid use together.
- ⚡ **ALERT** Assess the patient for evidence of rhabdomyolysis, including fatigue; muscle aches and weakness; joint pain; dark, red, or cola-colored urine; weight gain; seizures; and greatly increased CK level.
- If the patient may have rhabdomyolysis, notify the prescriber and obtain renal function tests and serum potassium, sodium, calcium, lactic acid, and myoglobin levels.
- Pravastatin is less likely than other HMG-CoA reductase inhibitors to interact with diltiazem and may be the best choice for combined use.
- Urge the patient to report muscle pain, tenderness, or weakness.

---

lovastatin ➤◄ fibric acids
Mevacor   fenofibrate, gemfibrozil

Risk rating: 1
Severity: Major   Onset: Delayed   Likelihood: Suspected

Cause
The mechanism of this interaction is unknown.

Effect
Severe myopathy or rhabdomyolysis may occur.

Nursing considerations
- Avoid use together.

■ If the patient has severe hyperlipidemia, combined therapy may be an option, but only with careful monitoring.

▨ ALERT Assess the patient for evidence of rhabdomyolysis, including fatigue; muscle aches and weakness; joint pain; dark, red, or cola-colored urine; weight gain; seizures; and greatly increased CK level.

■ Watch for evidence of acute renal failure, including decreased urine output, elevated BUN and creatinine levels, edema, dyspnea, tachycardia, distended neck veins, nausea, vomiting, poor appetite, weakness, fatigue, confusion, and agitation.

■ Urge the patient to report muscle pain, tenderness, or weakness.

---

lovastatin ▰▰▰▰►◄▰▰▰▰ grapefruit juice
Mevacor

Risk rating: 2
Severity: **Moderate**   Onset: **Rapid**   Likelihood: **Suspected**

Cause
Grapefruit juice may inhibit CYP3A4 metabolism of certain HMG-CoA reductase inhibitors, such as lovastatin.

Effect
HMG-CoA reductase inhibitor level may increase, raising the risk of adverse effects.

Nursing considerations
■ Avoid giving lovastatin with grapefruit juice.

▨ ALERT Fluvastatin and pravastatin are metabolized by other enzymes and may be less affected by grapefruit juice.

■ Caution the patient to take the drug with a liquid other than grapefruit juice.

■ Urge the patient to report muscle pain, tenderness, or weakness.

---

lovastatin ▰▰▰▰►◄▰▰▰▰ macrolide antibiotics
Mevacor   azithromycin, clarithromycin,
                               erythromycin, telithromycin

Risk rating: 1
Severity: **Major**   Onset: **Delayed**   Likelihood: **Probable**

Cause
CYP3A4 metabolism of certain HMG-CoA reductase inhibitors such as lovastatin may be decreased.

Effect
HMG-CoA reductase inhibitor level may increase, raising the risk of severe myopathy or rhabdomyolysis.

Nursing considerations
■ If lovastatin is given with a macrolide antibiotic, watch for evidence of rhabdomyolysis, especially 5 to 21 days after macrolide antibiotic starts. Evidence may include fatigue; muscle aches and weakness; joint pain; dark, red, or cola-colored urine; weight gain; seizures; and greatly increased serum CK level.
■ Fluvastatin and pravastatin are metabolized by other enzymes and may be better choices when used with a macrolide antibiotic.
■ It may be safe to give atorvastatin with azithromycin.
■ Urge the patient to report muscle pain, tenderness, or weakness.

---

lovastatin ➤◀ protease inhibitors
Mevacor

atazanavir, darunavir
nelfinavir, ritonavir

Risk rating: 1
Severity: Major   **Onset: Delayed**   **Likelihood: Suspected**

Cause
Protease inhibitors may inhibit CYP3A4 metabolism of lovastatin.

Effect
Lovastatin level may increase.

Nursing considerations
◣ ALERT Use of lovastatin with nelfinavir is contraindicated.
■ Avoid using lovastatin with ritonavir or atazanavir.
■ If a protease inhibitor is added to a regimen that includes lovastatin, monitor the patient closely.
◣ ALERT Watch for evidence of rhabdomyolysis, which may include fatigue; muscle aches and weakness; joint pain; dark, red, or cola-colored urine; weight gain; seizures; and greatly increased serum CK level.
■ Urge the patient to immediately report any unexplained muscle weakness.

lovastatin ▶◀ warfarin
Mevacor   Coumadin

Risk rating: 2
Severity: Moderate   Onset: Delayed   Likelihood: Probable

Cause
Hepatic metabolism of warfarin may be inhibited.

Effect
Anticoagulant effects may increase.

Nursing considerations
- Monitor PT and INR closely when starting or stopping lovastatin.
- Atorvastatin and pravastatin, other HMG-CoA reductase inhibitors, don't appear to have this interaction with warfarin and may be better treatment options.
- Tell the patient to report unusual bruising or bleeding.
- Remind the patient that warfarin interacts with many drugs and that he should report any change in drug regimen.
- Advise the patient to keep all follow-up medical appointments for proper monitoring and dosage adjustments.

magnesium salts, oral ▶◀ tetracyclines

magaldrate, magnesium carbonate, magnesium citrate, magnesium gluconate, magnesium hydroxide, magnesium oxide, magnesium sulfate, magnesium trisilicate

doxycycline, minocycline, oxytetracycline, tetracycline

Risk rating: 2
Severity: Moderate   Onset: Delayed   Likelihood: Probable

Cause
Magnesium salts form an insoluble complex with tetracyclines, which lowers tetracycline absorption.

Effect
Tetracycline level and efficacy decrease.

Nursing considerations
- Separate administration of tetracyclines from magnesium salts by at least 3 to 4 hours.

- Monitor efficacy of tetracycline in resolving infection. Notify the prescriber if the patient's infection isn't responding to treatment.
- Teach patients to separate the tetracycline dose from magnesium-based antacids, laxatives, and supplements by 3 to 4 hours.

---

magnesium sulfate ➤◄ nondepolarizing muscle relaxants

pancuronium, vecuronium

Risk rating: 2
Severity: Moderate   **Onset: Rapid**   **Likelihood: Suspected**

Cause
Magnesium probably potentiates the action of nondepolarizing muscle relaxants.

Effect
Risk of profound, severe respiratory depression increases.

Nursing considerations
- Use these drugs together cautiously.
- Nondepolarizing muscle relaxant dosage may need to be adjusted.
- Monitor the patient for respiratory distress.
- Provide ventilatory support as needed.
- Make sure the patient is adequately sedated when receiving a nondepolarizing muscle relaxant.

---

mefloquine ➤◄ ziprasidone

Lariam   Geodon

Risk rating: 1
Severity: Major   **Onset: Delayed**   **Likelihood: Suspected**

Cause
Synergistic or additive prolongation of the QT interval may occur.

Effect
Risk of life-threatening arrhythmias, including torsades de pointes, increases.

Nursing considerations
🔔 **ALERT** Use of mefloquine with ziprasidone is contraindicated.
- Monitor the patient for other risk factors for torsades de pointes, including bradycardia, hypokalemia, and hypomagnesmia.

- Ask the patient if he or anyone in his family has a history of prolonged QT interval or arrhythmias.
- Monitor the patient for bradycardia.
- Measure QTc interval at baseline and throughout therapy.

---

megestrol ━━━━▶◀ dofetilide
Megace   Tikosyn

Risk rating: 1
Severity: Major   **Onset: Delayed**   **Likelihood: Suspected**

Cause
Dofetilide renal elimination may be inhibited.

Effect
Dofetilide level and risk of ventricular arrhythmias, including torsades de pointes, increase.

Nursing considerations
◪ **ALERT** Use of dofetilide with megestrol is contraindicated.
- Monitor ECG for prolonged QTc interval and development of ventricular arrhythmias.
- Monitor renal function every 3 months during dofetilide therapy.
- Monitor the patient for prolonged diarrhea, sweating, and vomiting during dofetilide therapy. Alert the prescriber because electrolyte imbalance may increase risk of arrhythmias.
- Urge the patient to tell the prescriber about increased adverse effects.

---

meperidine ━━━━▶◀ chlorpromazine
Demerol   Thorazine

Risk rating: 2
Severity: Moderate   **Onset: Rapid**   **Likelihood: Probable**

Cause
Combined use may produce additive CNS depressant and cardiovascular effects.

Effect
Excessive sedation and hypotension may occur.

Nursing considerations
- Avoid using meperidine with phenothiazines, such as chlorpromazine.

■ These drugs have been used together to minimize opioid dosage and control nausea and vomiting, but the risks may outweigh the benefits.
■ Watch for more severe and extended respiratory depression.

---

meperidine ◄►◄ MAO inhibitors
Demerol   phenelzine, selegiline, tranylcypromine

Risk rating: 1
Severity: Major   **Onset: Rapid**   **Likelihood: Probable**

Cause
The mechanism of this interaction is unknown.

Effect
The combination increases the risk of severe adverse reactions.

Nursing considerations
■ If possible, avoid giving these drugs together.
■ Monitor the patient; report agitation, seizures, diaphoresis, and fever.
■ Reaction may progress to coma, apnea, and death.
■ Reaction may occur several weeks after stopping the MAO inhibitor.
🟦 ALERT Give opioid analgesics other than meperidine cautiously. It isn't known if similar reactions occur.

---

meperidine ◄►◄ ritonavir
Demerol   Norvir

Risk rating: 1
Severity: Major   **Onset: Delayed**   **Likelihood: Suspected**

Cause
Ritonavir inhibits the metabolism of meperidine.

Effect
Meperidine levels increase significantly, increasing the risk of toxicity.

Nursing considerations
🟦 ALERT Use of these drugs together is contraindicated.
■ Toxic effects of meperidine include CNS side effects, seizures, and cardiac arrhythmias.
■ This interaction is based on pharmacokinetics, not actual patient studies.

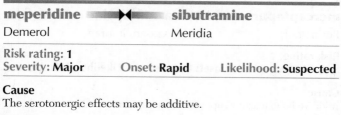

meperidine ◄► sibutramine
Demerol   Meridia

Risk rating: 1
Severity: Major   **Onset: Rapid**   **Likelihood: Suspected**

Cause
The serotonergic effects may be additive.

Effect
Serotonin syndrome may occur.

Nursing considerations
- Avoid using these drugs together.
- Monitor the patient for evidence of serotonin syndrome, including CNS irritability, motor weakness, shivering, muscle twitching, and altered consciousness.

◄ALERT Serotonin syndrome may be fatal and warrants immediate medical attention.

mercaptopurine ◄► allopurinol
Purinethol   Aloprim, Zyloprim

Risk rating: 1
Severity: Major   **Onset: Delayed**   **Likelihood: Established**

Cause
Allopurinol inhibits the first-pass metabolism of thiopurines such as mercaptopurine.

Effect
Pharmacologic and toxic effects of orally administered thiopurines are increased.

Nursing considerations
- When administering mercaptopurine with allopurinol, decrease the dose of mercaptopurine by 25% to 33%.

◄ ALERT Monitor the patient for toxic effects, which include thrombocytopenia and hepatotoxicity.

- Monitor the patient's hematologic and hepatic function tests.
- Advise the patient to report increased bleeding, yellow skin or eyes, or dark-colored urine.

mercaptopurine ━━►◄━━ azathioprine
Purinethol   Azasan, Imuran

Risk rating: 1
Severity: Major   **Onset: Delayed**   **Likelihood: Suspected**

Cause
Additive bone marrow suppression may occur.

Effect
Risk of developing life-threatening myelosuppression may be increased.

Nursing considerations
◼ **ALERT** Avoid administering these drugs together.
■ Myelosuppression may occur with either drug alone, or in combination.
■ Monitor the patient for toxic effects of azathioprine, including leukopenia, thrombocytopenia, and bone marrow suppression.

mercaptopurine ━━►◄━━ warfarin
Purinethol   Coumadin

Risk rating: 2
Severity: Moderate   **Onset: Delayed**   **Likelihood: Suspected**

Cause
The mechanism of the interaction is unknown. Thiopurines such as mercaptopurine may increase the synthesis of prothrombin and decrease plasma warfarin levels.

Effect
The effects of warfarin may be decreased.

Nursing considerations
■ Monitor PT and INR when starting, changing, or stopping mercaptopurine therapy in a patient who takes warfarin.
■ Maintain INR at 2 to 3 for an acute MI, atrial fibrillation, treatment of pulmonary embolism, prevention of systemic embolism, tissue heart valves, valvular heart disease, or prophylaxis or treatment of venous thrombosis. Maintain INR at 3 to 4.5 for mechanical prosthetic valves or recurrent systemic embolism.
■ Warfarin dose may need to be adjusted.
■ Tell the patient to report unusual bruising or bleeding.
■ Remind the patient that warfarin interacts with many drugs, and tell the patient to report any change in drug regimen.

meropenem ◄►► valproic acid
Merrem   Depakote

Risk rating: 2
Severity: Moderate   **Onset: Delayed**   **Likelihood: Suspected**

Cause
The mechanism of this interaction is unknown.

Effect
Valproic acid plasma levels may be decreased.

Nursing considerations
- Monitor the patient's valproic acid levels, and observe the patient for seizure activity when starting a carbapenem antibiotic such as meropenem.
- Consider giving an alternative antibiotic if an interaction is suspected.
- If the patient is taking either imipenem or cilastatin and stops the drug, it may be necessary to decrease the dose of valproic acid.

methadone ◄►► diazepam
Dolophine, Methadose   Valium

Risk rating: 2
Severity: Moderate   **Onset: Rapid**   **Likelihood: Suspected**

Cause
Additive or synergistic effects are involved.

Effect
Strength and drug effects of methadone are increased.

Nursing considerations
- Monitor the patient for increased sedation.
- Instruct the patient not to perform tasks such as driving or operating machinery.
- The interaction appears to be dose- and time-related, with the most increase in adverse effects coming 1 to 2 hours after taking the diazepam.

methadone ━━━▶◀━━━ efavirenz
Dolophine, Methadose   Sustiva

Risk rating: 2
Severity: Moderate   Onset: Delayed   Likelihood: Probable

Cause
Increased CYP3A4 hepatic metabolism of methadone may occur.

Effect
Action of methadone may be reduced, resulting in opiate withdrawal symptoms.

Nursing considerations
■ When starting a patient on a non-nucleoside reverse transcriptase inhibitor such as efavirenz, carefully monitor the patient's clinical response to methadone.
■ Be prepared to increase methadone dose.
■ Monitor the patient for methadone overdose when efavirenz therapy is stopped.
■ Monitor the patient for dilated pupils, diarrhea, abdominal pain, sweating, agitation, nausea, and vomiting.
■ Instruct the patient not to change the dose of his medications before consulting with the prescriber or pharmacist.

methadone ━━━▶◀━━━ phenytoin
Dolophine,   Dilantin
Methadose

Risk rating: 2
Severity: Moderate   Onset: Delayed   Likelihood: Suspected

Cause
The mechanism of this interaction is unknown but probably involves altered metabolic process.

Effect
Methadone level and effects may decrease.

Nursing considerations
■ Methadone dosage may need adjustment.
■ If hydantoin therapy starts while the patient is taking methadone, watch for signs of opioid withdrawal.
■ Urge the patient to tell the prescriber about a loss of methadone effect.

methadone ▰▰▰▶◀ protease inhibitors
Dolophine, Methadose

lopinavir/ritonavir, nelfinavir, ritonavir

Risk rating: 2
Severity: Moderate   **Onset: Delayed**   **Likelihood: Suspected**

Cause
Protease inhibitors may increase metabolism of methadone.

Effect
Pharmacologic effects of methadone may decrease. Patients on maintenance methadone treatment may experience opiate withdrawal symptoms.

Nursing considerations
- Methadone dosage may need adjustment.
- If protease inhibitor therapy starts while the patient is taking methadone, watch for signs of opioid withdrawal.
- If protease inhibitor is stopped, methadone dosage may need to be decreased.
- Urge the patient to tell the prescriber about loss of methadone effect.

methadone ▰▰▰▶◀ rifampin
Dolophine, Methadose

Rifadin, Rimactane

Risk rating: 2
Severity: Moderate   **Onset: Delayed**   **Likelihood: Established**

Cause
Rifampin increases hepatic and intestinal metabolism of methadone.

Effect
Pharmacologic effects of methadone may decrease. Patients on maintenance methadone treatment may experience opiate withdrawal symptoms.

Nursing considerations
- Methadone dosage may need adjustment.
- If rifampin therapy starts while the patient is taking methadone, watch for signs of opioid withdrawal.
- If rifampin is stopped, methadone dosage may need to be decreased.
- Urge the patient to tell the prescriber about loss of methadone effect.

methadone ►◄ zidovudine

Dolophine, Methadose   AZT, Retrovir

Risk rating: 2
Severity: Moderate   **Onset: Delayed**   **Likelihood: Probable**

Cause
The mechanism of this interaction is unknown.

Effect
Zidovudine levels and risk of adverse effects increase.

Nursing considerations
■ Monitor clinical response to zidovudine therapy.
■ If adverse effects to zidovudine increase, discuss a lower dosage with the prescriber.
■ Monitor the patient for anemia, neutropenia, leukopenia, muscle aches, and fever.

methamphetamine ►◄ MAO inhibitors

Desoxyn   phenelzine, tranylcypromine

Risk rating: 1
Severity: Major   **Onset: Rapid**   **Likelihood: Suspected**

Cause
This interaction probably stems from increased norepinephrine level at the synaptic cleft.

Effect
Anorexiant effects increase.

Nursing considerations
■ If possible, avoid giving these drugs together.
■ Headache and severe hypertension may occur rapidly if an amphetamine such as methamphetamine is given to a patient who takes an MAO inhibitor.
◪ **ALERT** Several deaths have resulted from hypertensive crisis and cerebral hemorrhage.
■ Monitor the patient for hypotension, hyperpyrexia, and seizures.
■ Hypertensive reaction may occur for several weeks after stopping an MAO inhibitor.

methamphetamine ➤◄ urinary acidifiers
Desoxyn

Risk rating: 3
Severity: Minor   **Onset: Rapid**   **Likelihood: Established**

Cause
Acidification of the urine decreases renal absoprtion of methamphetamine, thereby increasing excretion of methamphetamine.

Effect
Duration of methampetamine effects decreases.

Nursing considerations
- No special precautions are necessary with this interaction.
- This interaction has been used to therapeutic benefit in patients with amphetamine poisoning.

---

methamphetamine ➤◄ urine alkalinizers
Desoxyn

potassium citrate, sodium acetate, sodium bicarbonate, sodium citrate, sodium lactate, tromethamine

Risk rating: 2
Severity: Moderate   **Onset: Rapid**   **Likelihood: Established**

Cause
Alkaline urine prolongs clearance of amphetamines such as methamphetamine.

Effect
In amphetamine overdose, the toxic period is extended, increasing the risk of injury.

Nursing considerations
- **ALERT** Avoid drugs that may alkalinize the urine, particularly during amphetamine overdose.
- Watch for evidence of amphetamine toxicity, such as dermatoses, marked insomnia, irritability, hyperactivity, and personality changes.
- If the patient takes an anorexiant, advise against excessive use of sodium bicarbonate as an antacid.

methimazole ▶◀ theophyllines
Tapazole   aminophylline, theophylline

Risk rating: 2
Severity: **Moderate**   Onset: **Delayed**   Likelihood: **Suspected**

Cause
Methimazole and other thioamines increase theophylline clearance in a hyperthyroid patient.

Effect
Theophylline level and effects decrease.

Nursing considerations
- Watch closely for decreased theophylline efficacy while abnormal thyroid status continues.
- ◤ ALERT Assess the patient for return to a euthyroid state, when interaction no longer occurs.
- Explain that hyperthyroidism and hypothyroidism can affect theophylline efficacy and toxicity; tell the patient to immediately report evidence of either one.
- Urge patients to have TSH and theophylline levels tested regularly.

methimazole ▶◀ warfarin
Tapazole   Coumadin

Risk rating: 1
Severity: **Major**   Onset: **Delayed**   Likelihood: **Suspected**

Cause
The mechanism of this interaction is unknown.

Effect
Anticoagulant effects may be altered.

Nursing considerations
- Monitor coagulation values closely.
- Monitor the patient for inadequate response to anticoagulant.
- Tell the patient to report unusual bruising or bleeding.
- Remind the patient that warfarin interacts with many other drugs, and tell the patient to report any change in drug regimen.

methotrexate ▬▬►◄▬▬ cyclosporine
Trexall   Gengraf, Neoral, Sandimmune

Risk rating: 2
Severity: Moderate   **Onset: Delayed**   **Likelihood: Suspected**

Cause
Cyclosporine blocks the metabolism of methotrexate.

Effect
Methotrexate levels and pharmacologic and adverse effects increase.

Nursing considerations
■ Closely monitor clinical response to methotrexate when starting or stopping cyclosporine.
■ Adjust the dose of methotrexate as needed.
■ No effect is seen on cyclosporine.
■ Monitor the patient for methotrexate toxicity, including renal failure, neutropenia, leukopenia, thrombocytopenia, increased liver function tests, and skin ulcers.
■ Monitor the patient for mouth sores. This may be the first outward appearance of methotrexate toxicity; however, in some patients, bone marrow suppression coincides with or precedes mouth sores.

methotrexate ▬▬►◄▬▬ NSAIDs
Trexall   diclofenac, flurbiprofen,
                                           ibuprofen, indomethacin,
                                           ketoprofen, naproxen, tolmetin

Risk rating: 1
Severity: Major   **Onset: Delayed**   **Likelihood: Suspected**

Cause
Renal clearance of methotrexate may decrease.

Effect
Methotrexate toxicity may occur.

Nursing considerations
■ Monitor the patient for renal impairment that may predispose him to methotrexate toxicity.
■ Monitor the patient for mouth sores. This may be the first outward appearance of methotrexate toxicity; however, in some patients, bone marrow suppression coincides with or precedes mouth sores.

■ Methotrexate toxicity is less likely to occur with weekly low-dose methotrexate regimens for rheumatoid arthritis and other inflammatory diseases.
■ Longer leucovorin rescue should be considered when giving NSAIDs and methotrexate at antineoplastic doses.
■ Watch for other signs and symptoms of methotrexate toxicity, such as hematemesis, diarrhea with melena, nausea, and weakness.

---

methotrexate ➤◄ penicillins
Trexall   amoxicillin, oxacillin, piperacillin,

Risk rating: 1
Severity: Major   **Onset: Delayed**   **Likelihood: Probable**

Cause
Methotrexate secretion in the renal tubules is inhibited.

Effect
Methotrexate level and risk of toxicity increase.

Nursing considerations
■ Monitor the patient for methotrexate toxicity, including renal failure, neutropenia, leukopenia, thrombocytopenia, increased liver function tests, and skin ulcers.
■ Monitor the patient for mouth sores. This may be the first outward appearance of methotrexate toxicity; however, in some patients, bone marrow suppression coincides with or precedes mouth sores.
■ Obtain methotrexate level twice weekly for the first 2 weeks.
■ Dose and duration of leucovorin rescue may need to be increased.

---

methotrexate ➤◄ phenytoin
Trexall   Dilantin

Risk rating: 2
Severity: Moderate   **Onset: Delayed**   **Likelihood: Suspected**

Cause
Phenytoin absorption may be decreased or metabolism may be increased.

Effect
Phenytoin level and effects may decrease.

Nursing considerations
■ Monitor phenytoin level closely. Dosage may need to be adjusted.

- Therapeutic range for phenytoin is 10 to 20 mcg/ml.
- Toxic effects can occur at therapeutic level. Adjust the measured level for hypoalbuminemia or renal impairment, which can increase free drug level.
- Monitor the patient for seizure activity.
- Carefully monitor phenytoin level between courses of chemotherapy. Phenytoin dose may need to be reduced.
- Signs and symptoms of phenytoin toxicity include nystagmus, slurred speech, ataxia, blurred or double vision, confusion, drowsiness, and lethargy.

methotrexate ◄ probenecid
Trexall   Probalan

Risk rating: 1
Severity: **Major**   Onset: **Rapid**   Likelihood: **Probable**

Cause
Probenecid may impair renal excretion of methotrexate.

Effect
Methotrexate level, effects, and risk of toxicity may increase.

Nursing considerations
- Monitor the patient for methotrexate toxicity, including renal failure, neutropenia, leukopenia, thrombocytopenia, increased liver function tests, and skin ulcers.
- Monitor the patient for mouth sores. This may be the first outward appearance of methotrexate toxicity; however, in some patients, bone marrow suppression coincides with or precedes mouth sores.
- Notify the prescriber if signs of toxicity appear; the methotrexate dose may need to be reduced.

methotrexate ◄ salicylates
Trexall   aspirin, choline salicylate,
                                sodium salicylate

Risk rating: 1
Severity: **Major**   Onset: **Rapid**   Likelihood: **Suspected**

Cause
Renal clearance and plasma protein binding of methotrexate may be decreased by salicylates.

Effect
Methotrexate toxicity may occur.

Nursing considerations
■ Monitor the patient for methotrexate toxicity, including renal failure, neutropenia, leukopenia, thrombocytopenia, increased liver function tests, and skin ulcers.
■ Monitor the patient for mouth sores. This may be the first outward appearance of methotrexate toxicity; however, in some patients, bone marrow suppression coincides with or precedes mouth sores.
■ Notify the prescriber if signs of toxicity appear; the methotrexate dose may need to be reduced.

methotrexate ➤◄ trimethoprim
Trexall   Proloprim

Risk rating: 1
Severity: Major   **Onset: Delayed**   **Likelihood: Suspected**

Cause
Methotrexate and trimethoprim may have a synergistic effect on folate metabolism.

Effect
Methotrexate toxicity may occur.

Nursing considerations
■ Avoid using methotrexate with trimethoprim if possible.
■ Monitor the patient for methotrexate-induced bone marrow suppression and megaloblastic anemia.
■ Consider use of leucovorin to treat megaloblastic anemia and neutropenia resulting from folic acid deficiency.

methsuximide ➤◄ primidone
Celontin   Mysoline

Risk rating: 2
Severity: Moderate   **Onset: Delayed**   **Likelihood: Suspected**

Cause
The cause of this interaction is unknown.

Effect
Primidone levels and pharmacologic effects may be reduced.

Nursing considerations
- Monitor serum primidone levels.
- Adjustments to methsuximide dosage may necessitate a change in primidone.
- Monitor the patient for increased seizure activity.
- Therapeutic level of primidone is 5 to 12 mcg/ml.

---

methyclothiazide ➤◀ lithium
Enduron   Eskalith

Risk rating: 2
Severity: Moderate   Onset: Delayed   Likelihood: Established

Cause
Thiazide diuretics such as methyclothiazide may decrease lithium clearance.

Effect
Lithium level, effects, and risk of toxicity may increase.

Nursing considerations
- Despite this interaction, lithium and thiazide diuretics may be used together safely, with close monitoring of the lithium level.
- Reduction in lithium clearance may depend on thiazide dose.
- Monitor lithium level, and adjust dose as needed.
- Monitor the patient for evidence of lithium toxicity, such as diarrhea, vomiting, dehydration, drowsiness, muscle weakness, tremor, fever, and ataxia.

---

methyldopa ➤◀ norepinephrine
Aldomet   Levophed

Risk rating: 2
Severity: Moderate   Onset: Rapid   Likelihood: Suspected

Cause
The mechanism of this interaction is unknown.

Effect
Pressor response of norepinephrine may be increased, resulting in hypertension.

Nursing considerations
- Monitor the patient's blood pressure closely.
- If the patient takes methyldopa, explain that many OTC products contain drugs that can raise blood pressure. Urge the patient to read

labels carefully or check with the prescriber before using a new product.
- Teach the patient to monitor his blood pressure at home.

methylergonovine ➡◀ itraconazole
Methergine   Sporanox

Risk rating: 1
Severity: Major   **Onset: Delayed**   **Likelihood: Suspected**

Cause
Itraconazole inhibits CYP3A4 metabolism of ergot derivatives such as methylergonovine.

Effect
Risk of ergot toxicity may increase.

Nursing considerations
⚠ **ALERT** Use of these drugs together is contraindicated.
- Signs of ergot toxicity include peripheral vasospasm and ischemia.
- Caution the patient against using ergot derivatives (for migraine, for example) while taking itraconazole; advise him to consult the prescriber about alternatives.

methylergonovine ➡◀ protease inhibitors
Methergine   amprenavir, atazanavir,
                                    darunavir, indinavir, lopinavir-
                                    ritonavir, nelfinavir, ritonavir,
                                    saquinavir

Risk rating: 1
Severity: Major   **Onset: Delayed**   **Likelihood: Probable**

Cause
Protease inhibitors may interfere with CYP3A4 metabolism of ergot derivatives such as methylergonovine.

Effect
Risk of ergot-induced peripheral vasospasm and ischemia may increase.

Nursing considerations
⚠ **ALERT** Use of ergot derivatives with protease inhibitors is contraindicated.
- Monitor the patient for evidence of peripheral ischemia, including pain in limb muscles while exercising and later at rest; numbness and

tingling of fingers and toes; cool, pale, or cyanotic limbs; red or violet blisters on hands or feet; and gangrene.
■ Sodium nitroprusside may be given for ergot-induced vasospasm.
■ If the patient takes a protease inhibitor, consult the prescriber or pharmacist about alternative treatments for migraine pain.
■ Urge the patient to tell the prescriber about increased adverse effects.

methylphenidate ➤◀ tranylcypromine

Concerta, Ritalin   Parnate

Risk rating: 1
Severity: Major   **Onset: Delayed**   **Likelihood: Suspected**

Cause
The mechanism of this interaction is unknown.

Effect
Risk of hypertensive crisis increases.

Nursing considerations
🖳 ALERT Use of methylphenidate with MAO inhibitors such as tranylcypromine is contraindicated.
■ Don't use methylphenidate within 14 days after stopping an MAO inhibitor.
■ Monitor blood pressure closely if methylphenidate is given with an MAO inhibitor.
■ Teach the patient and parents to monitor blood pressure at home.

methylprednisolone ➤◀ aprepitant

Medrol   Emend

Risk rating: 2
Severity: Moderate   **Onset: Delayed**   **Likelihood: Suspected**

Cause
Aprepitant may inhibit first-pass metabolism of certain corticosteroids such as methylprednisolone.

Effect
Corticosteroid level may be increased and half-life prolonged.

Nursing considerations
■ Corticosteroid dosage may need to be decreased.
■ When starting or stopping aprepitant, adjust corticosteroid dosage as needed.

■ Watch closely for evidence of increased corticosteroid level, such as insomnia, euphoria, increased appetite, mood changes, and increased blood glucose level.
■ Tell the patient to report symptoms of increased blood glucose level, including increased thirst, hunger, and frequency of urination.

methylprednisolone ▶◀ azole antifungals
Medrol   itraconazole, ketoconazole

Risk rating: 2
Severity: Moderate   Onset: Delayed   Likelihood: Suspected

Cause
Inhibition of CYP3A4 metabolism of methylprednisolone and decrease in elimination.

Effect
Corticosteroid effects and toxicity may be increased.

Nursing considerations
■ Monitor the patient for increased adverse effects to methylprednisolone and adjust dose as needed.
■ Monitor the patient taking corticosteroids such as methylprednisolone with azole antifungals for Cushing's syndrome.
■ Carefully monitor the patient for infection, edema, and increased serum glucose level.
■ Instruct the patient not to abruptly stop methylprednisolone; it should be tapered gradually to prevent withdrawal symptoms.

methylprednisolone ▶◀ barbiturates
Medrol   pentobarbital, phenobarbital, primidone

Risk rating: 2
Severity: Moderate   Onset: Delayed   Likelihood: Established

Cause
Barbiturates induce liver enzymes, which stimulate metabolism of corticosteroids such as methylprednisolone.

Effect
Corticosteroid effects may be decreased.

Nursing considerations
■ Avoid giving barbiturates with corticosteroids.

- If the patient takes a corticosteroid, watch for worsening symptoms when a barbiturate is started or stopped.
- During barbiturate treatment, corticosteroid dosage may need to be increased.

methylprednisolone ▪◀ cholinesterase inhibitors
Medrol   neostigmine, pyridostigmine

Risk rating: 1
Severity: Major   **Onset: Delayed**   **Likelihood: Probable**

Cause
In myasthenia gravis, methylprednisolone and other corticosteroids antagonize the effects of cholinesterase inhibitors by an unknown mechanism.

Effect
The patient may develop severe muscular depression refractory to cholinesterase inhibitor.

Nursing considerations
- Corticosteroids may have long-term benefits in myasthenia gravis.
- Combined therapy may be attempted under strict supervision.
- In myasthenia gravis, monitor the patient for severe muscle deterioration.
- **ALERT** Be prepared to provide respiratory support and mechanical ventilation if needed.
- Consult the prescriber or pharmacist about safe corticosteroid delivery to maximize improvement in muscle strength.

methylprednisolone ▪◀ diltiazem
Medrol   Cardizem

Risk rating: 2
Severity: Moderate   **Onset: Delayed**   **Likelihood: Suspected**

Cause
Methylprednisolone CYP3A4 metabolism may be inhibited.

Effect
Methylprednisolone effects and risk of toxicity may increase.

Nursing considerations
- Corticosteroids other than methylprednisolone may have a similar interaction with diltiazem. If you suspect a drug interaction, consult the prescriber or pharmacist.

■ Monitor the patient's response to methylprednisolone.
■ Monitor the patient for signs of methylprednisolone toxicity, including nervousness, sleepiness, depression, psychoses, weakness, decreased hearing, leg edema, skin disorders, hypertension, muscle weakness, and seizures.
■ Methylprednisolone dosage may need adjustment.
■ Advise the patient to report increased adverse effects.

methylprednisolone ▶◀ macrolide antibiotics
Medrol   clarithromycin, erythromycin

Risk rating: 2
Severity: Moderate   Onset: Delayed   Likelihood: Established

Cause
The mechanism of this interaction is unclear.

Effect
Methylprednisolone effects, including toxic effects, may increase.

Nursing considerations
■ This interaction may be used for therapeutic benefit because it may be possible to reduce methylprednisolone dosage.
■ Methylprednisolone dosage may need adjustment.
■ Monitor the patient for adverse or toxic effects, such as euphoria, insomnia, peptic ulceration, and cushingoid effects.

methylprednisolone ▶◀ phenytoin
Medrol   Dilantin

Risk rating: 2
Severity: Moderate   Onset: Delayed   Likelihood: Established

Cause
Hydantoins such as phenytoin induce liver enzymes, which stimulate metabolism of corticosteroids such as methylprednisolone.

Effect
Corticosteroid effects may be decreased.

Nursing considerations
■ Avoid giving hydantoins with corticosteroids if possible.
■ Monitor the patient for decreased corticosteroid effects. Also monitor phenytoin level, and adjust the dosage of either drug as needed.

- Corticosteroid effects may decrease within days of starting phenytoin and may stay decreased for 3 weeks after the patient stops taking
the phenytoin.
- Dosage of either or both drugs may need to be increased.

methylprednisolone ➤◀ primidone
Medrol   Mysoline

Risk rating: 2
Severity: Moderate   Onset: Delayed   Likelihood: Established

Cause
Primidone and other barbiturates induce liver enzymes, which stimulate metabolism of corticosteroids such as methylprednisolone.

Effect
Corticosteroid effects may decrease.

Nursing considerations
- Avoid giving barbiturates with corticosteroids if possible.
- If the patient takes a corticosteroid such as methylprednisolone with
a barbiturate such as primidone, watch for worsening symptoms when
the barbiturate is started or stopped.
- During barbiturate treatment, corticosteroid dosage may need to be
increased.

methylprednisolone ➤◀ rifampin
Medrol   Rifamycin, Rimactane

Risk rating: 1
Severity: Major   Onset: Delayed   Likelihood: Established

Cause
Rifampin increases hepatic metabolism of corticosteroids such as
methylprednisolone.

Effect
Corticosteroid effects may decrease.

Nursing considerations
- If possible, avoid giving rifampin with corticosteroids.
- Monitor the patient for decreased corticosteroid effects, including
loss of disease control.
- Watch for symptom control after increasing rifampin dose. Drug
may need to be stopped to regain control of disease.

■ Corticosteroid effects may decrease within days of starting rifampin and may stay at those lower levels for 2 to 3 weeks after the patient stops taking the corticosteroid.
■ Corticosteroid dose may need to be doubled after adding rifampin.

methyltestosterone ➡◀ cyclosporine
Virilon   Gengraf, Neoral, Sandimmune

Risk rating: 2
Severity: Moderate   Onset: Delayed   Likelihood: Suspected

Cause
Cyclosporine metabolism is inhibited.

Effect
Cyclosporine level and risk of toxicity may increase.

Nursing considerations
■ Monitor the patient for signs and symptoms of cyclosporine toxicity, such as nephrotoxicity and neurotoxicity.
■ Monitor BUN and creatinine levels and urine output.
■ Monitor cyclosporine level.
■ Adjust cyclosporine dosage as needed. It may need to be reduced 20% to 50%.
■ Check urine for increased proteins, cells, or casts.
■ If renal insufficiency develops, notify the prescriber.

methyltestosterone ➡◀ warfarin
Virilon   Coumadin

Risk rating: 1
Severity: Major   Onset: Delayed   Likelihood: Probable

Cause
The mechanism of this interaction is unknown.

Effect
Anticoagulant effects increase.

Nursing considerations
■ If possible, avoid this combination.
■ Monitor coagulation values carefully. Warfarin dosage will be decreased.
■ Tell the patient to report unusual bleeding or bruising,
■ Remind the patient that warfarin interacts with many drugs; tell him to report any change in drug regimen to the prescriber or pharmacist.

metoclopramide ◄►► cyclosporine
Reglan   Gengraf, Neoral, Sandimmune

Risk rating: 2
Severity: Moderate   Onset: Delayed   Likelihood: Suspected

Cause
Metoclopramide increases gastric emptying time, which may increase cyclosporine absorption.

Effect
Cyclosporine level and risk of toxicity may increase.

Nursing considerations
- Monitor cyclosporine level closely.
- Watch for cyclosporine toxicity, including hepatotoxicity, nephrotoxicity, nausea, vomiting, tremors, and seizures.
- Consider decreasing cyclosporine dose as needed.
- It isn't known whether altering dosage or schedule of metoclopramide would decrease risk or severity of interaction.

metoclopramide ◄►► digoxin
Reglan   Lanoxin

Risk rating: 2
Severity: Moderate   Onset: Delayed   Likelihood: Probable

Cause
Metoclopramide increases GI motility and may decrease digoxin absorption.

Effect
Serum digoxin level and effects may decrease.

Nursing considerations
- Monitor the patient for decreased digoxin level; therapeutic range is 0.8 to 2 nanograms/ml.
- Monitor the patient for expected digoxin effects, including decreased heart rate, arrhythmia conversion, maintenance of converted rhythm, and improvement of heart failure symptoms.
- Digoxin dosage may need adjustment if effect or level decreases.
- **⚠ ALERT** This interaction may not occur with high-bioavailability digoxin preparations, including capsule, elixir, and tablet with a high dissolution rate.
- Urge the patient to tell the prescriber about increased adverse effects.

metolazone ◄► loop diuretics

Zaroxolyn

bumetanide, furosemide

Risk rating: 2
Severity: Moderate   **Onset: Rapid**   **Likelihood: Probable**

Cause
The mechanism of this interaction is unclear.

Effect
Because these drugs work synergistically, they may cause profound diuresis and serious electrolyte abnormalities.

Nursing considerations
- This drug combination may be used for therapeutic benefit.
- Expect increased sodium, potassium, and chloride excretion and greater diuresis.
- Monitor the patient for dehydration and electrolyte abnormalities.
- Carefully adjust drugs, using small or intermittent doses.

metoprolol ◄► aluminum salts

Lopressor

aluminum carbonate, aluminum hydroxide, aluminum phosphate, kaolin

Risk rating: 3
Severity: Minor   **Onset: Rapid**   **Likelihood: Suspected**

Cause
Rate of gastric emptying is decreased, leading to reduced bioavailability of metoprolol.

Effect
Pharmacologic effects of beta-adrenergic blockers such as metoprolol may be decreased.

Nursing considerations
- Separate administration of aluminum salts and beta-adrenergic blockers by at least 2 hours.
- Monitor the patient's blood pressure and heart rate.
- Tell the patient to notify the prescriber if he notices an increase in his heart rate.

metoprolol ━━━━▶◀━━━ cimetidine

Lopressor   Tagamet

Risk rating: 2
Severity: Moderate   Onset: Rapid   Likelihood: Probable

Cause
By inhibiting CYP pathway, cimetidine reduces first-pass metabolism of certain beta-adrenergic blockers such as metoprolol.

Effect
Clearance of metoprolol is decreased and its action is increased.

Nursing considerations
- Monitor the patient for severe bradycardia and hypotension.
- If interaction occurs, notify the prescriber; beta-adrenergic blocker dosage may be decreased.
- Teach the patient to monitor pulse rate. If it's significantly lower than usual, tell him to withhold beta-adrenergic blocker and to contact the prescriber.
- Instruct the patient to change positions slowly to reduce effects of orthostatic hypotension.
- Other beta-adrenergic blockers may interact with cimetidine. If you suspect an interaction, consult the prescriber or pharmacist.

metoprolol ━━━━▶◀━━━ hydralazine

Lopressor   Apresoline

Risk rating: 2
Severity: Moderate   Onset: Rapid   Likelihood: Probable

Cause
Hydralazine may cause transient increase in visceral blood flow and decreased first-pass hepatic metabolism of some oral beta-adrenergic blockers such as metoprolol.

Effect
Effects of both drugs may increase.

Nursing considerations
- Monitor blood pressure regularly, and tailor dosages of both drugs to the patient's response.
- Other beta-adrenergic blockers may interact with hydralazine. If you suspect an interaction, consult the prescriber or pharmacist.

■ Explain that both drugs can affect blood pressure. Urge the patient to report evidence of hypotension, such as light-headedness and dizziness when changing positions.

metoprolol 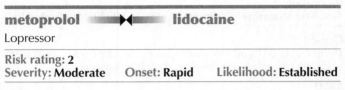 lidocaine
Lopressor

Risk rating: 2
Severity: Moderate   **Onset: Rapid**   **Likelihood: Established**

Cause
Metoprolol and other beta-adrenergic blockers reduce hepatic metabolism of lidocaine.

Effect
Lidocaine level and risk of toxicity may increase.

Nursing considerations
■ Check for normal therapeutic level of lidocaine: 2 to 5 mcg/ml.
■ Monitor the patient closely for evidence of lidocaine toxicity, including dizziness, somnolence, confusion, paresthesia, and seizures.
■ Slow the I.V. bolus rate of lidocaine to decrease risk of high peak level and toxic reaction.
■ Explain warning signs of toxicity to the patient and family, and tell them to contact the prescriber if they have concerns.

metoprolol 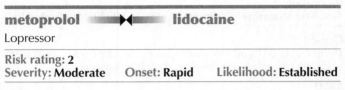 propafenone
Lopressor   Rythmol

Risk rating: 2
Severity: Moderate   **Onset: Rapid**   **Likelihood: Probable**

Cause
Propafenone inhibits first-pass metabolism of certain beta-adrenergic blockers such as metoprolol, and reduces their systemic clearance.

Effect
Beta-adrenergic blocker effects may be increased.

Nursing considerations
■ Monitor blood pressure, pulse, and cardiac complaints.
■ Notify the prescriber about abnormally low blood pressure or change in heart rate; beta-adrenergic blocker dosage may be decreased.
■ Tell the patient to promptly report nightmares or other CNS complaints.

■ To minimize effects of orthostatic hypotension, tell the patient to change positions slowly.

metoprolol ━━━━►◄━━━ quinidine
Lopressor

Risk rating: 2
Severity: Moderate   **Onset: Rapid**   **Likelihood: Suspected**

Cause
Quinidine may inhibit metabolism of certain beta-adrenergic blockers such as metoprolol.

Effect
Beta-adrenergic blocker effects may increase.

Nursing considerations
■ Monitor pulse and blood pressure more often during combined use.
■ Teach the patient how to check blood pressure and pulse rate; tell him to do so regularly.
■ Tell the patient to consult the prescriber if his pulse slows or blood pressure falls. Beta-adrenergic blocker dosage may need to be decreased.

metoprolol ━━━━►◄━━━ rifampin
Lopressor   Rifadin, Rimactane

Risk rating: 2
Severity: Moderate   **Onset: Delayed**   **Likelihood: Suspected**

Cause
Rifampin increases hepatic metabolism of beta-adrenergic blockers such as metoprolol.

Effect
Beta-adrenergic blocker effects are reduced.

Nursing considerations
■ Monitor blood pressure and heart rate closely to assess beta-adrenergic blocker efficacy.
■ If beta-adrenergic blocker effects are decreased, consult the prescriber; the dosage may need to be increased.
■ Teach the patient how to monitor blood pressure and heart rate and when to contact the prescriber.
■ Other beta-adrenergic blockers may interact with rifampin. If you suspect an interaction, consult the prescriber or pharmacist.

metoprolol ━━━▶◀━━━ verapamil
Lopressor   Calan

Risk rating: 1
Severity: **Major**   Onset: **Rapid**   Likelihood: **Probable**

Cause
Verapamil may inhibit metabolism of beta-adrenergic blockers such as metoprolol.

Effect
Effects of both drugs may increase.

Nursing considerations
- Combination therapy is common in patients with hypertension and unstable angina.
- ⚡ **ALERT** Giving these drugs together increases risk of adverse effects, including heart failure, conduction disturbances, arrhythmias, and hypotension.
- Assess the patient for adverse effects, including left ventricular dysfunction and AV conduction defects.
- Risk of interaction is greater when drugs are given I.V.
- Dosages of both drugs may need to be decreased.

metronidazole ━━━▶◀━━━ alcohol
Flagyl

Risk rating: 2
Severity: **Moderate**   Onset: **Rapid**   Likelihood: **Suspected**

Cause
Metronidazole may inhibit aldehyde dehydrogenase, which causes an accumulation of acetaldehyde.

Effect
Disulfiram-like reaction may occur.

Nursing considerations
- Monitor the patient for flushing, palpitations, tachycardia, nausea, and vomiting.
- Warn the patient about the interaction and instruct him to avoid alcohol ingestion.
- This interaction has been noted with the oral, injectable, and suppository forms of metronidazole.
- If the patient takes metronidazole, explain that many OTC products contain alcohol. Urge the patient to read labels carefully or check with the prescriber before using a new product.

metronidazole ➤◀ busulfan
Flagyl   Mylyan

Risk rating: 1
Severity: Major   **Onset: Delayed**   **Likelihood: Suspected**

Cause
The mechanism of the interaction is unknown.

Effect
Busulfan trough level may be elevated, increasing the risk of serious toxicity, including veno-occlusive disease and hemorrhagic cystitis.

Nursing considerations
⚠ **ALERT** The use of these two drugs together is contraindicated.
■ If a patient taking busulfan is started on metronidazole, the dose of busulfan may need to be decreased.
■ Monitor the patient for persistent cough, labored breathing, thrombocytopenia, and signs of infection.
■ Tell the patient to call the prescriber if he notices increased bleeding or bruising, jaundice, fever, sore throat, or fatigue.

metronidazole ➤◀ disulfiram
Flagyl   Antabuse

Risk rating: 2
Severity: Moderate   **Onset: Delayed**   **Likelihood: Suspected**

Cause
Excess dopaminergic activity may occur.

Effect
Acute psychosis or confusion may occur.

Nursing considerations
■ Combined use of these drugs should be avoided, if possible.
■ Watch for adverse effects, including paranoid delusions and visual and auditory hallucinations.
■ Symptoms may develop at 10th to 14th day of combined use.
■ Notify the prescriber if acute psychosis or confusion occurs; one or both drugs may need to be stopped.
■ Symptoms may continue or increase for a few days after drugs are stopped.
■ Assure family members that full recovery usually occurs within 2 weeks.

metronidazole ━━►◄━━ warfarin
Flagyl   Coumadin

Risk rating: 1
Severity: Major   **Onset: Delayed**   **Likelihood: Established**

Cause
May decrease hepatic metabolism of warfarin.

Effect
Anticoagulant effects and risk of bleeding increase.

Nursing considerations
- Monitor the patient for signs of bleeding.
- Warfarin dose may need to be reduced during metronidazole use.
- Tell the patient to report unusual bruising or bleeding.
- Remind the patient that warfarin interacts with many drugs; tell him to report any change in drug regimen.

metyrapone ━━►◄━━ cyproheptadine
Metopirone   Periactin

Risk rating: 2
Severity: Moderate   **Onset: Rapid**   **Likelihood: Probable**

Cause
Cyproheptadine decreases the expected adrenocorticotropic hormone secretion seen after administering metyrapone.

Effect
Decreased pituitary-adrenal response to metyrapone.

Nursing considerations
◼ ALERT Discontinue cyproheptadine before assessment of pituitary-adrenal axis with metyrapone.
- Tell the patient how important it is to tell his health care practitioners about all the drugs he's taking.

metyrapone ━━►◄━━ phenytoin
Metopirone   Dilantin

Risk rating: 2
Severity: Moderate   **Onset: Delayed**   **Likelihood: Established**

Cause
Phenytoin increases first-pass metabolism of metyrapone.

Effect
This causes a decreased pituitary-adrenal response to oral metyrapone.

Nursing considerations
■ Two times the normal dosage of metyrapone may be needed for pituitary-adrenal axis assessment.
■ If possible, stop phenytoin before administering metyrapone.
■ Administering metyrapone I.V. bypasses first-pass metabolism and doesn't have this interaction.

---

mexiletine ▶◀ phenytoin
Mexitil   Dilantin

Risk rating: 2
Severity: Moderate   Onset: Delayed   Likelihood: Established

Cause
Phenytoin increases hepatic metabolism of mexiletine.

Effect
Mexiletine levels and effectiveness decrease.

Nursing considerations
■ Monitor clinical response to mexiletine.
■ Mexiletine dosage may need to be increased.
■ Monitor ECG for recurrence of arrhythmias; notify the prescriber if increase in arrhythmias is noted.

---

mexiletine ▶◀ propafenone
Mexitil   Rythmol

Risk rating: 2
Severity: Moderate   Onset: Delayed   Likelihood: Established

Cause
Propafenone inhibits CYP2D6 metabolism of mexiletine.

Effect
Mexiletine levels and risk of adverse effects increase.

Nursing considerations
■ Monitor blood levels of mexiletine when propafenone therapy is started or stopped.
■ If both medications are started together, carefully titrate the dose of both medications.
■ Monitor ECG for new or increased arrhythmias.

■ Instruct the patient to notify the prescriber if he experiences chest pain, palpitations, or angina.

---

mexiletine ▶◀ theophyllines

Mexitil

aminophylline, theophylline

Risk rating: 2
Severity: Moderate   Onset: Delayed   Likelihood: Established

Cause
Mexiletine inhibits CYP metabolism of theophylline.

Effect
Theophylline level and risk of toxicity may increase.

Nursing considerations
■ When adding mexiletine, monitor theophylline level closely. Therapeutic range is 10 to 20 mcg/ml for adults and 5 to 15 mcg/ml for children.
■ Interaction usually occurs within 2 days of combining these drugs. Theophylline dosage may be decreased when mexiletine starts.
■ Watch for evidence of toxicity, such as ventricular tachycardia, anorexia, nausea, vomiting, diarrhea, seizures, restlessness, irritability, and headache.
■ Describe adverse effects of theophylline and signs of toxicity, and tell the patient to report them immediately to the prescriber.

---

micafungin ▶◀ cyclosporine

Mycamine

Gengraf, Neoral, Sandimmune

Risk rating: 2
Severity: Moderate   Onset: Delayed   Likelihood: Suspected

Cause
Micafungin inhibits CYP3A metabolism of cyclosporine.

Effect
Cyclosporine level and risk of adverse reactions may increase.

Nursing considerations
■ Cyclosporine dose may need to be adjusted when starting or stopping micafungin therapy.
■ Monitor cyclosporine level closely.
■ Watch for signs and symptoms of toxicity including shakiness, headaches, tremor, hypertension, and fatigue.
■ Decrease cyclosporine dose as needed.

midazolam ━━━▶◀━━━ azole antifungals
fluconazole, itraconazole,
ketoconazole, voriconazole

Risk rating: 2
Severity: Moderate   Onset: Delayed   Likelihood: Established

Cause
Azole antifungals decrease CYP3A4 metabolism of certain benzodiazepines such as midazolam.

Effect
Benzodiazepine effects are increased and prolonged, which may
cause CNS depression and psychomotor impairment.

Nursing considerations
■ If the patient takes an azole antifungal, talk with the prescriber
about giving a lower benzodiazepine dose or a drug not metabolized
by CYP3A4, such as temazepam or lorazepam.
■ Caution that the effects of this interaction may last several days after
stopping the azole antifungal.
■ Explain that taking these drugs together may increase sedative effects; tell the patient to report such effects promptly.
■ Teach the patient alternative methods for inducing sleep or relieving anxiety.
■ Various benzodiazepine–azole antifungal combinations may interact. If you suspect an interaction, consult the prescriber or pharmacist.

midazolam ━━━━▶◀━━━ carbamazepine
Tegretol

Risk rating: 2
Severity: Moderate   Onset: Delayed   Likelihood: Suspected

Cause
The metabolism of benzodiazepines such as midazolam is increased.

Effect
The pharmacologic effects of benzodiazepines may be decreased.

Nursing considerations
■ Carbamazepine may cause decreased effectiveness of benzodiazepines.
■ If the patient is taking carbamazepine and midazolam together,
monitor the patient for a decreased response to midazolam.

■ Consult with the prescriber for an increased dose of midazolam, if needed.

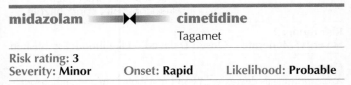

midazolam ▶◀ cimetidine
Tagamet

Risk rating: 3
Severity: Minor   **Onset: Rapid**   **Likelihood: Probable**

Cause
Hepatic metabolism of benzodiazepines such as midazolam may be decreased.

Effect
Serum levels of midazolam may be increased, causing increased sedation.

Nursing considerations
◆ **ALERT** Carefully monitor the patient for increased sedation after taking cimetidine and a benzodiazepine.
■ Warn the patient about the risk of increased sedation when taking cimetidine and midazolam together.
■ If the patient has increased sedation, discuss the possibility of decreasing the dose of midazolam with the prescriber.
◆ **ALERT** Elderly patients are at a higher risk for increased levels of sedation.
■ Monitor serum benzodiazepine levels while the patient is taking cimetidine and a benzodiazepine together.

midazolam ▶◀ diltiazem
Cardizem

Risk rating: 2
Severity: Moderate   **Onset: Rapid**   **Likelihood: Probable**

Cause
Diltiazem may decrease metabolism of some benzodiazepines such as midazolam.

Effect
Benzodiazepine effects may increase.

Nursing considerations
■ Watch for signs of increased CNS depression: sedation, dizziness, confusion, asthenia, ataxia, altered level of consciousness, hypoactive reflexes, hypotension, bradycardia, and respiratory depression.

- A lower midazolam dose may be needed.
- Explain the risk of increased and prolonged CNS effects.
- Warn the patient to avoid hazardous activites until effects of this combination are clear.
- Other benzodiazepines may interact with diltiazem. If you suspect an interaction, consult the prescriber or pharmacist.

midazolam ━━━━▶◀━━━━ grapefruit juice

Risk rating: 2
Severity: Moderate   Onset: Rapid   Likelihood: Probable

Cause
Grapefruit juice inhibits first-pass CYP3A4 metabolism of certain benzodiazepines such as midazolam.

Effect
Benzodiazepine onset is delayed and effects are increased, causing CNS depression and psychomotor impairment.

Nursing considerations
⚠ ALERT Tell the patient not to take a benzodiazepine with grape-fruit juice.
- If the patient uses grapefruit juice to take a benzodiazepine, explain that oversedation may last up to 72 hours.
- This interaction is increased in patients with cirrhosis of the liver.
- Instruct the patient to tell the prescriber about increased sedation or trouble walking or using limbs.

midazolam ━━━━▶◀━━━━ macrolide antibiotics
clarithromycin, erythromycin, telithromycin

Risk rating: 2
Severity: Moderate   Onset: Rapid   Likelihood: Suspected

Cause
Macrolide antibiotics may decrease metabolism of certain benzodi-azepines such as midazolam.

Effect
Sedative effects of benzodiazepines may be increased or prolonged.

Nursing considerations
- Consult the prescriber about decreasing benzodiazepine dosage during antibiotic therapy.
- Lorazepam, oxazepam, and temazepam probably don't interact with macrolide antibiotics; substitution may be possible.
- Azithromycin doesn't alter midazolam metabolism but may delay its absorption.
- Urge the patient to promptly report oversedation.

---

midazolam ━━━►◄━━━ nonnucleoside reverse-transcriptase inhibitors
delavirdine, efavirenz

Risk rating: 2
Severity: Moderate   Onset: Delayed   Likelihood: Suspected

Cause
Nonnucleoside reverse-transcriptase inhibitors may inhibit CYP3A4 metabolism of certain benzodiazepines such as midazolam.

Effect
Sedative effects of benzodiazepines may be increased or prolonged, leading to respiratory depression.

Nursing considerations
- **⚠ ALERT** Don't combine midazolam with delavirdine or efavirenz.
- Other benzodiazepines and nonnucleoside reverse-transcriptase inhibitors may interact. If you suspect an interaction, consult the prescriber or pharmacist.
- Explain the risk of oversedation and respiratory depression.
- Urge the patient to promptly report any suspected interaction.

---

midazolam ━━━►◄━━━ phenytoin
Dilantin

Risk rating: 2
Severity: Moderate   Onset: Delayed   Likelihood: Suspected

Cause
Metabolism of phenytoin and benzodiazepines such as midazolam is altered.

Effect
Phenytoin levels and risk of toxicity may increase.

Nursing considerations
■ Monitor phenytoin level closely. Dosage may need to be adjusted. Therapeutic range for phenytoin is 10 to 20 mcg/ml.
■ Toxic effects can occur at a therapeutic level. Adjust the measured level for hypoalbuminemia or renal impairment, which can increase free drug level.
■ Signs and symptoms of phenytoin toxicity include nystagmus, slurred speech, ataxia, blurred or double vision, confusion, drowsiness, and lethargy.
■ In some cases, the efficacy of midazolam may decrease, resulting in the need for a larger dose.

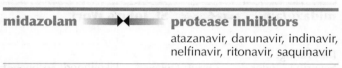

midazolam ━━━◄►━━━ protease inhibitors
atazanavir, darunavir, indinavir, nelfinavir, ritonavir, saquinavir

Risk rating: 1
Severity: Major   **Onset: Delayed**   **Likelihood: Suspected**

Cause
Protease inhibitors may inhibit CYP3A4 metabolism of certain benzodiazepines such as midazolam.

Effect
Sedative effects may be increased and prolonged.

Nursing considerations
◼ **ALERT** Don't combine midazolam with protease inhibitors.
◼ **ALERT** Midazolam is contraindicated in patients taking atazanavir.
■ If the patient takes any benzodiazepine–protease inhibitor combination, notify the prescriber. Interaction could involve other drugs in the class.
■ Watch for evidence of oversedation and respiratory depression.
■ Teach the patient and family about the risks of combined use.

midazolam ━━━◄►━━━ rifampin
Rifadin, Rimactane

Risk rating: 2
Severity: Moderate   **Onset: Delayed**   **Likelihood: Suspected**

Cause
Rifampin may increase CYP3A4 metabolism of benzodiazepines such as midazolam.

Effect
Antianxiety, sedative, and sleep-inducing effects may decrease.

Nursing considerations
- Watch for expected benzodiazepine effects and lack of efficacy.
- If benzodiazepine efficacy is reduced, notify the prescriber; dosage may be changed.
- Other benzodiazepines may interact with rifampin. If you suspect an interaction, consult the prescriber or pharmacist.
- For insomnia, temazepam may be more effective because it doesn't undergo CYP3A4 metabolism.

---

midazolam ◄► St. John's Wort

Risk rating: 2
Severity: Moderate   Onset: Delayed   Likelihood: Suspected

Cause
Hepatic and intestinal metabolism of benzodiazepines such as midazolam may be increased.

Effect
Pharmacologic effects of midazolam may be decreased.

Nursing considerations
- If possible, avoid administering St. John's Wort and benzodiazepines together.
- Monitor the patient for a decreased plasma level of benzodiazepines.
- If the patient is taking midazolam and St. John's Wort together, monitor him for a decreased response to the midazolam.
- Consult with the prescriber about adjusting the dose of midazolam if a decreased response is noted.
- Tell patients who are taking an herbal supplement to inform their health care providers of all the prescription and nonprescription medications they're taking.

minocycline ▸◂ iron salts
Minocin

ferrous fumarate, ferrous gluconate, ferrous sulfate, iron polysaccharide

Risk rating: 2
Severity: Moderate   Onset: Delayed   Likelihood: Probable

Cause
Minocycline and other tetracyclines form insoluble chelates with iron salts, which may reduce absorption of both substances.

Effect
Tetracycline and iron salt levels and effects may decrease.

Nursing considerations
⚠ **ALERT** If possible, avoid giving tetracyclines with iron salts.
- If both tetracyclines and iron salts must be taken, tell the patient to separate doses by 3 to 4 hours.
- If you suspect an interaction, consult the prescriber or pharmacist; an enteric-coated or sustained-release iron salt may reduce interaction.
- Monitor the patient for expected response to tetracycline.
- Assess the patient for evidence of iron deficiency, including fatigue, dyspnea, tachycardia, palpitations, dizziness, and orthostatic hypotension.

mirtazapine ▸◂ phenytoin
Remeron

Dilantin

Risk rating: 2
Severity: Moderate   Onset: Delayed   Likelihood: Suspected

Cause
Phenytoin may increase CYP3A3 and CYP3A4 metabolism of mirtazapine.

Effect
Mirtazapine level and effects may decrease.

Nursing considerations
- Assess the patient for expected mirtazapine effects, including improvement of depression and stabilization of mood.
- Record mood changes, and monitor the patient for suicidal tendencies.
- If hydantoin therapy starts, mirtazapine dosage may be increased.

■ If hydantoin therapy stops, watch for mirtazapine toxicity, including disorientation, drowsiness, impaired memory, tachycardia, severe hypotension, heart failure, seizures, CNS depression, and coma.
■ Urge the patient to tell the prescriber about loss of drug effect and increased adverse effects.

modafinil ➤◄ estrogens
Provigil   ethinyl estradiol

Risk rating: 2
Severity: Moderate   Onset: Delayed   Likelihood: Suspected

Cause
Modafinil induces GI and hepatic metabolism of estrogens.

Effect
Estrogen level and efficacy may be reduced.

Nursing considerations
■ Inform the patient of the increased risk of hormonal contraceptive failure when taking modafinil.
■ The patient should consider an alternative nonhormonal contraceptive or an additional method of contraception while taking modafinil.
■ Watch for menstrual disturbances, such as spotting, intermenstrual bleeding, or amenorrhea.
■ Estrogen dose may need to be increased; consult the prescriber.

modafinil ➤◄ hormonal contraceptives
Provigil

Risk rating: 2
Severity: Moderate   Onset: Delayed   Likelihood: Suspected

Cause
Modafinil induces GI and hepatic metabolism of estrogens.

Effect
Effectiveness of hormonal contraceptive is decreased.

Nursing considerations
■ Inform the patient of the increased risk of hormonal contraceptive failure when taking modafinil.
■ The patient should consider an alternative nonhormonal contraceptive or an additional method of contraception while taking modafinil.
■ Watch for menstrual disturbances, such as spotting, intermenstrual bleeding, or amenorrhea.

- The patient should continue alternative contraception method for at least one month after stopping modafinil.

modafinil ━━━━━►◄ triazolam
Provigil   Halcion

Risk rating: 2
Severity: Moderate   **Onset: Delayed**   **Likelihood: Suspected**

Cause
Modafinil induces GI and hepatic metabolism of triazolam.

Effect
Triazolam levels and efficacy are reduced.

Nursing considerations
- Monitor clinical response to triazolam.
- Dose of triazolam may need to be adjusted when starting or stopping modafinil therapy.
- If triazolam efficacy is reduced, notify the prescriber; dosage may be changed.
- Tell the patient to notify the prescriber about increased anxiety and restlessness.

moexipril ━━━━━►◄ potassium-sparing diuretics
Univasc   amiloride, spironolactone

Risk rating: 1
Severity: Major   **Onset: Delayed**   **Likelihood: Probable**

Cause
The mechanism of this interaction is unknown.

Effect
Serum potassium level may increase.

Nursing considerations
- Use cautiously in patients at high risk for hyperkalemia, especially those with renal impairment.
- Monitor BUN, creatinine, and serum potassium levels as needed.
- ACE inhibitors other than moexipril may interact with potassium-sparing diuretics. If you suspect an interaction, consult the prescriber or pharmacist.
- Urge the patient to immediately report an irregular heartbeat, a slow pulse, weakness, and other evidence of hyperkalemia.

moricizine ▶◀ diltiazem
Ethmozine   Cardizem

Risk rating: 2
Severity: Moderate   Onset: Delayed   Likelihood: Suspected

Cause
Moricizine metabolism may decrease; diltiazem metabolism may increase.

Effect
Therapeutic and adverse effects of moricizine may increase; therapeutic effects of diltiazem may decrease.

Nursing considerations
■ Monitor the patient for expected effects of diltiazem, such as control of angina or hypertension.
■ Advise the patient to report increased episodes of angina or symptoms of hypertension, including headache, dizziness, and blurred vision.
■ Monitor the patient for increased moricizine adverse effects, including headache, dizziness, and paresthesia.
■ Advise the patient to avoid hazardous activities if adverse CNS reactions or blurred vision occurs. These adverse effects may be more common with increased moricizine level.
■ Dosage adjustments may be needed when either drug is started, changed, or stopped.

moricizine ▶◀ vardenafil
Ethmozine   Levitra

Risk rating: 1
Severity: Major   Onset: Rapid   Likelihood: Suspected

Cause
The mechanism of this interaction is unknown.

Effect
QTc interval may be prolonged, particularly in patients with previous QT-interval prolongation and those taking certain antiarrhythmics, increasing the risk of such life-threatening arrhythmias as torsades de pointes.

Nursing considerations
⚑ ALERT Use of vardenafil with a class IA or class III antiarrhythmic, such as moricizine, is contraindicated.

- Monitor ECG before and periodically after the patient starts vardenafil.
- Urge the patient to report light-headedness, faintness, palpitations, and chest pain or pressure while taking vardenafil.
- To reduce risk of adverse effects, patients age 65 and older should start with 5 mg vardenafil, one-half the usual starting dose.

moxifloxacin ▶◀ antiarrhythmics

Avelox

amiodarone, bretylium, disopyramide, procainamide, quinidine, sotalol

Risk rating: 1
Severity: Major   **Onset: Delayed**   **Likelihood: Suspected**

Cause
The mechanism of this interaction is unknown.

Effect
Risk of life-threatening arrhythmias, including torsades de pointes, increases.

Nursing considerations
- Avoid giving class IA or class III antiarrhythmics with the quinolone moxifloxacin.
- Monitor ECG for prolonged QTc interval.
- Quinolones that aren't metabolized by CYP3A4 isoenzymes or that don't prolong the QT interval may be given with antiarrhythmics.
- Tell the patient to report a rapid heartbeat, shortness of breath, dizziness, fainting, and chest pain.

moxifloxacin ▶◀ erythromycin

Avelox

E-mycin, Eryc

Risk rating: 1
Severity: Major   **Onset: Delayed**   **Likelihood: Suspected**

Cause
The mechanism of this interaction is unknown.

Effect
Risk of life-threatening arrhythmias, including torsades de pointes, increases.

Nursing considerations
- Use erythromycin cautiously with moxifloxacin.

■ Monitor QTc interval closely.
■ Tell the patient to report palpitations, dizziness, shortness of breath, and chest pain.

---

moxifloxacin ▬▬►◄▬▬ imipramine
Avelox   Tofranil

Risk rating: 1
Severity: Major   **Onset: Delayed**   **Likelihood: Suspected**

Cause
The mechanism of this interaction if unknown.

Effect
Life-threatening arrhythmias, including torsades de pointes, may increase when certain of these drugs are used together.

Nursing considerations
■ Use the quinolone moxifloxacin cautiously with a tricyclic antidepressant.
■ If possible, use other quinolone antibiotics that don't prolong the QTc interval or aren't metabolized by the CYP3A4 isoenzyme.

---

moxifloxacin ▬▬►◄▬▬ iron salts
Avelox   ferrous fumarate, ferrous
                                          gluconate, ferrous sulfate

---

Risk rating: 2
Severity: Moderate   **Onset: Rapid**   **Likelihood: Probable**

Cause
Formation of an iron-quinolone complex decreases GI absorption of moxifloxacin.

Effect
Effects of quinolones such as moxifloxacin decrease.

Nursing considerations
■ Tell the patient to separate moxifloxacin from iron by at least 2 hours.
■ Help the patient develop a daily plan to ensure proper intervals between drug doses.
■ Other quinolones may interact with iron.

moxifloxacin ►◄ sucralfate

Avelox   Carafate

Risk rating: 2
Severity: Moderate   **Onset: Rapid**   **Likelihood: Probable**

Cause
Sucralfate decreases GI absorption of quinolones such as moxifloxacin.

Effect
Quinolone effects decrease.

Nursing considerations
- Avoid use together. If it's unavoidable, give sucralfate at least 6 hours after the quinolone.
- Monitor the patient for resolving infection.
- Help the patient develop a plan to ensure proper dosage intervals.

moxifloxacin ►◄ warfarin

Avelox   Coumadin

Risk rating: 2
Severity: Moderate   **Onset: Delayed**   **Likelihood: Suspected**

Cause
The mechanism of the interaction is unknown.

Effect
Anticoagulant effects may increase.

Nursing considerations
- Monitor PT and INR closely.
- Tell the patient to report unusual bleeding or bruising.
- Remind the patient that warfarin interacts with many drugs, and tell the patient to report any change in drug regimen.

moxifloxacin ►◄ ziprasidone

Avelox   Geodon

Risk rating: 1
Severity: Major   **Onset: Delayed**   **Likelihood: Suspected**

Cause
The mechanism of this interaction is unknown.

Effect
Risk of life-threatening arrhythmias, including torsades de pointes, increases.

Nursing considerations
⚠ **ALERT** Use of ziprasidone with a quinolone such as moxifloxacin is contraindicated.
■ Monitor the patient for other risk factors for torsades de pointes, including bradycardia, hypokalemia, and hypomagnesemia.
■ Ask the patient if he or anyone in his family has a history of prolonged QT interval or arrhythmias.
■ Monitor the patient for bradycardia.
■ Measure the QTc interval at baseline and throughout therapy.

---

mycophenolate ➤◄ iron salts mofetil

CellCept

ferrous fumarate, ferrous gluconate, ferrous sulfate, iron polysaccharide

---

Risk rating: 2
Severity: Moderate   **Onset: Rapid**   **Likelihood: Suspected**

Cause
Mycophenolate mofetil absorption may decrease because drug may form a complex with iron salts in the GI tract.

Effect
Mycophenolate mofetil level and effects may decrease.

Nursing considerations
⚠ **ALERT** Avoid giving iron salts with mycophenolate mofetil.
■ If you must give both, separate doses as much as possible.
■ Watch for evidence of rejection or decreased drug effect if iron salts are given with mycophenolate mofetil.
■ Urge the patient to report signs of organ rejection, such as decreased urine output in kidney transplant patients or shortness of breath in heart transplant patients.
■ Help the patient develop a plan to ensure proper dosage intervals.

mycophenolate ■■■►◄■■ rifampin
mofetil

CellCept   Rifadin, Rimactane

Risk rating: 2
Severity: Moderate   Onset: Delayed   Likelihood: Suspected

Cause
Multiple factors work together to inhibit the amount of mycophenolate mofetil that recirculates.

Effect
Mycophenolate mofetil level and effects may decrease.

Nursing considerations
- Mycophenolate mofetil dosage may need to be adjusted when starting or stopping rifampin therapy.
- Watch for evidence of rejection or decreased drug effect if rifampin is given with mycophenolate mofetil.
- Urge the patient to report signs of organ rejection, such as decreased urine output in kidney transplant patients or shortness of breath in heart transplant patients.

mycophenolate ■■■►◄■■ sirolimus
mofetil

CellCept   Rapamune

Risk rating: 2
Severity: Moderate   Onset: Delayed   Likelihood: Suspected

Cause
The mechanism of the interaction is unknown.

Effect
Mycophenolate mofetil level and risk of adverse effects may increase.

Nursing considerations
- Mycophenolate mofetil dosage may need to be adjusted when starting or stopping sirolimus therapy.
- Monitor mycophenolate mofetil drug levels throughout therapy.
- Watch the patient for increased adverse effects, such as hypertension, headache, hematuria, constipation, diarrhea, anemia, cough, and peripheral edema.

mycophenolate ▸◂ tacrolimus
mofetil
CellCept   Prograf

Risk rating: 2
Severity: Moderate   Onset: Delayed   Likelihood: Suspected

Cause
The mechanism of the interaction is unknown.

Effect
Mycophenolate mofetil level and risk of adverse effects may increase.

Nursing considerations
■ Mycophenolate mofetil dosage may need to be adjusted when starting or stopping tacrolimus therapy.
■ Monitor mycophenolate mofetil drug levels throughout therapy.
■ Watch the patient for increased adverse effects, such as hypertension, headache, hematuria, constipation, diarrhea, anemia, cough,
and peripheral edema.

nadolol ▸◂ epinephrine
Corgard

Risk rating: 1
Severity: Major   Onset: Rapid   Likelihood: Established

Cause
Alpha-receptor effects of epinephrine supersede effects of nonselective beta-adrenergic blockers such as nadolol, increasing vascular resistance.

Effect
Initial marked hypertensive effect is followed by reflex bradycardia.

Nursing considerations
◤ **ALERT** Three days before planned use of epinephrine, stop the
beta-adrenergic blocker. Or, if possible, don't use epinephrine.
■ If drugs must be combined, monitor blood pressure and pulse
closely. If interaction occurs, give I.V. chlorpromazine, hydralazine,
aminophylline, or atropine if needed.
■ Explain the risks of this interaction, and tell the patient to carry
medical identification at all times.
■ Other beta-adrenergic blockers may interact with epinephrine. If
you suspect an interaction, consult the prescriber or pharmacist.

nadolol ◄► lidocaine
Corgard

Risk rating: 2
Severity: Moderate   **Onset: Rapid**   **Likelihood: Established**

Cause
Nadolol and other beta-adrenergic blockers reduce hepatic metabolism of lidocaine.

Effect
Lidocaine level and risk of toxicity may increase.

Nursing considerations
- Check for therapeutic lidocaine level: 2 to 5 mcg/ml.
- Slow I.V. bolus rate to decrease the risk of high peak level and toxic reaction.
- Monitor the patient closely for evidence of lidocaine toxicity: dizziness, somnolence, confusion, paresthesias and seizures.
- Explain the warning signs of toxicity to the patient and family, and tell them to contact the prescriber if they have concerns.

nafcillin ◄► food

Risk rating: 2
Severity: Moderate   **Onset: Delayed**   **Likelihood: Suspected**

Cause
Food may delay or reduce GI absorption of penicillins such as nafcillin.

Effect
Nafcillin efficacy may decrease.

Nursing considerations
- Food may affect nafcillin absorption and peak level.
- Penicillin V and amoxicillin don't have this interaction and may be given without regard to meals.
- Tell the patient to take nafcillin 1 hour before or 2 hours after a meal.
- If the patient took nafcillin with food, watch for lack of drug efficacy.

nafcillin 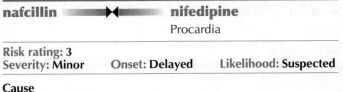 nifedipine
Procardia

Risk rating: 3
Severity: Minor   **Onset: Delayed**   **Likelihood: Suspected**

Cause
Nafcillin induces CYP3A4 metabolism of nifedipine.

Effect
Nifedipine levels and therapeutic effects decrease.

Nursing considerations
- Monitor the patient's clinical response to nifedipine when starting or stopping nafcillin.
- If necessary, adjust the dose of nifedipine.
- Nifedipine may interact with other penicillins.

nafcillin 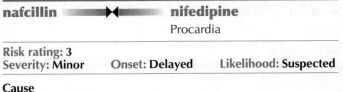 warfarin
Coumadin

Risk rating: 2
Severity: Moderate   **Onset: Delayed**   **Likelihood: Suspected**

Cause
Warfarin induces hypoprothrombinemia, and nafcillin inhibits platelet aggregation.

Effect
Bleeding time is prolonged. Warfarin resistance may also occur.

Nursing considerations
- Monitor PT and INR closely during combined use.
- Risk of interaction increases with large doses of I.V. penicillins.
- Monitor coagulation values before starting nafcillin and for at least 3 weeks after stopping to check for warfarin resistance.
- Tell the patient to report unusual bleeding or bruising.
- Remind the patient that warfarin interacts with many drugs and that he should report any change in drug regimen.
- Advise the patient to keep all follow-up medical appointments for proper monitoring and dosage adjustments.

naratriptan ▶◀ ergot derivatives
Amerge   dihydroergotamine, ergotamine

Risk rating: 1
Severity: Major   **Onset: Rapid**   **Likelihood: Suspected**

Cause
Combined use may have additive effects.

Effect
Risk of vasospastic effects increases.

Nursing considerations
⚠ ALERT Use of these drugs within 24 hours of each other is contraindicated.
■ Combined use may cause severe vasospastic effects, including sustained coronary artery vasospasm that triggers MI.
■ Warn patients not to mix migraine headache drugs within 24 hours
of each other, but to call the prescriber if a drug isn't effective.

nefazodone ▶◀ carbamazepine
Serzone   Carbatrol, Epitol, Equetro,
                                Tegretol

Risk rating: 1
Severity: Major   **Onset: Delayed**   **Likelihood: Suspected**

Cause
Nefazodone may inhibit CYP3A4 hepatic metabolism of carbamazepine. Carbamazepine may induce nefazodone metabolism.

Effect
Carbamazepine level and risk of adverse effects may increase. Nefazodone level and effects may decrease.

Nursing considerations
⚠ ALERT Use of carbamazepine with nefazodone is contraindicated.
■ Monitor carbamazepine level; therapeutic range is 4 to 12 mcg/ml.
■ Watch for signs of anorexia or subtle appetite changes, which may
indicate excessive carbamazepine level.
■ Watch for signs of carbamazepine toxicity: dizziness, ataxia, respira-
tory depression, tachycardia, arrhythmias, blood pressure changes,
impaired consciousness, abnormal reflexes, nystagmus, seizures, nau-
sea, vomiting, and urine retention.
■ Monitor the patient for adequate nefazodone clinical effects.
■ Urge the patient to tell the prescriber about increased adverse effects.

nefazodone ▰▰▰►◄ cyclosporine
Serzone   Gengraf, Neoral, Sandimmune

Risk rating: 2
Severity: Moderate   Onset: Delayed   Likelihood: Probable

Cause
Nefazodone may inhibit cyclosporine metabolism.

Effect
Cyclosporine level and risk of toxicity may increase.

Nursing considerations
- Patients who take cyclosporine may need an alternative antidepressant to nefazodone.
- Monitor cyclosporine level closely when starting or stopping nefazodone.
- Toxicity may cause shakiness, headaches, tremor, hypertension, and fatigue.
- Cyclosporine dosage may need to be reduced.

nefazodone ▰▰▰►◄ eplerenone
Serzone   Inspra

Risk rating: 1
Severity: Major   Onset: Delayed   Likelihood: Suspected

Cause
Nefazodone inhibits the CYP3A4 metabolism of eplerenone.

Effect
Eplerenone level increases, which may increase risk of hyperkalemia and serious arrhythmias.

Nursing considerations
⚠ **ALERT** Administration of nefazodone and eplerenone is contraindicated.
- The basis for this interaction is the risk of hyperkalemia from eplerenone therapy.
- The interaction is based on pharmacodynamics, not actual patient studies.

nefazodone ━━━━▶◀━━━━ pimozide
Serzone   Orap

Risk rating: 1
Severity: Major   **Onset: Delayed**   **Likelihood: Suspected**

Cause
Nefazodone may inhibit CYP3A4 metabolism of pimozide.

Effect
Risk of life-threatening arrhythmias may increase.

Nursing considerations
◪ ALERT Combined use of these drugs is contraindicated.
▪ Arrhythmias are related to prolonged QT interval, a known risk of pimozide.
▪ Interaction warning is based on pharmacokinetics of these drugs, not actual patient studies.

nefazodone ━━━━▶◀━━━━ St. John's wort
Serzone

Risk rating: 2
Severity: Moderate   **Onset: Rapid**   **Likelihood: Suspected**

Cause
St. John's wort may cause additive inhibition of serotonin reuptake.

Effect
Sedative-hypnotic effects of serotonin reuptake inhibitors such as nefazodone may increase.

Nursing considerations
◪ ALERT Discourage use of a serotonin reuptake inhibitor with St. John's wort.
▪ In addition to oversedation, mild serotonin-like symptoms may occur, including anxiety, dizziness, nausea, restlessness, and vomiting.
▪ Inform the patient about the dangers of this combination.
▪ Urge the patient to consult the prescriber before taking any herb.

nelfinavir ■■■■▶◀ amiodarone
Viracept   Pacerone, Cordarone

Risk rating: 1
Severity: Major   **Onset: Delayed**   **Likelihood: Suspected**

Cause
Protease inhibitors such as nelfinavir inhibit the CYP3A4 metabolism of amiodarone.

Effect
Amiodarone level increases, increasing the risk of toxicity.

Nursing considerations
- Use other protease inhibitors cautiously; they may have similar effects.
- Increased amiodarone level may prolong the QT interval and cause life-threatening arrhythmias.
- Monitor ECG and QTc interval closely during combined therapy.
- Tell the patient to immediately report slowed pulse or fainting.

nelfinavir ■■■■▶◀ benzodiazepines
Viracept   alprazolam, clorazepate,
                                  diazepam, estazolam,
                                  flurazepam, midazolam,
                                  triazolam

Risk rating: 1
Severity: Major   **Onset: Delayed**   **Likelihood: Suspected**

Cause
Nelfinavir and other protease inhibitors may inhibit CYP3A4 metabolism of certain benzodiazepines.

Effect
Sedative effects may be increased and prolonged.

Nursing considerations
- ◼ **ALERT** Don't combine these benzodiazepines with protease inhibitors.
- If the patient takes any protease inhibitor–benzodiazepine combination, notify the prescriber. Interaction could involve other drugs in the class.
- Watch for evidence of oversedation and respiratory depression.
- Teach the patient and family about the risks of combined use.

nelfinavir ━━━━▶◀━━━━ carbamazepine
Viracept

Carbatrol, Epitol, Equetro, Tegretol

Risk rating: 2
Severity: Moderate   **Onset: Rapid**   **Likelihood: Suspected**

Cause
Nelfinavir may inhibit hepatic metabolism (CYP3A4) of carbamazepine. Carbamazepine may induce metabolism (CYP3A4) of nelfinavir.

Effect
Carbamazepine levels and risk of toxicity may increase. Nelfinavir levels may decrease.

Nursing considerations
- Closely monitor carbamazepine levels when starting, stopping, or changing the dose of nelfinavir.
- Observe the patient's clinical response to nelfinavir therapy. Adjust the dose as needed.
- **ALERT** If nelfinavir level decreases, antiretroviral treatment therapy may fail.
- Monitor carbamazepine level; therapeutic range is 4 to 12 mcg/ml.
- **ALERT** Watch for signs of anorexia or subtle appetite changes, which may indicate excessive carbamazepine level.
- Monitor the patient for evidence of carbamazepine toxicity, including dizziness, ataxia, respiratory depression, tachycardia, arrhythmias, blood pressure changes, impaired consciousness, abnormal reflexes, nystagmus, seizures, nausea, vomiting, and urine retention.

nelfinavir ━━━━▶◀━━━━ eplerenone
Viracept

Inspra

Risk rating: 1
Severity: Major   **Onset: Delayed**   **Likelihood: Suspected**

Cause
Protease inhibitors such as nelfinavir inhibit metabolism of eplerenone.

Effect
Eplerenone level rises, causing hyperkalemia and increasing the risk of life-threatening arrhythmias.

Nursing considerations
- **ALERT** Use of nelfinavir with eplerenone is contraindicated.

■ Potent CYP3A4 inhibitors increase the eplerenone level and the risk of hyperkalemia-induced arrhythmias—some fatal.
■ Monitor the patient's serum potassium level.
■ Tell the patient to report nausea, irregular heartbeat, and slowed pulse to the prescriber.

---

nelfinavir ►◄ ergot derivatives

Viracept

dihydroergotamine, ergonovine, ergotamine, methylergonovine

Risk rating: 1
Severity: Major   **Onset: Delayed**   **Likelihood: Probable**

Cause
Protease inhibitors such as nelfinavir may interfere with CYP3A4 metabolism of ergot derivatives.

Effect
Risk of ergot-induced peripheral vasospasm and ischemia may be increased.

Nursing considerations
◣ ALERT Use of ergot derivatives with protease inhibitors is contraindicated.
■ Monitor the patient for evidence of peripheral ischemia, including pain in limb muscles while exercising and later at rest; numbness and tingling of fingers and toes; cool, pale, or cyanotic limbs; red or violet blisters on hands or feet; and gangrene.
■ Sodium nitroprusside may be given for ergot-induced vasospasm.
■ If the patient takes a protease inhibitor, consult the prescriber or pharmacist about other treatments for migraine pain.
■ Urge the patient to tell the prescriber about increased adverse effects.

---

nelfinavir ►◄ lovastatin

Viracept

Mevacor, Altoprev

Risk rating: 1
Severity: Major   **Onset: Delayed**   **Likelihood: Suspected**

Cause
Protease inhibitors such as nelfinavir inhibit the CYP3A4 metabolism of lovastatin.

Effect
Lovastatin level may increase.

Nursing considerations
◼ **ALERT** Nelfinavir and lovastatin shouldn't be used together.
■ Use other protease inhibitors cautiously; they may have similar effect.
■ If a protease inhibitor is added to a regimen that includes lovastatin, monitor the patient closely.
◼ **ALERT** Watch for evidence of rhabdomyolysis, including dark or red urine, muscle weakness, and myalgia.
■ Urge the patient to immediately report unexplained muscle weakness.

---

nelfinavir ▶◀ **methadone**
Viracept   Reyataz

Risk rating: 2
Severity: Moderate   **Onset: Delayed**   **Likelihood: Suspected**

Cause
Protease inhibitors such as nelfinavir may increase metabolism of methadone.

Effect
Pharmacologic effects of methadone may decrease. Patients on maintenance methadone treatment may experience opiate withdrawal symptoms.

Nursing considerations
■ Methadone dosage may need adjustment.
■ If protease inhibitor therapy starts while the patient is taking methadone, watch for signs of opioid withdrawal.
■ If protease inhibitor is stopped, methadone dosage may need to be decreased.
■ Urge the patient to tell the prescriber about loss of methadone effect.

nelfinavir ━━━━►◄	nonnucleoside reverse-transcriptase inhibitors
Viracept	efavirenz, nevirapine

Risk rating: 2
Severity: Moderate   Onset: Delayed   Likelihood: Suspected

Cause
Nonnucleoside reverse transcriptase (NNRT) inhibitors may increase hepatic metabolism of protease inhibitors such as nelfinavir.

Effect
Protease inhibitor level and effects decrease.

Nursing considerations
■ If NNRT inhibitor therapy is started or stopped, monitor protease inhibitor level.
■ Protease inhibitor dosage may need adjustment.
■ Monitor CD4+ and T-cell counts; tell the prescriber if they decrease.
■ Urge the patient to report opportunistic infections.
■ Tell the patient not to change an HIV regimen without consulting the prescriber.

nelfinavir ━━━━►◄	pimozide
Viracept	Orap

Risk rating: 1
Severity: Major   Onset: Delayed   Likelihood: Suspected

Cause
Protease inhibitors such as nelfinavir may inhibit CYP3A4 metabolism of pimozide.

Effect
Risk of life-threatening arrhythmias may increase.

Nursing considerations
◘ **ALERT** Combined use of these drugs is contraindicated
■ Arrhythmias are related to prolonged QT interval, a known risk of pimozide.
■ Interaction warning is based on pharmacokinetics of these drugs, not actual patient studies.

nelfinavir ▰▰▰◀ quinidine
Viracept

Risk rating: 1
Severity: Major   **Onset: Delayed**   **Likelihood: Suspected**

Cause
CYP3A4 metabolism of quinidine may be inhibited.

Effect
Quinidine level and risk of toxicity may increase.

Nursing considerations
▪ **ALERT** Use of nelfinavir with quinidine is contraindicated.
▪ Monitor ECG for prolonged QT interval and arrhythmias.
▪ **ALERT** Quinidine toxicity may cause GI irritation, arrhythmias, hypotension, vertigo, and rash.

nelfinavir ▰▰▰◀ simvastatin
Viracept   Zocor

Risk rating: 1
Severity: Major   **Onset: Delayed**   **Likelihood: Suspected**

Cause
First-pass metabolism of simvastatin by CYP3A4 in the GI tract may be inhibited.

Effect
Simvastatin level may increase.

Nursing considerations
▪ **ALERT** Combined use of these drugs is contraindicated.
▪ If a protease inhibitor such as nelfinavir is added to simvastatin, monitor the patient closely.
▪ **ALERT** Watch for evidence of rhabdomyolysis, including dark or red urine, muscle weakness, and myalgia.
▪ Urge the patient to immediately report unexplained muscle weakness.

nelfinavir ◄► St. John's wort

Viracept

Risk rating: 1
Severity: Major   **Onset: Delayed**   **Likelihood: Suspected**

Cause
Hepatic metabolism of protease inhibitor such as nelfinavir may increase.

Effect
Protease inhibitor level and effects may decrease.

Nursing considerations
■ If the patient starts or stops St. John's wort, monitor protease inhibitor level closely.
■ Monitor CD4+ and T-cell counts; tell the prescriber if they decrease.
■ Urge the patient to report opportunistic infections.
■ Tell the patient not to change an HIV regimen without consulting the prescriber.
■ Urge the patient to tell prescribers about all drugs, supplements, and alternative therapies he uses.

neomycin ◄► nondepolarizing muscle relaxants

Neo-Fradin

atracurium, doxacurium, mivacurium, pancuronium, rocuronium, vecuronium

Risk rating: 1
Severity: Major   **Onset: Rapid**   **Likelihood: Probable**

Cause
These drugs may be synergistic.

Effect
Effects of nondepolarizing muscle relaxants may increase.

Nursing considerations
■ Give these drugs together only when needed.
■ The nondepolarizing muscle relaxant dose may need adjustment based on neuromuscular response.
■ Monitor the patient for prolonged respiratory depression.
■ Provide ventilatory support as needed.

neomycin 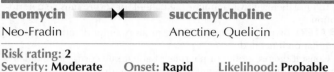 succinylcholine

Neo-Fradin   Anectine, Quelicin

Risk rating: 2
Severity: Moderate   Onset: Rapid   Likelihood: Probable

Cause
Neomycin and other aminoglycosides may stabilize the postjunctional membrane and disrupt prejunctional calcium influx and acetylcholine output, thereby causing a synergistic interaction with succinylcholine.

Effect
Aminoglycosides potentiate the neuromuscular effects of succinylcholine.

Nursing considerations
- After succinylcholine use, delay aminoglycoside delivery as long as
possible after adequate respirations return.
- If drugs must be given together, use extreme caution and monitor
respiratory status closely.
- ◤ ALERT Patients with renal impairment and those receiving aminoglycosides by peritoneal instillation have an increased risk of prolonged neuromuscular blockade.
- If respiratory depression occurs, the patient may need mechanical
ventilation. Give I.V. calcium or a cholinesterase inhibitor if needed.

neostigmine 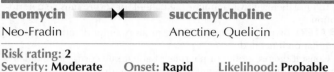 corticosteroids

Prostigmin   corticotropin, cortisone,
                                    hydrocortisone, methylpred-
                                    nisolone, prednisone

Risk rating: 1
Severity: Major   Onset: Delayed   Likelihood: Probable

Cause
In myasthenia gravis, corticosteroids antagonize the effects of
cholinesterase inhibitors such as neostigmine by an unknown mechanism.

Effect
Patients may develop severe muscular depression refractory to
cholinesterase inhibitor.

Nursing considerations
- Corticosteroids may have long-term benefits in myasthenia gravis.
- Combined therapy may be attempted under strict supervision.

■ In myasthenia gravis, monitor the patient for severe muscle deterioration.
⚠ ALERT Be prepared to provide respiratory support and mechanical ventilation if needed.
■ Consult the prescriber or pharmacist about safe corticosteroid delivery to maximize improvement in muscle strength.

neostigmine ▬▬▶◀▬▬ succinylcholine
Prostigmin   Anectine, Quelicin

Risk rating: 2
Severity: Moderate   Onset: Rapid   Likelihood: Probable

Cause
Anticholinesterases such as neostigmine inhibit plasma cholinesterase which delays the breakdown of succinylcholine. Also, increased levels of acetylcholine may increase the neuromuscular blockade.

Effect
The neuromuscular blockade is prolonged.

Nursing considerations
■ Use this combination with caution.
■ This interaction is more likely in patients receiving succinylcholine by continuous infusion.
⚠ALERT Provide respiratory support and mechanical ventilation if needed.

nevirapine ▬▬▶◀▬▬ methadone
Viramune   Methadose

Risk rating: 2
Severity: Moderate   Onset: Delayed   Likelihood: Probable

Cause
Increased CYP3A4 hepatic metabolism of methadone.

Effect
Action of methadone may be reduced, resulting in opiate withdrawal symptoms.

Nursing considerations
■ When starting a patient on a nonnucleoside reverse transcriptase inhibitor such as nevirapine, carefully monitor the patient's clinical response to methadone.

- Be prepared to increase methadone dose.
- Monitor the patient for methadone overdose when nevirapine therapy is stopped.
- Monitor the patient for dilated pupils, diarrhea, abdominal pain, sweating, agitation, nausea, and vomiting.
- Instruct the patient not to change the dose of his medications before consulting with the prescriber or pharmacist.

nevirapine ▶◀ protease inhibitors

Viramune

atazanavir, fosamprenavir, indinavir, lopinavir-ritonavir, nelfinavir, ritonavir

Risk rating: 2
Severity: Moderate   Onset: Delayed   Likelihood: Suspected

Cause
Nevirapine may increase hepatic metabolism of protease inhibitors.

Effect
Protease inhibitor level and effects decrease.

Nursing considerations
- If nevirapine is started or stopped, monitor protease inhibitor level.
- Protease inhibitor dosage may need adjustment.
- Monitor CD4+ and T-cell counts; tell the prescriber if they decrease.
- Urge the patient to report opportunistic infections.
- Tell the patient not to change an HIV regimen without consulting the prescriber.

nicardipine ▶◀ cyclosporine

Cardene

Gengraf, Neoral, Sandimmune

Risk rating: 2
Severity: Moderate   Onset: Delayed   Likelihood: Suspected

Cause
Nicardipine probably inhibits cyclosporine metabolism in the liver.

Effect
Cyclosporine level and renal toxicity may increase.

Nursing considerations
- Check cyclosporine level. Trough level may be elevated.
- Monitor renal function.
- Assess the patient for evidence of toxicity.
- Adjust cyclosporine dose as needed.
- If nicardipine is stopped, consider increasing cyclosporine dose to prevent rejection.

---

nifedipine ▶◀ cimetidine
Procardia   Tagamet

Risk rating: 2
Severity: Moderate   **Onset: Delayed**   **Likelihood: Suspected**

Cause
The exact mechanism of this interaction is unknown; hepatic metabolism of nifedipine may be reduced.

Effect
Nifedipine effects, including adverse effects, may increase.

Nursing considerations
- Monitor the patient for increased adverse effects, including hypotension, dizziness, light-headedness, syncope, peripheral edema, flushing, and nausea.
- Adjust the nifedipine dose as ordered.
- H_2-receptor antagonists other than cimetidine may interact with nifedipine. Calcium channel blockers other than nifedipine may interact with cimetidine. If you suspect an interaction, consult the prescriber or pharmacist.

---

nifedipine ▶◀ diltiazem
Procardia   Cardizem

Risk rating: 3
Severity: Minor   **Onset: Rapid**   **Likelihood: Suspected**

Cause
Possible reduction of hepatic clearance.

Effect
Levels, effects, and risk of toxicity of digoxin and nifedipine increase.

Nursing considerations
- Monitor the patient for increased adverse effects, including hypotension and dizziness.

- Dosage of nifedipine or diltiazem may need to be decreased.
- Diltiazem may interact with other calcium-channel blockers in the same way.

---

nifedipine ━━━▶◀━━━ food, grapefruit juice
Procardia

Risk rating: 2
Severity: Moderate   **Onset: Rapid**   **Likelihood: Suspected**

Cause
Food slows the absorption of nifedipine. Grapefruit juice inhibits CYP3A4 metabolism of nifedipine.

Effect
Grapefruit juice increases bioavailability and activity of nifedipine.

Nursing considerations
- Nifedipine may be administered without regard to meals.
- Nifedipine and grapefruit shouldn't be administered together.
- Instruct the patient to take nifedipine with liquid other than grapefruit juice.

---

nifedipine ━━━▶◀━━━ nafcillin
Procardia

Risk rating: 3
Severity: Minor   **Onset: Delayed**   **Likelihood: Suspected**

Cause
Nafcillin induces CYP3A4 metabolism of nifedipine.

Effect
Nifedipine levels and therapeutic effects decrease.

Nursing considerations
- Monitor the patient's clinical response to nifedipine when starting or stopping nafcillin.
- If necessary, adjust the dose of nifedipine.
- Nifedipine may interact with other penicillins.

nisoldipine ▶◀ ketoconazole
Sular   Nizoral

Risk rating: 2
Severity: Moderate   **Onset: Delayed**   **Likelihood: Suspected**

Cause
Azole antifungals such as ketoconazole inhibit CYP3A4, which is needed for nisoldipine metabolism.

Effect
Nisoldipine level, effects, and adverse effects may increase.

Nursing considerations
■ Notify the prescriber if the patient takes both drugs; an alternative may be available.
■ If drugs must be taken together, watch for orthostatic hypotension from increased nisoldipine effect.
■ Tell the patient to report adverse effects, such as chest pain, dizziness, headache, weight gain, nausea, palpitations, and peripheral edema.

nitroglycerin ▶◀ alteplase
Minitran, Nitro-Dur,   Activase, tPA
NitroQuick, Nitrostat

Risk rating: 1
Severity: Major   **Onset: Rapid**   **Likelihood: Probable**

Cause
Nitroglycerin may enhance hepatic blood flow, thereby increasing alteplase metabolism.

Effect
Alteplase level and thrombolytic effects may decrease.

Nursing considerations
■ Don't use together, if possible.
■ If use together is unavoidable, maintain nitroglycerin at the lowest effective dose.
■ Monitor the patient for inadequate thrombolytic effects.
■ Tell the patient that other reperfusion therapies may be needed.

nitroglycerin ➡◀ dihydroergotamine

Minitran, Nitro-Dur,
NitroQuick, Nitrostat

Risk rating: 2
Severity: Moderate   **Onset: Rapid**   **Likelihood: Suspected**

Cause
Metabolism of dihydroergotamine decreases, increasing its availability, which antagonizes nitrates.

Effect
Increased dihydroergotamine availability may increase systolic blood pressure and decrease the antianginal effects of nitrates.

Nursing considerations
- Use these drugs together cautiously in patients with angina.
- I.V. dihydroergotamine may antagonize coronary vasodilation.
- Monitor the patient for evidence of ergotism, such as peripheral ischemia, paresthesia, headache, nausea, and vomiting.
- Teach the patient to immediately report indicators of peripheral ischemia, such as numbness or tingling in fingers and toes or red blisters on hands or feet. Dihydroergotamine dosage may need to be decreased.

nitroglycerin ➡◀ phosphodiesterase-5 inhibitors

Minitran, Nitro-Dur,   sildenafil, tadalafil, vardenafil
NitroQuick, Nitrostat

Risk rating: 1
Severity: Major   **Onset: Rapid**   **Likelihood: Suspected**

Cause
Phosphodiesterase-5 (PDE-5) inhibitors potentiate the hypotensive effects of nitroglycerin.

Effect
Risk of severe hypotension increases.

Nursing considerations
- ⚡ **ALERT** Use of nitroglycerin with PDE-5 inhibitors may be fatal and is contraindicated.
- Carefully screen the patient for PDE-5 inhibitor use before giving a nitroglycerin.

■ Even during an emergency, before giving a nitroglycerin, find out if a patient with chest pain has taken an erectile dysfunction drug during the previous 24 hours.
■ Monitor the patient for orthostatic hypotension, dizziness, sweating, and headache.

---

norepinephrine ➤◄ methyldopa
Levophed   Aldomet

Risk rating: 2
Severity: Moderate   **Onset: Rapid**   **Likelihood: Suspected**

Cause
The mechanism of this interaction is unknown.

Effect
Pressor response of sympathomimetics and the risk of hypertension may increase.

Nursing considerations
■ Monitor the patient's blood pressure closely.
■ The hypertensive response may increase two to five times over norepinephrine alone.

---

norepinephrine ➤◄ reserpine
Levophed   Serpalan

Risk rating: 2
Severity: Moderate   **Onset: Rapid**   **Likelihood: Suspected**

Cause
Receptor sensitivity to sympathomimetics such as norepinephrine is increased.

Effect
Pressor response of norepinephrine may increase, resulting in hypertension. The pressor response may be decreased.

Nursing considerations
■ Monitor the patient's blood pressure closely.
■ The dose of norepinephrine may need to be increased or decreased depending on the patient's clinical response.

norepinephrine ▬▶◀▬ tricyclic antidepressants

Levophed

amitriptyline, desipramine, imipramine, nortriptyline, protriptyline

Risk rating: 2
Severity: Moderate   Onset: Rapid   Likelihood: Established

Cause
Tricyclic antidepressants (TCAs) increase the effects of direct-acting sympathomimetics such as norepinephrine.

Effect
When sympathomimetic effects increase, the risk of hypertension and arrhythmias increases.

Nursing considerations
- If possible, avoid using these drugs together.
- Watch the patient closely for hypertension and heart rhythm changes; they may warrant reduction of sympathomimetic dosage.
- Other TCAs and sympathomimetics may interact. If you suspect an interaction, consult the prescriber or pharmacist.

norfloxacin ▬▶◀▬ food

Noroxin

Risk rating: 2
Severity: Moderate   Onset: Rapid   Likelihood: Suspected

Cause
GI absorption of certain quinolones such as norfloxacin decreases.

Effect
Quinolone effects may decrease.

Nursing considerations
- Advise the patient not to take the drug with milk and to lengthen the time as much as possible between milk ingestion and the quinolone dose.
- This interaction doesn't affect all quinolones.
- Monitor the patient for quinolone efficacy.

norfloxacin ▶◀ iron salts

Noroxin

ferrous fumarate, ferrous gluconate, ferrous sulfate, iron polysaccharide

Risk rating: 2
Severity: Moderate   **Onset: Rapid**   **Likelihood: Probable**

Cause
Formation of an iron-quinolone complex decreases GI absorption of quinolones such as norfloxacin.

Effect
Quinolone effects decrease.

Nursing considerations
- Monitor the patient for quinolone efficacy.
- Tell the patient to separate quinolone dose from iron by at least 2 hours.
- Help the patient develop a plan to ensure proper dosage intervals.
- Other quinolones may interact with iron.

norfloxacin ▶◀ sucralfate

Noroxin

Carafate

Risk rating: 2
Severity: Moderate   **Onset: Rapid**   **Likelihood: Probable**

Cause
GI absorption of quinolones such as norfloxacin decreases.

Effect
Quinolone effects decrease.

Nursing considerations
- Avoid use together. If it's unavoidable, give sucralfate at least 6 hours after the quinolone.
- Monitor the patient for resolving infection.
- Help the patient develop a plan to ensure proper dosage intervals.

norfloxacin ▰▰▰▶◀▰▰▰ theophyllines
Noroxin   aminophylline, theophylline

Risk rating: 2
Severity: Moderate   **Onset: Delayed**   **Likelihood: Established**

Cause
Hepatic metabolism of theophyllines is decreased.

Effect
Theophylline levels may increase, causing toxicity.

Nursing considerations
■ Monitor theophylline level closely. Therapeutic range is 10 to 20 mcg/ml for adults and 5 to 15 mcg/ml for children.
■ Interaction doesn't appear to affect ciprofloxacin or other quinolones.
■ Watch for evidence of toxicity, such as ventricular tachycardia, anorexia, nausea, vomiting, diarrhea, seizures, restlessness, irritability, and headache.
■ Describe adverse effects of theophylline and signs of toxicity, and tell the patient to report them immediately to the prescriber.

norfloxacin ▰▰▰▶◀▰▰▰ warfarin
Noroxin   Coumadin

Risk rating: 2
Severity: Moderate   **Onset: Delayed**   **Likelihood: Suspected**

Cause
The mechanism of the interaction is unknown.

Effect
Anticoagulant effects may increase.

Nursing considerations
■ Monitor PT and INR closely.
■ Tell the patient to report unusual bleeding or bruising.
■ Remind the patient that warfarin interacts with many drugs and that he should report any change in drug regimen.

nortriptyline ━━━▶◀━━━ azole antifungals
Pamelor   fluconazole, ketoconazole

Risk rating: 2
Severity: Moderate   Onset: Delayed   Likelihood: Suspected

Cause
Azole antifungals may inhibit metabolism of nortriptyline and other tricyclic antidepressants (TCAs) by CYP pathways.

Effect
TCA level and risk of toxicity may increase.

Nursing considerations
■ When starting or stopping an azole antifungal, monitor serum TCA level and adjust dosage as needed.
■ After starting an azole antifungal, check sitting and standing blood pressure for changes.
■ Assess symptoms and behavior for evidence of adverse reactions, such as increased drowsiness, dizziness, confusion, heart rate or rhythm changes, and urine retention.

nortriptyline ━━━▶◀━━━ carbamazepine
Pamelor   Carbatrol, Epitol, Equetro,
                                 Tegretol

Risk rating: 2
Severity: Moderate   Onset: Delayed   Likelihood: Probable

Cause
Tricyclic antidepressants (TCAs) such as nortriptyline may compete with carbamazepine for hepatic metabolism. Carbamazepine may induce hepatic metabolism.

Effect
TCA level and effects may decrease. Carbamazepine levels and risk of toxicity may increase.

Nursing considerations
■ Other TCAs may interact with carbamazepine. If you suspect a drug interaction, consult the prescriber or pharmacist.
■ Monitor carbamazepine level; therapeutic range is 4 to 12 mcg/ml.
■ Watch for evidence of carbamazepine toxicity, including dizziness, ataxia, respiratory depression, tachycardia, arrhythmias, blood pressure changes, impaired consciousness, abnormal reflexes, nystagmus, seizures, nausea, vomiting, and urine retention.

nortriptyline ◄► chlorpromazine
Pamelor   Thorazine

Risk rating: 3
Severity: Minor   **Onset: Delayed**   **Likelihood: Probable**

Cause
Competitive inhibition of tricyclic antidepressant (TCA) metabolism.

Effect
Increased levels of TCAs.

Nursing considerations
■ Monitor the patient's clinical response to TCAs and decrease the dose if needed.
■ No toxic effects were noted from this interaction.

nortriptyline ◄► cimetidine
Pamelor   Tagamet

Risk rating: 2
Severity: Moderate   **Onset: Rapid**   **Likelihood: Probable**

Cause
Cimetidine may interfere with metabolism of tricyclic antidepressants (TCAs) such as nortriptyline.

Effect
TCA level and bioavailability increase.

Nursing considerations
■ When starting or stopping cimetidine, monitor serum TCA level and adjust dosage as needed.
■ Tell the prescriber if TCA level or effect increases; dosage may need to be decreased.
■ If needed, consult the prescriber about possible change from cimetidine to ranitidine.
■ Urge the patient and family to watch for and report increased anticholinergic effects, dizziness, drowsiness, and psychosis.

nortriptyline ▸◂ fluoxetine
Pamelor   Prozac, Sarafem

Risk rating: 2
Severity: Moderate   **Onset: Delayed**   **Likelihood: Probable**

Cause
Fluoxetine may inhibit hepatic metabolism of tricyclic antidepressants (TCAs) such as nortriptyline.

Effect
Serum TCA level and toxicity may increase.

Nursing considerations
■ Monitor serum TCA level and watch closely for evidence of toxicity, such as increased anticholinergic effects, delirium, dizziness, drowsiness, and psychosis.
■ Report evidence of increased TCA level or toxicity; dosage may need to be decreased.
■ If TCA starts when the patient already takes fluoxetine, TCA dosage may need to be decreased by up to 75% to avoid interaction.
■ Other TCAs may interact with fluoxetine. If you suspect an interaction, consult the prescriber or pharmacist.

nortriptyline ▸◂ paroxetine
Pamelor   Paxil

Risk rating: 2
Severity: Moderate   **Onset: Delayed**   **Likelihood: Suspected**

Cause
Paroxetine may decrease nortriptyline metabolism in some people and increase it in others.

Effect
Therapeutic and toxic effects of certain tricyclic antidepressants (TCAs) such as nortriptyline may increase.

Nursing considerations
⚠ **ALERT** TCAs other than nortriptyline may have this interaction.
■ When starting or stopping paroxetine, monitor TCA level and adjust dosage as needed.
■ Watch for adverse reactions, such as increased drowsiness, dizziness, confusion, heart rate or rhythm changes, and urine retention.
■ Watch closely for evidence of serotonin syndrome, such as delirium, bizarre movements, and tachycardia. Alert the prescriber if they occur; TCA may need to be stopped.

■ Symptoms of serotonin syndrome may resolve within 24 hours of stopping a TCA and starting a short course of cyproheptadine.

nortriptyline ▶◀ rifampin
Pamelor   Rifadin, Rimactane

Risk rating: 2
Severity: Moderate   **Onset: Delayed**   **Likelihood: Suspected**

Cause
Hepatic metabolism of tricyclic antidepressants (TCAs) such as nortriptyline may increase.

Effect
TCA level and efficacy may decrease.

Nursing considerations
■ When starting or stopping rifampin or changing its dosage, monitor serum TCA level to maintain therapeutic range.
■ Watch for resolution of depression as TCA dosage is adjusted to therapeutic level during rifampin therapy.
■ Urge the patient and family to watch for and promptly report adverse reactions, including increased drowsiness and dizziness, for several weeks after rifampin stops.
■ Other TCAs may interact with rifampin. If you suspect an interaction, consult the prescriber or pharmacist.

nortriptyline ▶◀ sertraline
Pamelor   Zoloft

Risk rating: 2
Severity: Moderate   **Onset: Delayed**   **Likelihood: Suspected**

Cause
Sertraline may decrease metabolism of nortriptyline and other tricyclic antidepressants (TCAs) in some people and increase it in others.

Effect
Therapeutic and toxic effects of certain TCAs may increase.

Nursing considerations
■ If possible, avoid this drug combination.
■ Monitor serum TCA level and watch closely for evidence of toxicity, such as drowsiness, dizziness, confusion, delirium, heart rate or rhythm changes, urine retention, and psychosis.

■ Report evidence of increased TCA level or serotonin syndrome; dosage may need to be decreased or drug stopped.
■ Symptoms of serotonin syndrome may resolve within 24 hours of stopping a TCA and starting a short course of an antiserotonergic drug.
■ Other TCAs may interact. If you suspect an interaction, consult the prescriber or pharmacist.

nortriptyline ▶◀ sympathomimetics

Pamelor

epinephrine, norepinephrine, phenylephrine

Risk rating: 2
Severity: **Moderate**   Onset: **Rapid**   Likelihood: **Established**

Cause
Tricyclic antidepressants (TCAs) such as nortriptyline increase the effects of direct-acting sympathomimetics and decrease the effects of indirect-acting sympathomimetics.

Effect
When sympathomimetic effects increase, the risk of hypertension and arrhythmias increases. When sympathomimetic effects decrease, blood pressure control decreases.

Nursing considerations
■ If possible, avoid using these drugs together.
■ Watch the patient closely for hypertension and heart rhythm changes; they may warrant reduction of sympathomimetic dosage.
■ If the patient takes a mixed-acting sympathomimetic, watch for negative effects; dosage may need to be altered.
■ Other TCAs and sympathomimetics may interact. If you suspect an interaction, consult the prescriber or pharmacist.

nortriptyline ▶◀ terbinafine

Pamelor

Lamisil

Risk rating: 2
Severity: **Moderate**   Onset: **Delayed**   Likelihood: **Suspected**

Cause
Hepatic metabolism of tricyclic antidepressants (TCAs) such as nortriptyline may be inhibited.

Effect
Therapeutic and toxic effects of certain TCAs may increase.

Nursing considerations
- Check for toxic TCA level, and report abnormal level.
- TCA dosage may need to be decreased.
- Adverse effects or toxicity may include vertigo, fatigue, loss of appetite, ataxia, muscle twitching, or trouble swallowing.
- Terbinafine's inhibitory effects may take several weeks to dissipate after drug is stopped.
- Describe signs and symptoms the patient should look for.

ofloxacin	►◄	antiarrhythmics
Floxin		amiodarone, bretylium, disopyramide, procainamide, quinidine, sotalol

Risk rating: 1
Severity: **Major**   Onset: **Delayed**   Likelihood: **Suspected**

Cause
The mechanism of this interaction is unknown.

Effect
Risk of life-threatening arrhythmias, including torsades de pointes, increases when certain quinolones such as ofloxacin are combined with antiarrhythmics.

Nursing considerations
- Avoid giving class IA or class III antiarrhythmics with ofloxacin.
- Quinolones that aren't metabolized by CYP3A4 isoenzymes or that don't prolong the QT interval may be given with antiarrhythmics.
- Monitor ECG for prolonged QTc interval.
- Tell the patient to report a rapid heartbeat, shortness of breath, dizziness, fainting, and chest pain.

ofloxacin	►◄	iron salts
Floxin		ferrous fumarate, ferrous gluconate, ferrous sulfate, iron polysaccharide

Risk rating: 2
Severity: **Moderate**   Onset: **Rapid**   Likelihood: **Probable**

Cause
Formation of an iron-quinolone complex decreases GI absorption of quinolone antibiotics such as ofloxacin.

Effect
Quinolone effects decrease.

Nursing considerations
- Other quinolones may interact with iron.
- Monitor the patient for quinolone efficacy.
- Tell the patient to separate quinolone dose from iron dose by at least 2 hours.
- Help the patient develop a plan to ensure proper dosage intervals.

---

ofloxacin ◀▶ sucralfate
Floxin   Carafate

Risk rating: 2
Severity: Moderate   **Onset: Rapid**   **Likelihood: Probable**

Cause
Sucralfate decreases GI absorption of quinolones such as ofloxacin.

Effect
Quinolone effects decrease.

Nursing considerations
- Don't use together. If that's unavoidable, give sucralfate at least 6 hours after the quinolone.
- Monitor the patient to make sure his infection is resolved.
- Help the patient develop a plan to ensure proper dosage intervals.

---

ofloxacin ◀▶ warfarin
Floxin   Coumadin

Risk rating: 2
Severity: Moderate   **Onset: Delayed**   **Likelihood: Suspected**

Cause
The mechanism of the interaction is unknown.

Effect
Anticoagulant effects may increase.

Nursing considerations
- Monitor PT and INR closely.
- Tell the patient to report unusual bleeding or bruising.
- Remind the patient that warfarin interacts with many drugs. Tell him to report any change in drug regimen to the prescriber or pharmacist.

olanzapine ▶◀ carbamazepine

Zyprexa, Symbyax

Carbatrol, Epitol, Equetro, Tegretol

Risk rating: 3
Severity: Minor   **Onset: Delayed**   **Likelihood: Suspected**

Cause
Carbamazepine increases hepatic metabolism.

Effect
Olanzapine level and effects decrease.

Nursing considerations
- Observe the patient's clinical response to olanzapine.
- If an interaction is suspected, adjust the dose of olanzapine as needed.
- Monitor the patient for increased agitation, manic or depressed episodes, or schizophrenic activity.

olanzapine ▶◀ fluoxetine

Zyprexa, Symbyax

Prozac, Sarafem

Risk rating: 3
Severity: Minor   **Onset: Delayed**   **Likelihood: Suspected**

Cause
Fluoxetine inhibits CYP2D6 metabolism of olanzapine.

Effect
Olanzapine levels may be increased.

Nursing considerations
- Use together cautiously. Adjust olanzapine dose if an interaction is suspected.
- Observe the patient's response to olanzapine when starting, stopping, or adjusting the dose.
- Monitor olanzapine levels.
- No significant adverse effects were reported due to this interaction.

omeprazole ━━▶◀━━ azole antifungals
Prilosec   itraconazole, ketoconazole

Risk rating: 2
Severity: Moderate   **Onset: Rapid**   **Likelihood: Suspected**

Cause
Proton pump inhibitors such as omeprazole increase gastric pH, which may impair dissolution of azole antifungals.

Effect
Efficacy of azole antifungals may decrease.

Nursing considerations
■ Notify the prescriber if the patient takes both drugs; an alternative may be available.
■ If no alternative is possible, advise the patient to take the azole anti-fungal with an acidic beverage such as cola.
■ Monitor the patient for lack of response to the antifungal drug.
■ If the patient can't tolerate acidic beverages and antifungal therapy appears to be ineffective, antifungal dosage may need to be increased.
■ Other drugs that increase gastric pH may interact with azole anti-fungals. If you suspect an interaction, consult the prescriber or pharmacist.

omeprazole ━━▶◀━━ benzodiazepines
Prilosec   diazepam, flurazepam, triazolam

Risk rating: 3
Severity: Minor   **Onset: Delayed**   **Likelihood: Suspected**

Cause
Metabolism of benzodiazepine may be decreased.

Effect
Half-life of benzodiazepines may be increased, leading to increased levels. Sedation or ataxia may be enhanced.

Nursing considerations
■ Monitor the patient for increased sedation or CNS impairment.
■ Consult the prescriber about reducing benzodiazepine dosage.
■ Other benzodiazepines, such as alprazolam, may not have this inter-action.

omeprazole ◄► cilostazol
Prilosec   Pletal

Risk rating: 2
Severity: Moderate   Onset: Delayed   Likelihood: Suspected

Cause
Omeprazole may inhibit CYP2C19 metabolism of cilostazol.

Effect
Cilostazol effects, including adverse effects, may increase.

Nursing considerations
- Cilostazol dose may need to be decreased during combined therapy; consider cilostazol 50 mg b.i.d.
- Watch for evidence of cilostazol toxicity, including severe headache, diarrhea, hypotension, tachycardia, and arrhythmias.
- Urge the patient to tell the prescriber about all drugs and supplements he takes and about any increase in adverse effects.

omeprazole ◄► clarithromycin
Prilosec   Biaxin

Risk rating: 3
Severity: Minor   Onset: Delayed   Likelihood: Suspected

Cause
Clarithromycin inhibits the metabolism of omeprazole. Omeprazole increases clarithromycin absorption.

Effect
Omeprazole and clarithromycin levels may increase. Gastric mucus concentration of clarithromycin may increase.

Nursing considerations
- This interaction may be beneficial in the treatment of *Helicobacter pylori* infections.
- No special action is needed with this interaction.

omeprazole ▸◂ protease inhibitors
Prilosec   atazanavir, indinavir,
                                   saquinavir

Risk rating: 1
Severity: Major   **Onset: Delayed**   **Likelihood: Suspected**

Cause
GI absorption of protease inhibitors may be decreased.

Effect
Antiviral activity of protease inhibitors may be reduced.

Nursing considerations
- Use of protease inhibitors and proton pump inhibitors isn't recommended.
- Monitor the patient for a decrease in antiviral activity.
- Adjust the dose of the protease inhibitor as needed.

omeprazole ▸◂ St. John's wort
Prilosec

Risk rating: 2
Severity: Moderate   **Onset: Delayed**   **Likelihood: Suspected**

Cause
St. John's wort may increase omeprazole metabolism.

Effect
Omeprazole level and effects may decrease.

Nursing considerations
- Discourage use of St. John's wort while taking omeprazole.
- If use together is unavoidable, monitor the patient for loss of GI symptom control.
- Tell the patient not to change the omeprazole regimen without consulting the prescriber.

orlistat ▶◀ cyclosporine

Xenical   Gengraf, Neoral, Sandimmune

Risk rating: 1
Severity: Major   **Onset: Delayed**   **Likelihood: Probable**

Cause
Orlistat may decrease cyclosporine absorption.

Effect
Cyclosporine level may decrease.

Nursing considerations
- Don't administer orlistat to patients who are taking cyclosporine.
- If the drugs must be used together, monitor cyclosporine level.
- Increasing the cyclosporine dose may not result in elevated level of cyclosporine.

orphenadrine ▶◀ phenothiazines

                 chlorpromazine,
                 perphenazine,
                 thioridazine

Risk rating: 2
Severity: Moderate   **Onset: Delayed**   **Likelihood: Suspected**

Cause
Anticholinergics such as orphenadrine may antagonize phenothiazines. Also, phenothiazine metabolism may increase.

Effect
Phenothiazine efficacy may decrease.

Nursing considerations
- Data regarding this interaction conflict.
- Monitor the patient for decreased phenothiazine efficacy.
- The phenothiazine dosage may need adjustment.
- Anticholinergic adverse effects may increase.
- Monitor the patient for adynamic ileus, hyperpyrexia, hypoglycemia, and neurologic changes.

oxacillin  food

Risk rating: 2
Severity: Moderate   Onset: Delayed   Likelihood: Suspected

Cause
Food may delay or reduce GI absorption of penicillins, including oxacillin.

Effect
Oxacillin efficacy may decrease.

Nursing considerations
- Food may affect penicillin absorption and peak level.
- Penicillin V and amoxicillin don't have this interaction and may be given without regard to meals.
- Tell the patient to take oxacillin 1 hour before or 2 hours after a meal.
- If the patient takes oxacillin with food, watch for lack of drug effect.

oxacillin  methotrexate
Trexall

Risk rating: 1
Severity: Major   Onset: Delayed   Likelihood: Probable

Cause
Methotrexate secretion in the renal tubules is inhibited.

Effect
Methotrexate level and risk of toxicity increase.

Nursing considerations
- Monitor the patient for methotrexate toxicity, including renal failure, neutropenia, leukopenia, thrombocytopenia, increased liver function tests, and skin ulcers.
- Monitor the patient for mouth sores. This may be the first outward appearance of methotrexate toxicity; however, in some patients, bone marrow suppression coincides with or precedes mouth sores.
- Obtain methotrexate level twice weekly for the first 2 weeks.
- Dose and duration of leucovorin rescue may need to be increased.
- Consider using ceftazidime instead of a penicillin if the patient needs a broad-spectrum antibiotic.

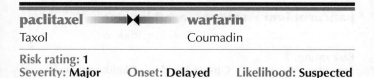

paclitaxel ◄ warfarin
Taxol   Coumadin

Risk rating: 1
Severity: Major   **Onset: Delayed**   **Likelihood: Suspected**

Cause
Warfarin metabolism, clotting factor synthesis, and possibly protein displacement may be inhibited.

Effect
Anticoagulant effects increase.

Nursing considerations
- Monitor PT and INR closely during and after chemotherapy.
- Tell the patient to report unusual bruising or bleeding.
- Remind the patient that warfarin interacts with many drugs, and tell the patient to report any change in drug regimen.

pancuronium ◄ aminoglycosides
                         gentamicin, neomycin,
                         streptomycin, tobramycin

Risk rating: 1
Severity: Major   **Onset: Rapid**   **Likelihood: Probable**

Cause
These drugs may be synergistic.

Effect
Effects of nondepolarizing muscle relaxants such as pancuronium may increase.

Nursing considerations
- Give these drugs together only when needed.
- Nondepolarizing muscle relaxant dosage may need adjustment based on neuromuscular response.
- Monitor the patient for prolonged respiratory depression.
- Provide ventilatory support as needed.

pancuronium ━━━▶◀━━━ azathioprine
Azasan, Imuran

Risk rating: 2
Severity: Moderate   **Onset: Rapid**   **Likelihood: Suspected**

Cause
Phosphodiesterase is inhibited in the motor nerve terminal.

Effect
Effects of nondepolarizing muscle relaxants such as pancuronium may decrease.

Nursing considerations
- Closely monitor the patient's respiratory status.
- Dosage reduction may be needed with combination therapy.
- Provide ventilatory support as needed.

pancuronium ━━━▶◀━━━ carbamazepine
Carbatrol, Epitol, Equetro, Tegretol

Risk rating: 2
Severity: Moderate   **Onset: Rapid**   **Likelihood: Probable**

Cause
The mechanism of this interaction is unknown.

Effect
Effects or duration of a nondepolarizing muscle relaxant such as pancuronium may decrease.

Nursing considerations
- Monitor the patient for decreased efficacy of muscle relaxant.
- Dosage of nondepolarizing muscle relaxant may be increased.
- Make sure the patient is adequately sedated when receiving a nondepolarizing muscle relaxant.

pancuronium 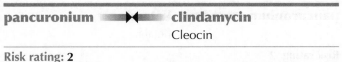 clindamycin
Cleocin

Risk rating: 2
Severity: Moderate   **Onset: Rapid**   **Likelihood: Suspected**

Cause
Clindamycin may potentiate the actions of nondepolarizing muscle relaxants such as pancuronium.

Effect
Nondepolarizing muscle relaxant action may increase.

Nursing considerations
- If possible, avoid using clindamycin or other lincosamides with non-depolarizing muscle relaxants.
- Monitor the patient for respiratory distress.
- Combined use may lead to profound, severe respiratory depression.
- Provide ventilatory support as needed.
- Cholinesterase inhibitors or calcium may help reverse drug effects.
- Make sure the patient is adequately sedated when receiving a non-depolarizing muscle relaxant.

pancuronium 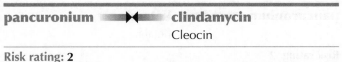 inhalation anesthetics
enflurane, isoflurane, nitrous oxide

Risk rating: 1
Severity: Major   **Onset: Rapid**   **Likelihood: Established**

Cause
These drugs potentiate pharmacologic actions.

Effect
The actions of nondepolarizing muscle relaxants such as pancuronium are potentiated.

Nursing considerations
- Closely monitor respiratory function.
- The dose of both the inhalation anesthetic and pancuronium may need to be adjusted.
- Provide ventilatory support as needed.
- The interaction is dose dependant.
- If the patient is receiving pancuronium continuously, the maintenance dose may need to be decreased 25% to 30%.

pancuronium 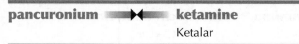 ketamine
Ketalar

Risk rating: 2
Severity: Moderate   **Onset: Rapid**   **Likelihood: Probable**

Cause
Increased acetylcholine release and decreased postsynaptic membrane sensitivity are suspected.

Effect
The actions of nondepolarizing muscle relaxants, including pancuronium, are enhanced, leading to profound and severe respiratory depression.

Nursing considerations
- Use these drugs together cautiously.
- The nondepolarizing muscle relaxant dosage may need adjustment.
- Provide ventilatory support as needed.
- The recovery time from pancuronium may also be increased.

pancuronium 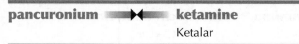 magnesium sulfate

Risk rating: 2
Severity: Moderate   **Onset: Rapid**   **Likelihood: Suspected**

Cause
Magnesium probably potentiates the action of nondepolarizing muscle relaxants such as pancuronium.

Effect
Risk of profound, severe respiratory depression increases.

Nursing considerations
- Use these drugs together cautiously.
- Nondepolarizing muscle relaxant dosage may need to be adjusted.
- Monitor the patient for respiratory distress.
- Provide ventilatory support as needed.
- Make sure the patient is adequately sedated when receiving a nondepolarizing muscle relaxant.

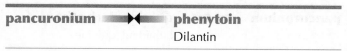

pancuronium ◄► phenytoin
Dilantin

Risk rating: 2
Severity: Moderate   **Onset: Rapid**   **Likelihood: Established**

Cause
Phenytoin has effects at prejunctional sites similar to those of nondepolarizing muscle relaxants such as pancuronium. Also, phenytoin alters the metabolism of pancuronium.

Effect
Effects or duration of nondepolarizing muscle relaxant may decrease.

Nursing considerations
■ Monitor the patient for decreased efficacy of the nondepolarizing muscle relaxant.
■ Dosage of nondepolarizing muscle relaxant may need to be increased.
■ Atracurium may be a suitable alternative to pancuronium because this interaction may not occur in all patients.
■ Make sure the patient is adequately sedated when receiving a nondepolarizing muscle relaxant.

pancuronium ◄► polypeptide antibiotics
bacitracin, polymyxin B, vancomycin

Risk rating: 2
Severity: Moderate   **Onset: Rapid**   **Likelihood: Probable**

Cause
Polypeptide antibiotics may act synergistically with nondepolarizing muscle relaxants such as pancuronium.

Effect
Neuromuscular blockade may increase.

Nursing considerations
■ If possible, avoid using polypeptide antibiotics with nondepolarizing muscle relaxants.
■ Monitor neuromuscular function closely.
■ Dosage of nondepolarizing muscle relaxant may need adjustment.
■ Provide ventilatory support, as needed.
■ Make sure the patient is adequately sedated when receiving a nondepolarizing muscle relaxant.

pancuronium ━━━▶◀━━━ quinine derivatives
quinidine, quinine

Risk rating: 2
Severity: Moderate   **Onset: Rapid**   **Likelihood: Suspected**

Cause
Quinine derivatives may act synergistically with nondepolarizing muscle relaxants such as pancuronium.

Effect
Effects of nondepolarizing muscle relaxants may increase.

Nursing considerations
◤ ALERT This interaction may be life-threatening. Monitor neuromuscular function closely.
- Intensity and duration of neuromuscular blockade may be affected.
- Dosage of nondepolarizing muscle relaxant may need adjustment.
- Provide ventilatory support as needed.
- Make sure the patient is adequately sedated when receiving a nondepolarizing muscle relaxant.

pancuronium ━━━▶◀━━━ theophyllines
aminophylline, theophylline

Risk rating: 2
Severity: Moderate   **Onset: Rapid**   **Likelihood: Suspected**

Cause
These drugs may act antagonistically.

Effect
Neuromuscular blockade may be reversed.

Nursing considerations
- Monitor the patient closely for lack of drug effect.
- Dosage of nondepolarizing muscle relaxant may need adjustment.
- This interaction is dose dependent.
- Make sure the patient is adequately sedated when receiving a nondepolarizing muscle relaxant.

pancuronium 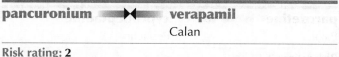 verapamil
Calan

Risk rating: 2
Severity: Moderate   **Onset: Rapid**   **Likelihood: Suspected**

Cause
This interaction may stem from a blockade of calcium channels in skeletal muscle.

Effect
Effects of nondepolarizing muscle relaxants such as pancuronium may increase.

Nursing considerations
- Avoid using verapamil with nondepolarizing muscle relaxants.
- Watch for prolonged respiratory depression.
- Provide ventilatory support as needed.
- Dosage of nondepolarizing muscle relaxant may be decreased.

pantoprazole 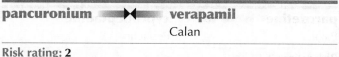 protease inhibitors
Protonix   atazanavir, indinavir, saquinavir

Risk rating: 1
Severity: Major   **Onset: Delayed**   **Likelihood: Suspected**

Cause
GI absorption of protease inhibitors may be decreased.

Effect
Antiviral activity of protease inhibitors may be reduced.

Nursing considerations
- Use of protease inhibitors and proton pump inhibitors isn't recommended.
- Monitor the patient for a decrease in antiviral activity.
- Adjust the dose of the protease inhibitor as needed.

paroxetine ━━━━▶◀ cyproheptadine
Paxil   Periactin

Risk rating: 2
Severity: Moderate   **Onset: Rapid**   **Likelihood: Suspected**

Cause
Because cyproheptadine is a serotonin antagonist, the interaction is thought to occur at the receptor level.

Effect
Pharmacologic effects of serotonin reuptake inhibitors (SRIs) decrease.

Nursing considerations
- Monitor the clinical response to SRIs such as paroxetine.
- If loss of antidepressant efficacy occurs, discuss discontinuing cyproheptadine.
- Depressive symptoms may resolve within 5 days of discontinuing this combination.

paroxetine ━━━━▶◀ digoxin
Paxil   Lanoxin

Risk rating: 1
Severity: Major   **Onset: Delayed**   **Likelihood: Suspected**

Cause
Renal excretion of digoxin is inhibited.

Effect
Digoxin level and risk of toxicity may increase.

Nursing considerations
- Monitor digoxin level. Therapeutic range is 0.8 to 2 nanograms/ml.
- Check ECG for digoxin toxicity: arrhythmias, such as bradycardia and AV blocks, ventricular ectopy, and shortened QTc interval.
- Watch other evidence of digoxin toxicity: lethargy, drowsiness, confusion, hallucinations, headaches, syncope, vision disturbances, nausea, anorexia, failure to thrive, vomiting, and diarrhea.
- If paroxetine starts or stops during digoxin therapy, digoxin dosage may need adjustment.
- Citalopram and venlafaxine don't have this interaction with digoxin and may be better alternatives than paroxetine.

paroxetine ▰▶◀▰ linezolid
Paxil   Zyvox

Risk rating: 1
Severity: Major   **Onset: Delayed**   **Likelihood: Suspected**

Cause
Serotonin may accumulate rapidly in the CNS.

Effect
The risk of serotonin syndrome increases.

Nursing considerations
⚠ **ALERT** Don't use these drugs together.
- Allow 2 weeks after stopping linezolid and administering paroxetine.
- Allow 2 weeks after stopping an SSRI such as paroxetine and administering linezolid.
- Describe the traits of serotonin syndrome, including confusion, restlessness, incoordination, muscle tremors and rigidity, fever, and sweating.
- Explain that serotonin-induced symptoms can be fatal if not treated immediately.

paroxetine ▰▶◀▰ risperidone
Paxil   Risperdal

Risk rating: 1
Severity: Major   **Onset: Rapid**   **Likelihood: Suspected**

Cause
SSRIs such as paroxetine may inhibit CYP2D6 metabolism of risperidone.

Effect
Risperidone level may increase, along with the risk of adverse reactions and rapid accumulation of serotonin in the CNS.

Nursing considerations
- Monitor the patient carefully if starting or stopping SSRI therapy or if the dosage changes during risperidone therapy.
- Assess the patient for CNS irritability, increased muscle tone, muscle twitching or jerking, and changes in level of consciousness.
- Advise the patient not to alter the dose of either drug without the advice of his prescriber.
- Average doses of paroxetine may cause this interaction.

paroxetine ━━━▶◀━━━ sibutramine
Paxil   Meridia

Risk rating: 1
Severity: Major   **Onset: Rapid**   **Likelihood: Suspected**

Cause
Serotonin may accumulate rapidly in the CNS.

Effect
Risk of serotonin syndrome increases.

Nursing considerations
⚡ **ALERT** If possible, don't give these drugs together.
■ Watch carefully for adverse effects, which require immediate medical attention.
■ Describe traits of serotonin syndrome: CNS irritability, motor weakness, shivering, muscle twitching, and altered consciousness.
■ Explain that serotonin syndrome can be fatal if not treated immediately.

paroxetine ━━━▶◀━━━ St. John's wort
Paxil

Risk rating: 2
Severity: Moderate   **Onset: Rapid**   **Likelihood: Suspected**

Cause
St. John's wort may cause additive inhibition of serotonin reuptake.

Effect
Sedative-hypnotic effects of SSRIs such as paroxetine may increase.

Nursing considerations
⚡ **ALERT** Discourage use of an SSRI with St. John's wort.
■ In addition to oversedation, mild serotonin-like symptoms may occur, including anxiety, dizziness, nausea, restlessness, and vomiting.
■ Inform the patient about the dangers of this combination.
■ Urge the patient to consult the prescriber before taking any herb.

paroxetine ◢◤ tricyclic antidepressants

Paxil

amitriptyline, desipramine,
imipramine, nortriptyline

Risk rating: 2
Severity: Moderate   Onset: Delayed   Likelihood: Suspected

Cause
Paroxetine may decrease tricyclic antidepressant (TCA) metabolism
in some people and increase it in others.

Effect
Therapeutic and toxic effects of certain TCAs may increase.

Nursing considerations
■ When starting or stopping paroxetine, monitor TCA level and adjust
dosage as needed.
■ Assess symptoms and behavior for evidence of adverse reactions,
such as increased drowsiness, dizziness, confusion, heart rate or
rhythm changes, and urine retention.
■ Watch closely for evidence of serotonin syndrome, such as delirium,
bizarre movements, and tachycardia. Alert the prescriber if they occur; the TCA may need to be stopped.
■ Symptoms of serotonin syndrome may resolve within 24 hours of
stopping a TCA and starting a short course of antiserotonergic drug.
◖ALERT Other TCAs may have this interaction.

penicillamine ◢◤ aluminum salts

Cuprimine, Depen

aluminum carbonate,
aluminum hydroxide,
attapulgite, kaolin,
magaldrate, sucralfate

Risk rating: 2
Severity: Moderate   Onset: Delayed   Likelihood: Probable

Cause
Formation of a physical or chemical complex with aluminum may decrease GI absorption of penicillamine.

Effect
Penicillamine efficacy may be reduced.

Nursing considerations
■ Separate administration times.

- If the patient must take these drugs together, notify the prescriber. Penicillamine dose may need adjustment.
- Help the patient develop a daily plan to ensure proper intervals between drug doses.

penicillins ━━━━━▶◀━━━ aminoglycosides

ampicillin, oxacillin, nafcillin, penicillin G, piperacillin, ticarcillin

amikacin, gentamicin, tobramycin

Risk rating: 2
Severity: Moderate   Onset: Delayed   Likelihood: Probable

Cause
The mechanism of this interaction is unknown.

Effect
Penicillins may inactivate certain aminoglycosides.

Nursing considerations
🔌 **ALERT** Check peak and trough aminoglycoside levels after third dose. For peak level, draw blood 30 minutes after I.V. or 60 minutes after I.M. dose. For trough level, draw blood just before a dose.
- Monitor the patient's renal function.
- Other aminoglycosides may interact with penicillins. If you suspect an interaction, consult the prescriber or pharmacist.
- Penicillins affect gentamicin and tobramycin more than amikacin.

penicillins ━━━━━▶◀━━━ food

ampicillin, cloxacillin, dicloxacillin, nafcillin, oxacillin, penicillin G

Risk rating: 2
Severity: Moderate   Onset: Delayed   Likelihood: Suspected

Cause
Food may delay or reduce GI absorption of penicillins.

Effect
Penicillin efficacy may decrease.

Nursing considerations
- Food may affect penicillin absorption and peak level.
- Penicillin V and amoxicillin don't have this interaction and may be given without regard to meals.

- If the patient took penicillin with food, watch for lack of drug effect.
- Tell the patient to take penicillin 1 hour before or 2 hours after a meal.

penicillins ▶◀ tetracycline

amoxicillin, ampi-
cillin, carbenicillin,
cloxacillin,
dicloxacillin,
nafcillin, oxacillin,
penicillin G,
penicillin V, pipera-
cillin, ticarcillin

Risk rating: 1
Severity: Major   **Onset: Delayed**   **Likelihood: Suspected**

Cause
Tetracyclines may adversely affect bactericidal activity of penicillins.

Effect
Penicillin efficacy may be reduced.

Nursing considerations
- If possible, avoid giving tetracyclines with penicillins.
- Monitor the patient closely for lack of penicillin effect.

perindopril ▶◀ potassium-sparing diuretics

Aceon   amiloride, spironolactone

Risk rating: 1
Severity: Major   **Onset: Delayed**   **Likelihood: Probable**

Cause
The mechanism of this interaction is unknown.

Effect
Serum potassium level may increase.

Nursing considerations
- Use cautiously in patients at high risk for hyperkalemia, especially those with renal impairment.
- Monitor BUN, creatinine, and serum potassium levels as needed.

■ ACE inhibitors other than perindopril may interact with potassium-sparing diuretics. If you suspect an interaction, consult the prescriber or pharmacist.
■ Urge the patient to immediately report an irregular heartbeat, a slow pulse, weakness, and other evidence of hyperkalemia.

perphenazine ➡◀ alcohol

Risk rating: 2
Severity: Moderate   Onset: Rapid   Likelihood: Probable

Cause
The mechanism of this interaction is unknown. It may be that these substances produce CNS depression by working on different sites in the brain. Also, alcohol may lower resistance to neurotoxic effects of phenothiazines such as perphenazine.

Effect
CNS depression may increase.

Nursing considerations
■ Watch for extrapyramidal reactions, such as dystonic reactions, and acute akathisia and restlessness.
■ If the patient takes a phenothiazine, warn that alcohol may worsen CNS depression and impair psychomotor skills.
■ Discourage alcohol intake during phenothiazine therapy.

perphenazine ➡◀ anticholinergics
benztropine, orphenadrine, procyclidine, trihexyphenidyl

Risk rating: 2
Severity: Moderate   Onset: Delayed   Likelihood: Suspected

Cause
Anticholinergics may antagonize phenothiazines such as per-phenazine. Also, phenothiazine metabolism may increase.

Effect
Phenothiazine efficacy may decrease.

Nursing considerations
■ Data regarding this interaction conflict.
■ Monitor the patient for decreased phenothiazine efficacy.
■ Phenothiazine dosage may need adjustment.

- Anticholinergic side effects may increase.
- Monitor the patient for adynamic ileus, hyperpyrexia, hypoglycemia, and neurologic changes.

---

phenelzine ◄►◄ anorexiants
Nardil

amphetamine, dextroamphetamine, methamphetamine

Risk rating: 1
Severity: Major   **Onset: Rapid**   **Likelihood: Suspected**

Cause
This interaction probably stems from increased norepinephrine levels at the synaptic cleft.

Effect
Anorexiant effects increase.

Nursing considerations
- If possible, avoid giving these drugs together.
- Headache and severe hypertension may occur rapidly if amphetamine is given to patients who take an MAO inhibitor such as phenelzine.
- ☒ ALERT Several deaths have been attributed to this combination after patients suffered a hypertensive crisis that led to cerebral hemorrhage.
- Monitor the patient for hypotension, hyperpyrexia, and seizures.
- Hypertensive reaction may occur for several weeks after stopping an MAO inhibitor.

---

phenelzine ◄►◄ atomoxetine
Nardil

Strattera

Risk rating: 1
Severity: Major   **Onset: Rapid**   **Likelihood: Suspected**

Cause
Level of monoamine in the brain may change.

Effect
Risk of serious or fatal reaction resembling neuroleptic malignant syndrome may increase.

Nursing considerations
☒ ALERT Use of atomoxetine and an MAO inhibitor such as

phenelzine, together or within 2 weeks of each other, is contraindicated.
■ Before starting atomoxetine, ask the patient when he last took an MAO inhibitor. Before starting an MAO inhibitor, ask the patient when he last took atomoxetine.
■ Monitor the patient for hyperthermia, rapid changes in vital signs, rigidity, muscle twitching, and mental status changes.

phenelzine ▶◀ bupropion
Wellbutrin, Zyban

Risk rating: 1
Severity: Major   **Onset: Delayed**   **Likelihood: Suspected**

Cause
The cause of this interaction is unknown.

Effect
Risk of acute bupropion toxicity is increased.

Nursing considerations
⚠ ALERT Administration of bupropion and MAO inhibitors together is contraindicated.
■ Allow at least 14 days between discontinuing an MAO inhibitor and starting bupropion.
■ Interaction warning is based on animal trials, not actual patient studies.

phenelzine ▶◀ carbamazepine
Nardil   Carbatrol, Epitol, Equetro, Tegretol

Risk rating: 1
Severity: Major   **Onset: Delayed**   **Likelihood: Suspected**

Cause
The mechanism of this interaction is unknown.

Effect
Risk of severe adverse effects, including hyperpyrexia, hyperexcitability, muscle rigidity, and seizures, may increase.

Nursing considerations
⚠ ALERT Use of carbamazepine with an MAO inhibitor such as phenelzine is contraindicated.
⚠ ALERT Carbamazepine is structurally related to tricyclic antide-

pressants, which may cause hypertensive crisis, seizures, and death when given with MAO inhibitors.
■ MAO inhibitor should be stopped at least 14 days before carbamazepine starts.
■ Urge the patient to tell the prescriber about all drugs and supplements he takes and about any increase in adverse effects.

phenelzine ━━━━▶◀━━━━ dextromethorphan
Nardil   Robitussin DM

Risk rating: 1
Severity: Major   **Onset: Rapid**   **Likelihood: Suspected**

Cause
MAO inhibitors such as phenelzine may decrease serotonin metabolism. Dextromethorphan may decrease synaptic reuptake of serotonin.

Effect
Risk of serotonin syndrome increases.

Nursing considerations
■ If possible, avoid giving these drugs together.
◼ **ALERT** Combined use may cause hyperpyrexia, abnormal muscle movement, hypotension, coma, and death.
■ If the patient takes an MAO inhibitor, caution against taking OTC cough and cold medicines that contain dextromethorphan.

phenelzine ━━━━▶◀━━━━ foods that contain amines
Nardil   aged, fermented, and overripe foods and drinks: broad beans, caviar, fermented sausage, liver, pickled herring, red wines, various cheeses, yeast extract

Risk rating: 1
Severity: Major   **Onset: Rapid**   **Likelihood: Established**

Cause
MAO inhibition interferes with metabolism of tyramine and other amines in certain foods.

Effect
Risk of marked hypertension increases.

Nursing considerations
■ Give the patient a list of foods to avoid while taking an MAO inhibitor such as phenelzine.
■ Urge the patient to avoid high-amine foods for 4 or more weeks after stopping an MAO inhibitor.
■ Monitor blood pressure closely; marked hypertension, hypertensive crisis, and hemorrhagic stroke are possible.
■ If the patient takes an MAO inhibitor, explain that yeast-containing supplements and cocoa-containing chocolates may cause this interaction.

phenelzine ◄►◄ insulin
Nardil

Risk rating: 2
Severity: Moderate   Onset: Delayed   Likelihood: Established

Cause
MAO inhibitors stimulate insulin secretion and inhibit gluconeogenesis (glucose formation).

Effect
Hypoglycemic response to insulin may be increased and prolonged.

Nursing considerations
■ Monitor glucose level closely if MAO inhibitor starts or dosage changes.
■ The extent of MAO inhibitor effect on glucose level may not be known for several weeks.
■ Watch for evidence of hypoglycemia: tachycardia, palpitations, anxiety, diaphoresis, nausea, hunger, dizziness, restlessness, headache, confusion, tremors, and speech and motor dysfunction.
■ Consult the prescriber if the patient experiences hypoglycemia; insulin dosage may need to be decreased.
■ Treat hypoglycemia as needed, such as with fast-acting oral carbohydrates, parenteral glucagon, or I.V. $D_{50}W$ bolus.
■ Make sure the patient and family can recognize hypoglycemia and respond appropriately.

phenelzine ◄► levodopa
Nardil   Larodopa

Risk rating: 1
Severity: Major   **Onset: Rapid**   **Likelihood: Established**

Cause
Peripheral metabolism of levodopa-derived dopamine is inhibited, increasing level at dopamine receptors.

Effect
Risk of hypertensive reaction increases.

Nursing considerations
- If possible, avoid giving these drugs together.
- If they're given together, an interaction—if it's going to occur—will occur within 1 hour. It appears to be dose related.
- Monitor the patient for flushing, light-headedness, and palpitations.
- Selegiline doesn't cause hypertensive reaction and may be used instead of phenelzine and other MAO inhibitors in patients taking levodopa.

phenelzine ◄► L-tryptophan
Nardil

Risk rating: 1
Severity: Major   **Onset: Rapid**   **Likelihood: Suspected**

Cause
Giving these drugs together may cause additive serotonergic effects.

Effect
Risk of serotonin syndrome increases.

Nursing considerations
⚡ ALERT Combined use of these drugs is contraindicated.
- They may cause CNS irritability, motor weakness, shivering, muscle twitching, and altered consciousness.

phenelzine ━━━▶◀━━━ meperidine

Nardil   Demerol

Risk rating: 1
Severity: Major   **Onset: Rapid**   **Likelihood: Probable**

Cause
The mechanism of this interaction is unknown.

Effect
Risk of severe adverse reactions increases.

Nursing considerations
- If possible, avoid giving these drugs together.
- If given together, monitor the patient and report agitation, seizures, diaphoresis, and fever.
- Reaction may progress to coma, apnea, and death.
- Reaction may occur several weeks after stopping an MAO inhibitor such as phenelzine.

🔋 **ALERT** Give opioid analgesics other than meperidine cautiously. It isn't known if similar reactions occur.

phenelzine ━━━▶◀━━━ selective 5-HT$_1$ receptor agonists

Nardil   rizatriptan, sumatriptan, zolmitriptan

Risk rating: 1
Severity: Major   **Onset: Rapid**   **Likelihood: Suspected**

Cause
Monoamine oxidase subtype-A inhibitors such as phenelzine may inhibit metabolism of selective 5-HT$_1$ receptor agonists.

Effect
Serum level of—and risk of cardiac toxicity from—certain selective 5HT$_1$ receptor agonists may increase.

Nursing considerations
🔋 **ALERT** Use of certain selective 5-HT$_1$ receptor agonists with or within 2 weeks of stopping an MAO inhibitor is contraindicated.
- If these drugs must be used together, naratriptan is less likely to interact with an MAO inhibitor.
- Cardiac toxicity may include coronary artery vasospasm and transient myocardial ischemia.

phenelzine ━━━━▶◀━━━ serotonin reuptake inhibitors

Nardil

citalopram, duloxetine, fluoxetine, sertraline, venlafaxine

Risk rating: 1
Severity: Major   **Onset: Rapid**   **Likelihood: Suspected**

Cause
Serotonin may accumulate rapidly in the CNS.

Effect
Risk of serotonin syndrome increases.

Nursing considerations
☒ **ALERT** Don't use these drugs together.
- Allow 1 week after stopping venlafaxine (2 weeks after stopping citalopram or sertraline; 5 weeks after stopping fluoxetine) before giving an MAO inhibitor such as phenelzine.
- Allow 2 weeks after stopping an MAO inhibitor before giving a serotonin reuptake inhibitor.
- The selective MAO type-B inhibitor selegiline has been given with fluoxetine, paroxetine, or sertraline to patients with Parkinson's disease without negative effects.
- Describe the traits of serotonin syndrome, including CNS irritability, motor weakness, shivering, myoclonus, and altered consciousness.
- Urge the patient to promptly report adverse effects to the prescriber.

---

phenelzine ━━━━▶◀━━━ sulfonylureas

Nardil

chlorpropamide, tolbutamide

Risk rating: 2
Severity: Moderate   **Onset: Rapid**   **Likelihood: Suspected**

Cause
The mechanism of this interaction is unknown.

Effect
Phenelzine and other MAO inhibitors increase the hypoglycemic effects of sulfonylureas.

Nursing considerations
- If the patient takes a sulfonylurea, start MAO inhibitor carefully, monitoring the patient for hypoglycemia.

■ Consult the prescriber about adjustments to either drug to control glucose level and mental status.
■ Describe signs and symptoms of hypoglycemia: diaphoresis, fatigue, headache, hunger, irritability, malaise, nervousness, rapid heart rate, tension, and trembling.
■ Instruct the patient to eat a small carbohydrate snack or meal if hypoglycemia develops, preferably after checking blood glucose level.

---

phenelzine ◄► sympathomimetics
Nardil   dopamine, ephedrine,
                          phenylephrine,
                          pseudoephedrine

Risk rating: 1
Severity: Major   **Onset: Rapid**   **Likelihood: Established**

Cause
When MAO is inhibited, as by phenelzine and other MAO inhibitors, norepinephrine accumulates and is released by indirect and mixed-acting sympathomimetics, increasing the pressor response at receptor sites.

Effect
Risk of severe headaches, hypertension, high fever, and hypertensive crisis increases.

Nursing considerations
■ Avoid giving indirect or mixed-acting sympathomimetics with an MAO inhibitor.
■ Phentolamine can be administered to block epinephrine- and norepinephrine-induced vasoconstriction and reduce blood pressure.
■ Direct-acting sympathomimetics interact minimally.
⚑ **ALERT** Warn the patient that OTC medicines such as decongestants may cause this interaction.

---

phenelzine ◄► tricyclic antidepressants
Nardil   amitriptyline, clomipramine,
                          desipramine, imipramine

Risk rating: 1
Severity: Major   **Onset: Rapid**   **Likelihood: Suspected**

Cause
The mechanism of this interaction is unknown.

Effect
Risk of hyperpyretic crisis, seizures, and death increase.

Nursing considerations
🔋 **ALERT** Don't give a tricyclic antidepressant with or within 2 weeks of an MAO inhibitor such as phenelzine.
■ Imipramine and clomipramine may be more likely to interact with MAO inhibitors.
■ Watch for adverse effects, including confusion, hyperexcitability, rigidity, seizures, increased temperature, increased pulse, increased respiration, sweating, mydriasis, flushing, headache, coma, and DIC.

---

phentermine ▶️◀ SSRIs
Adipex-P

citalopram, fluoxetine, venlafaxine

Risk rating: 2
Severity: Moderate   **Onset: Rapid**   **Likelihood: Suspected**

Cause
The mechanism of this interaction is unknown.

Effect
Sympathomimetic effects and risk of serotonin syndrome increase.

Nursing considerations
■ Watch closely for increased CNS effects, such as anxiety, jitteriness, agitation, and restlessness.
■ Mild serotonin-like symptoms may develop, including anxiety, dizziness, restlessness, nausea, and vomiting.
■ Explain the risk of interaction and the need to avoid amphetamines such as phentermine.
■ Describe the traits of serotonin syndrome, including CNS irritability, motor weakness, shivering, myoclonus, and altered consciousness.

---

phenylephrine ▶️◀ MAO inhibitors
Neo-Synephrine

phenelzine, tranylcypromine

Risk rating: 1
Severity: Major   **Onset: Rapid**   **Likelihood: Established**

Cause
When MAO is inhibited, norepinephrine accumulates and is released by indirect and mixed-acting sympathomimetics such as phenylephrine, increasing the pressor response at receptor sites.

Effect
Risk of severe headaches, hypertension, high fever, and hypertensive crisis increases.

Nursing considerations
■ Avoid giving indirect or mixed-acting sympathomimetics with an MAO inhibitor.
■ Phentolamine can be administered to block epinephrine- and nor-epinephrine-induced vasoconstriction and reduce blood pressure.
■ Direct-acting sympathomimetics interact minimally.
⚡ **ALERT** Warn the patient that OTC medicines such as deconges-tants may cause this interaction.

---

phenylephrine ■■■▶◀■■■ **tricyclic antidepressants**
Neo-Synephrine   amitriptyline, desipramine,
                                        imipramine, nortriptyline,
                                        trimipramine

Risk rating: 2
Severity: Moderate   Onset: Rapid   Likelihood: Established

Cause
Tricyclic antidepressants (TCAs) increase the effects of direct-acting sympathomimetics such as phenylephrine.

Effect
When sympathomimetic effects increase, the risk of hypertension and arrhythmias increases.

Nursing considerations
■ If possible, avoid using these drugs together.
■ Watch the patient closely for hypertension and heart rhythm changes; they may warrant reduction of sympathomimetic dosage.
■ Other TCAs and sympathomimetics may interact. If you suspect an interaction, consult the prescriber or pharmacist.

---

phenytoin ■■■▶◀■■■ **acetaminophen**
Dilantin   Acephen, NeoPAP, Tylenol

Risk rating: 2
Severity: Moderate   Onset: Delayed   Likelihood: Suspected

Cause
Phenytoin may induce hepatic microsomal enzymes, accelerating the metabolism of acetaminophen.

Effect

An abnormally high rate of acetaminophen metabolism may lead to higher level of hepatotoxic metabolites, increasing the risk of hepatic impairment.

Nursing considerations

- Hydantoins other than phenytoin may have a similar interaction with acetaminophen. Discuss concerns with the prescriber.

ALERT The hepatotoxic risk is greatest after acetaminophen overdose in patients who use phenytoin regularly.

- No special monitoring or dosage adjustment is required at the usual therapeutic dosages.
- Advise patients who take phenytoin to avoid regular use of acetaminophen.
- Tell the patient to notify the prescriber about abdominal pain, yellowing of skin or eyes, or darkened urine.

---

phenytoin ⧓ amiodarone

Dilantin | Cordarone, Pacerone

Risk rating: 2
Severity: Moderate **Onset: Delayed** **Likelihood: Probable**

Cause

Metabolism of hydantoins such as phenytoin may decrease. Amiodarone metabolism may increase.

Effect

Serum hydantoin level and risk of toxicity increase; amiodarone level decreases.

Nursing considerations

- Therapeutic range of phenytoin is 10 to 20 mcg/ml. Patients with decreased protein binding may show signs of toxicity despite a "normal" phenytoin level. Free phenytoin level is a better indicator in these patients (range: 1 to 2 mcg/ml).

ALERT Signs and symptoms of toxicity may progress in the following manner: nystagmus, ataxia, slurred speech, nausea, vomiting, lethargy, confusion, seizures, and coma.

- After adjusting dosage of either drug, the patient will need long-term monitoring because effects may be delayed several weeks.
- Watch for loss of amiodarone effect and return of symptoms, such as palpitations, shortness of breath, dizziness, and chest pain.

phenytoin ━━▶◀━━ antineoplastics
Dilantin   bleomycin, carboplatin, carmustine, cisplatin, methotrexate, vinblastine

Risk rating: 2
Severity: Moderate   Onset: Delayed   Likelihood: Suspected

Cause
Phenytoin absorption may be decreased or metabolism may be increased.

Effect
Phenytoin level and effects may decrease.

Nursing considerations
- Monitor phenytoin level closely. Dosage may need to be adjusted.
- Therapeutic range for phenytoin is 10 to 20 mcg/ml.
- Toxic effects can occur at therapeutic levels. Adjust the measured level for hypoalbuminemia or renal impairment, which can increase free drug level.
- Monitor the patient for seizure activity.
- Carefully monitor phenytoin level between courses of chemotherapy. Phenytoin dose may need to be reduced.
- Signs and symptoms of phenytoin toxicity include nystagmus, slurred speech, ataxia, blurred or double vision, confusion, drowsiness, and lethargy.

phenytoin ━━▶◀━━ benzodiazepines
Dilantin   chlordiazepoxide, diazepam, midazolam

Risk rating: 2
Severity: Moderate   Onset: Delayed   Likelihood: Suspected

Cause
Metabolism of phenytoin and benzodiazepines may be altered.

Effect
Phenytoin level and risk of toxicity increase, but there are conflicting data.

Nursing considerations
- Monitor phenytoin level closely. Dosage may need to be adjusted.
- Therapeutic range for phenytoin is 10 to 20 mcg/ml.

■ Toxic effects can occur at therapeutic levels. Adjust the measured level for hypoalbuminemia or renal impairment, which can increase free drug level.
■ Signs and symptoms of phenytoin toxicity include nystagmus, slurred speech, ataxia, blurred or double vision, confusion, drowsiness, and lethargy.
■ Monitor the patient's response to chlordiazepoxide; a larger dose may be needed.

---

phenytoin ▶◀ carbamazepine
Dilantin   Carbatrol, Epitol, Equetro, Tegretol

Risk rating: 2
Severity: Moderate   Onset: Delayed   Likelihood: Suspected

Cause
Carbamazepine metabolism may increase. Carbamazepine may also decrease phenytoin availability.

Effect
Carbamazepine level and effects decrease. The effect of carbamazepine on phenytoin is variable.

Nursing considerations
■ Monitor serum levels of both drugs as appropriate, especially when starting or stopping either one.
■ Therapeutic carbamazepine level is 4 to 12 mcg/ml.
■ Therapeutic phenytoin level is 10 to 20 mcg/ml.
■ Dosage adjustments may be needed to maintain therapeutic effects and avoid toxicity.
■ Monitor the patient for loss of carbamazepine effect (loss of seizure control).

---

phenytoin ▶◀ cimetidine
Dilantin   Tagamet

Risk rating: 2
Severity: Moderate   Onset: Delayed   Likelihood: Established

Cause
The hepatic metabolism of phenytoin is inhibited.

Effect
Phenytoin level and risk of toxicity may increase.

Nursing considerations
- Hydantoins other than phenytoin may have a similar interaction with cimetidine.
- Monitor phenytoin level closely. Dosage may need to be adjusted.
- Therapeutic range for phenytoin is 10 to 20 mcg/ml.
- Toxic effects can occur at therapeutic levels. Adjust the measured level for hypoalbuminemia or renal impairment, which can increase free drug level.
- Signs and symptoms of phenytoin toxicity include nystagmus, slurred speech, ataxia, blurred or double vision, confusion, drowsiness, and lethargy.
- Ranitidine and felodipine may be better alternatives than cimetidine.

---

phenytoin ▶◀ chloramphenicol
Dilantin   Chloromycetin

Risk rating: 2
Severity: Moderate   Onset: Delayed   Likelihood: Suspected

Cause
Metabolism of phenytoin is altered.

Effect
Phenytoin level and risk of toxicity increase. Chloramphenicol concentration may also change.

Nursing considerations
- Monitor drug levels closely. Dosage may need to be adjusted.
- Therapeutic range for phenytoin is 10 to 20 mcg/ml.
- Toxic effects of phenytoin can occur at therapeutic levels. Adjust the measured level for hypoalbuminemia or renal impairment.
- Signs and symptoms of phenytoin toxicity include nystagmus, slurred speech, ataxia, blurred or double vision, confusion, drowsiness, and lethargy.

---

phenytoin ▶◀ corticosteroids
Dilantin   dexamethasone, fludrocorti-
                            sone, hydrocortisone, methyl-
                            prednisolone, prednisolone

Risk rating: 2
Severity: Moderate   Onset: Delayed   Likelihood: Established

Cause
Phenytoin and other hydantoins induce liver enzymes, which stimulate corticosteroid metabolism. Corticosteroids may enhance hepatic clearance of phenytoin.

Effect
The effects of corticosteroids may decrease.

Nursing considerations
■ Avoid giving hydantoins with corticosteroids if possible.
■ Monitor the patient for decreased corticosteroid effects. Also monitor phenytoin level, and adjust dosage of either drug as needed.
■ Corticosteroid effects may decrease within days of starting phenytoin and may stay at those lower levels for 3 weeks after the patient stops phenytoin.
■ Dosage of either or both drugs may need to be increased.

---

phenytoin ◄► **cyclosporine**
Dilantin   Gengraf, Neoral, Sandimmune

Risk rating: 1
Severity: Major   **Onset: Delayed**   **Likelihood: Probable**

Cause
Cyclosporine absorption may decrease or metabolism may increase.

Effect
Cyclosporine level may decrease.

Nursing considerations
■ Patients may be at risk for transplant rejection when cyclosporine is given with phenytoin.
■ Cyclosporine level decreases within 48 hours of phenytoin treatment and returns to normal within 1 week of stopping phenytoin.
■ Monitor cyclosporine level closely.
■ Adjust cyclosporine dose as needed.

---

phenytoin ◄► **disopyramide**
Dilantin   Norpace

Risk rating: 2
Severity: Moderate   **Onset: Delayed**   **Likelihood: Suspected**

Cause
Hepatic metabolism of disopyramide is increased.

Effect
Disopyramide levels and effects may be decreased. Anticholinergic actions may be increased.

Nursing considerations
- Monitor the clinical response to disopyramide. The dose may need to be increased.
- This interaction may continue for several days after discontinuing phenytoin.
- Monitor the patient for increase or return of arrhythmias.
- If increased anticholinergic effects are seen, consider using another antiarrhythmic agent besides disopyramide.

---

phenytoin ▶◀ disulfiram
Dilantin   Antabuse

Risk rating: 2
Severity: Moderate   **Onset: Rapid**   **Likelihood: Established**

Cause
Disulfiram inhibits hepatic metabolism of the hydantoin, phenytoin, and may also interfere with the rate of elimination.

Effect
Phenytoin level, effects, and risk of toxicity may increase.

Nursing considerations
- Other hydantoins may have a similar interaction with disulfiram. If you suspect a drug interaction, consult the prescriber or pharmacist.
- Monitor phenytoin level; therapeutic range is 10 to 20 mcg/ml.
- Monitor the patient for signs of phenytoin toxicity, including nystagmus, slurred speech, ataxia, blurred or double vision, confusion, drowsiness, and lethargy.
- Watch for loss of phenytoin effects (for example, loss of seizure control) if disulfiram therapy is stopped.
- Adjust phenytoin dose as ordered.

---

phenytoin ▶◀ dopamine
Dilantin   Intropin

Risk rating: 1
Severity: Major   **Onset: Rapid**   **Likelihood: Suspected**

Cause
Hypotension may result from phenytoin-induced myocardial depression and dopamine-related depletion of catecholamines.

Effect
Profound, life-threatening hypotension may occur.

Nursing considerations
■ Use extreme caution and frequent blood pressure monitoring when administering both drugs to a patient.
◤ **ALERT** Life-threatening hypotension can occur in a few minutes of coadministration. Cardiac arrest and death may occur.
■ Stop phenytoin infusion at the first sign of hypotension.
■ It isn't known if phenytoin reacts similarly to sympathomimetics other than dopamine. Use cautiously.

---

phenytoin ▸◂ doxycycline
Dilantin   Vibramycin

Risk rating: 2
Severity: Moderate   Onset: Delayed   Likelihood: Probable

Cause
Phenytoin increases doxycycline metabolism. In addition, doxycycline may be displaced from plasma proteins.

Effect
Doxycycline elimination may increase and its effects may decrease.

Nursing considerations
■ Monitor the patient for expected doxycycline effects (absence of infection) when given with the hydantoin phenytoin.
■ Doxycycline dose may need to be doubled to maintain therapeutic serum level.
■ Consult the prescriber or pharmacist about using a tetracycline (other than doxycycline) that doesn't interact with phenytoin.
■ Urge the patient to tell the prescriber if signs and symptoms don't improve.
■ Other hydantoins may have a similar interaction with doxycycline. If you suspect an interaction, consult the prescriber or pharmacist.

---

phenytoin ▸◂ estrogens
Dilantin   conjugated estrogens, esterified estrogens, estradiol, estrone, estropipate, ethinyl estradiol

Risk rating: 2
Severity: Moderate   Onset: Delayed   Likelihood: Suspected

Cause
Phenytoin may induce hepatic metabolism of estrogens. Estrogens may increase water retention, worsen seizures, and alter phenytoin protein-binding.

Effect
Risk of spotting, breakthrough bleeding, and pregnancy increases. Seizure control may decrease.

Nursing considerations
- Estrogen dose may need to be altered to obtain cycle control.
- **⚡ ALERT** Advise the patient that breakthrough bleeding, spotting, and amenorrhea are signs of contraceptive failure.
- There is anecdotal evidence, not yet confirmed, that seizures may worsen in patients who take estrogens.
- Monitor the patient for increased seizure activity when estrogen therapy starts.
- Hydantoins other than phenytoin may interact with estrogens. If you suspect an interaction, consult the prescriber or pharmacist.
- If the patient takes phenytoin, suggest a nonhormonal contraceptive.

---

phenytoin ➤◄ felbamate
Dilantin   Felbatol

Risk rating: 2
Severity: Moderate   Onset: Delayed   Likelihood: Probable

Cause
The mechanism of this interaction is unknown. Possibly felbamate inhibits metabolism of phenytoin. Phenytoin may increase the metabolism of felbamate.

Effect
Phenytoin levels, pharmacologic effects, and risk of toxicity may increase. Felbamate levels may decrease.

Nursing considerations
- Monitor the patient for change in seizure control.
- If felbamate is added, consider reducing phenytoin dosage by 20%.
- Monitor phenytoin level; therapeutic range is 10 to 20 mcg/ml.
- Monitor the patient for signs of phenytoin toxicity, which include nystagmus, slurred speech, ataxia, blurred or double vision, confusion, drowsiness, and lethargy.
- Toxic effects can occur at therapeutic levels. Adjust the measured level for hypoalbuminemia or renal impairment, which can increase free drug level.

phenytoin ━━━━▶◀━━━━ felodipine
Dilantin   Plendil

Risk rating: 2
Severity: Moderate   Onset: Delayed   Likelihood: Suspected

Cause
Phenytoin may increase felodipine metabolism and decrease its availability.

Effect
Felodipine effects may decrease.

Nursing considerations
- Felodipine dose may need to be increased.
- Watch for loss of blood pressure control if the patient who takes felodipine starts phenytoin.
- Watch for evidence of felodipine toxicity (peripheral vasodilation, hypotension, bradycardia, and palpitations) if phenytoin is stopped.
- Urge the patient to have blood pressure monitored if phenytoin therapy starts. Remind the patient that hypertension may cause no symptoms.
- Urge the patient to tell the prescriber about increased adverse effects.

phenytoin ━━━━▶◀━━━━ fluconazole
Dilantin   Diflucan

Risk rating: 2
Severity: Moderate   Onset: Delayed   Likelihood: Probable

Cause
Fluconazole may inhibit hepatic metabolism of phenytoin.

Effect
Phenytoin levels, pharmacologic effects, and risk of toxicity may increase.

Nursing considerations
- Monitor phenytoin levels and patient response if fluconazole therapy is started or stopped. Therapeutic range for phenytoin is 10 to 20 mcg/ml.
- Phenytoin dose may need to be adjusted when fluconazole therapy is started or stopped.
- Toxic effects can occur at therapeutic levels. Adjust the measured level for hypoalbuminemia or renal impairment, which can increase free drug level.
- Monitor the patient for signs and symptoms of phenytoin toxicity, which include nystagmus, slurred speech, ataxia, blurred or double vision, confusion, drowsiness, and lethargy.

phenytoin ▶◀ fluoxetine
Dilantin   Prozac, Sarafem

Risk rating: 2
Severity: Moderate   Onset: Delayed   Likelihood: Suspected

Cause
Fluoxetine may inhibit phenytoin metabolism.

Effect
Serum phenytoin level, effects, and risk of toxicity may increase.

Nursing considerations
■ Monitor serum phenytoin level. Therapeutic range for phenytoin is 10 to 20 mcg/ml.
■ Phenytoin dosage may need adjustment.
■ Watch for evidence of phenytoin toxicity: nystagmus, slurred speech, ataxia, blurred or double vision, confusion, drowsiness, and lethargy.
■ Urge the patient to tell the prescriber about increased adverse effects.

phenytoin ▶◀ fluvoxamine
Dilantin   Luvox

Risk rating: 2
Severity: Moderate   Onset: Delayed   Likelihood: Suspected

Cause
Fluvoxamine may inhibit CYP2C9 and CYP2C19 metabolism of hydantoins such as phenytoin.

Effect
Hydantoin level and risk of toxic effects may increase.

Nursing considerations
■ Monitor serum hydantoin level. Therapeutic range for phenytoin is 10 to 20 mcg/ml.
■ Hydantoin dosage may need adjustment.
■ When fluvoxamine is started, watch for hydantoin toxicity: drowsiness, nausea, vomiting, nystagmus, ataxia, dysarthria, tremor, slurred speech, hypotension, arrhythmias, respiratory depression, and coma.
■ When fluvoxamine stops, watch for loss of anticonvulsant effect and increased seizure activity.

phenytoin ━━━━━►◄━━━━ folic acid
Dilantin   Folvite

Risk rating: 2
Severity: Moderate   Onset: Delayed   Likelihood: Suspected

Cause
The mechanism of this interaction is unknown but probably involves altered metabolic process.

Effect
Level and effects of hydantoins, such as phenytoin, may decrease.

Nursing considerations
■ Monitor hydantoin level. Therapeutic range for phenytoin is 10 to 20 mcg/ml.
■ Hydantoin dosage may need adjustment.
■ If folic acid is started during hydantoin therapy, watch for loss of anticonvulsant effect and increased seizure activity.
■ If folic acid is stopped during hydantoin therapy, watch for signs of hydantoin toxicity, such as nystagmus, slurred speech, ataxia, blurred or double vision, confusion, drowsiness, and lethargy.
■ Urge the patient to tell the prescriber about increased adverse effects.

phenytoin ━━━━━►◄━━━━ furosemide
Dilantin   Lasix

Risk rating: 3
Severity: Minor   Onset: Delayed   Likelihood: Suspected

Cause
Reduced oral absorption of furosemide may occur.

Effect
Phenytoin may reduce furosemide effects.

Nursing considerations
■ Patients taking phenytoin may need to have an increase in furosemide dose.
■ Monitor diuretic response.
■ Monitor the patient for expected furosemide effects: reduction in peripheral edema, resolution of pulmonary edema, or decreased blood pressure in hypertensive patients.

phenytoin 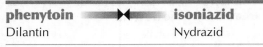 isoniazid
Dilantin   Nydrazid

Risk rating: 2
Severity: Moderate   Onset: Delayed   Likelihood: Established

Cause
Hepatic microsomal enzyme metabolism of phenytoin is inhibited.

Effect
Phenytoin level, effects, and risk of toxicity increase.

Nursing considerations
■ Monitor phenytoin level closely. Dosage may need to be adjusted. Therapeutic range for phenytoin is 10 to 20 mcg/ml.
■ Toxic effects can occur at therapeutic levels. Adjust the measured level for hypoalbuminemia or renal impairment, which can increase free drug level.
■ Signs and symptoms of phenytoin toxicity include nystagmus, slurred speech, ataxia, blurred or double vision, confusion, drowsiness, and lethargy.
■ If the patient's phenytoin level has been stabilized with isoniazid and isoniazid is stopped, watch for loss of seizure control.
■ Hydantoins other than phenytoin may have a similar interaction with isoniazid.

phenytoin 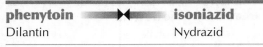 itraconazole
Dilantin   Sporanox

Risk rating: 2
Severity: Moderate   Onset: Delayed   Likelihood: Suspected

Cause
Metabolism of itraconazole increases and phenytoin metabolism is inhibited.

Effect
Efficacy of itraconazole may decrease; phenytoin effects increase.

Nursing considerations
■ Avoid use of these drugs together.
■ More research is being done on this interaction.
■ Monitor the patient for lack of response to antifungal drug.
■ Monitor phenytoin level closely. Dosage may need to be adjusted. Therapeutic range for phenytoin is 10 to 20 mcg/ml.
■ Signs and symptoms of phenytoin toxicity include nystagmus, slurred speech, ataxia, blurred or double vision, confusion, drowsiness, and lethargy.

phenytoin ━━━▶◀━━━ levodopa
Dilantin

Risk rating: 2
Severity: Moderate   **Onset: Delayed**   **Likelihood: Suspected**

Cause
The exact mechanism of interaction is unknown.

Effect
Levodopa effects may decrease.

Nursing considerations
- Avoid this combination if possible.
- If these drugs are used together, watch for recurring or worsening Parkinson symptoms: increased tremors, muscle rigidity, bradykinesia (slowing of voluntary movement), shuffling gait, loss of facial expression, speech disturbances, and drooling.
- In the patient treated for chronic manganese poisoning, watch for recurring or worsening symptoms of manganese toxicity: muscle weakness, difficulty walking, tremors, salivation, and psychological disturbances, such as irritability, aggressiveness, and hallucinations.
- If you suspect a drug interaction, consult the prescriber or pharmacist; an alternative therapy may need to be considered.
- Warn the patient or caregiver not to change levodopa dosage without consulting the prescriber.

phenytoin ━━━▶◀━━━ methadone
Dilantin   Dolophine, Methadose

Risk rating: 2
Severity: Moderate   **Onset: Delayed**   **Likelihood: Suspected**

Cause
The mechanism of this interaction is unknown but probably involves altered metabolic processes.

Effect
Level and effects of methadone may decrease.

Nursing considerations
- Methadone dosage may need adjustment.
- If phenytoin is started during methadone therapy, watch for signs and symptoms of opioid withdrawal.
- Urge the patient to tell the prescriber about return of withdrawal symptoms.

phenytoin ▶◀ metyrapone
Dilantin   Metopirone

Risk rating: 2
Severity: Moderate   Onset: Delayed   Likelihood: Established

Cause
Phenytoin increases first-pass metabolism of metyrapone.

Effect
Pituitary-adrenal response to oral metyrapone is decreased.

Nursing considerations
■ Two times the normal dosage of metyrapone may be needed for
pituitary-adrenal axis assessment.
■ If possible, stop phenytoin before administering metyrapone.
■ Administering metyrapone I.V. bypasses first-pass metabolism and
doesn't have this interaction.

phenytoin ▶◀ mexiletine
Dilantin   Mexitil

Risk rating: 2
Severity: Moderate   Onset: Delayed   Likelihood: Established

Cause
Phenytoin increases hepatic metabolism of mexiletine.

Effect
Mexiletine levels and effectiveness decrease.

Nursing considerations
■ Monitor clinical response to mexiletine.
■ Mexiletine dosage may need to be increased.
■ Monitor ECG for recurrence of arrhythmias; notify the prescriber if
increase in arrhythmias is noted.

phenytoin ▶◀ mirtazapine
Dilantin   Remeron

Risk rating: 2
Severity: Moderate   Onset: Delayed   Likelihood: Suspected

Cause
Phenytoin and other hydantoins may increase CYP3A3 and CYP3A4
metabolism of mirtazapine.

Effect
Mirtazapine level and effects may decrease.

Nursing considerations
- Assess the patient for expected mirtazapine effects, including improvement of depression and stabilization of mood.
- Record mood changes and monitor the patient for suicidal tendencies.
- If a hydantoin starts, mirtazapine dosage may need to be increased.
- If a hydantoin stops, watch for mirtazapine toxicity, including disorientation, drowsiness, impaired memory, tachycardia, severe hypotension, heart failure, seizures, CNS depression, and coma.
- Urge the patient to tell the prescriber about loss of drug effect and increased adverse effects.

---

phenytoin ◄►	nondepolarizing muscle relaxants
Dilantin	atracurium, cisatracurium, pancuronium, vecuronium

Risk rating: 2
Severity: Moderate   Onset: Rapid   Likelihood: Established

Cause
Phenytoin has effects at prejunctional sites similar to those of non-depolarizing muscle relaxants. Phenytoin also alters the metabolism of pancuronium.

Effect
Effect or duration of nondepolarizing muscle relaxant may decrease.

Nursing considerations
- Monitor the patient for decreased efficacy of the muscle relaxant.
- Dosage of nondepolarizing muscle relaxant may need to be increased.
- Atracurium may be a suitable alternative because this interaction may not occur in all patients.
- Make sure the patient is adequately sedated when receiving a non-depolarizing muscle relaxant.

---

phenytoin ◄►	quetiapine
Dilantin	Seroquel

Risk rating: 2
Severity: Moderate   Onset: Delayed   Likelihood: Suspected

Cause
Quetiapine metabolism increases.

Effect
Pharmacologic response to quetiapine may decrease.

Nursing considerations
■ Monitor the patient for loss of symptom control for bipolar disorder or schizophrenia.
■ The dose of quetiapine may need to be changed when starting, stopping, or changing the dose of phenytoin.
■ Tell the patient that, although no serious side effects have been noted from this interaction, he should report unusual or bothersome adverse effects to the prescriber.

phenytoin ◄►◄ quinidine
Dilantin

Risk rating: 2
Severity: Moderate   **Onset: Delayed**   **Likelihood: Suspected**

Cause
Phenytoin stimulates the hepatic enzyme system, which increases quinidine metabolism.

Effect
Quinidine level decreases.

Nursing considerations
■ Monitor quinidine level during combined use.
■ Therapeutic range of quinidine is 2 to 6 mcg/ml. More specific assays have levels of less than 1 mcg/ml.
■ Monitor the patient for loss of arrhythmia control if phenytoin is started.
■ Tell the patient to report palpitations, shortness of breath, dizziness or fainting, and chest pain.
■ If the patient's quinidine level is stable on combined therapy and phenytoin is stopped, monitor the patient for quinidine toxicity.
⚡ **ALERT** Quinidine toxicity may cause GI irritation, arrhythmias, hypotension, vertigo, and rash.

phenytoin ◄►◄ sertraline
Dilantin   Zoloft

Risk rating: 2
Severity: Moderate   **Onset: Delayed**   **Likelihood: Suspected**

Cause
Sertraline may inhibit metabolism of hydantoins such as phenytoin.

Effect
Hydantoin level, effects, and risk of toxicity may increase.

Nursing considerations
- Monitor hydantoin level. Therapeutic range for phenytoin is 10 to 20 mcg/ml.
- Hydantoin dosage may need adjustment.
- If sertraline is started during hydantoin therapy, watch for evidence of hydantoin toxicity, including drowsiness, nausea, vomiting, nystagmus, ataxia, dysarthria, tremor, slurred speech, hypotension, arrhythmias, respiratory depression, and coma.
- If sertraline stops during hydantoin therapy, watch for decreased anticonvulsant effect and increased seizure activity.
- Urge the patient to tell the prescriber about loss of drug effect and increased adverse effects.

---

phenytoin ◄► sulfadiazine
Dilantin

Risk rating: 2
Severity: Moderate   Onset: Delayed   Likelihood: Probable

Cause
Sulfadiazine may inhibit hepatic metabolism of hydantoins such as phenytoin.

Effect
Hydantoin level, effects, and risk of toxicity may increase.

Nursing considerations
- Monitor hydantoin level. Therapeutic range for phenytoin is 10 to 20 mcg/ml.
- Hydantoin dosage may need adjustment.
- If sulfadiazine is started during hydantoin therapy, watch for evidence of hydantoin toxicity, including nystagmus, slurred speech, ataxia, blurred or double vision, confusion, drowsiness, and lethargy.
- If sulfadiazine is stopped during hydantoin therapy, watch for decreased anticonvulsant effect and increased seizure activity.
- Consult the prescriber and pharmacist about other anti-infective drugs if the patient takes a hydantoin.

phenytoin ━━━━▶◀━━━━ tacrolimus
Dilantin   Prograf

Risk rating: 2
Severity: Moderate   **Onset: Delayed**   **Likelihood: Suspected**

Cause
CYP3A4 metabolism of tacrolimus may increase.

Effect
Tacrolimus level may decrease; phenytoin level may increase.

Nursing considerations
■ Monitor levels of both drugs. Expected trough level of tacrolimus is 6 to 10 mcg/L; expected phenytoin level is 10 to 20 mcg/ml.
■ Watch closely for signs of neurotoxicity or syncope; adjust doses of both drugs as needed.
■ This effect may occur with fosphenytoin as well.
■ If one drug is stopped, continue to monitor serum level of remaining drug; dosage may need to be changed.

phenytoin ━━━━▶◀━━━━ theophyllines
Dilantin   aminophylline, theophylline

Risk rating: 2
Severity: Moderate   **Onset: Delayed**   **Likelihood: Probable**

Cause
Metabolism of both drugs increases.

Effect
Theophylline or phenytoin efficacy may decrease.

Nursing considerations
■ Monitor levels of both drugs carefully. Normal phenytoin level is 10 to 20 mcg/ml. Normal theophylline level is 10 to 20 mcg/ml for adults and 5 to 15 mcg/ml for children.
■ Assess the patient for recurrence of seizures and increased respiratory distress, and report findings to the prescriber promptly; dosages may need adjustment.
■ Interaction typically occurs within 5 days after adding one of these drugs while the patient is taking the other.

phenytoin ━━━━▶◀ ticlopidine
Dilantin   Ticlid

Risk rating: 2
Severity: Moderate   **Onset: Delayed**   **Likelihood: Probable**

Cause
Ticlopidine may inhibit hepatic metabolism of hydantoins such as phenytoin.

Effect
Hydantoin level may increase, raising the risk of adverse effects.

Nursing considerations
- Monitor hydantoin level. Therapeutic range for phenytoin is 10 to 20 mcg/ml.
- Hydantoin level may increase gradually over a month.
- Hydantoin dosage may need adjustment.
- If ticlopidine starts during hydantoin therapy, monitor the patient for adverse CNS effects of hydantoins, including vertigo, ataxia, and somnolence.
- If ticlopidine is stopped during hydantoin therapy, watch for decreased anticonvulsant effect and increased seizure activity.

phenytoin ━━━━▶◀ valproic acid
Dilantin   divalproex sodium,
                                valproic acid

Risk rating: 2
Severity: Moderate   **Onset: Delayed**   **Likelihood: Suspected**

Cause
Valproic acid metabolism increases; phenytoin metabolism decreases.

Effect
Phenytoin effects may increase; valproic acid effects may decrease. Phenytoin toxicity may occur despite therapeutic total serum level.

Nursing considerations
- Watch for altered seizure control and evidence of phenytoin toxicity: nystagmus, slurred speech, ataxia, blurred or double vision, confusion, drowsiness, and lethargy.
- Monitor serum levels of free phenytoin and valproic acid. The amount of free phenytoin may be more important than the therapeutic range of 10 to 20 mcg/ml.
- Be prepared to alter the dosage of either drug as needed.
- Other hydantoins may interact with valproic acid. If you suspect an interaction, consult the prescriber or pharmacist.

phenytoin ━━━▶◀━━━ warfarin
Dilantin   Coumadin

Risk rating: 2
Severity: Moderate   Onset: Delayed   Likelihood: Suspected

Cause
Phenytoin level may increase and half-life may lengthen. Phenytoin may increase PT when added to warfarin therapy.

Effect
Risk of phenytoin toxicity and severe bleeding increases.

Nursing considerations
- Monitor the patient for signs or symptoms of phenytoin toxicity or for altered anticoagulant effects.
- Therapeutic range for phenytoin is 10 to 20 mcg/ml.
- Toxic effects can occur at therapeutic levels. Adjust the measured level for hypoalbuminemia or renal impairment, which can increase free drug level.
- Signs and symptoms of phenytoin toxicity include nystagmus, slurred speech, ataxia, blurred or double vision, confusion, drowsiness, and lethargy.
- Monitor phenytoin level 7 to 10 days after therapy starts or changes.
- Tell the patient to report unusual bruising or bleeding.

pimozide ━━━▶◀━━━ aprepitant
Orap   Emend

Risk rating: 1
Severity: Major   Onset: Delayed   Likelihood: Suspected

Cause
Aprepitant may inhibit CYP3A4 metabolism of pimozide.

Effect
Risk of life-threatening arrhythmias may increase.

Nursing considerations
- ⚡ **ALERT** Combined use of these drugs is contraindicated.
- Arrhythmias are related to prolonged QT intervals, a known risk of pimozide.
- Interaction warning is based on pharmacokinetics of these drugs, not actual patient studies.

pimozide ◄ azole antifungals
Orap

itraconazole, ketoconazole,
voriconazole

Risk rating: 1
Severity: Major   **Onset: Delayed**   **Likelihood: Suspected**

Cause
Azole antifungals may inhibit CYP3A4 metabolism of pimozide.

Effect
Risk of life-threatening arrhythmias may increase.

Nursing considerations
⚠ ALERT Combined use of these drugs is contraindicated.
- Interaction warning is based on pharmacokinetics of these drugs,
not actual patient studies.
- Prolonged QT intervals are a known risk of pimozide; arrhythmias
are related to prolonged QT intervals.

pimozide ◄ macrolide antibiotics
Orap

azithromycin, clarithromycin,
erythromycin, telithromycin

Risk rating: 1
Severity: Major   **Onset: Delayed**   **Likelihood: Probable**

Cause
Macrolide antibiotics may inhibit CYP3A4 metabolism of pimozide.

Effect
Risk of life-threatening arrhythmias may increase.

Nursing considerations
⚠ ALERT Combined use of these drugs is contraindicated.
- Arrhythmias are related to prolonged QT intervals, a known risk
of pimozide.
⚠ ALERT People with normal baseline ECG and no history have
died of pimozide blood levels 2.5 times the upper limit of normal
from this interaction.

pimozide ━━━▶◀━━━ nefazodone
Orap

Risk rating: 1
Severity: Major   **Onset: Delayed**   **Likelihood: Suspected**

Cause
Nefazodone may inhibit CYP3A4 metabolism of pimozide.

Effect
Risk of life-threatening arrhythmias may increase.

Nursing considerations
⚠ ALERT Combined use of these drugs is contraindicated.
▪ Arrhythmias are related to prolonged QT intervals, a known risk of pimozide.
▪ Interaction warning is based on pharmacokinetics of these drugs, not actual patient studies.

pimozide ━━━▶◀━━━ protease inhibitors
Orap   amprenavir, atazanavir,
                    darunavir, fosamprenavir,
                    indinavir, lopinavir/ritonavir,
                    nelfinavir, ritonavir, saquinavir

Risk rating: 1
Severity: Major   **Onset: Delayed**   **Likelihood: Suspected**

Cause
Protease inhibitors may inhibit CYP3A4 metabolism of pimozide.

Effect
Risk of life-threatening arrhythmias may increase.

Nursing considerations
⚠ ALERT Combined use of these drugs is contraindicated.
▪ Arrhythmias are related to prolonged QT interval, a known risk of pimozide.
▪ Interaction warning is based on pharmacokinetics of these drugs, not actual patient studies.

pimozide ◄► SSRIs
Orap   citalopram, sertraline

Risk rating: 1
Severity: Major   **Onset: Delayed**   **Likelihood: Suspected**

Cause
The mechanism of this interaction is unknown.

Effect
Risk of life-threatening arrhythmias, including torsades de pointes, may increase.

Nursing considerations
◼ **ALERT** Combined use of these drugs is contraindicated.
◼ Arrhythmias are related to prolonged QT intervals, a known risk of pimozide.
◼ Interaction warning is based on actual patient experience with these drugs as well as pharmacokinetics.

pimozide ◄► thioridazine
Orap

Risk rating: 1
Severity: Major   **Onset: Delayed**   **Likelihood: Suspected**

Cause
Thioridazine may have additive effects on prolongation of the QTc interval.

Effect
Risk of life-threatening arrhythmias may increase.

Nursing considerations
◼ **ALERT** Combined use of these drugs is contraindicated.
◼ Life-threatening torsades de pointes may result.
◼ Bradycardia, hypokalemia, and congenital prolongation of the QTc are added risk factors for torsades de pointes or sudden death.
◼ Prolongation of the QTc interval depends on the dose of thioridazine, becoming more pronounced as the dose increases.

pimozide ═══►◄═══ zileuton
Orap   Zyflo

Risk rating: 1
Severity: Major   **Onset: Delayed**   **Likelihood: Suspected**

Cause
Zileuton may inhibit CYP3A4 metabolism of pimozide.

Effect
Risk of life-threatening arrhythmias may increase.

Nursing considerations
◙ **ALERT** Combined use of these drugs is contraindicated.
■ Arrhythmias are related to prolonged QT intervals, a known risk of pimozide.
■ Interaction warning is based on known pharmacokinetics of these drugs, not actual patient studies.

pimozide ═══►◄═══ ziprasidone
Orap   Geodon

Risk rating: 1
Severity: Major   **Onset: Delayed**   **Likelihood: Suspected**

Cause
Ziprasidone may have additive effects on QT-interval prolongation.

Effect
Risk of life-threatening arrhythmias, including torsades de pointes, may increase.

Nursing considerations
◙ **ALERT** Combined use of these drugs is contraindicated.
■ Arrhythmias are related to prolonged QT intervals, a known risk of pimozide.
■ Interaction warning is based on known pharmacokinetics of these drugs, not actual patient studies.

pindolol 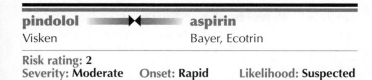 aspirin
Visken   Bayer, Ecotrin

Risk rating: 2
Severity: Moderate   Onset: Rapid   Likelihood: Suspected

Cause
Salicylates inhibit synthesis of prostaglandins, which pindolol and other beta-adrenergic blockers need to reduce blood pressure. In patients with heart failure, the mechanism of this interaction is unknown.

Effect
Beta-adrenergic blocker's effect is reduced.

Nursing considerations
■ Watch closely for signs of heart failure and hypertension, and notify provider if they occur.
■ Talk with the prescriber about switching the patient to a different antihypertensive or antiplatelet drug.
■ Other beta-adrenergic blockers may interact with salicylates. If you suspect an interaction, consult the prescriber or pharmacist.
■ Explain signs and symptoms of heart failure, and tell the patient when to contact the prescriber.

pindolol 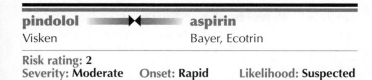 lidocaine
Visken   Xylocaine

Risk rating: 2
Severity: Moderate   Onset: Rapid   Likelihood: Established

Cause
Pindolol and other beta-adrenergic blockers reduce hepatic metabolism of lidocaine.

Effect
Lidocaine level and risk of toxicity may increase.

Nursing considerations
■ Check for normal therapeutic level of lidocaine: 2 to 5 mcg/ml.
■ Monitor the patient closely for evidence of lidocaine toxicity, including dizziness, somnolence, confusion, paresthesias, and seizures.
■ Slow I.V. bolus rate to decrease risk of high peak level and toxic reaction.
■ Explain warning signs of toxicity to the patient and his family, and tell them to contact the prescriber if they have concerns.

pindolol 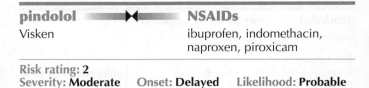 NSAIDs
Visken

ibuprofen, indomethacin,
naproxen, piroxicam

Risk rating: 2
Severity: Moderate   **Onset: Delayed**   **Likelihood: Probable**

Cause
NSAIDs may inhibit renal prostaglandin synthesis, allowing pressor
systems to be unopposed.

Effect
Pindolol and other beta-adrenergic blockers may not be able to lower
blood pressure.

Nursing considerations
- Avoid using these drugs together if possible.
- Monitor blood pressure and related signs and symptoms of hypertension closely.
- Consult the prescriber about ways to minimize interaction, such as
adjusting beta-adrenergic blocker dosage or switching to sulindac as
the NSAID.
- Explain the risks of using these drugs together, and teach the patient
how to monitor his blood pressure.
- Other NSAIDs may interact with beta-adrenergic blockers. If you
suspect an interaction, consult the prescriber or pharmacist.

pindolol 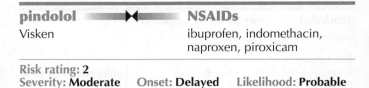 phenothiazines
Visken

chlorpromazine, thioridazine

Risk rating: 1
Severity: Major   **Onset: Delayed**   **Likelihood: Probable**

Cause
Pindolol inhibits phenothiazine metabolism.

Effect
Effects of both drugs and the risk of serious adverse reactions may
increase.

Nursing considerations
⚠ **ALERT** Combined use of these drugs is contraindicated.
- Educate the patient and his family about the risk of drug interaction.
- Beta-adrenergic blockers other than pindolol may interact with
phenothiazines. If you suspect an interaction, consult the prescriber
or pharmacist.

pindolol ◄ verapamil

Visken   Calan

Risk rating: 1
Severity: Major   **Onset: Rapid**   **Likelihood: Probable**

Cause
Verapamil may inhibit metabolism of beta-adrenergic blockers such as pindolol.

Effect
Effects of both drugs may be increased.

Nursing considerations
◄ ALERT Giving these drugs together increases the risk of adverse effects, including heart failure, conduction disturbances, arrhythmias, and hypotension.
■ Combination therapy is, in general, effective and acceptable in patients with hypertension and unstable angina.
■ Monitor the patient for adverse effects, including left ventricular dysfunction and AV conduction defects.
■ Risk of interaction is greater when drugs are given I.V.
■ Dosages of both drugs may need to be decreased.

piperacillin ◄ aminoglycosides

amikacin, gentamicin,
tobramycin

Risk rating: 2
Severity: Moderate   **Onset: Delayed**   **Likelihood: Probable**

Cause
The mechanism of this interaction is unknown.

Effect
Piperacillin and other penicillins may inactivate certain aminoglycosides, decreasing their effects.

Nursing considerations
◄ ALERT Check peak and trough aminoglycoside levels after the third dose. For peak level, draw blood 30 minutes after I.V. or 60 minutes after I.M. dose. For trough level, draw blood just before a dose.
■ Monitor the patient's renal function.
■ Other aminoglycosides may interact with penicillins. If you suspect an interaction, consult the prescriber or pharmacist.

piperacillin 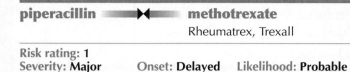 methotrexate
Rheumatrex, Trexall

Risk rating: 1
Severity: Major **Onset: Delayed** **Likelihood: Probable**

Cause
Methotrexate secretion in the renal tubules is inhibited.

Effect
Methotrexate level and risk of toxicity increase.

Nursing considerations
- Monitor the patient for methotrexate toxicity, including renal failure, neutropenia, leukopenia, thrombocytopenia, increased liver function test results, and skin ulcers.
- Monitor the patient for mouth sores. This may be the first outward appearance of methotrexate toxicity; however, in some patients, bone marrow suppression coincides with or precedes mouth sores.
- Obtain methotrexate level twice weekly for the first 2 weeks.
- Dose and duration of leucovorin rescue may need to be increased.

piperacillin ➤◀ tetracycline

Risk rating: 1
Severity: Major **Onset: Delayed** **Likelihood: Suspected**

Cause
Tetracyclines may adversely affect the bactericidal activity of penicillins such as piperacillin.

Effect
Penicillin efficacy may be reduced.

Nursing considerations
- If possible, avoid giving tetracyclines with penicillins.
- Monitor the patient closely for lack of penicillin effect.

polymyxin B ━━━▶◀━━━ nondepolarizing muscle relaxants

atracurium, pancuronium, vecuronium

Risk rating: 2
Severity: Moderate   **Onset: Rapid**   **Likelihood: Probable**

Cause
Polymyxin B and other polypeptide antibiotics may act synergistically with nondepolarizing muscle relaxants.

Effect
Neuromuscular blockade may increase.

Nursing considerations
■ If possible, avoid using polypeptide antibiotics with nondepolarizing muscle relaxants.
■ Monitor neuromuscular function closely.
■ Dosage of nondepolarizing muscle relaxant may need adjustment.
■ Provide ventilatory support as needed.
■ Make sure the patient is adequately sedated when receiving a nondepolarizing muscle relaxant.

pravastatin ━━━▶◀━━━ azole antifungals

Pravachol   fluconazole, itraconazole, ketoconazole

Risk rating: 2
Severity: Moderate   **Onset: Rapid**   **Likelihood: Probable**

Cause
Azole antifungals may inhibit hepatic metabolism of HMG-CoA reductase inhibitors, such as pravastatin.

Effect
Pravastatin level and adverse effects may increase.

Nursing considerations
■ If possible, avoid use together.
■ Pravastatin dosage may need to be decreased.
■ Monitor serum cholesterol and lipid levels to assess the patient's response to therapy.
⚡ ALERT Assess the patient for evidence of rhabdomyolysis: fatigue, muscle aches and weakness, joint pain, weight gain, seizures, greatly increased serum CK level, and dark, red, or cola-colored urine.
■ Pravastatin is the HMG-CoA reductase inhibitor least affected by this interaction and may be preferable for use with azole antifungals.

pravastatin ━━━━▶◀━━━ cyclosporine
Pravachol   Gengraf, Neoral, Sandimmune

Risk rating: 1
Severity: Major   **Onset: Delayed**   **Likelihood: Probable**

Cause
Metabolism of certain HMG-CoA reductase inhibitors, such as
pravastatin, may decrease.

Effect
Pravastatin level and adverse effects may increase.

Nursing considerations
- If possible, avoid use together.
- Pravastatin dosage may need to be decreased.
- Monitor serum cholesterol and lipid levels.

⚡ ALERT Assess the patient for evidence of rhabdomyolysis: fatigue,
muscle aches and weakness, joint pain, weight gain, seizures, greatly
increased serum CK level, and dark, red, or cola-colored urine.
- Urge the patient to report muscle pain, tenderness, or weakness.

pravastatin ━━━━▶◀━━━ fibric acids
Pravachol   fenofibrate, gemfibrozil

Risk rating: 1
Severity: Major   **Onset: Delayed**   **Likelihood: Suspected**

Cause
The mechanism of this interaction is unknown.

Effect
Severe myopathy or rhabdomyolysis may occur.

Nursing considerations
- Avoid use together.
- If the patient has severe hyperlipidemia, combined therapy may be
an option, but only with careful monitoring.

⚡ ALERT Assess the patient for evidence of rhabdomyolysis: fatigue,
muscle aches and weakness, joint pain, weight gain, seizures, greatly
increased serum CK level, and dark, red, or cola-colored urine.
- Watch for evidence of acute renal failure, including decreased
urine output, elevated BUN and creatinine levels, edema, dyspnea,
tachycardia, distended jugular veins, nausea, vomiting, poor appetite,
weakness, fatigue, confusion, and agitation.
- Urge the patient to report muscle pain, tenderness, or weakness.

pravastatin ━━━━▶◀━━━ rifampin
Pravachol   Rifadin, Rimactane

Risk rating: 2
Severity: Moderate   Onset: Delayed   Likelihood: Suspected

Cause
Rifampin may induce CYP3A4 metabolism of pravastatin and other HMG-CoA reductase inhibitors in the intestine and liver.

Effect
Pravastatin effects may decrease.

Nursing considerations
■ Assess the patient for expected response to therapy. If you suspect an interaction, consult the prescriber or pharmacist.
■ Check serum cholesterol and lipid levels.
■ Obtain liver function test results at start of therapy and periodically thereafter. If ALT or AST level stays three times or more above the upper limit of normal, pravastatin will need to be stopped.
◪ **ALERT** Withhold HMG-CoA reductase inhibitor temporarily if the patient's risk of myopathy or rhabdomyolysis increases, as from sepsis, hypotension, major surgery, trauma, uncontrolled seizures, or a severe metabolic, endocrine, or electrolyte disorder.
■ Pravastatin is the HMG-CoA reductase inhibitor least likely to interact with rifampin and may be the best choice for combined use.

praziquantel ━━━━▶◀━━━ cimetidine
Biltricide   Tagamet

Risk rating: 2
Severity: Moderate   Onset: Delayed   Likelihood: Probable

Cause
Cimetidine may inhibit first-pass metabolism of praziquantel.

Effect
Praziquantel levels and effects, including adverse effects, may be increased.

Nursing considerations
■ Observe for increased effects of praziquantel.
■ Praziquantel dosage may need adjustment.
■ Ranitidine may be a better alternative than cimetidine.

prazosin ━━━━▶◀━━━━ propranolol
Minipress   Inderal

Risk rating: 2
Severity: Moderate   Onset: Rapid   Likelihood: Probable

Cause
The mechanism of this interaction is unknown.

Effect
Effect of these drugs on orthostatic hypotension increases.

Nursing considerations
▪ Assess the patient's lying, sitting, and standing blood pressures closely, especially when combined therapy starts.
▪ Adjust dosages of either drug based on patient effects.
▪ To minimize effects of orthostatic hypotension, teach the patient to change positions slowly.
▪ Interaction is confirmed only with propranolol but may occur with other beta-adrenergic blockers as well.

prazosin ━━━━▶◀━━━━ tadalafil
Minipress   Cialis

Risk rating: 1
Severity: Major   Onset: Rapid   Likelihood: Suspected

Cause
The cause of the interaction is unknown.

Effect
The hypotensive effects of alpha$_1$-adrenergic blockers, such as prazosin, may be increased.

Nursing considerations
◤ **ALERT** Administering tadalafil and an alpha$_1$-adrenergic blocker together is contraindicated.
▪ If the patient has taken tadalafil and an alpha$_1$-adrenergic blocker, carefully monitor his blood pressure and cardiac output.
▪ Alert the prescriber that the patient is taking tadalafil and an alpha$_1$-adrenergic blocker and that their use together is contraindicated.
▪ Make sure the patient has ready I.V. access to administer fluids if needed for hypotension.

prazosin ━━━━━━▶◀━━━━━━ vardenafil
Minipress   Levitra

Risk rating: 2
Severity: Moderate   Onset: Rapid   Likelihood: Suspected

Cause
Vardenafil causes an additive pharmacologic action.

Effect
The risk of hypotension may be increased.

Nursing considerations
◤ **ALERT** Administering vardenafil with an alpha$_1$-adrenergic blocker such as prazosin is contraindicated.
▪ If the patient has taken vardenafil and an alpha$_1$-adrenergic blocker, carefully monitor his blood pressure and cardiac output.
▪ Alert the prescriber that the patient is taking vardenafil and an alpha$_1$-adrenergic blocker and that their use together is contraindicated.
▪ Make sure the patient has ready I.V. access to administer fluids if needed for hypotension.

prednisolone ━━━━━━▶◀━━━━━━ phenytoin
                                                 Dilantin

Risk rating: 2
Severity: Moderate   Onset: Delayed   Likelihood: Established

Cause
Hydantoins, such as phenytoin, induce liver enzymes, which stimulate metabolism of corticosteroids, such as prednisolone.

Effect
Corticosteroid effects may decrease.

Nursing considerations
▪ Avoid giving hydantoins with corticosteroids if possible.
▪ Monitor the patient for decreased corticosteroid effects. Also monitor phenytoin level and adjust the dosage of either drug as needed.
▪ Corticosteroid effects may decrease within days of starting phenytoin and may stay decreased for 3 weeks after it's stopped.
▪ Dosage of either or both drugs may need to be increased.

prednisolone ━━▶◀━━ salicylates
aspirin, choline salicylate, sodium salicylate

Risk rating: 2
Severity: Moderate   **Onset: Delayed**   **Likelihood: Probable**

Cause
Prednisolone, and other corticosteroids stimulate hepatic metabolism of salicylates and may increase renal excretion.

Effect
Salicylate level and effects decrease.

Nursing considerations
■ Monitor salicylate level and efficacy; dosage may need adjustment.
◪ **ALERT** Giving a salicylate while tapering a corticosteroid may result in salicylate toxicity.
■ Watch for evidence of salicylate toxicity, including diaphoresis, nausea, vomiting, tinnitus, hyperventilation, and CNS depression.
■ Patients with renal impairment may be at greater risk.

prednisolone, ━━▶◀━━ azole antifungals
prednisone
itraconazole, ketoconazole

Risk rating: 2
Severity: Moderate   **Onset: Delayed**   **Likelihood: Suspected**

Cause
CYP3A4 metabolism of corticosteroid is inhibited and elimination is decreased.

Effect
Corticosteroid effects and toxicity may be increased.

Nursing considerations
■ Monitor the patient for increased adverse effects to corticosteroids and adjust dose as needed.
■ Monitor the patient taking corticosteroid and itraconazole for Cushing syndrome.
■ Carefully monitor the patient for infection, edema, and increased serum glucose level.
■ Instruct the patient not to abruptly stop the corticosteroid; it should be gradually tapered to prevent withdrawal symptoms.

prednisolone, ━━▶◀━━ estrogens
prednisone

conjugated estrogens, esterified estrogens, estradiol, estrone, estropipate, ethinyl estradiol

Risk rating: 2
Severity: Moderate   Onset: Delayed   Likelihood: Suspected

Cause
Estrogens may inhibit hepatic metabolism of corticosteroids, such as prednisolone and prednisone.

Effect
Therapeutic and toxic corticosteroid effects may increase.

Nursing considerations
- Assess the patient's response to corticosteroid.
- Watch for evidence of corticosteroid toxicity: nervousness, sleepiness, depression, psychosis, weakness, decreased hearing, leg edema, skin disorders, hypertension, muscle weakness, and seizures.
- If given with estrogens, corticosteroid dosage may need adjustment.
- Estrogen may continue to affect corticosteroid therapy for an unknown length of time after estrogen is stopped.
- Other corticosteroids may interact with estrogens. If you suspect an interaction, consult the prescriber or pharmacist.
- Tell the patient to report increased adverse effects.

prednisolone, ━━▶◀━━ primidone
prednisone

Mysoline

Risk rating: 2
Severity: Moderate   Onset: Delayed   Likelihood: Established

Cause
Primidone and other barbiturates induce liver enzymes, which stimulate corticosteroid metabolism.

Effect
Corticosteroid effects may decrease.

Nursing considerations
- Avoid giving barbiturates with corticosteroids if possible.
- If the patient takes a corticosteroid with a barbiturate, watch for worsening symptoms when the barbiturate is started or stopped.
- During barbiturate treatment, corticosteroid dosage may need to be increased.

prednisolone, prednisone ⧓ rifamycins

rifabutin, rifampin, rifapentine

Risk rating: 1
Severity: Major **Onset: Delayed** **Likelihood: Established**

Cause
Rifamycins increase hepatic metabolism of corticosteroids, such as prednisolone and prednisone.

Effect
Corticosteroid effects may decrease.

Nursing considerations
- If possible, avoid giving rifamycins with corticosteroids.
- Monitor the patient for decreased corticosteroid effects, including loss of disease control.
- Monitor the patient closely for symptom control after increasing rifamycin dose. Drug may need to be stopped to regain control of disease.
- Corticosteroid effects may decrease within days of starting rifampin and may stay decreased 2 to 3 weeks after it is stopped.
- Corticosteroid dose may need to be doubled after adding rifampin.

prednisone ⧓ cholinesterase inhibitors

neostigmine, pyridostigmine

Risk rating: 1
Severity: Major **Onset: Delayed** **Likelihood: Probable**

Cause
In myasthenia gravis, prednisone and other corticosteroids antagonize the effects of cholinesterase inhibitors.

Effect
The patient may develop severe muscular depression refractory to cholinesterase inhibitors.

Nursing considerations
- Corticosteroids may have long-term benefits in myasthenia gravis.
- Combined therapy may be attempted under strict supervision.
- In myasthenia gravis, monitor the patient for severe muscle deterioration.

ALERT Be prepared to provide respiratory support and mechanical ventilation if needed.

- Consult the prescriber or pharmacist about safe corticosteroid delivery to maximize improvement in muscle strength.

primidone ━━━━►◄━━━━ carbamazepine

Mysoline

Carbatrol, Epitol, Equetro, Tegretol

Risk rating: 2
Severity: Moderate   Onset: Delayed   Likelihood: Suspected

Cause
Hepatic metabolism is altered.

Effect
Carbamazepine and primidone levels decrease.

Nursing considerations
- Monitor serum levels of both drugs as appropriate, especially when starting or stopping either one.
- Therapeutic carbamazepine level is 4 to 12 mcg/ml.
- Dosage adjustments may be needed to maintain therapeutic effects.
- Monitor the patient for loss of drug effect (loss of seizure control).

primidone ━━━━►◄━━━━ corticosteroids

Mysoline

dexamethasone, hydrocortisone, methylprednisolone, prednisolone, prednisone

Risk rating: 2
Severity: Moderate   Onset: Delayed   Likelihood: Established

Cause
Primidone and other barbiturates induce liver enzymes, which stimulate corticosteroid metabolism.

Effect
Corticosteroid effects may decrease.

Nursing considerations
- Avoid giving barbiturates with corticosteroids if possible.
- If the patient takes a corticosteroid with a barbiturate, watch for worsening symptoms when the barbiturate is started or stopped.
- During barbiturate treatment, corticosteroid dosage may need to be increased.

primidone ▬▬▶◀▬▬ doxycycline
Mysoline   Vibramycin

Risk rating: 2
Severity: Moderate   **Onset: Delayed**   **Likelihood: Suspected**

Cause
Barbiturates such as primidone may increase hepatic metabolism of doxycycline, a tetracycline.

Effect
Doxycycline level and effects may decrease.

Nursing considerations
- Monitor the patient for expected doxycycline effects.
- Doxycycline dose may need to be increased.
- Effects of barbiturates on doxycycline may persists for weeks after barbiturate is stopped.
- Consult the prescriber or pharmacist about using a tetracycline that doesn't interact with barbiturates, such as demeclocycline, oxytetracycline, or tetracycline.
- Urge the patient to tell the prescriber if he isn't improving with doxycycline.

primidone ▬▬▶◀▬▬ hormonal contraceptives
Mysoline

Risk rating: 1
Severity: Major   **Onset: Delayed**   **Likelihood: Suspected**

Cause
Primidone and other barbiturates may induce hepatic metabolism of contraceptives and synthesis of sex-hormone–binding protein.

Effect
Risk of breakthrough bleeding and pregnancy may increase.

Nursing considerations
- Consult the prescriber about increasing contraceptive dosage during barbiturate therapy.
- Consult the prescriber about alternative treatments for seizures or sleep disturbance.
- Instruct the patient to also use barrier contraception.

primidone ━━━━▶◀━━━━ griseofulvin
Mysoline   Grisactin

Risk rating: 2
Severity: Moderate   Onset: Delayed   Likelihood: Suspected

Cause
Primidone may decrease griseofulvin absorption and increase hepatic metabolism.

Effect
Griseofulvin levels decrease.

Nursing considerations
- Separate drug administration times.
- Give primidone in divided doses.
- Griseofulvin dose may need to be increased.
- Consider stopping either drug; alternative therapy may be needed.

primidone ━━━━▶◀━━━━ succinimide
Mysoline   ethosuximide, methsuximide

Risk rating: 2
Severity: Moderate   Onset: Delayed   Likelihood: Suspected

Cause
The cause of this interaction is unknown.

Effect
Primidone levels and pharmacologic effects may be reduced.

Nursing considerations
- Monitor serum primidone levels.
- Adjustments to succinimide dosage may necessitate a change in primidone dose.
- Monitor the patient for increased seizure activity.
- Therapeutic level of primidone is 5 to 12 mcg/ml

---

probenecid ━━━▶◀━━━ aspirin
Probalan   Bayer, Ecotrin

Risk rating: 2
Severity: Moderate   **Onset: Delayed**   **Likelihood: Probable**

Cause
The mechanism of this interaction is unknown. It may stem from altered renal filtration of uric acid.

Effect
Combined use inhibits uricosuric action of both drugs.

Nursing considerations
▧ **ALERT** Typically, combining probenecid and a salicylate is contra-indicated.
■ Occasional use of aspirin at low doses may not interfere with urico-suric action of probenecid.
■ Monitor serum urate level; the usual goal of probenecid therapy is about 6 mg/dl.
▧ **ALERT** Remind the patient to carefully read the labels of OTC medicines because many contain salicylates.
■ If an analgesic or antipyretic is needed during probenecid therapy, suggest acetaminophen.
■ Advise the patient to maintain adequate fluid intake to prevent formation of uric acid kidney stones.

---

probenecid ━━━━▶◀━━━ methotrexate
Probalan   Rheumatrex, Trexall

Risk rating: 1
Severity: Major   **Onset: Rapid**   **Likelihood: Probable**

Cause
Probenecid may impair excretion of methotrexate by the kidneys.

Effect
Methotrexate level, effects, and toxicity may increase.

Nursing considerations
■ Monitor the patient for methotrexate toxicity, including renal failure, neutropenia, leukopenia, thrombocytopenia, increased liver function tests results, and skin ulcers.
■ Check the patient for mouth sores. This may be the first outward appearance of methotrexate toxicity; however, in some patients, bone marrow suppression coincides with or precedes mouth sores.
■ Notify the patient if signs of toxicity appear; the methotrexate dose may need to be reduced.

probenecid ▶◀ zidovudine
Probalan   AZT, Retrovir

Risk rating: 2
Severity: Moderate   **Onset: Delayed**   **Likelihood: Suspected**

Cause
Zidovudine glucuronidation decreases and level increases.

Effect
Risk of rash increases, possibly with malaise, myalgia, and fever.

Nursing considerations
- Monitor the patient for rash.
- Zidovudine dosage interval may need to be doubled.
- Tell the patient to report muscle aches, fever, and general illness.

procainamide ▶◀ amiodarone
Procanbid, Pronestyl   Cordarone, Pacerone

Risk rating: 2
Severity: Moderate   **Onset: Rapid**   **Likelihood: Probable**

Cause
The mechanism of the interaction is unknown.

Effect
Amiodarone may increase serum procainamide levels.

Nursing considerations
- Monitor serum procainamide levels after starting or adjusting amiodarone dosages.
- Some patients may experience severe nausea and transient hypotension, necessitating a reduction in procainamide dosage.

procainamide ▶◀ cimetidine
Procanbid, Pronestyl   Tagamet

Risk rating: 2
Severity: Moderate   **Onset: Rapid**   **Likelihood: Established**

Cause
Cimetidine may reduce procainamide renal clearance.

Effect
Procainamide level and risk of toxicity may increase.

Nursing considerations
⚡ **ALERT** Avoid combined use if possible.
- Monitor levels of procainamide and its active metabolite N-acetylprocainamide (NAPA). Therapeutic range for procainamide is 4 to 8 mcg/ml; therapeutic level of NAPA is 10 to 30 mcg/ml.
- Monitor the patient for increased adverse effects, including severe hypotension, widening QRS complex, arrhythmias, seizures, oliguria, confusion, lethargy, nausea, and vomiting.
- Procainamide dosage may need adjustment.
- H_2-receptor antagonists other than cimetidine may interact. If you suspect an interaction, consult the prescriber or pharmacist.

---

procainamide ➤◀ macrolide antibiotics
Procanbid, Pronestyl   azithromycin, clarithromycin, erythromycin, telithromycin

---

Risk rating: 1
Severity: Major   **Onset: Delayed**   **Likelihood: Suspected**

Cause
An additive increase in the QT interval is seen when administering macrolide antibiotics and antiarrhythmic agents.

Effect
The risk of life-threatening cardiac arrhythmias, including torsades de pointes is increased.

Nursing considerations
⚡ **ALERT** Monitor the patient for prolonged QT interval and torsades de pointes.
- This interaction may be more likely with telithromycin; avoid administering with antiarrhythmics.
- This interaction appears to be dose related.
- Instruct the patient to let the prescriber know if he experiences dizziness, palpitations, or light-headedness.
- The QT interval returns to normal within 3 days of stopping the medications.

procainamide ━━━▶◀━━━ quinolones

Procanbid, Pronestyl

gatifloxacin, levofloxacin,
moxifloxacin, sparfloxacin

Risk rating: 1
Severity: **Major**   Onset: **Delayed**   Likelihood: **Suspected**

Cause
The mechanism of this interaction is unknown.

Effect
Risk of life-threatening arrhythmias, including torsades de pointes,
increases.

Nursing considerations
⚠ ALERT Giving sparfloxacin with antiarrhythmics such as procainamide
is contraindicated.
▪ Quinolones that aren't metabolized by CYP3A4 isoenzymes or that
don't prolong the QT interval may be given with antiarrhythmics.
▪ Avoid giving class IA or class III antiarrhythmics with gatifloxacin,
levofloxacin, and moxifloxacin.
▪ Monitor ECG for prolonged QTc interval.
▪ Tell the patient to report a rapid heartbeat, shortness of breath,
dizziness, fainting, and chest pain.

procainamide ━━━▶◀━━━ quinolones

Procanbid, Pronestyl

ciprofloxacin, levofloxacin,
ofloxacin

Risk rating: 2
Severity: **Moderate**   Onset: **Rapid**   Likelihood: **Suspected**

Cause
Tubular secretion of procainamide decreases.

Effect
Procainamide levels may increase.

Nursing considerations
▪ Monitor levels of procainamide and its active metabolite NAPA.
Therapeutic range for procainamide is 4 to 8 mcg/ml; therapeutic
level of NAPA is 10 to 30 mcg/ml.
▪ Monitor the patient for increased adverse effects, including severe
hypotension, widening QRS complex, arrhythmias, seizures, oliguria,
confusion, lethargy, nausea, and vomiting.
▪ Procainamide dosage may need adjustment.

procainamide ◣▶ vardenafil
Procanbid, Pronestyl   Levitra

Risk rating: 1
Severity: Major   **Onset: Rapid**   **Likelihood: Suspected**

Cause
The mechanism of this interaction is unknown.

Effect
QTc interval may be prolonged, particularly in patients with previous QT-interval prolongation and those taking certain antiarrhythmics (such as procainamide), increasing the risk of such life-threatening arrhythmias as torsades de pointes.

Nursing considerations
❧ ALERT Avoid use of vardenafil with a class IA or class III antiarrhythmics.
- Monitor ECG before and periodically after the patient starts vardenafil.
- Urge the patient to report light-headedness, faintness, palpitations, and chest pain or pressure while taking vardenafil.
- To reduce risk of adverse effects, patients age 65 and older should start with 5 mg of vardenafil, half the usual starting dose.

procainamide ▶◣ ziprasidone
Procanbid, Pronestyl   Geodon

Risk rating: 1
Severity: Major   **Onset: Delayed**   **Likelihood: Suspected**

Cause
The mechanism of this interaction is unknown.

Effect
Risk of life-threatening arrhythmias, including torsades de pointes, increases.

Nursing considerations
❧ ALERT Use of ziprasidone with certain antiarrhythmics is contraindicated.
- Monitor the patient for other risk factors of torsades de points, including bradycardia, hypokalemia, and hypomagnesemia.
- Ask the patient if he or anyone in his family has a history of prolonged QT interval or arrhythmias.
- Monitor the patient for bradycardia.
- Measure the QTc interval at baselines and throughout therapy.

procarbazine ━━►◄━━ alcohol
Matulane

Risk rating: 3
Severity: Minor   **Onset: Rapid**   **Likelihood: Suspected**

Cause
The mechanism of this interaction is unknown.

Effect
Flushing of the face may occur.

Nursing considerations
- Discourage the patient from ingesting alcohol if he's taking procarbazine.
- The flushing lasts a short while.
- Warn the patient about this interaction.

prochlorperazine ━━►◄━━ alcohol
Compazine

Risk rating: 2
Severity: Moderate   **Onset: Rapid**   **Likelihood: Probable**

Cause
The mechanism of this interaction is unknown. It may be that these substances produce CNS depression by working on different sites in the brain. Also, alcohol may lower resistance to neurotoxic effects of phenothiazines, such as prochlorperazine.

Effect
CNS depression may increase.

Nursing considerations
- Watch for extrapyramidal reactions, such as dystonic reactions, acute akathisia, and restlessness.
- If the patient takes a phenothiazine, warn that alcohol may worsen CNS depression and impair psychomotor skills.
- Discourage the patient from drinking alcohol when taking a phenothiazine.

prochlorperazine ━━▶◀━━ dofetilide
Compazine   Tikosyn

Risk rating: 1
Severity: Major   **Onset: Rapid**   **Likelihood: Suspected**

Cause
Dofetilide renal elimination may be inhibited.

Effect
Dofetilide level and risk of ventricular arrhythmias, including torsades de pointes, may increase.

Nursing considerations
▪ **ALERT** Combined use of these drugs is contraindicated.
▪ Monitor ECG for prolonged QTc interval and ventricular arrhythmias.
▪ Monitor renal function and QTc interval every 3 months during dofetilide therapy.
▪ Consult the prescriber or pharmacist for alternative to prochlorperazine to control nausea, vomiting, and psychoses.

procyclidine ━━━▶◀━━━ haloperidol
Kemadrin   Haldol

Risk rating: 2
Severity: Moderate   **Onset: Delayed**   **Likelihood: Suspected**

Cause
The mechanism of this interaction is unknown. It may involve central cholinergic pathways rather than a true pharmacokinetic interaction.

Effect
Effects may vary and include decreased haloperidol level, worsened schizophrenic symptoms, and development of tardive dyskinesia.

Nursing considerations
▪ **ALERT** If the patient takes haloperidol, avoid anticholinergics such as procyclidine, if possible.
▪ Watch for signs of worsening schizophrenia, including delusions, hallucinations, disorganized speech or behavior, inappropriate affect, and abnormal psychomotor activity.
▪ Watch for development of tardive dyskinesia—involuntary abnormal repetitive movements, including lip smacking, cheek puffing, chewing motions, tongue thrusting, finger flicking, and trunk twisting.

- Consult the prescriber if adverse effects occur; procyclidine may need to be stopped, or haloperidol dosage may need adjustment.
- Other anticholinergics may interact with haloperidol. If you suspect an interaction, consult the prescriber or pharmacist.

---

procyclidine ➤◄ phenothiazines

Kemadrin

chlorpromazine, per-
phenazine, thioridazine

Risk rating: 2
Severity: Moderate   **Onset: Delayed**   **Likelihood: Suspected**

Cause
Anticholinergics such as procyclidine may antagonize phenothiazines. Also, phenothiazine metabolism may increase.

Effect
Phenothiazine efficacy may decrease.

Nursing considerations
- Data regarding this interaction conflict.
- Monitor the patient for decreased phenothiazine efficacy.
- The phenothiazine dosage may need adjustment.
- Anticholinergic side effects may increase.
- Monitor the patient for adynamic ileus, hyperpyrexia, hypoglycemia, and neurologic changes.

---

propafenone ➤◄ beta-adrenergic blockers

Rythmol

metoprolol, propranolol

Risk rating: 2
Severity: Moderate   **Onset: Rapid**   **Likelihood: Probable**

Cause
Propafenone inhibits first-pass metabolism of certain beta-adrenergic blockers and reduces their systemic clearance.

Effect
Beta-adrenergic blocker effects may increase.

Nursing considerations
- Monitor blood pressure, pulse, and cardiac complaints.
- Notify the prescriber about abnormally low blood pressure or change in heart rate; beta-adrenergic dosage may be decreased.
- If the patient takes metoprolol and propafenone, tell him to promptly report nightmares or other CNS complaints.
- To minimize effects of orthostatic hypotension, tell the patient to change positions slowly.

propafenone ━━━►◄━━━ digoxin
Rythmol   Lanoxin

Risk rating: 1
Severity: Major   **Onset: Delayed**   **Likelihood: Established**

Cause
Exact cause of this interaction is unknown; decreased digoxin distribution and renal and nonrenal clearance of digoxin may be involved.

Effect
Digoxin level and risk of toxicity may increase.

Nursing considerations
- Monitor digoxin level. Therapeutic range is 0.8 to 2 nanograms/ml.
- Monitor ECG for signs of digoxin toxicity: arrhythmias (such as bradycardia and AV blocks), ventricular ectopy, and shortened QTc interval.
- Watch for other signs of digoxin toxicity, including lethargy, drowsiness, confusion, hallucinations, headaches, syncope, visual disturbances, nausea, anorexia, failure to thrive, vomiting, and diarrhea.
- Digoxin dosage may need adjustment if propafenone is started or stopped.

propafenone ━━━►◄━━━ fluoxetine
Rythmol   Prozac

Risk rating: 2
Severity: Moderate   **Onset: Delayed**   **Likelihood: Suspected**

Cause
Certain serotonin reuptake inhibitors such as fluoxetine may inhibit CYP2D6 metabolism of propafenone.

Effect
Serum propafenone level and risk of adverse effects may increase.

Nursing considerations
- Monitor cardiac function closely during combined therapy.
- Citalopram doesn't inhibit CYP2D6 and may be a safer choice than fluoxetine.
- Tell the patient to promptly report dizziness, drowsiness, ataxia, tremor, palpitations, chest pain, edema, dyspnea, and other new symptoms.

propafenone ▶◀ mexiletine
Rythmol   Mexitil

Risk rating: 2
Severity: Moderate   Onset: Delayed   Likelihood: Established

Cause
Propafenone inhibits CYP2D6 metabolism of mexiletine.

Effect
Mexiletine levels and risk of adverse effects increase.

Nursing considerations
■ Monitor blood levels of mexiletine when propafenone therapy is
started or stopped.
■ If both medications are started together, carefully titrate the dose of
both medications.
■ Monitor ECG for new or increased arrhythmias.
■ Instruct the patient to notify the prescriber if he experiences chest
pain, palpitations, or angina.

propafenone ▶◀ rifampin
Rythmol   Rifadin, Rimactane

Risk rating: 2
Severity: Moderate   Onset: Delayed   Likelihood: Probable

Cause
Rifampin may enhance hepatic metabolism of propafenone.

Effect
Propafenone clearance is increased and effects may decrease.

Nursing considerations
■ Consult the prescriber about alternative anti-infective drugs for
patients stabilized on propafenone.
■ If this combination can't be avoided, monitor propafenone level and
watch for loss of effect.
■ Propafenone dosage may need adjustment while the patient takes
rifampin.
■ This effect was seen less readily with I.V. propafenone than with the
oral form.

propafenone ➤◀ ritonavir
Rythmol   Norvir

Risk rating: 1
Severity: Major   **Onset: Delayed**   **Likelihood: Suspected**

Cause
Ritonavir may inhibit CYP2D6 metabolism of propafenone.

Effect
Propafenone level and risk of toxicity may increase.

Nursing considerations
⚠ **ALERT** Combined use of these drugs is contraindicated.
■ Monitor the patient for new or worsened arrhythmias, including an increase in premature ventricular contractions, ventricular tachycardia, ventricular fibrillation, and torsades de pointes.
■ Monitor ECG for AV block and QTc interval prolongation.
■ Advise the patient to report a rapid heartbeat, shortness of breath, dizziness or fainting, and chest pain.

propoxyphene ➤◀ carbamazepine
Darvon   Carbatrol, Epitol, Equetro,
                           Tegretol

Risk rating: 2
Severity: Moderate   **Onset: Rapid**   **Likelihood: Suspected**

Cause
Hepatic metabolism of carbamazepine is inhibited, decreasing drug clearance.

Effect
Carbamazepine level and risk of toxicity may increase.

Nursing considerations
⚠ **ALERT** Avoid combined use if possible.
■ Consult the prescriber or pharmacist about alternative analgesics.
■ Monitor carbamazepine level; therapeutic range is 4 to 12 mcg/ml.
■ Monitor the patient for signs of carbamazepine toxicity, including dizziness, ataxia, respiratory depression, tachycardia, arrhythmias, blood pressure changes, impaired consciousness, abnormal reflexes, nystagmus, seizures, nausea, vomiting, and urine retention.
■ Carbamazepine dosage may need adjustment.

propranolol ━━━►◄━━━ aluminum salts
Inderal

aluminum carbonate,
aluminum hydroxide,
aluminum phosphate, kaolin

Risk rating: 3
Severity: Minor   **Onset: Rapid**   **Likelihood: Suspected**

Cause
Rate of gastric emptying is decreased, leading to reduced bioavailability of atenolol.

Effect
Pharmacologic effects of beta-adrenergic blockers such as propranolol may be decreased.

Nursing considerations
■ Separate administration of aluminium salts and beta-adrenergic blockers by at least 2 hours.
■ Monitor the patient's blood pressure and heart rate.
■ Tell the patient to notify the prescriber if he notices an increase in his heart rate.

propranolol ━━━►◄━━━ aspirin
Inderal

Bayer, Ecotrin

Risk rating: 2
Severity: Moderate   **Onset: Rapid**   **Likelihood: Suspected**

Cause
Salicylates inhibit synthesis of prostaglandins, which propranolol and other beta-adrenergic blockers need to reduce blood pressure. In patients with heart failure, the mechanism of this interaction is unknown.

Effect
Beta-adrenergic blocker effects decrease.

Nursing considerations
■ Watch closely for signs of heart failure and hypertension, and notify the provider if they occur.
■ Consult the prescriber about a different antihypertensive or antiplatelet drug.
■ Other beta-adrenergic blockers may interact with salicylates. If you suspect an interaction, consult the prescriber or pharmacist.
■ Explain signs and symptoms of heart failure, and tell the patient when to contact the prescriber.

propranolol ━━━━►◄━━━━ cimetidine
Inderal   Tagamet

Risk rating: 2
Severity: Moderate   **Onset: Rapid**   **Likelihood: Probable**

Cause
By inhibiting CYP450, cimetidine reduces first-pass metabolism of certain beta-adrenergic blockers such as propranolol.

Effect
Clearance of propranolol is decreased, increasing its action.

Nursing considerations
■ Monitor the patient for severe bradycardia and hypotension.
■ If interaction occurs, notify the prescriber; beta-adrenergic blocker dosage may need to be decreased.
■ Teach the patient to monitor pulse rate. If it's significantly lower than usual, tell him to withhold beta-adrenergic blocker and to contact his prescriber.
■ Instruct the patient to change positions slowly to reduce effects of orthostatic hypotension.
■ Other beta-adrenergic blockers may interact with cimetidine. If you suspect an interaction, consult the prescriber or pharmacist.

propranolol ━━━━►◄━━━━ clonidine
Inderal   Catapres

Risk rating: 1
Severity: Major   **Onset: Delayed**   **Likelihood: Suspected**

Cause
The mechanism of this interaction is unclear.

Effect
Potentially life-threatening hypertension may occur.

Nursing considerations
■ Life-threatening hypertension may occur after simultaneously stopping clonidine and a beta-adrenergic blocker such as propanolol.
■ It's unknown whether hypertension is caused by an interaction or withdrawal syndrome linked to each drug.
■ Closely monitor blood pressure after starting or stopping the propranolol or clonidine.
■ When stopping combined therapy, gradually withdraw propranolol first to minimize adverse reactions.

propranolol ━━━▶◀━━━ digoxin
Inderal   Lanoxin

Risk rating: 2
Severity: Moderate   **Onset: Rapid**   **Likelihood: Probable**

Cause
Propranolol increases digoxin bioavailability. Renal excretion of digoxin may be decreased and additive depression of myocardial conduction may occur.

Effect
Digoxin level may increase and risk of toxicity may occur. Synergistic bradycardia may occur.

Nursing considerations
◪ **ALERT** Carefully monitor patients receiving propranolol and digoxin for bradycardia.
- Monitor digoxin level. Therapeutic range is 0.8 to 2 nanograms/ml
- Watch for evidence of digoxin toxicity: arrhythmias (bradycardia, AV block, and ventricular ectopy), lethargy, drowsiness, confusion, hallucinations, headaches, syncope, visual disturbances, nausea, anorexia, vomiting, and diarrhea
- Digoxin dosage may need to be decreased.
- Patients with higher serum digoxin levels have an increased risk of toxicity.

propranolol ━━━▶◀━━━ epinephrine
Inderal   Adrenalin

Risk rating: 1
Severity: Major   **Onset: Rapid**   **Likelihood: Established**

Cause
Alpha-receptor effects of epinephrine supersede the effects of nonselective beta-adrenergic blockers, such as propranolol, increasing vascular resistance.

Effect
Initial marked hypertensive effect is followed by reflex bradycardia.

Nursing considerations
◪ **ALERT** Three days before planned use of epinephrine, stop the beta-adrenergic blocker. Or, if possible, don't use epinephrine.
- Monitor blood pressure and pulse. If interaction occurs, give I.V. chlorpromazine, hydralazine, aminophylline, or atropine, if needed.

- Explain the risks of this interaction and tell the patient to carry medical identification at all times.
- Other beta-adrenergic blockers may interact with epinephrine. If you suspect an interaction, consult the prescriber or pharmacist.

propranolol ▶◀ ergot derivatives
Inderal   dihydroergotamine, ergotamine

Risk rating: 2
Severity: Moderate   **Onset: Delayed**   **Likelihood: Suspected**

Cause
Vasoconstriction and blockade of peripheral beta$_2$ receptors allows unopposed ergot action.

Effect
Vasoconstrictive effects of ergot derivatives increase, causing peripheral ischemia, cold extremities, and possible gangrene.

Nursing considerations
- Watch for evidence of peripheral ischemia.
- If needed, stop propranolol and adjust ergot derivative.
- Other ergot derivatives may interact with propranolol and other beta-adrenergic blockers. If you suspect an interaction, consult the prescriber or pharmacist.

propranolol ▶◀ hydralazine
Inderal   Apresoline

Risk rating: 2
Severity: Moderate   **Onset: Rapid**   **Likelihood: Probable**

Cause
Hydralazine may cause transient increase in visceral blood flow and decreased first-pass hepatic metabolism of some oral beta-adrenergic blockers such as propranolol.

Effect
Effects of both drugs may increase.

Nursing considerations
- Monitor blood pressure regularly and tailor dosages of both drugs to the patient's response.
- With propranolol, interaction involves only oral, immediate-release form and not extended-release or I.V. drug.

■ Other beta-adrenergic blockers may interact with hydralazine. If you suspect an interaction, consult the prescriber or pharmacist.
■ Explain that both drugs can affect blood pressure. Urge the patient to report evidence of hypotension, such as light-headedness or dizziness when changing positions.

---

propranolol ━━━▶◀━━━ lidocaine
Inderal   Xylocaine

Risk rating: 2
Severity: Moderate   Onset: Rapid   Likelihood: Established

Cause
Propranolol and other beta-adrenergic blockers reduce hepatic metabolism of lidocaine.

Effect
Lidocaine level and risk of toxicity may increase.

Nursing considerations
■ Check for normal therapeutic level of lidocaine, which is 2 to 5 mcg/ml.
■ Monitor the patient closely for evidence of lidocaine toxicity, including dizziness, somnolence, confusion, paresthesias, and seizures.
■ Slow the I.V. bolus rate to decrease the risk of high peak level and toxic reaction.
■ Explain the warning signs of toxicity to the patient and his family, and tell them to contact the prescriber if they have concerns.

---

propranolol ━━━▶◀━━━ NSAIDs
Inderal   ibuprofen, indomethacin,
                               naproxen, piroxicam

Risk rating: 2
Severity: Moderate   Onset: Delayed   Likelihood: Probable

Cause
NSAIDs may inhibit renal prostaglandin synthesis, allowing pressor systems to be unopposed.

Effect
Propranolol and other beta-adrenergic blockers may not be able to lower blood pressure.

Nursing considerations
■ Avoid using these drugs together if possible.
■ Monitor blood pressure and related signs and symptoms of hypertension closely.

■ Talk with the prescriber about ways to minimize interaction, such as adjusting beta-adrenergic blocker dosage or switching to sulindac as the NSAID.
■ Explain the risks of using these drugs together and teach the patient how to monitor his blood pressure.
■ Other NSAIDs may interact with beta-adrenergic blockers. If you suspect an interaction, consult the prescriber or pharmacist.

---

propranolol ➤◀ phenothiazines
Inderal   chlorpromazine, thioridazine

Risk rating: 1
Severity: Major   **Onset: Delayed**   **Likelihood: Probable**

Cause
Chlorpromazine may inhibit first-pass hepatic metabolism of propranolol. Propranolol inhibits thioridazine metabolism.

Effect
Effects of both drugs and the risk of serious adverse reactions may increase.

Nursing considerations
⚑ ALERT Use of thioridazine with propranolol is contraindicated.
■ Assess the patient for fatigue, lethargy, dizziness, nausea, heart failure, and agranulocytosis, all adverse reactions to propranolol.
■ Educate the patient and his family about the risk of drug interactions.
■ Beta-adrenergic blockers other than propranolol may interact with phenothiazines. If you suspect an interaction, consult the prescriber or pharmacist.

---

propranolol ➤◀ prazosin
Inderal   Minipress

Risk rating: 2
Severity: Moderate   **Onset: Rapid**   **Likelihood: Probable**

Cause
The mechanism of this interaction is unknown.

Effect
Effect of these drugs on orthostatic hypotension is increased.

Nursing considerations
■ Assess the patient's lying, sitting, and standing blood pressures closely, especially when concurrent therapy starts.
■ Adjust dosages of either drug based on patient effects.

■ To minimize effects of orthostatic hypotension, teach the patient to change positions slowly.
■ Interaction is confirmed only with propranolol but may occur with other beta-adrenergic blockers as well.

---

propranolol ➤◄ propafenone
Inderal   Rythmol

Risk rating: 2
Severity: Moderate   Onset: Rapid   Likelihood: Probable

Cause
Propafenone inhibits first-pass metabolism of certain beta-adrenergic blockers, such as propranolol, and reduces their systemic clearance.

Effect
Beta-adrenergic blocker effects may be increased.

Nursing considerations
■ Monitor blood pressure, pulse, and cardiac complaints.
■ Notify the prescriber about abnormally low blood pressure or change in heart rate; beta-adrenergic blocker dosage may be decreased.
■ To minimize effects of orthostatic hypotension, tell the patient to change positions slowly.

---

propranolol ➤◄ quinidine
Inderal

Risk rating: 2
Severity: Moderate   Onset: Rapid   Likelihood: Suspected

Cause
Quinidine may inhibit metabolism of certain beta-adrenergic blockers, such as propranolol, in patients who are extensive metabolizers of debrisoquin.

Effect
Beta-adrenergic blocker effects may be increased.

Nursing considerations
■ Monitor pulse and blood pressure more often during combined use.
■ If pulse slows or blood pressure falls, consult the prescriber. Beta-adrenergic blocker dosage may need to be decreased.
■ Teach the patient how to check blood pressure and pulse rate; tell him to do so regularly.

propranolol ━━▶◀━━ rifampin
Inderal   Rifadin, Rimactane

Risk rating: 2
Severity: Moderate   Onset: Delayed   Likelihood: Suspected

Cause
Rifampin increases hepatic metabolism of beta-adrenergic blockers such as propranolol.

Effect
Beta-adrenergic blocker effects are reduced.

Nursing considerations
■ Monitor blood pressure and heart rate closely to assess beta-adrenergic blocker efficacy.
■ If beta-adrenergic blocker effects are decreased, consult the prescriber; dosage may need to be increased.
■ Teach the patient how to monitor blood pressure and heart rate and when to contact the prescriber.
■ Other beta-adrenergic blockers may interact with rifampin. If you suspect an interaction, consult the prescriber or pharmacist.

propranolol ━━▶◀━━ theophyllines
Inderal   aminophylline, theophylline

Risk rating: 2
Severity: Moderate   Onset: Rapid   Likelihood: Probable

Cause
Theophylline clearance may be reduced up to 50%.

Effect
Theophylline efficacy may decrease.

Nursing considerations
■ Watch for decreased theophylline efficacy.
■ Monitor serum theophylline level closely and notify the prescriber about subtherapeutic level. Therapeutic range for theophylline is 10 to 20 mcg/ml for adults and 5 to 15 mcg/ml for children.
■ Selective beta-adrenergic blockers may be preferred for patients who take theophylline, but interaction still occurs with high doses of beta-adrenergic blockers.
■ Other beta-adrenergic blockers may interact with theophyllines. If you suspect an interaction, consult the prescriber or pharmacist.

propranolol ━━━▶◀━━━ verapamil
Inderal   Calan

Risk rating: 1
Severity: Major   **Onset: Rapid**   **Likelihood: Probable**

Cause
Verapamil may inhibit metabolism of beta-adrenergic blockers such as propranolol.

Effect
Effects of both drugs may be increased.

Nursing considerations
■ Combination therapy is common in patients with hypertension and unstable angina.
🔔 **ALERT** Giving these drugs together increases risk of adverse effects, including heart failure, conduction disturbances, arrhythmias, and hypotension.
■ Assess the patient for increased risk of adverse effects, including left ventricular dysfunction and AV conduction defects.
■ Risk of interaction is greater when drugs are given I.V.
■ Monitor cardiac function.
■ Dosages of both drugs may need to be decreased.

protriptyline ━━━▶◀━━━ fluoxetine
Vivactil   Prozac, Sarafem

Risk rating: 2
Severity: Moderate   **Onset: Delayed**   **Likelihood: Probable**

Cause
Fluoxetine may inhibit hepatic metabolism of tricyclic antidepressants (TCAs), such as protriptyline.

Effect
Serum TCA level and toxicity may increase.

Nursing considerations
■ Monitor TCA level; watch for evidence of toxicity, such as increased anticholinergic effects, delirium, dizziness, drowsiness, and psychosis.
■ If TCA is started when the patient already takes fluoxetine, TCA dosage may need to be decreased by up to 75% to avoid interaction.
■ Other TCAs may interact with fluoxetine. If you suspect an interaction, consult the prescriber or pharmacist.

protriptyline ➤◄ sympathomimetics
Vivactil

epinephrine, norepinephrine, phenylephrine

Risk rating: 2
Severity: Moderate   Onset: Rapid   Likelihood: Established

Cause
Tricyclic antidepressants (TCAs), such as protriptyline, increase the effects of direct-acting sympathomimetics and decrease the effects of indirect-acting sympathomimetics.

Effect
When sympathomimetic effects increase, the risk of hypertension and arrhythmias increases. When sympathomimetic effects decrease, blood pressure control decreases.

Nursing considerations
■ If possible, avoid using these drugs together.
■ Watch the patient closely for hypertension and heart rhythm changes; they may warrant reduction of sympathomimetic dosage.
■ If the patient takes a mixed-acting sympathomimetic, watch for negative effects; dosage may need to be altered.
■ Other TCAs and sympathomimetics may interact. If you suspect an interaction, consult the prescriber or pharmacist.

pseudoephedrine ➤◄ MAO inhibitors
Sudafed

phenelzine, tranylcypromine

Risk rating: 1
Severity: Major   Onset: Rapid   Likelihood: Established

Cause
When MAO is inhibited, norepinephrine accumulates and is released by indirect-acting sympathomimetics, such as pseudoephedrine, increasing the pressor response at receptor sites.

Effect
Risk of severe headaches, hypertension, high fever, and hypertensive crisis increases.

Nursing considerations
■ Avoid giving indirect-acting sympathomimetic with MAO inhibitor.
◪ ALERT Warn the patient that OTC medicines such as decongestants may cause this interaction.

pyridostigmine ▶◀ corticosteroids

Mestinon

corticotropin, cortisone, hydrocortisone, methylprednisolone,
prednisone

Risk rating: 1
Severity: Major   **Onset: Delayed**   **Likelihood: Probable**

Cause
In myasthenia gravis, corticosteroids antagonize cholinesterase inhibitors,
such as pyridostigmine, by an unknown mechanism.

Effect
The patient may develop severe muscular depression refractory to
cholinesterase inhibitors.

Nursing considerations
- Corticosteroids may have long-term benefits in myasthenia gravis.
- Combined therapy may be attempted under strict supervision.
- In myasthenia gravis, monitor the patient for severe muscle
deterioration.

⚠ ALERT Be prepared to provide respiratory support and mechanical
ventilation if needed.

- Consult the prescriber or pharmacist about safe corticosteroid
delivery to maximize improvement in muscle strength.

pyridoxine ▶◀ levodopa
(vitamin B$_6$)

Aminoxin

Larodopa

Risk rating: 2
Severity: Moderate   **Onset: Rapid**   **Likelihood: Established**

Cause
Pyridoxine increases peripheral metabolism of levodopa, decreasing
level available for penetration into the CNS.

Effect
Pyridoxine reduces levodopa efficacy in Parkinson disease.

Nursing considerations
- Avoid combined use of pyridoxine and levodopa in patients taking
levodopa alone.
- Watch for recurring or worsening Parkinson symptoms: increased
tremors, muscle rigidity, bradykinesia (slowing of voluntary movement), shuffling gait, loss of facial expression, speech disturbances,
and drooling.

■ Advise the patient and caregivers that multivitamins, fortified cereals, and certain OTC drugs may contain pyridoxine.
⚠ ALERT The effect of pyridoxine is minimal or negligible in patients taking levodopa-carbidopa combination products.

---

quazepam ▪▪▪▪▶◀ azole antifungals
Doral   fluconazole, itraconazole,
                           ketoconazole

Risk rating: 2
Severity: Moderate   Onset: Delayed   Likelihood: Established

Cause
Azole antifungals decrease CYP3A4 metabolism of certain benzodiazepines such as quazepam.

Effect
Benzodiazepine effects are increased and prolonged, which may cause CNS depression and psychomotor impairment.

Nursing considerations
■ Various benzodiazepine–azole antifungal combinations may interact. If you suspect an interaction, consult the prescriber or pharmacist.
■ If the patient takes fluconazole, consult the prescriber about giving a lower benzodiazepine dose or a drug not metabolized by CYP3A4, such as temazepam or lorazepam.
■ Caution that the effects of this interaction may last several days after stopping the azole antifungal.
■ Explain that taking these drugs together may increase sedative effects; tell the patient to report such effects promptly.

---

quetiapine ▪▪▪▪▶◀ phenytoin
Seroquel   Dilantin

Risk rating: 2
Severity: Moderate   Onset: Delayed   Likelihood: Suspected

Cause
Quetiapine metabolism increases.

Effect
Pharmacologic response to quetiapine may decrease.

Nursing considerations
■ Monitor the patient for loss of symptom control for bipolar disorder or schizophrenia.

- The dose of quetiapine may need to be changed when starting, stopping, or changing the dose of phenytoin.
- Tell the patient that, although no serious side effects have been noted from this interaction, he should report unusual or bothersome adverse effects to the prescriber.

---

quinidine ➤◄ amiloride
Midamor

Risk rating: 1
Severity: Major   **Onset: Delayed**   **Likelihood: Suspected**

Cause
This interaction may result from a synergistic increase in myocardial sodium channel blockade.

Effect
Quinidine effects may be reversed, contributing to a pro-arrhythmic state.

Nursing considerations
- If possible, avoid combining quinidine and amiloride.
- If used together, monitor ECG closely.
- Therapeutic range of quinidine is 2 to 6 mcg/ml. More specific assays have levels of less than 1 mcg/ml.
- Monitor the patient for loss of arrhythmia control.
- Advise the patient to report palpitations, shortness of breath, dizziness or fainting, and chest pain.

---

quinidine ➤◄ amiodarone
Cordarone, Pacerone

Risk rating: 1
Severity: Major   **Onset: Rapid**   **Likelihood: Probable**

Cause
The mechanism of this interaction is unknown.

Effect
Risk of potentially fatal arrhythmias increases.

Nursing considerations
- If possible, avoid combining quinidine and amiodarone.
- If taken together, monitor ECG closely for prolonged QTc interval, increasing ventricular ectopy, and torsades de pointes.

■ Therapeutic range of quinidine is 2 to 6 mcg/ml. More specific assays have levels of less than 1 mcg/ml.

■ Monitor the patient for signs and symptoms of quinidine toxicity, including GI irritation, arrhythmias, hypotension, vertigo, and rash.

■ Advise the patient to report palpitations, shortness of breath, dizziness or fainting, and chest pain.

■ If amiodarone is stopped in a patient stabilized on combined therapy, quinidine dosage may need to be increased.

---

quinidine ▶◀ antacids
aluminum hydroxide,
aluminum-magnesium
hydroxide, magnesium
hydroxide, sodium bicarbonate

Risk rating: 2
Severity: Moderate   Onset: Delayed   Likelihood: Suspected

Cause
Interaction may result from a pH-related decrease in urinary quinidine excretion.

Effect
Quinidine level and risk of toxicity may increase.

Nursing considerations
■ Monitor quinidine level closely during combined use.

■ Therapeutic range of quinidine is 2 to 6 mcg/ml. More specific assays have levels of less than 1 mcg/ml.

■ Monitor the patient for evidence of quinidine toxicity, including GI irritation, arrhythmias, hypotension, vertigo, and rash.

■ Advise the patient to report palpitations, shortness of breath, dizziness or fainting, and chest pain.

■ Aluminum-only antacid may be a suitable alternative.

---

quinidine ▶◀ aripiprazole
Abilify

Risk rating: 2
Severity: Moderate   Onset: Delayed   Likelihood: Suspected

Cause
Quinidine may inhibit CYP3A4 metabolism of aripiprazole.

Effect
Plasma concentrations of aripiprazole may be increased, increasing pharmacologic and adverse effects.

Nursing considerations
■ When quinidine is administered with aripiprazole, reduce the dose of aripiprazole by 50%.
■ The dose of aripiprazole will need to be increased when quinidine is discontinued.
■ Instruct the patient to notify the prescriber of increased adverse effects, such as anxiety, insomnia, nausea, vomiting, and flu-like symptoms.

quinidine ◄ azole antifungals
itraconazole, voriconazole

Risk rating: 1
Severity: Major   **Onset: Delayed**   **Likelihood: Probable**

Cause
Azole antifungals may inhibit the CYP3A4 metabolism and renal excretion of quinidine.

Effect
Increased quinidine level may cause serious arrhythmias.

Nursing considerations
■ **ALERT** Use of quinidine with itraconazole is contraindicated.
■ **ALERT** Monitor the patient for evidence of quinidine toxicity, including GI irritation, arrhythmias, hypotension, vertigo, and rash.
■ Advise the patient to report palpitations, shortness of breath, dizziness or fainting, and chest pain.

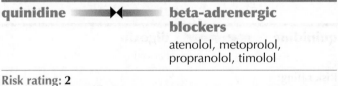

quinidine ◄ beta-adrenergic blockers
atenolol, metoprolol, propranolol, timolol

Risk rating: 2
Severity: Moderate   **Onset: Rapid**   **Likelihood: Suspected**

Cause
Quinidine may inhibit metabolism of certain beta-adrenergic blockers in patients who are extensive metabolizers of debrisoquin.

Effect
Beta-adrenergic blocker effects may increase.

Nursing considerations
■ Monitor pulse and blood pressure more often during combined use.

■ If pulse slows or blood pressure falls, consult the prescriber. Beta-adrenergic blocker dosage may need to be decreased.
■ Teach the patient how to check blood pressure and pulse rate; tell him to do so regularly.
■ If the patient uses timolol eye drops, warn about possible systemic effects, including slow pulse and low blood pressure. Urge the patient to notify the prescriber promptly if they occur.

---

quinidine ▶◀ cimetidine
Tagamet

Risk rating: 2
Severity: Moderate   Onset: Delayed   Likelihood: Probable

Cause
Interaction may result from increased quinidine absorption, decreased quinidine metabolism, or both.

Effect
Quinidine effects and risk of toxicity increase.

Nursing considerations
■ If possible, use of quinidine with cimetidine should be avoided.
■ Monitor quinidine level closely; dose may need to be reduced.
■ Therapeutic range of quinidine is 2 to 6 mcg/ml. More specific assays have levels of less than 1 mcg/ml.
⊠ ALERT Monitor the patient for evidence of quinidine toxicity, including GI irritation, arrhythmias, hypotension, vertigo, and rash.
■ Advise the patient to report palpitations, shortness of breath, dizziness or fainting, and chest pain.

---

quinidine ▶◀ digoxin
Lanoxin

Risk rating: 1
Severity: Major   Onset: Delayed   Likelihood: Established

Cause
Total renal and biliary digoxin clearance and distribution decrease.

Effect
Digoxin level and risk of toxicity may increase.

Nursing considerations
■ Monitor digoxin level. Therapeutic range is 0.8 to 2 nanograms/ml.
■ For some patients, digoxin toxicity may occur even within therapeutic range.

■ Watch for evidence of digoxin toxicity, including arrhythmias (such as bradycardia, AV blocks, and ventricular ectopy), lethargy, drowsiness, confusion, hallucinations, headaches, syncope, visual disturbances, nausea, anorexia, vomiting, and diarrhea.
■ Digoxin dosage may need adjustment (up to 50% reduction in some patients) if quinidine is started.

quinidine ➤◀ diltiazem
Cardizem

Risk rating: 2
Severity: Moderate   Onset: Delayed   Likelihood: Suspected

Cause
Hepatic metabolism of quinidine may be inhibited.

Effect
Quinidine effects, including toxic effects, may increase.

Nursing considerations
■ Check serum quinidine level; therapeutic range is 2 to 6 mcg/ml.
■ Monitor ECG for widened QRS complexes, prolonged QT and PR intervals, and ventricular arrhythmias, including torsades de pointes.
■ Watch for evidence of quinidine toxicity: hypotension, seizures, ataxia, anuria, respiratory distress, irritability, and hallucinations.
■ Advise the patient that adverse GI effects, especially diarrhea, may be an indicator of quinidine toxicity. Tell the patient to alert the prescriber.
■ Adjust the quinidine dosage as ordered.

quinidine ➤◀ macrolide antibiotics
azithromycin, clarithromycin, erythromycin, telithromycin

Risk rating: 1
Severity: Major   Onset: Delayed   Likelihood: Suspected

Cause
An additive increase in the QT interval is seen when administering macrolide antibiotics and antiarrhythmic agents, such as quinidine.

Effect
The risk of life-threatening cardiac arrhythmias, including torsades de pointes is increased.

Nursing considerations
⚠ **ALERT** Monitor the patient for prolonged QT interval and torsades de pointes.
- This interaction appears to be dose related.
- Instruct the patient to let the prescriber know if he experiences dizziness, palpitations, or light-headedness.
- The QT interval returns to normal within 3 days of stopping the medications.

---

quinidine ▶◀ phenytoin
Dilantin

Risk rating: 2
Severity: Moderate   **Onset: Delayed**   **Likelihood: Suspected**

Cause
Phenytoin stimulates the hepatic enzyme system, which increases quinidine metabolism.

Effect
Quinidine level decreases.

Nursing considerations
- Monitor quinidine level during combined use.
- Therapeutic range of quinidine is 2 to 6 mcg/ml. More specific assays have levels of less than 1 mcg/ml.
- Monitor the patient for loss of arrhythmia control if phenytoin starts.
- Tell the patient to report palpitations, shortness of breath, dizziness or fainting, and chest pain.
- If the patient's quinidine level is stable on combined therapy, and phenytoin is stopped, monitor the patient for toxicity.
⚠ **ALERT** Quinidine toxicity may cause GI irritation, arrhythmias, hypotension, vertigo, and rash.

---

quinidine ▶◀ protease inhibitors
nelfinavir, ritonavir

Risk rating: 1
Severity: Major   **Onset: Delayed**   **Likelihood: Suspected**

Cause
CYP3A4 metabolism of quinidine may be inhibited.

Effect
Quinidine level and risk of toxicity may increase.

Nursing considerations
■ **ALERT** Use of ritonavir or nelfinavir with quinidine is contraindicated.
■ Monitor ECG for prolonged QT interval and arrhythmias.
■ **ALERT** Quinidine toxicity may cause GI irritation, arrhythmias, hypotension, vertigo, and rash.

---

quinidine ◀▶ quinolones
gatifloxacin, levofloxacin, moxifloxacin, ofloxacin

Risk rating: 1
Severity: Major   **Onset: Delayed**   **Likelihood: Suspected**

Cause
The mechanism of this interaction is unknown.

Effect
Risk of life-threatening arrhythmias, including torsades de pointes, increases.

Nursing considerations
■ **ALERT** Giving sparfloxacin with antiarrhythmics such as quinidine is contraindicated.
■ Quinolones that aren't metabolized by CYP3A4 isoenzymes or that don't prolong the QT interval may be given with antiarrhythmics.
■ Avoid giving class IA or class III antiarrhythmics with gatifloxacin, levofloxacin, and moxifloxacin.
■ Monitor ECG for prolonged QTc interval.
■ Tell the patient to report a rapid heartbeat, shortness of breath, dizziness, fainting, and chest pain.

---

quinidine ◀▶ thioridazine

Risk rating: 1
Severity: Major   **Onset: Delayed**   **Likelihood: Suspected**

Cause
Synergistic or additive prolongation of the QTc interval.

Effect
Risk of life-threatening arrhythmias, including torsades de pointes, increases.

Nursing considerations
■ **ALERT** The use of thioridazine and antiarrhythmic agents together is contraindicated.

- If the patient is receiving thioridazine and quinidine, notify the prescriber immediately.
- Monitor the patient for other risk factors for torsades de points, including bradycardia, hypokalemia, and hypomagnesemia.
- Ask the patient if he or anyone in his family has a history of prolonged QT interval or arrhythmias.
- Monitor the patient for bradycardia.

quinidine ➤◀ verapamil
Calan

Risk rating: 1
Severity: Major   **Onset: Rapid**   **Likelihood: Suspected**

Cause
Verapamil may interfere with quinidine clearance and prolong its half-life.

Effect
Serious cardiac events may result.

Nursing considerations
- Use together only when there are no other alternatives.
- Monitor the patient for hypotension, bradycardia, ventricular tachycardia, and AV block.
- Tell the patient to report diaphoresis, dizziness, fainting, blurred vision, palpitations, shortness of breath, and chest pain.
- Notify the prescriber if arrhythmias occur. One or both drugs may need to be stopped.
- The complications of this interaction may be noticed in a little as 1 day or after as long as 5 months of combined use.

quinidine ➤◀ ziprasidone
Geodon

Risk rating: 1
Severity: Major   **Onset: Delayed**   **Likelihood: Suspected**

Cause
The mechanism of this interaction is unknown.

Effect
Risk of life-threatening arrhythmias, including torsades de pointes, increases.

Nursing considerations
◣ ALERT Use of ziprasidone with certain antiarrhythmics is contraindicated.
- Monitor the patient for other risk factors for torsades de points, including bradycardia, hypokalemia, and hypomagnesemia.
- Ask the patient if he or anyone in his family has a history of prolonged QT interval or arrhythmias.
- Monitor the patient for bradycardia.
- Measure the QTc interval at baselines and throughout therapy.

---

quinine derivatives ━━━━►◄━━━━ ketoconazole
quinidine, quinine   Nizoral

Risk rating: 2
Severity: Moderate   **Onset: Delayed**   **Likelihood: Probable**

Cause
Hepatic CYP3A4 metabolism of quinine derivative is inhibited.

Effect
Quinine derivative level may increase, resulting in toxicity.

Nursing considerations
- When starting or stopping ketoconazole, monitor quinidine level.
- Therapeutic range of quinidine is 2 to 6 mcg/ml. More specific assays have levels of less than 1 mcg/ml.
- Monitor ECG for conduction disturbances, prolonged QTc interval, and increased ventricular ectopy.
- Urge the patient to report palpitations, chest pain, dizziness, and shortness of breath.

---

quinine derivatives ━━━━►◄━━━━ pancuronium
quinidine, quinine

Risk rating: 2
Severity: Moderate   **Onset: Rapid**   **Likelihood: Suspected**

Cause
Quinine derivatives may act synergistically with nondepolarizing muscle relaxants.

Effect
Effects of nondepolarizing muscle relaxants may increase.

Nursing considerations
⚡ ALERT This interaction may be life-threatening. Monitor neuro-muscular function closely.
- The intensity and duration of neuromuscular blockade may be affected.
- The dosage of nondepolarizing muscle relaxant may need adjustment.
- Provide ventilatory support as needed.
- Make sure the patient is adequately sedated when receiving a non-depolarizing muscle relaxant.

---

quinine derivatives ▶◀ rifampin
quinidine, quinine   Rifadin, Rimactane

Risk rating: 2
Severity: Moderate   Onset: Delayed   Likelihood: Probable

Cause
Rifampin is a potent inducer of hepatic enzymes and increases quinidine clearance.

Effect
Quinine derivative level and effects may decrease.

Nursing considerations
- Therapeutic range of quinidine is 2 to 6 mcg/ml. More specific assays have levels of less than 1 mcg/ml.
- Monitor the patient for loss of arrhythmia control.
- If rifampin is added to a stable quinidine regimen, rifampin dosage may be increased.
⚡ ALERT Stopping rifampin during quinidine therapy may cause dose-related toxicity. Monitor quinidine level and ECG closely.
- Enzyme induction may persist for several days after rifampin stops.
- Urge the patient to report palpitations, chest pain, dizziness, and shortness of breath.

---

quinine derivatives ▶◀ warfarin
quinidine, quinine   Coumadin

Risk rating: 1
Severity: Major   Onset: Delayed   Likelihood: Suspected

Cause
Quinidine derivatives may inhibit clotting factors synthesized in the liver.

Effect
Anticoagulant effects and risk of bleeding may increase.

Nursing considerations
- Monitor PT and INR closely.
- Tell the patient to report unusual bruising or bleeding.
- Remind the patient that warfarin interacts with many drugs and that he should report any change in drug regimen.

---

rabeprazole ▶◀ protease inhibitors

Aciphex   atazanavir, indinavir,
                                 saquinavir

Risk rating: 1
Severity: Major   **Onset: Delayed**   **Likelihood: Suspected**

Cause
GI absorption of protease inhibitors may be decreased.

Effect
Antiviral activity of protease inhibitors may be reduced.

Nursing considerations
- Use of protease inhibitors and proton pump inhibitors is not recommended.
- Monitor the patient for a decrease in antiviral activity.
- Adjust the dose of the protease inhibitor as needed.

---

ramipril ▶◀ aspirin

Altace   Bayer, Ecotrin

Risk rating: 2
Severity: Moderate   **Onset: Rapid**   **Likelihood: Suspected**

Cause
Salicylates such as aspirin inhibit synthesis of prostaglandins, which ramipril and other ACE inhibitors need to lower blood pressure.

Effect
ACE inhibitor's hypotensive effect will be reduced.

Nursing considerations
- This interaction is more likely in people with hypertension, coronary artery disease, and possibly heart failure.

ramipril ◀▶ potassium-sparing diuretics

Altace   amiloride, spironolactone

Risk rating: 1
Severity: Major   **Onset: Delayed**   **Likelihood: Probable**

Cause
The mechanism of this interaction is unknown.

Effect
Serum potassium level may increase.

Nursing considerations
- Use cautiously in patients at high risk for hyperkalemia, especially those with renal impairment.
- Monitor BUN, creatinine, and serum potassium levels, as needed.
- ACE inhibitors other than ramipril may interact with potassium-sparing diuretics. If you suspect an interaction, consult the prescriber or pharmacist.
- Urge the patient to immediately report an irregular heartbeat, a slow pulse, weakness, and other evidence of hyperkalemia.

ranitidine ◀▶ azole antifungals

Zantac   itraconazole, ketoconazole

Risk rating: 2
Severity: Moderate   **Onset: Delayed**   **Likelihood: Suspected**

Cause
Azole antifungal availability may decrease because elevated gastric pH may reduce tablet dissolution.

Effect
Azole antifungal effects may decrease.

Nursing considerations
- If possible, don't administer an azole antifungal with an H_2 antagonist, such as ranitidine.
- If combined use is needed, give 680 mg of glutamic acid hydrochloride 15 minutes before ketoconazole.
- Watch for expected antifungal effects.
- Explain that other drugs that increase gastric pH, such as antacids, may also decrease azole antifungal absorption.

repaglinide ━━━━▶◀━━━━ clarithromycin
Prandin   Biaxin

Risk rating: 2
Severity: Moderate   Onset: Delayed   Likelihood: Suspected

Cause
Certain macrolide antibiotics, such as clarithromycin, may inhibit repaglinide metabolism.

Effect
Repaglinide level and effects, including adverse effects, may increase.

Nursing considerations
- Monitor blood glucose level closely when starting or stopping a macrolide antibiotic.
- Adjust repaglinide dose as needed.
- Monitor the patient for evidence of hypoglycemia, including hunger, dizziness, shakiness, sweating, confusion, and light-headedness.
- Advise the patient to carry glucose tablets or another simple sugar in case of hypoglycemia.
- Make sure the patient and his family know what to do about hypoglycemia.

repaglinide ━━━━▶◀━━━━ cyclosporine
Prandin   Gengraf, Neoral, Sandimmune

Risk rating: 2
Severity: Moderate   Onset: Delayed   Likelihood: Suspected

Cause
Cyclosporine may inhibit repaglinide metabolism.

Effect
Repaglinide level and effects, including adverse effects, may increase.

Nursing considerations
- Monitor blood glucose level closely.
- Repaglinide dose should be adjusted as needed.
- Monitor the patient for evidence of hypoglycemia, including hunger, dizziness, shakiness, sweating, confusion, and light-headedness.
- Advise the patient to carry glucose tables or another simple sugar in case of hypoglycemia.
- Make sure the patient and his family know what to do if hypoglycemia occurs.

reserpine ━━━━▶◀━━━━ sympathomimetics
Serpalan   norepinephrine, ephedrine

Risk rating: 2
Severity: Moderate   Onset: Rapid   Likelihood: Suspected

Cause
Receptor sensitivity to sympathomimetics is increased.

Effect
Pressor response of sympathomimetics may increase, resulting in hypertension. The pressor response may be decreased.

Nursing considerations
- Monitor the patient's blood pressure closely.
- The dose of sympathomimetics may need to be increased or decreased depending on the patient's clinical response.

rifabutin ━━━━▶◀━━━━ amprenavir
Agenerase

Risk rating: 2
Severity: Moderate   Onset: Delayed   Likelihood: Suspected

Cause
Amprenavir may decrease CYP3A4 metabolism of rifabutin. Rifabutin may increase CYP3A4 metabolism of amprenavir.

Effect
Amprenavir level, effects, and risk of adverse effects may increase.

Nursing considerations
- **⚠ ALERT** Use of amprenavir with rifabutin is contraindicated.
- If the patient takes amprenavir with rifabutin, watch for adverse reactions.
- When administering amprenavir and rifabutin, consider decreasing the dose of rifabutin by 50%.
- Tell the patient he may develop diarrhea, fever, headache, muscle pain, or nausea, but not to alter the regimen without consulting the prescriber.
- To minimize interactions, urge the patient to tell the prescriber about all drugs and supplements he takes.

rifabutin ◄► **macrolide antibiotics**
clarithromycin, telithromycin

Risk rating: 2
Severity: Moderate   Onset: Delayed   Likelihood: Probable

Cause
Metabolism of rifabutin may be inhibited. Metabolism of macrolide antibiotics may be increased.

Effect
Adverse effects of rifabutin may increase. Antimicrobial effects of macrolide antibiotic may decrease.

Nursing considerations
■ Monitor the patient for increased rifabutin adverse effects, such as abdominal pain, anorexia, nausea, vomiting, diarrhea, and rash.
■ Monitor the patient for decreased response to antibiotics.
■ Rifabutin and clarithromycin usually cause nausea, vomiting, or diarrhea. This interaction doesn't occur with azithromycin or dirithromycin; these drugs may be better choices.
■ Giving a macrolide antibiotic with rifabutin may increase the risk of neutropenia.

---

rifampin ◄► **amprenavir**
Rifadin, Rimactane   Agenerase

Risk rating: 2
Severity: Moderate   Onset: Delayed   Likelihood: Suspected

Cause
Amprenavir may decrease CYP3A4 metabolism of rifampin. Rifampin may increase CYP3A4 metabolism of amprenavir.

Effect
Amprenavir level, effects, and risk of adverse effects may increase.

Nursing considerations
◣ **ALERT** Use of amprenavir with rifampin is contraindicated.
■ When administering amprenavir and rifampin, considering decreasing the dose of rifampin by 50%.
■ Tell the patient he may develop diarrhea, fever, headache, muscle pain, or nausea, but not to alter regimen without consulting the prescriber.
■ To minimize interactions, urge the patient to tell the prescriber about all drugs and supplements he takes.

rifampin ━━━━▶◀━━━━ benzodiazepines

Rifadin, Rimactane   diazepam, midazolam, triazolam

Risk rating: 2
Severity: Moderate   Onset: Delayed   Likelihood: Suspected

Cause
Rifampin may increase CYP3A4 metabolism of benzodiazepines.

Effect
Antianxiety, sedative, and sleep-inducing effects of benzodiazepines may be decreased.

Nursing considerations
■ Watch for expected benzodiazepine effects and lack of efficacy.
■ If benzodiazepine efficacy is reduced, notify the prescriber; dosage may be changed.
■ Other benzodiazepines may interact with rifampin. If you suspect an interaction, consult the prescriber or pharmacist.
■ For insomnia, temazepam may be more effective because it doesn't undergo CYP3A4 metabolism.

rifampin ━━━━▶◀━━━━ beta-adrenergic blockers

Rifadin, Rimactane   bisoprolol, metoprolol, propranolol

Risk rating: 2
Severity: Moderate   Onset: Delayed   Likelihood: Suspected

Cause
Rifampin increases hepatic metabolism of beta-adrenergic blockers.

Effect
Beta-adrenergic blocker effects are reduced.

Nursing considerations
■ Monitor blood pressure and heart rate closely to assess beta-adrenergic blocker efficacy.
■ If beta-adrenergic blocker effects are decreased, consult the prescriber; dosage may need to be increased.
■ Teach the patient how to monitor blood pressure and heart rate and when to contact the prescriber.
■ Other beta-adrenergic blockers may interact with rifampin. If you suspect an interaction, consult the prescriber or pharmacist.

rifampin ▸◂ buspirone

Rifadin, Rimactane   BuSpar

Risk rating: 2
Severity: Moderate   Onset: Delayed   Likelihood: Probable

Cause
Buspirone metabolism may be increased via induction of CYP3A4 metabolism by rifampin.

Effect
Buspirone effects may decrease.

Nursing considerations
■ Other rifamycins may interact. If you suspect an interaction, consult the prescriber or pharmacist.
■ Watch for expected buspirone effects when rifampin is started or stopped or the dosage changes.
■ Advise the patient to report increases or changes in anxiety if rifampin is started.
■ Urge the patient to tell prescribers about all drugs and supplements he takes and about any increase in adverse effects.

rifampin ▸◂ corticosteroids

Rifadin, Rimactane   cortisone, fludrocortisone, hydrocortisone, methylpred-nisolone, prednisolone, prednisone

Risk rating: 1
Severity: Major   Onset: Delayed   Likelihood: Established

Cause
Rifampin increases hepatic metabolism of corticosteroid.

Effect
Corticosteroid effects may be decreased.

Nursing considerations
■ If possible, avoid giving rifampin with corticosteroids.
■ Monitor the patient for decreased corticosteroid effects, including loss of disease control.
■ Monitor the patient closely for symptom control after increasing rifampin dose. Drug may need to be stopped to regain control of disease.
■ Corticosteroid effects may decrease within days of starting rifampin and may stay decreased 2 to 3 weeks after it stops.
■ Corticosteroid dose may need to be doubled after adding rifampin.

rifampin ▰▰▰►◄▰▰▰ disopyramide

Rifadin, Rimactane   Norpace

Risk rating: 2
Severity: Moderate   Onset: Delayed   Likelihood: Suspected

Cause
Hepatic metabolism of disopyramide is increased.

Effect
Disopyramide levels are decreased. Levels of an active metabolite may be increased, so it isn't known if decreased effects occur.

Nursing considerations
- Monitor the patient's ECG while he's taking rifampin.
- An increase in disopyramide dose may be necessary.

rifampin ▰▰▰►◄▰▰▰ doxycycline

Rifadin, Rimactane   Vibramycin

Risk rating: 2
Severity: Moderate   Onset: Delayed   Likelihood: Suspected

Cause
Rifampin may increase hepatic metabolism of doxycycline.

Effect
Doxycycline level and effects may decrease.

Nursing considerations
- Monitor the patient for expected doxycycline effects.
- Doxycycline dose may need to be increased.
- Consult the prescriber or pharmacists about using a tetracycline that doesn't interact with rifampins, such as streptomycin.
- Urge the patient to tell the prescriber if he isn't improving with doxycycline.

rifampin ▰▰▰►◄▰▰▰ estrogens

Rifadin, Rimactane   conjugated estrogens, esterified estrogens, estradiol, estrone, estropipate, ethinyl estradiol

Risk rating: 2
Severity: Moderate   Onset: Delayed   Likelihood: Suspected

Cause
Rifampin induces hepatic metabolism of estrogens, leading to increased estrogen elimination and decreased estrogen levels.

Effect

Estrogen efficacy may be reduced.

Nursing considerations

▪ If the patient takes rifampin and estrogen, watch for menstrual disturbances, such as spotting, intermenstrual bleeding, and amenorrhea.

▪ Estrogen dose may need to be increased during rifampin therapy; consult the prescriber or pharmacist.

▪ If the patient takes rifampin, suggest using a nonhormonal contraceptive.

▪ Explain that contraception may fail during combined therapy.

▪ Urge the patient to take the full course of rifampin exactly as prescribed to minimize risk of continued infection.

rifampin ▸◂ fentanyl

Rifadin, Rimactane   Sublimaze

Risk rating: 2

Severity: Moderate   Onset: Rapid   Likelihood: Suspected

Cause

Rifampin may induce CYP3A4 metabolism of fentanyl.

Effect

Fentanyl level and pharmacologic effects may decrease.

Nursing considerations

▪ Monitor the patient response when rifampin is started or discontinued. Be prepared to adjust fentanyl dosage as needed.

▪ Explain that taking these drugs together may decrease therapeutic effects of fentanyl.

▪ Monitor for adequate pain relief.

rifampin ▸◂ gefitinib

Rifadin, Rimactane   Iressa

Risk rating: 2

Severity: Moderate   Onset: Delayed   Likelihood: Suspected

Cause

Rifamycins such as rifampin may increase the metabolism of gefitinib.

Effect

Gefitinib levels and efficacy may be reduced.

Nursing considerations
■ Monitor clinical response to gefitinib when starting or stopping rifampin therapy.
■ Adjust the gefitinib dose as needed.
■ Encourage the patient to report signs and symptoms of adverse reactions including: eye problems such as pain, redness, or vision changes; diarrhea; rash; vomiting; itching; loss of appetite; weakness; weight loss; and liver damage.
⚡ ALERT The FDA has limited the use of gefitinib to certain patient populations. New clinical trials are being developed to determine future benefits of this drug.

---

rifampin ▶◀	haloperidol
Rifadin, Rimactane	Haldol

Risk rating: 2
Severity: Moderate   Onset: Delayed   Likelihood: Suspected

Cause
Haloperidol metabolism may increase.

Effect
Haloperidol level and effects may decrease.

Nursing considerations
■ Watch for expected haloperidol effects if the patient starts or stops a rifamycin.
■ Monitor haloperidol level (therapeutic ranger: 5 to 20 nanograms/ml).
■ Watch for loss of haloperidol effects: psychomotor agitation, obsessive-compulsive rituals, withdrawn behavior, auditory hallucinations, delusions, and delirium.
■ Consult the prescriber if haloperidol effects decline; haloperidol dosage may need adjustment.
■ Advise the patient to tell the prescriber about increased adverse effects.

---

rifampin ▶◀	HMG-CoA reductase inhibitors
Rifadin, Rimactane	atorvastatin, pravastatin, simvastatin

Risk rating: 2
Severity: Moderate   Onset: Delayed   Likelihood: Suspected

Cause
Rifampin may induce CYP3A4 metabolism of HMG-CoA reductase inhibitors in the intestine and liver.

Effect

HMG-CoA reductase inhibitor effects may decrease.

Nursing considerations

■ Assess the patient for expected response to therapy. If you suspect an interaction, consult the prescriber or pharmacist; the patient may need a different drug.

■ Check serum cholesterol and lipid levels.

■ Obtain liver function test results at start of therapy and periodically thereafter. If ALT or AST level stays three times or more above the upper limit of normal, HMG-CoA reductase inhibitor will need to be stopped.

■ Withhold HMG-CoA reductase inhibitor temporarily if the patient's risk of myopathy or rhabdomyolysis increases, as from sepsis, hypotension, major surgery, trauma, uncontrolled seizures, or a severe metabolic, endocrine, or electrolyte disorder.

◩ **ALERT** Pravastatin is less likely to interact with rifampin and may be the best choice for combined use.

---

rifampin ━━━▶◀━━━ imatinib

Rifadin, Rimactane   Gleevec

Risk rating: 2
Severity: Moderate   Onset: Delayed   Likelihood: Suspected

Cause

Rifampin increases CYP3A4 metabolism of imatinib.

Effect

Imatinib levels and therapeutic effect decrease.

Nursing considerations

■ Monitor the patient clinical response when rifampin therapy is started or stopped.

■ Consider alternative rifamycin therapy.

■ Use these drugs together cautiously.

---

rifampin ━━━▶◀━━━ isoniazid

Rifadin, Rimactane   Nydrazid

Risk rating: 1
Severity: Major   Onset: Delayed   Likelihood: Probable

Cause

Rifampin may alter isoniazid metabolism.

Effect
Risk of hepatotoxicity increases over either drug given alone.

Nursing considerations
- Monitor liver function tests in patients taking both drugs.
- Consult the prescriber about increased liver enzyme levels; one or both drugs may need to be stopped.
- Monitor the patient's liver enzymes and condition even after one or both drugs are stopped because of possible severity of reaction.
- **ALERT** Children may be more prone to hepatotoxicity.
- Advise the patient to report signs of hepatotoxicity: abdominal pain, appetite loss, fatigue, yellow skin or eye discoloration, and dark urine.

---

rifampin ▶◀ methadone
Rifadin, Rimactane   Methadose

Risk rating: 2
Severity: Moderate   Onset: Delayed   Likelihood: Established

Cause
Rifampin increases hepatic and intestinal metabolism of methadone.

Effect
Pharmacologic effects of methadone may decrease. The patient on maintenance methadone treatment may experience opiate withdrawal symptoms.

Nursing considerations
- Methadone dosage may need adjustment.
- If rifampin therapy is started while the patient is taking methadone, watch for signs of opioid withdrawal.
- If rifampin is stopped, methadone dosage may need to be decreased.
- Urge the patient to tell the prescriber about loss of methadone effect.

---

rifampin ▶◀ mycophenolate mofetil
Rifadin, Rimactane   CellCept

Risk rating: 2
Severity: Moderate   Onset: Delayed   Likelihood: Suspected

Cause
Multiple factors work together to inhibit the amount of mycophenolate mofetil that recirculates.

Effect
Mycophenolate mofetil level and effects may decrease.

Nursing considerations
■ Mycophenolate mofetil dosage may need to be adjusted when starting or stopping rifampin therapy.
■ Watch for evidence of rejection or decreased drug effect if rifampin is given with mycophenolate mofetil.
■ Urge the patient to report signs of organ rejection, such as decreased urine output in kidney transplant patients or shortness of breath in heart transplant patients.

rifampin ◄► nortriptyline
Rifadin, Rimactane   Pamelor

Risk rating: 2
Severity: Moderate   Onset: Delayed   Likelihood: Suspected

Cause
Metabolism of tricyclic antidepressants (TCAs) such as nortriptyline in the liver may increase.

Effect
TCA level and efficacy may decrease.

Nursing considerations
■ When starting, stopping, or changing the dosage of rifampin, monitor serum TCA level to maintain therapeutic range.
■ Watch for resolution of depression as TCA dosage is adjusted to therapeutic level during rifampin therapy.
■ Urge the patient and his family to watch for adverse reactions, including increased drowsiness and dizziness, for several weeks after rifampin stops. Tell them to notify the prescriber promptly if reactions occur.
■ Other TCAs may interact with rifampin. If you suspect an interaction, consult the prescriber or pharmacist.

rifampin ◄► quinine derivatives
Rifadin, Rimactane   quinidine, quinine

Risk rating: 2
Severity: Moderate   Onset: Delayed   Likelihood: Probable

Cause
Rifampin is a potent inducer of hepatic enzymes and increases quinidine clearance.

Effect
Quinine derivative level and effects may decrease.

Nursing considerations
- Therapeutic range of quinidine is 2 to 6 mcg/ml. More specific assays have levels of less than 1 mcg/ml.
- Monitor the patient for loss of arrhythmia control.
- If rifampin is added to a stable quinidine regimen, rifampin dosage may be increased.

⚠ ALERT Stopping rifampin during quinidine therapy may cause dose-related toxicity. Monitor quinidine level and ECG closely.
- Enzyme induction may persist for several days after rifampin is stopped.
- Urge the patient to report palpitations, chest pain, dizziness, and shortness of breath.

---

rifampin ▬▬▶◀ propafenone
Rifadin, Rimactane   Rythmol

Risk rating: 2
Severity: Moderate   Onset: Delayed   Likelihood: Probable

Cause
Rifampin may enhance hepatic metabolism of propafenone.

Effect
Propafenone clearance is increased and effects may decrease.

Nursing considerations
- Consult the prescriber about alternative anti-infective drug for patients stabilized on propafenone.
- If this combination can't be avoided, monitor propafenone level and watch for loss of effect.
- Propafenone dosage may need adjustment while the patient takes rifampin.
- This effect was seen less readily with I.V. propafenone than with the oral dosage form.

---

rifampin ▬▬▶◀ sulfonylureas
Rifadin, Rimactane   chlorpropamide, glipizide,
                                    glyburide, tolbutamide

Risk rating: 2
Severity: Moderate   Onset: Delayed   Likelihood: Probable

Cause
Rifampin may increase hepatic metabolism of certain sulfonylureas.

Effect

Risk of hyperglycemia increases.

Nursing considerations

- Use these drugs together cautiously.
- Monitor blood glucose level regularly, and consult the prescriber about adjustments to either drug to maintain stable glucose level.
- Tell the patient to stay alert for increased fatigue, thirst, eating, or urination and possible blurred vision or dry skin and mucous membranes as evidence of high blood glucose level.

---

rifampin ⧓ tacrolimus

Rifadin, Rimactane — Prograf

Risk rating: 1
Severity: Major **Onset: Delayed** **Likelihood: Probable**

Cause

Rifampin increases CYP3A4 metabolism of tacrolimus.

Effect

Immunosuppressive effects of tacrolimus on organ transplant recipients may decrease.

Nursing considerations

- Monitor tacrolimus level closely when rifampin is started; it may decrease in as little as 2 days. Expected trough level is 6 to 10 mcg/L.
- Increase tacrolimus dosage to compensate for faster metabolism.
- Watch the patient closely and check serum level when rifampin is stopped so dosage can be adjusted upward.
- Watch for signs of organ rejection or infection during rifampin treatment.

---

rifampin ⧓ tamoxifen

Rifadin, Rimactane — Nolvadex

Risk rating: 2
Severity: Moderate **Onset: Delayed** **Likelihood: Suspected**

Cause

Rifampin increases CYP3A4 metabolism of tamoxifen.

Effect

Tamoxifen levels and antiestrogen effects may be decreased.

Nursing considerations
■ Monitor the patient response to tamoxifen; dosage may need to be increased.
■ Warn female patients of risk of increased uterine bleeding.
■ Instruct the patient not to change dosage unless instructed by the practitioner.

---

rifampin ▶◀ theophyllines
Rifadin, Rimactane   aminophylline, theophylline

Risk rating: 2
Severity: Moderate   Onset: Delayed   Likelihood: Established

Cause
Rifampin may induce GI and hepatic metabolism of theophyllines.

Effect
Theophylline efficacy may decrease.

Nursing considerations
■ Monitor serum theophylline level closely. Therapeutic range is 10 to 20 mcg/ml for adults and 5 to 15 mcg/ml for children.
■ After rifampin is started, watch for increased pulmonary signs and symptoms.
■ Tell the patient to immediately report all concerns about drug efficacy to the prescriber; dosage may need adjustment.

---

rifampin ▶◀ zolpidem
Rifadin, Rimactane   Ambien

Risk rating: 3
Severity: Minor   Onset: Delayed   Likelihood: Suspected

Cause
Rifampin may increase CYP3A4 metabolism of zolpidem.

Effect
Zolpidem levels and therapeutic effects may be decreased.

Nursing considerations
■ Monitor patient response to zolpidem.
■ Dose of zolpidem may need to be increased while the patient is taking rifampin.
■ Instruct the patient to notify the prescriber about increased sleep-lessness or insomnia.
■ Tell the patient not to increase zolpidem dose without discussing with the prescriber.

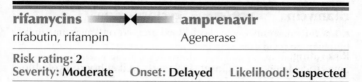

rifamycins ►◄ amprenavir

rifabutin, rifampin   Agenerase

Risk rating: 2
Severity: Moderate   **Onset: Delayed**   **Likelihood: Suspected**

Cause
Amprenavir may decrease CYP3A4 metabolism of rifabutin. Rifampin may increase CYP3A4 metabolism of amprenavir.

Effect
Amprenavir level, effects, and risk of adverse effects may increase.

Nursing considerations
🔰 **ALERT** Use of amprenavir with rifampin is contraindicated.
- If the patient takes amprenavir with rifabutin, watch for adverse reactions.
- When administering amprenavir and rifabutin, consider decreasing the dose of rifabutin by 50%.
- Tell the patient he may develop diarrhea, fever, headache, muscle pain, or nausea, but not to alter regimen without consulting the prescriber.
- To minimize interactions, urge the patient to tell the prescriber about all drugs and supplements he takes.

rifamycins ►◄ azole antifungals

rifabutin, rifampin,   fluconazole, itraconazole,
rifapentine   ketoconazole

Risk rating: 2
Severity: Moderate   **Onset: Delayed**   **Likelihood: Suspected**

Cause
Rifamycins may decrease azole antifungal levels. Also, ketoconazole may decrease rifampin level.

Effect
Infection may recur.

Nursing considerations
- Notify the prescriber if the patient takes both drugs; an alternative may be available.
- If drugs must be taken together and the antifungal appears ineffective, antifungal dosage may need to be increased.
- Teach the patient to recognize signs and symptoms of his infection and to contact the prescriber promptly if they occur.
- If ketoconazole and rifampin must be taken together, separate doses by 12 hours.

rifamycins ━━━▶◀━━━ cyclosporine

rifabutin, rifampin   Gengraf, Neoral, Sandimmune

Risk rating: 1
Severity: Major   **Onset: Delayed**   **Likelihood: Probable**

Cause
Rifamycins increase CYP3A4 cyclosporine metabolism.

Effect
Immunosuppressive effects of cyclosporine may decrease.

Nursing considerations
- Avoid using rifamycins during cyclosporine treatment if possible.
- Cyclosporine effects may decrease within 2 days after starting a rifamycin and may continue 1 to 3 weeks after it's stopped.
- Monitor cyclosporine level often during and after rifamycin treatment.
- Adjust cyclosporine dose as needed.
- Cyclosporine level may remain decreased despite dosage increases.
- Assess the patient for signs and symptoms of rejection.
- Monitor creatinine level during and after rifamycin treatment.

rifamycins ━━━▶◀━━━ dapsone

rifabutin, rifampin

Risk rating: 2
Severity: Moderate   **Onset: Delayed**   **Likelihood: Suspected**

Cause
Rifamycins increase the metabolism of dapsone.

Effect
Pharmacologic effects of dapsone may be decreased.

Nursing considerations
- Monitor for clinical failure of dapsone.
- Dosage of dapsone may need to be increased.
- If the patient is taking a rifamycin, consider using an alternative *Pneumocystis carinii* pneumonia prophylaxis.

rifamycins ━━━▶◀━━━ delavirdine
rifabutin, rifampin   Rescriptor

Risk rating: 2
Severity: Moderate   **Onset: Delayed**   **Likelihood: Suspected**

Cause
Rifamycins increase the metabolism of delavirdine.

Effect
Delavirdine levels decrease.

Nursing considerations
◪ **ALERT** Avoid concurrent use of delavirdine and rifamycins.
■ Monitor the patient for fever, fatigue, headache, nausea, abdominal pain, or cough.
■ Tell the patient not to alter drug regimen without notifying the prescriber or practitioner.

rifamycins ━━━▶◀━━━ erlotinib
rifabutin, rifampin   Tarceva

Risk rating: 2
Severity: Moderate   **Onset: Delayed**   **Likelihood: Suspected**

Cause
Rifamycins induce CYP3A4 metabolism of erlotinib.

Effect
Erlotinib level and effects may be reduced.

Nursing considerations
■ If possible, consider using another class of drug besides rifamycins if the patient is taking erlotinib.
■ If the patient must take a rifamycin and erlotinib, the dose of erlotinib may need to be increased.
■ Erlotinib dose may need to be increased to greater than 150 mg.

rifamycins ▰▰▰▰▶◀▰▰▰▰ indinavir
rifabutin, rifampin   Crixivan

Risk rating: 2
Severity: Moderate   Onset: Delayed   Likelihood: Probable

Cause
Indinavir decreases CYP3A4 metabolism of rifamycins, while rifamycins increase the metabolism of indinavir.

Effect
Antiviral activity of indinavir may be reduced. The rifamycin levels and risk of toxicity increase.

Nursing considerations
■ Decrease rifamycin dose to half the standard dose when administering together.
■ Use of these drugs together isn't recommended.
■ Adjust the dose of the protease inhibitor as needed.
■ Monitor CD4+ and T-cell counts; tell the prescriber if they decrease.
■ Tell the patient not to change an HIV regimen without consulting the prescriber.
■ Monitor the patient for increased rifamycin adverse effects, such as abdominal pain, anorexia, nausea, vomiting, diarrhea, and rash.

rifamycins ▰▰▰▰▶◀▰▰▰▰ warfarin
rifabutin, rifampin   Coumadin

Risk rating: 2
Severity: Moderate   Onset: Delayed   Likelihood: Established

Cause
Rifamycins increase hepatic metabolism of warfarin.

Effect
Anticoagulant effects decrease.

Nursing considerations
■ Monitor the patient for inadequate response to warfarin.
■ Warfarin dose may need to be increased during rifamycin therapy; monitor PT and INR often.
■ Blood tests may be needed for several weeks after stopping a rifamycin.
■ Tell the patient to report unusual bruising or bleeding.
■ Remind the patient that warfarin interacts with many drugs and that he should report any change in drug regimen.
■ Explain importance of following up with the prescriber for proper monitoring and dosage adjustments.

risperidone ►◄ SSRIs

Risperdal   fluoxetine, paroxetine, sertraline

Risk rating: 1
Severity: Major   **Onset: Rapid**   **Likelihood: Suspected**

Cause
SSRIs may inhibit CYP2D6 metabolism of risperidone.

Effect
Risperidone level and risk of adverse reactions and rapid accumulation of serotonin in the CNS may increase.

Nursing considerations
- Monitor the patient carefully if SSRI therapy is started or stopped or if the dosage changes during risperidone therapy.
- Assess the patient for CNS irritability, increased muscle tone, muscle twitching or jerking, and changes in level of consciousness.
- Advise the patient not to alter the dose of either drug without the advice of his prescriber.
- Average doses of fluoxetine and paroxetine may cause this interaction; higher doses of sertraline (greater than 100 mg daily) are needed.

ritonavir ►◄ amiodarone

Norvir   Cordarone, Pacerone

Risk rating: 1
Severity: Major   **Onset: Delayed**   **Likelihood: Suspected**

Cause
Protease inhibitors, such as ritonavir, inhibit the CYP3A4 metabolism of amiodarone.

Effect
Amiodarone level increases, increasing the risk of toxicity.

Nursing considerations
- **ALERT** Ritonavir is contraindicated for use with amiodarone because of large increase in amiodarone level.
- Use other protease inhibitors cautiously; they may have a similar effect.
- Increased amiodarone level may prolong the QT interval and cause life-threatening arrhythmias.
- Monitor ECG and QTc interval closely during combined therapy.
- Tell the patient to immediately report slowed pulse or fainting.

ritonavir ▬▬▬►◄ atorvastatin
Norvir   Lipitor

Risk rating: 2
Severity: Moderate   Onset: Delayed   Likelihood: Suspected

Cause
First-pass metabolism of atorvastatin by CYP3A4 in the GI tract may be inhibited.

Effect
Atorvastatin level may increase.

Nursing considerations
■ Monitor the patient closely if a protease inhibitor such as ritonavir, is added to atorvastatin therapy.
◤ **ALERT** Watch for evidence of rhabdomyolysis, including dark or red urine, muscle weakness, and myalgia.
■ This interaction may be more likely when ritonavir and saquinavir are used together.
■ Tell the patient to immediately report unexplained muscle weakness to the prescriber.

ritonavir ▬▬▬►◄ azole antifungals
Norvir   fluconazole, itraconazole,
                                          ketoconazole

Risk rating: 2
Severity: Moderate   Onset: Delayed   Likelihood: Suspected

Cause
Azole antifungals may inhibit metabolism of protease inhibitors such as ritonavir.

Effect
Protease inhibitor level may increase.

Nursing considerations
■ Protease inhibitor dosage may be decreased when therapy starts.
■ Monitor the patient for increased protease inhibitor effects, including hyperglycemia, onset of diabetes, rash, GI complaints, and altered liver function test results.
■ Advise the patient to report increased hunger or thirst, frequent urination, fatigue, and dry, itchy skin.
■ Tell the patient not to change dosage or stop either drug without consulting the prescriber.

ritonavir ◄► benzodiazepines

Norvir

alprazolam, clonazepam, diazepam, estazolam, flurazepam, midazolam, quazepam, triazolam

Risk rating: 2
Severity: Moderate   Onset: Delayed   Likelihood: Suspected

Cause
Protease inhibitors such as ritonavir may inhibit CYP3A4 metabolism of certain benzodiazepines.

Effect
Sedative effects of benzodiazepines may be increased and prolonged, leading to severe respiratory depression.

Nursing considerations
◼ ALERT Don't combine these benzodiazepines with protease inhibitors.
◼ ALERT Midazolam and triazolam are contraindicated in patients taking ritonavir.
■ If the patient takes any protease inhibitor–benzodiazepine combination, notify the prescriber. Interaction could involve other drugs in the class.
■ Watch for evidence of oversedation and respiratory depression.
■ Teach the patient and his family about the risks of combining these drugs.

ritonavir ◄► bupropion

Norvir

Wellbutrin

Risk rating: 2
Severity: Moderate   Onset: Delayed   Likelihood: Suspected

Cause
Ritonavir may inhibit bupropion metabolism.

Effect
Large increases in serum bupropion level may occur.

Nursing considerations
◼ ALERT Use of ritonavir with bupropion is contraindicated.
■ Risk of bupropion toxicity–induced seizures increases.
■ Increased seizure risk is associated with high bupropion doses.
■ Assess the patient for increased risk of seizures, including history of head trauma, seizures, CNS tumor, and use of other drugs that lower the seizure threshold.

ritonavir �▶◀ carbamazepine
Norvir

Carbatrol, Epitol, Equetro, Tegretol

Risk rating: 2
Severity: Moderate   **Onset: Rapid**   **Likelihood: Suspected**

Cause
Inhibition of CYP3A4 metabolism of carbamazepine. Carbamazepine may also induce CYP3A4 metabolism of protease inhibitors such as ritonavir.

Effect
Carbamazepine level and risk of toxicity increase. Protease inhibitor levels may decrease, resulting in antiretroviral treatment failure.

Nursing considerations
■ Closely monitor carbamazepine level when starting, stopping, or changing the dose of the protease inhibitor.
■ Therapeutic carbamazepine level is 4 to 12 mcg/ml.
■ Dosage adjustments may be needed to maintain therapeutic effects and avoid toxicity.
■ Monitor the clinical response to the protease inhibitor therapy.
■ Monitor the patient for evidence of carbamazepine toxicity, including dizziness, ataxia, respiratory depression, tachycardia, arrhythmias, blood pressure changes, impaired consciousness, abnormal reflexes, nystagmus, seizures, nausea, vomiting, and urine retention.
■ Monitor laboratory values for increased CD4+ T-cell count and a decreased HIV-1 RNA level.

ritonavir ◀▶◀ clozapine
Norvir

Clozaril

Risk rating: 1
Severity: Major   **Onset: Delayed**   **Likelihood: Suspected**

Cause
Ritonavir may inhibit clozapine metabolism.

Effect
Clozapine level and risk of toxicity may increase.

Nursing considerations
⚠ **ALERT** Use of clozapine with ritonavir is contraindicated.
■ Increased clozapine dose may increase risk of seizures.
■ Watch for evidence of clozapine toxicity, including agranulocytosis, ECG changes, and seizures.
■ Monitor ECG. Clozapine-induced ECG changes should normalize after drug is stopped.

ritonavir ◄ conivaptan

Norvir   Vaprisol

Risk rating: 1
Severity: Major   **Onset: Delayed**   **Likelihood: Suspected**

Cause
Protease inhibitors such as ritonavir may inhibit the CYP3A4 metabolism of conivaptan.

Effect
Conivaptan levels and adverse effects may be increased.

Nursing considerations
◼ **ALERT** Administration of protease inhibitors and conivaptan together is contraindicated.
■ The risk of increased conivaptan levels is unknown.
■ Further studies are needed to determine the total extent of this interaction.

ritonavir ◄ digoxin

Norvir   Lanoxin

Risk rating: 1
Severity: Major   **Onset: Delayed**   **Likelihood: Suspected**

Cause
Renal clearance of digoxin in the proximal tubules is decreased.

Effect
Digoxin level and risk of toxicity may increase.

Nursing considerations
■ Monitor digoxin level. Therapeutic range is 0.8 to 2 nanograms/ml.
■ Some patients may have toxicity even with serum digoxin level in therapeutic range.
■ Watch for signs of digoxin toxicity: arrhythmias (bradycardia, AV block, and ventricular ectopy), lethargy, drowsiness, confusion, hallucinations, headaches, syncope, visual disturbances, nausea, anorexia, vomiting, and diarrhea.
■ If ritonavir is started, digoxin dosage may need to be reduced.

ritonavir ━━━━▶◀━━━━ eplerenone

Norvir   Inspra

Risk rating: 1
Severity: Major   **Onset: Delayed**   **Likelihood: Suspected**

Cause
Protease inhibitors such as ritonavir inhibit eplerenone metabolism.

Effect
Eplerenone level rises, causing hyperkalemia and increasing the risk of life-threatening arrhythmias.

Nursing considerations
■ **ALERT** Use of ritonavir with eplerenone is contraindicated.
■ Potent CYP3A4 inhibitors increase eplerenone level and risk of hyperkalemia-induced arrhythmias—some fatal.
■ Monitor the patient's serum potassium level.
■ Tell the patient to report nausea, irregular heartbeat, or slowed pulse to the prescriber.

ritonavir ━━━━▶◀━━━━ ergot derivatives

Norvir   dihydroergotamine,
                                ergonovine, ergotamine,
                                methylergonovine

Risk rating: 1
Severity: Major   **Onset: Delayed**   **Likelihood: Probable**

Cause
Protease inhibitors such as ritonavir may interfere with CYP3A4 metabolism of ergot derivatives.

Effect
Risk of ergot-induced peripheral vasospasm and ischemia may increase.

Nursing considerations
■ **ALERT** Use of ergot derivatives with protease inhibitors is contraindicated.
■ Monitor the patient for evidence of peripheral ischemia, including pain in limb muscles while exercising and later at rest; numbness and tingling of fingers and toes; cool, pale, or cyanotic limbs; red or violet blisters on hands or feet; and gangrene.
■ Sodium nitroprusside may be given for ergot-induced vasospasm.
■ If the patient takes a protease inhibitor, consult the prescriber or pharmacist about alternative treatments for migraine pain.

ritonavir ━━━━▶◀━━━━ flecainide

Norvir   Tambocor

Risk rating: 1
Severity: Major   **Onset: Delayed**   **Likelihood: Suspected**

Cause
Ritonavir may inhibit CYP2D6 metabolism of flecainide.

Effect
Flecainide level and risk of toxicity may increase.

Nursing considerations
⚠ **ALERT** Ritonavir is contraindicated in patients taking flecainide.
■ Monitor serum flecainide level; therapeutic range is 0.2 to 1 mcg/ml.
■ Watch for flecainide toxicity: slowed or irregular pulse, palpitations, shortness of breath, hypotension, and new or worsened heart failure.
■ Monitor ECG for conduction disturbances (prolonged PR, QRS, and QT intervals), new or worsened arrhythmias, ventricular tachycardia, ventricular fibrillation, tachycardia, bradycardia, second- or third-degree AV block, and sinus arrest.

ritonavir ━━━━▶◀━━━━ fluoxetine

Norvir   Prozac, Sarafem

Risk rating: 2
Severity: Moderate   **Onset: Delayed**   **Likelihood: Suspected**

Cause
Fluoxetine and ritonavir may each inhibit the CYP2D6 metabolism of the other.

Effect
Ritonavir level may increase. Risk of serotonin syndrome increases.

Nursing considerations
■ If serotonin syndrome occurs, immediately stop fluoxetine.
■ The increased ritonavir level from this interaction doesn't increase the risk of adverse effects.
■ Ritonavir may increase fluoxetine level, causing cardiac and neurologic events, such as syncope, vasodilation, anxiety, depression, dizziness, and seizures.
■ Watch carefully for serotonin syndrome; it requires immediate attention.

■ Make the patient aware of the traits of serotonin syndrome: CNS irritability, motor weakness, shivering, muscle twitching, and altered consciousness.
■ Explain that serotonin syndrome can be fatal if not treated immediately.

---

ritonavir ━━━━━━◄► indinavir
Norvir   Crixivan

Risk rating: 2
Severity: Moderate   **Onset: Delayed**   **Likelihood: Probable**

Cause
Ritonavir may decrease CYP3A4 metabolism and clearance of indinavir.

Effect
Indinavir level, effects, and risk of adverse effects may increase.

Nursing considerations
🔛 **ALERT** Both drugs may need dosage adjustment.
■ Watch for increased indinavir adverse effects, including nausea, vomiting, diarrhea, and adverse renal effects.
■ Monitor the patient for nephrolithiasis; he may experience flank pain and hematuria.
■ Advise the patient to drink at least six 8-ounce glasses of fluid (1.5 L) daily.
■ Help the patient develop a plan to ensure proper dosage intervals.

---

ritonavir ━━━━━━◄► loperamide
Norvir   Imodium

Risk rating: 3
Severity: Minor   **Onset: Delayed**   **Likelihood: Suspected**

Cause
Ritonavir inhibits CYP3A4 metabolism of loperamide.

Effect
Loperamide level may increase.

Nursing considerations
■ The pharmacodynamics of loperamide aren't affected.
■ The dose of loperamide may be decreased.
■ No special precautions are needed for patients taking these drugs.

ritonavir ━━━━▸◂━━━━ lovastatin
Norvir   Mevacor, Altoprev

Risk rating: 1
Severity: Major   **Onset: Delayed**   **Likelihood: Suspected**

Cause
Protease inhibitors such as ritonavir inhibit CYP3A4 metabolism of lovastatin.

Effect
Lovastatin level may increase.

Nursing considerations
🔃 ALERT Ritonavir and lovastatin shouldn't be used together.
- Use other protease inhibitors cautiously; they may have similar effects.
- If a protease inhibitor is added to a regimen that includes lovastatin, monitor the patient closely.
🔃 ALERT Watch for evidence of rhabdomyolysis, including fatigue; muscle aches and weakness; joint pain; dark, red, or cola-colored urine; weight gain; seizures; and greatly increased CK level.
- Urge the patient to immediately report unexplained muscle weakness.

ritonavir ━━━━▸◂━━━━ meperidine
Norvir   Demerol

Risk rating: 1
Severity: Major   **Onset: Delayed**   **Likelihood: Suspected**

Cause
Ritonavir inhibits meperidine metabolism.

Effect
Meperidine levels increase significantly, increasing risk of toxicity.

Nursing considerations
🔃 ALERT Use of these drugs together is contraindicated.
- Toxic effects of meperidine include CNS side effects, seizures, and cardiac arrhythmias.
- This interaction is based on pharmacokinetics, not actual patient studies.

ritonavir ━━━━▶◀━━━━ **methadone**

Norvir

Risk rating: 2
Severity: Moderate   Onset: Delayed   Likelihood: Suspected

Cause
Protease inhibitors such as ritonavir may increase methadone metabolism.

Effect
Pharmacologic effects of methadone may decrease. The patient on maintenance methadone treatment may experience opioid withdrawal symptoms.

Nursing considerations
- Methadone dosage may need adjustment.
- If protease inhibitor therapy starts while the patient is taking methadone, watch for signs of opioid withdrawal.
- If the protease inhibitor is stopped, methadone dosage may need to be decreased.
- Urge the patient to tell the prescriber about loss of methadone effect.

ritonavir ━━━━▶◀━━━━ **non-nucleoside reverse transcriptase inhibitors**

Norvir   efavirenz, nevirapine

Risk rating: 2
Severity: Moderate   Onset: Delayed   Likelihood: Suspected

Cause
Non-nucleoside reverse transcriptase (NNRT) inhibitors may increase hepatic metabolism of protease inhibitors such as ritonavir.

Effect
Protease inhibitor level and effects decrease.

Nursing considerations
- If an NNRT inhibitor is started or stopped, monitor the protease inhibitor level closely.
- Protease inhibitor dosage may need adjustment.
- Monitor CD4+ and T-cell counts; tell the prescriber if they decrease.
- Urge the patient to report opportunistic infections.
- Tell the patient not to change an HIV regimen without consulting the prescriber.

ritonavir ━━━▶◀━━━ opioid analgesics
Norvir   buprenorphine, fentanyl

Risk rating: 2
Severity: Moderate   **Onset: Delayed**   **Likelihood: Suspected**

Cause
Metabolism of opioid analgesics in the GI tract and liver may be inhibited.

Effect
Opioid level may increase and half-life may lengthen.

Nursing considerations
◤ **ALERT** If the patient takes a protease inhibitor such as ritonavir watch closely for respiratory depression when an opioid analgesic is added.
- Because opioid half-life is prolonged, monitoring period should be extended, even after the opioid is stopped.
- Keep naloxone available to treat respiratory depression.
- If opioid is continuously infused, dosage should be decreased.

ritonavir ━━━▶◀━━━ pimozide
Norvir   Orap

Risk rating: 1
Severity: Major   **Onset: Delayed**   **Likelihood: Suspected**

Cause
Protease inhibitors such as ritonavir may inhibit CYP3A4 metabolism of pimozide.

Effect
Risk of life-threatening arrhythmias may increase.

Nursing considerations
◤ **ALERT** Use of ritonavir with pimozide is contraindicated.
- Arrhythmias are related to prolonged QT interval, a known risk of pimozide.
- Interaction warning is based on pharmacokinetics of these drugs, not actual patient studies.

ritonavir ◄ propafenone
Norvir   Rythmol

Risk rating: 1
Severity: Major   **Onset: Delayed**   **Likelihood: Suspected**

Cause
Ritonavir may inhibit CYP2D6 metabolism of propafenone.

Effect
Propafenone level and risk of toxicity may increase.

Nursing considerations
◆ **ALERT** Use of ritonavir with propafenone is contraindicated.
■ Monitor the patient for new or worsened arrhythmias, including an increase in premature ventricular contractions, ventricular tachycardia, ventricular fibrillation, and torsades de pointes.
■ Monitor ECG for AV block and prolonged QTc interval.
■ Advise the patient to report a rapid heartbeat, shortness of breath, dizziness or fainting, and chest pain.

ritonavir ◄ quinidine
Norvir

Risk rating: 1
Severity: Major   **Onset: Delayed**   **Likelihood: Suspected**

Cause
CYP3A4 metabolism of quinidine may be inhibited.

Effect
Quinidine level and risk of toxicity may increase.

Nursing considerations
◆ **ALERT** Use of ritonavir with quinidine is contraindicated.
■ Monitor ECG for prolonged QT interval and arrhythmias.
◆ **ALERT** Quinidine toxicity may cause GI irritation, arrhythmias, hypotension, vertigo, and rash.

ritonavir ◄ saquinavir
Norvir   Invirase

Risk rating: 3
Severity: Minor   **Onset: Rapid**   **Likelihood: Suspected**

Cause
First-pass metabolism and clearance of saquinavir decreases.

Effect
Saquinavir level and adverse effects may be increased.

Nursing considerations
- Typically, no interventions are needed with this interaction.
- The dose of saquinavir may be decreased.

---

ritonavir ▶◀ sildenafil
Norvir   Viagra

Risk rating: 1
Severity: Major   **Onset: Rapid**   **Likelihood: Suspected**

Cause
Sildenafil metabolism is inhibited.

Effect
Sildenafil level may increase, possibly leading to fatal hypotension.

Nursing considerations
- ◣ ALERT Tell the patient to take sildenafil exactly as prescribed.
- Dosage of sildenafil may be reduced and dosing interval lengthened.
- ◣ ALERT Warn the patient about potentially fatal low blood pressure if these drugs are taken together.
- Tell the patient to notify the prescriber about dizziness, fainting, or chest pain if the drugs are used together.

---

ritonavir ▶◀ simvastatin
Norvir   Zocor

Risk rating: 1
Severity: Major   **Onset: Delayed**   **Likelihood: Suspected**

Cause
First-pass metabolism of simvastatin by CYP3A4 in the GI tract may be inhibited.

Effect
Simvastatin level may increase.

Nursing considerations
- ◣ ALERT Use of ritonavir with simvastatin is contraindicated.
- If a protease inhibitor such as ritonavir is added to simvastatin, monitor the patient closely.
- ◣ ALERT Watch for evidence of rhabdomyolysis, including fatigue; muscle aches and weakness; joint pain; dark, red, or cola-colored urine; weight gain; seizures; and greatly increased CK level.
- Urge the patient to immediately report unexplained muscle weakness.

ritonavir ▰▰▰▰►◄▰▰▰▰   St. John's wort
Norvir

Risk rating: 1
Severity: Major   **Onset: Delayed**   **Likelihood: Suspected**

Cause
Hepatic metabolism of protease inhibitors such as ritonavir may increase.

Effect
Protease inhibitor level and effects may decrease.

Nursing considerations
■ If the patient starts or stops taking St. John's wort, monitor protease inhibitor level closely.
■ Monitor CD4+ and T-cell counts; tell the prescriber if they decrease.
■ Urge the patient to report opportunistic infections.
■ Tell the patient not to change an HIV regimen without consulting the prescriber.
■ Urge the patient to tell the prescribers about all drugs, supplements, and alternative therapies he uses.

ritonavir ▰▰▰▰►◄▰▰▰▰   tacrolimus
Norvir   Prograf

Risk rating: 2
Severity: Moderate   **Onset: Delayed**   **Likelihood: Suspected**

Cause
Hepatic metabolism of tacrolimus is inhibited.

Effect
Tacrolimus level and risk of toxicity may increase.

Nursing considerations
■ Monitor renal function and mental status closely.
■ Check tacrolimus level often. Normal trough level is 6 to 10 mcg/ml.
■ Tacrolimus dosage may need to be decreased when the patient takes a protease inhibitor such as ritonavir.
■ Other protease inhibitors may have this same interaction.
■ **ALERT** Watch for renal failure, nephrotoxicity, hyperkalemia, hyperglycemia, delirium, and other changes in mental status.

ritonavir ⧓ zolpidem

Norvir | Ambien

Risk rating: 2
Severity: Moderate **Onset: Delayed** **Likelihood: Suspected**

Cause
Hepatic metabolism of zolpidem is inhibited.

Effect
Severe sedation and respiratory depression may occur.

Nursing considerations
ALERT Combined use of these drugs is contraindicated.
- Monitor the patient's respiratory status closely.
- Have emergency respiratory equipment available.

rizatriptan ⧓ ergot derivatives

Maxalt | dihydroergotamine, ergotamine

Risk rating: 1
Severity: Major **Onset: Rapid** **Likelihood: Suspected**

Cause
Combined use may have additive effects.

Effect
Risk of vasospastic effects increases.

Nursing considerations
ALERT Use of these drugs within 24 hours of each other is contraindicated. Combined use may cause severe vasospastic effects, including sustained coronary artery vasospasm that triggers MI.
ALERT Similarly, use of another selective 5-HT_1 receptor agonist (such as frovatriptan, naratriptan, sumatriptan, or zolmitriptan) within 24 hours of rizatriptan is contraindicated.
- Warn patients not to mix migraine headache drugs within 24 hours of each other, but to call the prescriber if a drug isn't effective.

rizatriptan ━━━▶◀━━━ MAO inhibitors

Maxalt

isocarboxazid, phenelzine,
tranylcypromine

Risk rating: 1

Severity: **Major**	Onset: **Rapid**	Likelihood: **Suspected**

Cause
MAO inhibitors, subtype-A, may inhibit metabolism of selective
$5\text{-}HT_1$ receptor agonists such as rizatriptan.

Effect
Serum level of certain selective $5\text{-}HT_1$ receptor agonists may increase,
as may risk of cardiac toxicity.

Nursing considerations
◤ **ALERT** Use of certain selective $5\text{-}HT_1$ receptor agonists with an
MAO inhibitor or within 2 weeks of stopping an MAO inhibitor is
contraindicated.
■ If these drugs must be used together, naratriptan is less likely to
interact with an MAO inhibitor than rizatriptan.
■ Cardiac toxicity may include coronary artery vasospasm and
transient myocardial ischemia.

rocuronium ━━━▶◀━━━ aminoglycosides

Zemuron

gentamicin, neomycin,
streptomycin, tobramycin

Risk rating: 1

Severity: **Major**	Onset: **Rapid**	Likelihood: **Probable**

Cause
These drugs may be synergistic.

Effect
Effects of nondepolarizing muscle relaxants such as rocuronium may
increase.

Nursing considerations
■ The nondepolarizing muscle relaxant dose may need adjustment
based on neuromuscular response.
■ Monitor the patient for prolonged respiratory depression.
■ Provide ventilatory support as needed.

rocuronium ➤◄ carbamazepine

Zemuron

Carbatrol, Epitol,
Equetro, Tegretol

Risk rating: 2
Severity: Moderate   **Onset: Rapid**   **Likelihood: Probable**

Cause
The mechanism of this interaction is unknown.

Effect
Effects or duration of a nondepolarizing muscle relaxant such as rocuronium may decrease.

Nursing considerations
- Monitor the patient for decreased efficacy of muscle relaxant.
- Dosage of the nondepolarizing muscle relaxant may need to be increased.
- Make sure the patient is adequately sedated when receiving a nondepolarizing muscle relaxant.

rosuvastatin ➤◄ azole antifungals

Crestor

fluconazole, itraconazole, ketoconazole

Risk rating: 1
Severity: Major   **Onset: Rapid**   **Likelihood: Probable**

Cause
Azole antifungals may inhibit hepatic metabolism of HMG-CoA reductase inhibitors such as rosuvastatin.

Effect
HMG-CoA reductase inhibitor level and adverse effects may increase.

Nursing considerations
- If possible, avoid use together.
- If drugs must be taken together, HMG-CoA reductase inhibitor dosage may need to be decreased.
- Monitor serum cholesterol and lipid levels.
- **ALERT** Assess the patient for evidence of rhabdomyolysis, including fatigue; muscle aches and weakness; joint pain; dark, red, or cola-colored urine; weight gain; seizures; and greatly increased CK level.
- Pravastatin is the HMG-CoA reductase inhibitor least affected by this interaction; it may be the best choice for use with azole antifungals.

rosuvastatin ➤◄ cyclosporine

Crestor   Neoral

Risk rating: 1
Severity: Major   **Onset: Delayed**   **Likelihood: Probable**

Cause
Metabolism of certain HMG-CoA reductase inhibitors such as
rosuvastatin may decrease.

Effect
Plasma level and adverse effects of HMG-CoA reductase inhibitors
may increase.

Nursing considerations
◤ ALERT If possible, avoid use together.
- HMG-CoA reductase inhibitor dosage may need to be decreased.
- Monitor serum cholesterol and lipid levels.
◤ ALERT Assess the patient for evidence of rhabdomyolysis, including
fatigue; muscle aches and weakness; joint pain; dark, red, or cola-
colored urine; weight gain; seizures; and greatly increased CK level.
- Urge the patient to report muscle pain, tenderness, or weakness.

rosuvastatin ➤◄ fibric acids

Crestor   fenofibrate, gemfibrozil

Risk rating: 1
Severity: Major   **Onset: Delayed**   **Likelihood: Suspected**

Cause
The mechanism of this interaction is unknown.

Effect
Severe myopathy or rhabdomyolysis may occur.

Nursing considerations
- Avoid use together.
- If the patient has severe hyperlipidemia, combined therapy may be
an option, but only with careful monitoring.
◤ ALERT Assess the patient for evidence of rhabdomyolysis, including
fatigue; muscle aches and weakness; joint pain; dark, red, or cola-
colored urine; weight gain; seizures; and greatly increased CK level.
- Watch for evidence of acute renal failure, including decreased urine
output, elevated BUN and creatinine levels, edema, dyspnea, tachycardia, distended jugular veins, nausea, vomiting, poor appetite, weakness, fatigue, confusion, and agitation.
- Urge the patient to report muscle pain, tenderness, or weakness.

rosuvastatin ━━━▶◀━━━ warfarin
Crestor   Coumadin

Risk rating: 2
Severity: Moderate   Onset: Delayed   Likelihood: Probable

Cause
Hepatic metabolism of warfarin may be inhibited.

Effect
Anticoagulant effects may increase.

Nursing considerations
■ Monitor PT and INR closely when starting or stopping rosuvastatin.
■ Atorvastatin and pravastatin, other HMG-CoA reductase inhibitors, don't appear to have this interaction with warfarin and may be better treatment options.
■ Tell the patient to report unusual bruising or bleeding.
■ Remind the patient that warfarin interacts with many drugs and that he should report any change in his drug regimen to his prescriber or pharmacist.
■ Advise the patient to keep all follow-up medical appointments for proper monitoring and dosage adjustments.

saquinavir ━━━▶◀━━━ atorvastatin
Invirase   Lipitor

Risk rating: 2
Severity: Moderate   Onset: Delayed   Likelihood: Suspected

Cause
First-pass metabolism of atorvastatin by CYP3A4 in the GI tract may be inhibited.

Effect
Atorvastatin level may increase.

Nursing considerations
■ Monitor the patient closely if a protease inhibitor is added to atorvastatin therapy.
◣ **ALERT** Watch for evidence of rhabdomyolysis, including fatigue; muscle aches and weakness; joint pain; dark, red, or cola-colored urine; weight gain; seizures; and greatly increased CK level.
■ This interaction may be more likely when ritonavir and saquinavir are used together.
■ Tell the patient to immediately report unexplained muscle weakness to the prescriber.

saquinavir ━━━▶◀ azole antifungals

Invirase

fluconazole, itraconazole, ketoconazole

Risk rating: 2
Severity: Moderate **Onset: Delayed** **Likelihood: Suspected**

Cause
Azole antifungals may inhibit metabolism of protease inhibitors such as saquinavir.

Effect
Protease inhibitor plasma level may increase.

Nursing considerations
- Protease inhibitor dosage may be decreased when therapy starts.
- Monitor the patient for increased protease inhibitor effects, including hyperglycemia, onset of diabetes, rash, GI complaints, and altered liver function tests.
- Advise the patient to report increased hunger or thirst, frequent urination, fatigue, and dry, itchy skin.
- Tell the patient not to change dosage or stop either drug without consulting the prescriber.

saquinavir ━━━▶◀ benzodiazepines

Invirase

alprazolam, clorazepate, diazepam, estazolam, flurazepam, midazolam, triazolam

Risk rating: 1
Severity: Major **Onset: Delayed** **Likelihood: Suspected**

Cause
Protease inhibitors such as saquinavir may inhibit CYP3A4 metabolism of certain benzodiazepines.

Effect
Sedative effects of benzodiazepines may be increased and prolonged, leading to severe respiratory depression.

Nursing considerations
- **ALERT** Don't combine the benzodiazepines listed above with protease inhibitors.
- **ALERT** Midazolam and triazolam are contraindicated in patients taking saquinavir.

- If the patient takes any protease inhibitor–benzodiazepine combination, notify the prescriber. Interaction could involve other drugs in the class.
- Watch for evidence of oversedation and respiratory depression.
- Teach the patient and his family about risks of combining these drugs.

saquinavir ▶◀ carbamazepine

Invirase

Carbatrol, Epitol, Equetro, Tegretol

Risk rating: 2
Severity: Moderate   **Onset: Rapid**   **Likelihood: Suspected**

Cause
Saquinavir inhibits CYP3A4 metabolism of carbamazepine. Carbamazepine may also induce CYP3A4 metabolism of protease inhibitors such as saquinavir.

Effect
Carbamazepine level and risk of toxicity increase. Protease inhibitor levels may decrease, resulting in antiretroviral treatment failure.

Nursing considerations
- Closely monitor carbamazepine level when starting, stopping, or changing protease inhibitor dose.
- Therapeutic carbamazepine level is 4 to 12 mcg/ml.
- Dosage adjustments may be needed to maintain therapeutic effects and avoid toxicity.
- Monitor clinical response to protease inhibitor therapy.
- Monitor the patient for evidence of carbamazepine toxicity, including dizziness, ataxia, respiratory depression, tachycardia, arrhythmias, blood pressure changes, impaired consciousness, abnormal reflexes, nystagmus, seizures, nausea, vomiting, and urine retention.
- Monitor laboratory values for increased CD4+ T-cell count and a decreased HIV-1 RNA level.

saquinavir ▶◀ ergot derivatives

Invirase

dihydroergotamine, ergonovine, ergotamine, methylergonovine

Risk rating: 1
Severity: Major   **Onset: Delayed**   **Likelihood: Probable**

Cause
Protease inhibitors such as saquinavir may interfere with CYP3A4 metabolism of ergot derivatives.

Effect
Risk of ergot-induced peripheral vasospasm and ischemia may increase.

Nursing considerations
⚠ ALERT Combining ergot derivatives and protease inhibitors is contraindicated.
■ Monitor the patient for evidence of peripheral ischemia, including pain in limb muscles while exercising and later at rest; numbness and tingling of fingers and toes; cool, pale, or cyanotic limbs; red or violet blisters on hands or feet; and gangrene.
■ Sodium nitroprusside may be given for ergot-induced vasospasm.
■ If the patient takes a protease inhibitor, consult the prescriber or pharmacist about alternative treatments for migraine pain.
■ Advise the patient to tell the prescriber about increased adverse effects.

---

saquinavir ■■■■►◄■■■■ grapefruit juice
Invirase

Risk rating: 2
Severity: Moderate   Onset: Delayed   Likelihood: Suspected

Cause
Grapefruit juice may inhibit CYP3A4 GI metabolism of saquinavir.

Effect
Saquinavir level may increase.

Nursing considerations
■ Avoid giving saquinavir with grapefruit juice.
■ Teach the patient to separate grapefruit products as much as possible from saquinavir doses.

---

saquinavir ■■■■►◄■■■■ opioid analgesics
Invirase   buprenorphine, fentanyl

Risk rating: 2
Severity: Moderate   Onset: Delayed   Likelihood: Suspected

Cause
Metabolism of fentanyl in the GI tract and liver may be inhibited.

Effect
Fentanyl level may increase and half-life lengthen.

Nursing considerations
⚠ ALERT If the patient takes a protease inhibitor such as saquinavir watch closely for respiratory depression when an opioid analgesic is added.

■ Because fentanyl half-life is prolonged, monitoring period should be extended, even after fentanyl is stopped.
■ Keep naloxone available to treat respiratory depression.
■ If fentanyl is continuously infused, dosage should be decreased.

saquinavir ━━━━►◄━━━━ pimozide
Invirase   Orap

Risk rating: 1
Severity: Major   **Onset: Delayed**   **Likelihood: Suspected**

Cause
Protease inhibitors such as saquinavir may inhibit CYP3A4 metabolism of pimozide.

Effect
Risk of life-threatening arrhythmias may increase.

Nursing considerations
◖ **ALERT** Combined use of these drugs is contraindicated.
■ Arrhythmias are related to prolonged QT interval, a known risk of pimozide.
■ Interaction warning is based on pharmacokinetics of these drugs, not actual patient studies.

saquinavir ━━━━►◄━━━━ proton pump inhibitors
Invirase   esomeprazole, lansoprazole, omeprazole, pantoprazole, rabeprazole

Risk rating: 1
Severity: Major   **Onset: Delayed**   **Likelihood: Suspected**

Cause
GI absorption of protease inhibitors such as saquinavir may be decreased.

Effect
Antiviral activity of protease inhibitors may be reduced.

Nursing considerations
■ Use of protease inhibitors and proton pump inhibitors isn't recommended.
■ Monitor the patient for a decrease in antiviral activity.
■ Adjust protease inhibitor dose as needed.

saquinavir ━━━━▶◀ ritonavir

Invirase   Norvir

Risk rating: 3
Severity: Minor　　**Onset: Rapid**　　**Likelihood: Suspected**

Cause
This interaction causes decreased first-pass metabolism and clearance of saquinavir.

Effect
Saquinavir level and adverse effects may be increased.

Nursing considerations
- Typically, no interventions are needed with this interaction.
- The dose of saquinavir may be decreased.

saquinavir ━━━━▶◀ sildenafil

Invirase   Viagra

Risk rating: 1
Severity: Major　　**Onset: Rapid**　　**Likelihood: Suspected**

Cause
Phosphodiesterase-5 (PDE-5) inhibitor metabolism is inhibited.

Effect
PDE-5 inhibitor level may increase, possibly leading to fatal hypotension.

Nursing considerations
- Tell the patient to take PDE-5 inhibitors such as sildenafil exactly as prescribed.
- PDE-5 inhibitor dosage will be reduced and interval lengthened.
- ⚠ ALERT Warn the patient about potentially fatal low blood pressure.
- Tell the patient to notify his prescriber about dizziness, fainting, or chest pain if drugs are used together.

saquinavir ━━━━▶◀ simvastatin

Invirase   Zocor

Risk rating: 1
Severity: Major　　**Onset: Delayed**　　**Likelihood: Suspected**

Cause
Protease inhibitors such as saquinavir may inhibit CYP3A4 metabolism of HMG-CoA reductase inhibitors such as simvastatin.

Effect
HMG-CoA reductase inhibitor level may increase.

Nursing considerations
■ **ALERT** Watch for evidence of rhabdomyolysis, including fatigue; muscle aches and weakness; joint pain; dark, red, or cola-colored urine; weight gain; seizures; and greatly increased CK level.
■ Urge the patient to immediately report unexplained muscle weakness.

saquinavir ━━━━▶◀━━━━ St. John's wort
Invirase

Risk rating: 1
Severity: Major   **Onset: Delayed**   **Likelihood: Suspected**

Cause
Hepatic metabolism of protease inhibitors such as saquinavir may increase.

Effect
Protease inhibitor level and effects may decrease.

Nursing considerations
■ If the patient starts or stops taking St. John's wort, monitor protease inhibitor level closely.
■ Monitor CD4+ and T-cell counts; tell the prescriber if they decrease.
■ Urge the patient to report opportunistic infections.
■ Tell the patient not to change an HIV regimen without consulting the prescriber.
■ Urge the patient to tell the prescriber about all drugs, supplements, and alternative therapies he uses.

saquinavir ━━━━▶◀━━━━ tacrolimus
Invirase   Prograf

Risk rating: 2
Severity: Moderate   **Onset: Delayed**   **Likelihood: Suspected**

Cause
Hepatic metabolism of tacrolimus is inhibited.

Effect
Tacrolimus level and risk of toxicity may increase.

Nursing considerations
■ Monitor renal function and mental status closely.
■ Check tacrolimus level often. Normal trough level is 6 to 10 mcg/ml.

- Tacrolimus dosage may need to be decreased when the patient takes a protease inhibitor such as saquinavir.
- Other protease inhibitors may have this same interaction.

⚡ ALERT Watch for renal failure, nephrotoxicity, hyperkalemia, hyperglycemia, delirium, and other changes in mental status.

---

secobarbital ━━━━▶◀━━━━ theophylline
Seconal

Risk rating: 2
Severity: Moderate   Onset: Delayed   Likelihood: Suspected

Cause
Barbiturates such as secobarbital may stimulate theophylline clearance by inducing CYP pathway.

Effect
Theophylline level and efficacy may decrease.

Nursing considerations
- Monitor the patient closely to determine theophylline efficacy.
- Monitor serum theophylline level regularly. Therapeutic range is 10 to 20 mcg/ml for adults and 5 to 15 mcg/ml for children.
- When a barbiturate is added to drug regimen, theophylline dosage may need to be increased.
- Dyphylline undergoes renal elimination and may not be affected by this interaction.

---

selegiline ━━━━▶◀━━━━ bupropion
Eldepryl   Wellbutrin, Zyban

Risk rating: 1
Severity: Major   Onset: Delayed   Likelihood: Suspected

Cause
The cause of this interaction is unknown.

Effect
Risk of acute bupropion toxicity increases.

Nursing considerations
⚡ ALERT Administration of bupropion and MAO inhibitors such as selegiline together is contraindicated.
- Allow at least 14 days between discontinuing an MAO inhibitor and starting bupropion.
- Interaction warning is based on animal trials, not actual patient studies.

selegiline ➤◄ meperidine
Eldepryl   Demerol

Risk rating: 1
Severity: Major   **Onset: Rapid**   **Likelihood: Probable**

Cause
The mechanism of this interaction is unknown.

Effect
Risk of severe adverse reactions increases.

Nursing considerations
■ If possible, avoid giving these drugs together.
■ Monitor the patient and report agitation, seizures, diaphoresis, and fever.
■ **ALERT** Reaction may progress to coma, apnea, and death.
■ Reaction may occur several weeks after stopping an MAO inhibitor such as selegiline.
■ **ALERT** Give opioid analgesics other than meperidine cautiously. It isn't known if similar reactions occur.

selegiline ➤◄ serotonin reuptake inhibitors
Eldepryl   citalopram, duloxetine, fluoxetine, sertraline, venlafaxine

Risk rating: 1
Severity: Major   **Onset: Rapid**   **Likelihood: Probable**

Cause
Serotonin may accumulate rapidly in the CNS.

Effect
Risk of serotonin syndrome increases.

Nursing considerations
■ **ALERT** Don't use these drugs together.
■ Allow 1 week after stopping venlafaxine (2 weeks after stopping citalopram, duloxetine, or sertraline; 5 weeks after stopping fluoxetine) before giving an MAO inhibitor such as selegiline.
■ Allow 2 weeks after stopping an MAO inhibitor before giving a serotonin reuptake inhibitor.

- A selective MAO type-B inhibitor, selegiline has been given with fluoxetine or sertraline to patients with Parkinson's disease without negative effects.
- Describe the traits of serotonin syndrome: CNS irritability, motor weakness, shivering, muscle twitching, and altered consciousness.
- Urge the patient to promptly report adverse effects.

sertraline ━━━▶◀━━━ carbamazepine
Zoloft   Carbatrol, Epitol, Equetro, Tegretol

Risk rating: 2
Severity: Moderate   **Onset: Delayed**   **Likelihood: Suspected**

Cause
CYP3A4 metabolism of sertraline increases.

Effect
Carbamazepine may decrease or reverse therapeutic effect of sertraline.

Nursing considerations
- If the patient is receiving carbamazepine, consider administering an antidepressant that isn't affected by CYP3A4 metabolism such as paroxetine.
- Closely monitor the patient's response to sertraline.
- Be prepared to adjust sertraline dose when starting, stopping, or changing carbamazepine dose.
- Increasing sertraline dose may help decrease interaction.

sertraline ━━━▶◀━━━ clozapine
Zoloft   Clozaril

Risk rating: 1
Severity: Major   **Onset: Delayed**   **Likelihood: Established**

Cause
Serotonin reuptake inhibitors such as sertraline inhibit hepatic metabolism of clozapine.

Effect
Clozapine level and risk of toxicity increase.

Nursing considerations
- Not all serotonin reuptake inhibitors share this interaction. If you suspect an interaction, consult the prescriber or pharmacist.
- Monitor serum clozapine level.

■ Assess the patient for increased adverse effects or toxicity, including agranulocytosis, ECG changes, and seizures.
■ Adjust clozapine dose as needed when adding or withdrawing a serotonin reuptake inhibitor.

sertraline ▸◂ linezolid
Zoloft
Zyvox

Risk rating: 1
Severity: Major   **Onset: Delayed**   **Likelihood: Suspected**

Cause
Serotonin may accumulate rapidly in the CNS.

Effect
The risk of serotonin syndrome increases.

Nursing considerations
◖ **ALERT** Don't use these drugs together.
■ Allow 2 weeks after stopping linezolid and administering sertraline.
■ Allow 2 weeks after stopping an SSRI such as sertraline and administering linezolid.
■ Describe the traits of serotonin syndrome: CNS irritability, motor weakness, shivering, muscle twitching, and altered consciousness.
■ Explain that serotonin-induced symptoms can be fatal if not treated immediately.

sertraline ▸◂ MAO inhibitors
Zoloft
isocarboxazid, phenelzine, selegiline, tranylcypromine

Risk rating: 1
Severity: Major   **Onset: Rapid**   **Likelihood: Probable**

Cause
Serotonin may accumulate rapidly in the CNS.

Effect
Risk of serotonin syndrome increases.

Nursing considerations
◖ **ALERT** Don't use these drugs together.
■ Allow 2 weeks after stopping sertraline before giving an MAO inhibitor. Allow 2 weeks after stopping an MAO inhibitor before giving an SSRI such as sertraline.

■ The selective MAO type-B inhibitor selegiline has been given with fluoxetine, paroxetine, or sertraline to patients with Parkinson's disease without negative effects.
■ Describe the traits of serotonin syndrome: CNS irritability, motor weakness, shivering, muscle twitching, and altered consciousness.
■ Urge the patient to promptly report adverse effects.

sertraline ━━━►◄━━━ phenytoin
Zoloft   Dilantin

Risk rating: 2
Severity: Moderate   Onset: Delayed   Likelihood: Suspected

Cause
Sertraline may inhibit hydantoin metabolism.

Effect
Hydantoin level and effects may be increased, along with risk of toxic effects.

Nursing considerations
■ Monitor serum hydantoin level. Therapeutic range for phenytoin is 10 to 20 mcg/ml.
■ Hydantoin dosage may need adjustment.
⚠ ALERT If sertraline is started during hydantoin therapy, watch for evidence of hydantoin toxicity, including drowsiness, nausea, vomiting, nystagmus, ataxia, dysarthria, tremor, slurred speech, hypotension, arrhythmias, respiratory depression, and coma.
■ If sertraline stops during hydantoin therapy, watch for decreased anticonvulsant effect and increased seizure activity.
■ Urge the patient to tell the prescriber about loss of drug effect and increased adverse effects.

sertraline ━━━►◄━━━ pimozide
Zoloft   Orap

Risk rating: 1
Severity: Major   Onset: Delayed   Likelihood: Suspected

Cause
The mechanism of this interaction is unknown.

Effect
Risk of life-threatening arrhythmias, including torsades de pointes, may increase.

Nursing considerations
◪ **ALERT** Combined use of these drugs is contraindicated.
■ Arrhythmias are related to prolonged QT interval, a known risk of pimozide.
■ Interaction warning is based on actual patient experience with these drugs as well as pharmacokinetics.

---

sertraline ▶◀ **risperidone**
Zoloft   Risperdal

Risk rating: 1
Severity: Major   **Onset: Rapid**   **Likelihood: Suspected**

Cause
SSRIs such as sertraline may inhibit CYP2D6 metabolism of risperidone.

Effect
Risperidone level and risk of adverse reactions and rapid accumulation of serotonin in the CNS may increase.

Nursing considerations
■ Monitor the patient carefully if SSRI therapy starts or stops or if dosage changes during risperidone therapy.
■ Assess the patient for serotonin syndrome, including CNS irritability, motor weakness, shivering, muscle twitching, and altered consciousness.
■ Advise the patient not to alter the dose of either drug without the advice of his prescriber.
■ Average doses of sertraline may cause this interaction.

---

sertraline ▶◀ **sibutramine**
Zoloft   Meridia

Risk rating: 1
Severity: Major   **Onset: Rapid**   **Likelihood: Suspected**

Cause
Serotonin may accumulate rapidly in the CNS.

Effect
Risk of serotonin syndrome increases.

Nursing considerations
◪ **ALERT** If possible, don't give these drugs together.
■ Watch carefully for adverse effects, which require immediate medical attention.
■ Describe the traits of serotonin syndrome: CNS irritability, motor weakness, shivering, muscle twitching, and altered consciousness.
■ Explain that serotonin syndrome can be fatal if not treated immediately.

sertraline ▣━━━◄► St. John's wort
Zoloft

Risk rating: 2
Severity: Moderate   **Onset: Rapid**   **Likelihood: Suspected**

Cause
St. John's wort may cause additive inhibition of serotonin reuptake.

Effect
Sedative-hypnotic effects of SSRIs such as sertraline may increase.

Nursing considerations
■ **ALERT** Discourage use of an SSRI with St. John's wort.
■ In addition to oversedation, mild serotonin-like symptoms may occur, including anxiety, dizziness, nausea, restlessness, and vomiting.
■ Inform the patient about the dangers of this combination.
■ Urge the patient to consult the prescriber before taking any herb.

sertraline ▣━━━◄► sumatriptan
Zoloft   Imitrex

Risk rating: 1
Severity: Major   **Onset: Rapid**   **Likelihood: Suspected**

Cause
Serotonin may accumulate rapidly in the CNS.

Effect
Risk of serotonin syndrome increases.

Nursing considerations
■ If possible, avoid combined use of these drugs.
■ Start with lowest dosages possible, and assess the patient closely.
■ Stop the selective 5-HT_1 receptor agonist at the first sign of interaction, and start an antiserotonergic.
■ In some patients, migraine frequency may increase and anti-migraine drug efficacy may decrease when an SSRI such as sertraline is started.
■ Describe the traits of serotonin syndrome: CNS irritability, motor weakness, shivering, muscle twitching, and altered consciousness.
■ Explain that serotonin syndrome can be fatal if not treated immediately.

sertraline ▶◀ tramadol
Zoloft   Ultracet, Ultram

Risk rating: 1
Severity: Major   **Onset: Delayed**   **Likelihood: Suspected**

Cause
The interaction is caused by additive serotonergic effects.

Effect
Serotonin syndrome may occur.

Nursing considerations
- Watch closely for increased CNS effects, such as anxiety, jitteriness, agitation, and restlessness.
- If serotonin syndrome occurs, stop sertraline and obtain immediate medical attention for the patient.
- Describe the traits of traits of serotonin syndrome: CNS irritability, motor weakness, shivering, muscle twitching, and altered consciousness.
- Urge the patient to promptly report adverse effects.

sertraline ▶◀ tricyclic antidepressants
Zoloft   amitriptyline, desipramine,
                                                 imipramine, nortriptyline

Risk rating: 2
Severity: Moderate   **Onset: Delayed**   **Likelihood: Suspected**

Cause
Hepatic metabolism of tricyclic antidepressants (TCAs) by CYP2D6 may be inhibited.

Effect
Therapeutic and toxic effects of certain TCAs may increase.

Nursing considerations
- If possible, avoid this drug combination.
- **ALERT** Watch for evidence of TCA toxicity and serotonin syndrome.
- Signs of serotonin syndrome include delirium, bizarre movements, and tachycardia, along with CNS irritability, motor weakness, shivering, muscle twitching, and altered consciousness.
- Monitor serum TCA level when starting or stopping sertraline.
- If abnormalities occur, decrease TCA dosage or stop drug.

sertraline ▶◀ zolpidem
Zoloft   Ambien

Risk rating: 3
Severity: Minor   **Onset: Delayed**   **Likelihood: Suspected**

Cause
Sertraline inhibits zolpidem metabolism.

Effect
Onset of action of zolpidem decreases and pharmacologic effect increases.

Nursing considerations
- Monitor the patient for increased response to zolpidem.
- Watch the patient for excessive daytime sleepiness and sedation.

sevelamer ▶◀ ciprofloxacin
Renagel   Cipro

Risk rating: 2
Severity: Moderate   **Onset: Rapid**   **Likelihood: Suspected**

Cause
Decreased GI absorption of ciprofloxacin is suspected.

Effect
Ciprofloxacin effects decrease.

Nursing considerations
- Tell the patient to separate doses of ciprofloxacin from sevelamer by at least 4 hours.
- Help the patient develop a daily plan to ensure proper intervals between drug doses.
- Other quinolones may interact with sevelamer.

sibutramine ▶◀ dextromethorphan
Meridia   Robitussin

Risk rating: 1
Severity: Major   **Onset: Rapid**   **Likelihood: Suspected**

Cause
The interaction is caused by additive serotonergic effects.

Effect
Risk of serotonin syndrome increases.

Nursing considerations
- If possible, avoid giving these drugs together.
⚠ ALERT Combined use may cause hyperpyrexia, abnormal muscle movement, hypotension, coma, and death.
- This interaction is based on pharmacokinetics, not actual patient studies.

---

sibutramine ▬▬▬►◄▬▬▬ dihydroergotamine
Meridia

Risk rating: 1
Severity: Major   **Onset: Rapid**   **Likelihood: Suspected**

Cause
Drugs may have additive serotonergic effects.

Effect
Risk of serotonin syndrome may increase.

Nursing considerations
⚠ ALERT If possible, avoid giving an ergot derivative with sibutramine.
- Watch for evidence of serotonin syndrome, including CNS irritability, motor weakness, shivering, muscle twitching, and altered consciousness.
- If serotonin syndrome occurs, stop these drugs and provide supportive care as needed.
- Other ergot derivatives may interact with sibutramine. If you suspect an interaction, consult the prescriber or pharmacist.
- Advise the patient to tell the prescriber about increased adverse effects.

---

sibutramine ▬▬▬►◄▬▬▬ lithium
Meridia   Eskalith

Risk rating: 1
Severity: Major   **Onset: Rapid**   **Likelihood: Suspected**

Cause
Serotonergic effects of these drugs may be additive.

Effect
The combination can cause serotonin syndrome, which includes CNS irritability, motor weakness, shivering, muscle twitching, and altered consciousness.

Nursing considerations
- Use of these drugs together isn't recommended.
- If used together, monitor the patient for adverse effects.

■ **ALERT** If signs and symptoms of serotonin syndrome occur, provide immediate treatment. Although rare, interaction may be fatal.

---

sibutramine ▶◀ meperidine
Meridia   Demerol

Risk rating: 1
Severity: Major   **Onset: Rapid**   **Likelihood: Suspected**

Cause
Serotonergic effects may be additive.

Effect
Serotonin syndrome may occur.

Nursing considerations
- Use of these drugs together isn't recommended.
- Monitor the patient for serotonin syndrome. The traits include CNS irritability, motor weakness, shivering, muscle twitching, and altered consciousness.

■ **ALERT** If serotonin syndrome occurs, immediate medical attention is required. Serotonin syndrome may be fatal.

---

sibutramine ▶◀ serotonin reuptake inhibitors
Meridia   fluoxetine, fluvoxamine,
                                           paroxetine, sertraline,
                                           venlafaxine

Risk rating: 1
Severity: Major   **Onset: Rapid**   **Likelihood: Suspected**

Cause
Serotonin may accumulate rapidly in the CNS.

Effect
Risk of serotonin syndrome increases.

Nursing considerations
■ **ALERT** If possible, don't give these drugs together.
- Watch carefully for adverse effects, which require immediate medical attention.

■ Describe the traits of serotonin syndrome, which include CNS irritability, motor weakness, shivering, muscle twitching, and altered consciousness.
■ Explain that serotonin syndrome can be fatal if not treated immediately.

sibutramine ➤◄ sumatriptan
Meridia   Imitrex

Risk rating: 1
Severity: Major   **Onset: Rapid**   **Likelihood: Suspected**

Cause
Sibutramine inhibits serotonin reuptake, which may have an additive effect with drugs that have serotonergic activity.

Effect
Risk of serotonin syndrome increases.

Nursing considerations
◨ **ALERT** If possible, avoid giving these drugs together.
■ Monitor the patient closely for adverse effects, which require immediate medical attention.
■ Stop the selective 5-HT$_1$ receptor agonist at the first sign of interaction and start an antiserotonergic drug.
■ Describe the traits of serotonin syndrome, which include CNS irritability, motor weakness, shivering, muscle twitching, and altered consciousness.
■ Urge the patient to promptly report adverse effects.

sildenafil ➤◄ azole antifungals
Viagra   itraconazole, ketoconazole

Risk rating: 2
Severity: Moderate   **Onset: Delayed**   **Likelihood: Suspected**

Cause
Azole antifungals inhibit CYP3A4 metabolism of phosphodiesterase-5 (PDE-5) inhibitors such as sildenafil.

Effect
PDE-5 inhibitor level, pharmacologic effects, and risk of adverse effects may increase.

Nursing considerations
- PDE-5 inhibitor dosage may need to be decreased.
- Administer these drugs together cautiously.
- Instruct the patient to take PDE-5 inhibitor exactly as instructed.
- Warn the patient of adverse effects, including prolonged, painful erection.

sildenafil ➤◀ nitrates

Viagra

isosorbide mononitrate, nitroglycerin

Risk rating: 1
Severity: Major   **Onset: Rapid**   **Likelihood: Suspected**

Cause
Sildenafil potentiates hypotensive effects of nitrates.

Effect
Risk of severe hypotension increases.

Nursing considerations
⚠ **ALERT** Use of nitrates with sildenafil may be fatal and is contraindicated.
- Carefully screen the patient for sildenafil use before giving a nitrate. Even during an emergency, before giving a nitrate, find out if the patient with chest pain has taken sildenafil during the previous 24 hours.
- Monitor the patient for orthostatic hypotension, dizziness, sweating, and headache.

sildenafil ➤◀ protease inhibitors

Viagra

amprenavir, indinavir, ritonavir, saquinavir

Risk rating: 1
Severity: Major   **Onset: Rapid**   **Likelihood: Suspected**

Cause
Sildenafil metabolism is inhibited.

Effect
Sildenafil level may increase, possibly leading to fatal hypotension.

Nursing considerations
- Tell the patient to take sildenafil exactly as prescribed.
- Dosage may be reduced to 25 mg and an interval of at least 48 hours may be needed.
- ⚠ ALERT Warn the patient about potentially fatal low blood pressure.
- Tell the patient to notify the prescriber about dizziness, fainting, or chest pain.

---

simvastatin ▶◀ azole antifungals
Zocor   fluconazole, itraconazole, ketoconazole

Risk rating: 1
Severity: Major   **Onset: Rapid**   **Likelihood: Probable**

Cause
Azole antifungals may inhibit hepatic metabolism of HMG-CoA reductase inhibitors such as simvastatin.

Effect
Simvastatin level and adverse effects may increase.

Nursing considerations
- If possible, avoid using these drugs together.
- HMG-CoA reductase inhibitor dosage may need to be decreased.
- Monitor serum cholesterol and lipid levels.
- ⚠ ALERT Assess the patient for evidence of rhabdomyolysis, including fatigue; muscle aches and weakness; joint pain; dark, red, or cola-colored urine; weight gain; seizures; and greatly increased CK level.
- Pravastatin is the HMG-CoA reductase inhibitor least affected by this interaction and may be preferable for use with azole antifungals.

---

simvastatin ▶◀ carbamazepine
Zocor   Carbatrol, Epitol, Equetro, Tegretol

Risk rating: 2
Severity: Moderate   **Onset: Delayed**   **Likelihood: Suspected**

Cause
Carbamazepine may increase CYP3A4 metabolism of HMG-CoA reductase inhibitors such as simvastatin.

Effect
Simvastatin effects may be reduced.

Nursing considerations
- If possible, avoid using these drugs together.
- Monitor serum cholesterol and lipid levels.
- If hypercholesterolemia increases, notify the prescriber.
- Pravastatin and rosuvastatin may be less likely to interact with carbamazepine and may be better choices than simvastatin.
- Help the patient develop a plan to ensure proper dosage intervals.

simvastatin ▸◂ cyclosporine
Zocor   Neoral

Risk rating: 1
Severity: Major   **Onset: Delayed**   **Likelihood: Probable**

Cause
Metabolism of certain HMG-CoA reductase inhibitors such as simvastatin may decrease.

Effect
Simvastatin level and adverse effects may increase.

Nursing considerations
- If possible, avoid using these drugs together.
- HMG-CoA reductase inhibitor dosage may need to be decreased.
- Monitor serum cholesterol and lipid levels.
- **ALERT** Assess the patient for evidence of rhabdomyolysis, including fatigue; muscle aches and weakness; joint pain; dark, red, or cola-colored urine; weight gain; seizures; and greatly increased CK level.
- Urge the patient to report muscle pain, tenderness, or weakness.

simvastatin ▸◂ diltiazem
Zocor   Cardizem

Risk rating: 2
Severity: Moderate   **Onset: Delayed**   **Likelihood: Probable**

Cause
CYP3A4 metabolism of certain HMG-CoA reductase inhibitors such as simvastatin may be inhibited.

Effect
HMG-CoA reductase inhibitor level may increase, raising risk of toxicity, including myositis and rhabdomyolysis.

Nursing considerations
- If possible, avoid using these drugs together.

⚡ ALERT Assess the patient for evidence of rhabdomyolysis, including fatigue; muscle aches and weakness; joint pain; dark, red, or cola-colored urine; weight gain; seizures; and greatly increased CK level.
⚡ ALERT If the patient may have rhabdomyolysis, notify the prescriber and obtain renal function tests and serum potassium, sodium, calcium, lactic acid, and myoglobin levels.
■ Pravastatin is less likely to interact with diltiazem than other HMG-CoA reductase inhibitors and may be best choice for combined use.
■ Urge the patient to report muscle pain, tenderness, or weakness.

simvastatin ▶◀ fibric acids
Zocor   fenofibrate, gemfibrozil

Risk rating: 1
Severity: Major   **Onset: Delayed**   **Likelihood: Suspected**

Cause
The mechanism of this interaction is unknown.

Effect
Severe myopathy or rhabdomyolysis may occur.

Nursing considerations
■ Avoid using these drugs together.
■ If the patient has severe hyperlipidemia, combined therapy may be an option, but only with careful monitoring.
⚡ ALERT Assess the patient for evidence of rhabdomyolysis, including fatigue; muscle aches and weakness; joint pain; dark, red, or cola-colored urine; weight gain; seizures; and greatly increased CK level.
■ Watch for evidence of acute renal failure, including decreased urine output, elevated BUN and creatinine levels, edema, dyspnea, tachycardia, distended jugular veins, nausea, vomiting, poor appetite, weakness, fatigue, confusion, and agitation.
■ Urge the patient to report muscle pain, tenderness, or weakness.

simvastatin ▶◀ grapefruit juice
Zocor

Risk rating: 2
Severity: Moderate   **Onset: Rapid**   **Likelihood: Probable**

Cause
Grapefruit juice may inhibit CYP3A4 metabolism of certain HMG-CoA reductase inhibitors such as simvastatin.

Effect
HMG-CoA reductase inhibitor level may increase, raising risk of adverse effects.

Nursing considerations
■ Caution the patient to take drug with liquid other than grapefruit juice.
🗈 ALERT Watch for evidence of rhabdomyolysis, including fatigue; muscle aches and weakness; joint pain; dark, red, or cola-colored urine; weight gain; seizures; and greatly increased CK level.
■ Fluvastatin and pravastatin are metabolized by other enzymes and may be less affected by grapefruit juice.
■ Urge the patient to report muscle pain, tenderness, or weakness.

---

simvastatin ━━▶◀━━ macrolide antibiotics
Zocor   azithromycin, clarithromycin, erythromycin

Risk rating: 1
Severity: Major   **Onset: Delayed**   **Likelihood: Probable**

Cause
CYP3A4 metabolism of certain HMG-CoA reductase inhibitors such as simvastatin may decrease.

Effect
HMG-CoA reductase inhibitor level may increase, raising risk of severe myopathy or rhabdomyolysis.

Nursing considerations
🗈 ALERT Watch for evidence of rhabdomyolysis, especially 5 to 21 days after macrolide starts. Evidence may include fatigue; muscle aches and weakness; joint pain; dark, red, or cola-colored urine; weight gain; seizures; and greatly increased CK level.
■ Fluvastatin and pravastatin are metabolized by other enzymes and may be better choices when used with macrolide antibiotics.
■ Urge the patient to report muscle pain, tenderness, or weakness.

---

simvastatin ━━▶◀━━ protease inhibitors
Zocor   darunavir, nelfinavir, ritonavir, saquinavir

Risk rating: 1
Severity: Major   **Onset: Delayed**   **Likelihood: Suspected**

Cause
First-pass metabolism of simvastatin by CYP3A4 in the GI tract may be inhibited.

Effect
Simvastatin level may increase.

Nursing considerations
⚠ ALERT Use of nelfinavir with simvastatin is contraindicated.
- Avoid giving simvastatin and ritonavir together.
- If a protease inhibitor is added to simvastatin, monitor the patient closely.

⚠ ALERT Watch for evidence of rhabdomyolysis, including fatigue; muscle aches and weakness; joint pain; dark, red, or cola-colored urine; weight gain; seizures; and greatly increased CK level.
- Urge the patient to immediately report unexplained muscle weakness.

---

simvastatin ▶◀ rifampin
Zocor   Rifadin, Rimactane

Risk rating: 2
Severity: Moderate   Onset: Delayed   Likelihood: Suspected

Cause
Rifampin may induce CYP3A4 metabolism of HMG-CoA reductase inhibitors such as simvastatin in the intestine and liver.

Effect
HMG-CoA reductase inhibitor effects may decrease.

Nursing considerations
- Assess the patient for expected response to therapy. If you suspect an interaction, consult the prescriber; the patient may need a different drug.
- Check serum cholesterol and lipid levels.
- Obtain liver function test results at start of therapy and periodically thereafter. If ALT or AST level stays three times or more above upper limit of normal, simvastatin will need to be stopped.
- Withhold HMG-CoA reductase inhibitor temporarily if the patient's risk of myopathy or rhabdomyolysis increases, as from sepsis, hypotension, major surgery, trauma, uncontrolled seizures, or a severe metabolic, endocrine, or electrolyte disorder.
- Pravastatin is less likely to interact with rifampin and may be the best choice for combined use.

---

simvastatin ▶◀ verapamil
Zocor   Calan

Risk rating: 2
Severity: Moderate   Onset: Delayed   Likelihood: Probable

Cause
CYP3A4 metabolism of certain HMG-CoA reductase inhibitors such as simvastatin may decrease.

Effect

HMG-CoA reductase inhibitor level may increase, raising risk of adverse effects.

Nursing considerations

■ If possible, avoid giving simvastatin with verapamil. If the patient must take both drugs, consult the prescriber; HMG-CoA reductase inhibitor dosage may be decreased.

⚠ **ALERT** Watch for evidence of rhabdomyolysis, including fatigue; muscle aches and weakness; joint pain; dark, red, or cola-colored urine; weight gain; seizures; and greatly increased CK level.

■ Fluvastatin and pravastatin are metabolized by other enzymes and may be better choices for combined use.

■ Urge the patient to report muscle pain, tenderness, or weakness.

simvastatin ━━━►◄ warfarin
Zocor   Coumadin

Risk rating: 2
Severity: Moderate   Onset: Delayed   Likelihood: Probable

Cause

Hepatic metabolism of warfarin may be inhibited.

Effect

Anticoagulant effects may increase.

Nursing considerations

■ Monitor PT and INR closely when starting or stopping simvastatin.

■ Atorvastatin and pravastatin, other HMG-CoA reductase inhibitors, don't appear to have this interaction with warfarin and may be better treatment options.

■ Tell the patient to report unusual bruising or bleeding.

■ Remind the patient that warfarin interacts with many drugs and that he should report any change in drug regimen.

■ Advise the patient to keep all follow-up medical appointments for proper monitoring and dosage adjustments.

sirolimus ━━━►◄ azole antifungals
Rapamune   itraconazole, ketoconazole

Risk rating: 2
Severity: Moderate   Onset: Delayed   Likelihood: Probable

Cause

Azole antifungals inhibit CYP3A4, which is needed for sirolimus metabolism.

Effect
Sirolimus level, effects, and risk of toxicity may increase.

Nursing considerations
- Monitor trough sirolimus level in whole blood when starting or stopping an azole antifungal. Therapeutic level varies depending on which other drugs the patient receives—cyclosporine for example.
- Watch for signs of sirolimus toxicity, such as anemia, leukopenia, thrombocytopenia, hypokalemia, hyperlipemia, fever, interstitial lung disease, and diarrhea.
- Other CYP3A4 inhibitors may interact with sirolimus. If you suspect an interaction, consult the prescriber or pharmacist.
- Urge the patient to promptly report new onset of fever over 100° F (37.8° C), fatigue, shortness of breath, easy bruising, gum bleeding, muscle twitches, palpitations, or chest discomfort or pain.

---

sirolimus ◀▶ **cyclosporine**

Rapamune   Gengraf, Neoral, Sandimmune

Risk rating: 2
Severity: Moderate   Onset: Delayed   Likelihood: Probable

Cause
The mechanism of this interaction is unknown.

Effect
Sirolimus level and risk of toxicity may increase.

Nursing considerations
- Give sirolimus 4 hours after cyclosporine.
- Monitor the patient for evidence of sirolimus toxicity, such as anemia, leucopenia, thrombocytopenia, hypokalemia, hyperlipemia, fever, interstitial lung disease, and diarrhea.
- Sirolimus level may decrease when cyclosporine is stopped.
- Sirolimus dosage may be increased if cyclosporine is stopped.

---

sirolimus ◀▶ **diltiazem**

Rapamune   Cardizem

Risk rating: 2
Severity: Moderate   Onset: Delayed   Likelihood: Suspected

Cause
First-pass metabolism of sirolimus is inhibited.

Effect
Sirolimus level and side effects may increase.

Nursing considerations
- Monitor sirolimus level when starting, stopping, or changing diltiazem therapy.
- Adjust the dose of sirolimus as needed.
- The effects of diltiazem aren't affected in this interaction.

---

sirolimus ━━━━▶◀━━━━ mycophenolate mofetil
Rapamune   CellCept

Risk rating: 2
Severity: Moderate   **Onset: Delayed**   **Likelihood: Suspected**

Cause
The mechanism of this interaction is unknown.

Effect
Mycophenolate mofetil level and risk of adverse effects may increase.

Nursing considerations
- Mycophenolate mofetil dosage may need to be adjusted when starting or stopping sirolimus therapy.
- Monitor mycophenolate mofetil drug level throughout therapy.
- Watch the patient for increased adverse effects, such as hypertension, headache, hematuria, constipation, diarrhea, anemia, cough, and peripheral edema.

---

sirolimus ━━━━▶◀━━━━ voriconazole
Rapamune   Vfend

Risk rating: 2
Severity: Moderate   **Onset: Delayed**   **Likelihood: Suspected**

Cause
Voriconazole may increase CYP3A4 metabolism of sirolimus.

Effect
Sirolimus level and adverse effects may increase.

Nursing considerations
- ⚠ **ALERT** Use of these drugs together is contraindicated.
- The immunosuppressant benefits of sirolimus may be compromised by increased adverse effects, such as heart failure, toxic nephropathy, thrombocytopenia with hemorrhage, sepsis, and lung edema.

sotalol ━━━━▶◀━━━ aluminum salts

Betapace

aluminum carbonate,
aluminum hydroxide,
aluminum phosphate, kaolin

Risk rating: 3
Severity: Minor   **Onset: Rapid**   **Likelihood: Suspected**

Cause
Rate of gastric emptying is decreased, leading to reduced bioavailability
of sotalol.

Effect
Pharmacologic effects of beta-adrenergic blockers such as sotalol
may be decreased.

Nursing considerations
■ Separate administration of aluminium salts and beta-adrenergic
blockers by at least 2 hours.
■ Monitor the patient's blood pressure and heart rate.
■ Tell the patient to notify the prescriber if he notices an increase in
his heart rate.

sotalol ━━━━▶◀━━━ macrolide antibiotics

Betapace

azithromycin, clarithromycin,
erythromycin, telithromycin

Risk rating: 1
Severity: Major   **Onset: Delayed**   **Likelihood: Suspected**

Cause
An additive increase in the QT interval is seen when administering
macrolide antibiotics and antiarrhythmic agents such as sotalol.

Effect
The risk of life-threatening cardiac arrhythmias, including torsades
de pointes, increases.

Nursing considerations
⚠ **ALERT** Monitor the patient for prolonged QT interval and torsades
de pointes.
■ This interaction may be more likely with telithromycin; avoid
administering with antiarrhythmics.
■ This interaction appears to be dose related.
■ Instruct the patient to let the prescriber know if he experiences
dizziness, palpitations, or light-headedness.
■ The QT interval returns to normal within 3 days of stopping
medications.

sotalol ►◄ quinolones
Betapace

gatifloxacin, levofloxacin,
moxifloxacin, ofloxacin

Risk rating: 1
Severity: Major   **Onset: Delayed**   **Likelihood: Suspected**

Cause
The mechanism of this interaction is unknown.

Effect
Risk of life-threatening arrhythmias, including torsades de pointes,
increases.

Nursing considerations
◗ **ALERT** Giving ofloxacin with an antiarrhythmic such as sotalol is
contraindicated.
■ Quinolones that aren't metabolized by CYP3A4 isoenzymes or that
don't prolong the QT interval may be given with antiarrhythmics.
■ Avoid giving class IA or class III antiarrhythmics with gatifloxacin,
levofloxacin, and moxifloxacin.
■ Monitor ECG for prolonged QTc interval.
■ Tell the patient to report a rapid heartbeat, shortness of breath,
dizziness, fainting, and chest pain.

sotalol ►◄ thioridazine
Betapace

Risk rating: 1
Severity: Major   **Onset: Delayed**   **Likelihood: Suspected**

Cause
Synergistic or additive prolongation of the QTc interval may occur.

Effect
Risk of life-threatening arrhythmias, including torsades de pointes,
increases.

Nursing considerations
◗ **ALERT** The use of thioridazine and antiarrhythmic agents together
is contraindicated.
■ If the patient is receiving thioridazine and sotalol, notify the prescriber
immediately.
■ Monitor the patient for other risk factors of torsades de pointes,
including bradycardia, hypokalemia, and hypomagnesemia.
■ Ask the patient if he or anyone in his family has a history of prolonged
QT interval or arrhythmias.
■ Monitor the patient for bradycardia.

sotalol ◀▶ vardenafil
Betapace   Levitra

Risk rating: 1
Severity: Major   **Onset: Rapid**   **Likelihood: Suspected**

Cause
The mechanism of this interaction is unknown.

Effect
QTc interval may be prolonged, particularly in patients with previous QT-interval prolongation and those taking certain antiarrhythmics, increasing risk of such life-threatening arrhythmias as torsades de pointes.

Nursing considerations
◪ **ALERT** Use of vardenafil with a class IA or class III antiarrhythmic such as sotalol is contraindicated.
■ Monitor the patient's ECG before and periodically after he starts taking vardenafil.
■ Urge the patient to report light-headedness, faintness, palpitations, and chest pain or pressure while taking vardenafil.
■ To reduce risk of adverse effects, patients age 65 and older should start with 5 mg of vardenafil, half the usual starting dose.

sotalol ◀▶ ziprasidone
Betapace   Geodon

Risk rating: 1
Severity: Major   **Onset: Delayed**   **Likelihood: Suspected**

Cause
The mechanism of this interaction is unknown.

Effect
Risk of life-threatening arrhythmias, including torsades de pointes, increases.

Nursing considerations
◪ **ALERT** Use of ziprasidone with certain antiarrhythmics is contra-indicated.
■ Monitor the patient for other risk factors of torsades de pointes, including bradycardia, hypokalemia, and hypomagnesemia.
■ Ask the patient if he or anyone in his family has a history of pro-longed QT interval or arrhythmias.
■ Monitor the patient for bradycardia.
■ Measure QTc interval at baseline and throughout therapy.

spironolactone ➤◀ ACE inhibitors

Aldactone

benazepril, captopril, enalapril, lisinopril, moexipril, perindopril, ramipril

Risk rating: 1
Severity: Major   **Onset: Delayed**   **Likelihood: Probable**

Cause
The mechanism of this interaction is unknown.

Effect
Serum potassium level may increase.

Nursing considerations
■ Use cautiously in patients at high risk for hyperkalemia.
■ Monitor BUN, creatinine, and serum potassium levels as needed.
■ Other ACE inhibitors may interact with potassium-sparing diuretics such as spironolactone. If you suspect an interaction, consult the prescriber or pharmacist.
■ Urge the patient to immediately report an irregular heartbeat, a slow pulse, weakness, and other evidence of hyperkalemia.

spironolactone ➤◀ angiotensin II receptor antagonists

Aldactone

candesartan, irbesartan, losartan, telmisartan

Risk rating: 1
Severity: Major   **Onset: Delayed**   **Likelihood: Suspected**

Cause
Angiotensin II receptor antagonists and potassium-sparing diuretics, such as spironolactone, may increase serum potassium level.

Effect
Risk of hyperkalemia may increase, especially among high-risk patients.

Nursing considerations
■ High-risk patients include elderly people and those with renal impairment, type 2 diabetes, or decreased renal perfusion; monitor these patients closely.
■ Check serum potassium, BUN, and creatinine levels regularly. If they increase, notify the prescriber.

- Advise the patient to immediately report an irregular heartbeat, a slow pulse, weakness, or other evidence of hyperkalemia.
- Give the patient a list of foods high in potassium; stress the need to eat them only in moderate amounts.

spironolactone ➤◄ digoxin
Aldactone   Lanoxin

Risk rating: 2
Severity: Moderate   **Onset: Rapid**   **Likelihood: Suspected**

Cause
Spironolactone may lessen digoxin's ability to increase the strength of myocardial contraction. Spironolactone may also decrease renal clearance of digoxin, resulting in increased serum level.

Effect
Positive inotropic effect of digoxin may decrease. Serum digoxin level may increase.

Nursing considerations
- Monitor the patient for expected digoxin effects, especially in heart failure patients.
- Monitor digoxin level. Therapeutic range is 0.8 to 2 nanograms/ml.
- **ALERT** Spironolactone may interfere with determination of serum digoxin level, causing falsely elevated digoxin level.
- Digoxin dosage may need adjustment during spironolactone therapy; remember the possibility of a falsely elevated level.

spironolactone ➤◄ eplerenone
Aldactone   Inspra

Risk rating: 1
Severity: Major   **Onset: Delayed**   **Likelihood: Suspected**

Cause
Potassium-sparing diuretics such as spironolactone decrease renal elimination of potassium ions.

Effect
Serum potassium levels increase.

Nursing considerations
- **ALERT** Taking eplerenone and potassium-sparing diuretics together is contraindicated.
- If the patient is taking eplerenone and spironolactone together, notify the prescriber that this combination is contraindicated.

- Monitor the patient for signs of hyperkalemia, such as muscle weakness and cardiac arrhythmias.
- Monitor serum potassium level closely.
- Urge the patient to immediately report an irregular heartbeat, a slow pulse, weakness, or other evidence of hyperkalemia.

---

spironolactone ▶◀ potassium preparations

Aldactone

potassium acetate, potassium bicarbonate, potassium chloride, potassium citrate, potassium gluconate, potassium iodine, potassium phosphate

Risk rating: 1
Severity: Major   **Onset: Delayed**   **Likelihood: Established**

Cause
Renal elimination of potassium ions is decreased.

Effect
Risk of severe hyperkalemia increases.

Nursing considerations
⚠ **ALERT** Don't use this combination unless the patient has severe hypokalemia that isn't responding to either drug class alone.
- To avoid hyperkalemia, monitor potassium level when therapy starts and frequently thereafter.
- Tell the patient to avoid high-potassium foods, such as citrus juices, bananas, spinach, broccoli, beans, potatoes, and salt substitutes.
- Urge the patient to immediately report palpitations, chest pain, nausea, vomiting, paresthesia, muscle weakness, and other signs of potassium overload.

---

streptomycin ▶◀ loop diuretics

ethacrynic acid, furosemide

Risk rating: 1
Severity: Major   **Onset: Rapid**   **Likelihood: Suspected**

Cause
The mechanism of this interaction is unknown.

Effect
Synergistic ototoxicity may cause hearing loss of varying degrees, possibly permanent.

Nursing considerations
⚠ ALERT Patients with renal insufficiency are at increased risk for ototoxicity.
- Perform baseline and periodic hearing function tests.
- Aminoglycosides other than streptomycin may interact with loop diuretics. If you suspect an interaction, consult the prescriber or pharmacist.
- Tell the patient to immediately report ringing or roaring in the ears, muffled sounds, or any noticeable changes in hearing.
- Advise family members to stay alert for evidence of hearing loss.

---

streptomycin ━━━▶◀━━━ nondepolarizing muscle relaxants
atracurium, pancuronium, rocuronium

Risk rating: 1
Severity: Major   **Onset: Rapid**   **Likelihood: Probable**

Cause
These drugs may be synergistic.

Effect
Effects of nondepolarizing muscle relaxants may increase.

Nursing considerations
- Give these drugs together only when needed.
- The nondepolarizing muscle relaxant dose may need adjustment based on neuromuscular response.
- Monitor the patient for prolonged respiratory depression.
- Provide ventilatory support as needed.

---

streptomycin ━━━▶◀━━━ succinylcholine
Anectine, Quelicin

Risk rating: 2
Severity: Moderate   **Onset: Rapid**   **Likelihood: Probable**

Cause
Streptomycin and other aminoglycosides may stabilize the postjunctional membrane and disrupt prejunctional calcium influx and acetylcholine output, thereby causing a synergistic interaction with succinylcholine.

Effect
Aminoglycosides potentiate neuromuscular effects of succinylcholine.

Nursing considerations
■ After succinylcholine use, delay aminoglycoside delivery as long as possible after adequate respirations return.
■ If drugs must be given together, use extreme caution and monitor respiratory status closely.
⚠ **ALERT** Patients with renal impairment and those receiving aminoglycosides by peritoneal instillation have an increased risk of prolonged neuromuscular blockade.
■ If respiratory depression occurs, the patient may need mechanical ventilation. Give I.V. calcium or a cholinesterase inhibitor if needed.

---

succinylcholine ➤◀ aminoglycosides
Anectine, Quelicin   neomycin, streptomycin

Risk rating: 2
Severity: Moderate   **Onset: Rapid**   **Likelihood: Probable**

Cause
Aminoglycosides may stabilize postjunctional membrane and disrupt prejunctional calcium influx and acetylcholine output, thereby causing a synergistic interaction with succinylcholine.

Effect
Aminoglycosides potentiate the neuromuscular effects of succinylcholine.

Nursing considerations
■ After succinylcholine use, delay aminoglycoside delivery as long as possible after adequate respirations return.
■ If drugs must be given together, use extreme caution and monitor respiratory status closely.
⚠ **ALERT** Patients with renal impairment and those receiving aminoglycosides by peritoneal instillation have an increased risk of prolonged neuromuscular blockade.
■ If respiratory depression occurs, the patient may need mechanical ventilation. Give I.V. calcium or a cholinesterase inhibitor if needed.

---

succinylcholine ➤◀ anticholinesterases
Anectine, Quelicin   edrophonium, neostigmine,
                                  pyridostigmine

Risk rating: 2
Severity: Moderate   **Onset: Rapid**   **Likelihood: Probable**

Cause
Anticholinesterases inhibit plasma cholinesterase, which delays the breakdown of succinylcholine. Also, increased levels of acetylcholine may increase neuromuscular blockade.

Effect
The neuromuscular blockade is prolonged.

Nursing considerations
■ Use this combination with caution.
■ This interaction is more likely in patients receiving succinylcholine by continuous infusion.
◪ **ALERT** Provide respiratory support and mechanical ventilation if needed.

---

succinylcholine ➤◀ cyclophosphamide

Anectine   Cytoxan

Risk rating: 2
Severity: Moderate   **Onset: Rapid**   **Likelihood: Probable**

Cause
Cyclophosphamide decreases succinylcholine metabolism by inhibiting cholinesterase activity.

Effect
Prolonged neuromuscular blockade caused by succinylcholine may occur.

Nursing considerations
■ Avoid using succinylcholine in a patient who has been receiving cyclophosphamide, if possible.
■ Effect of cyclophosphamide on plasma cholinesterase level is dose dependent.
■ If succinylcholine is given, measure plasma cholinesterase level.
■ If cholinesterase level declines, succinylcholine dosage may need to be reduced.
■ Monitor the patient for prolonged neuromuscular blockade.

---

succinylcholine ➤◀ lidocaine

Anectine   Xylocaine

Risk rating: 2
Severity: Moderate   **Onset: Rapid**   **Likelihood: Suspected**

Cause
The mechanism of this interaction is unknown.

Effect
Neuromuscular blockade may increase.

Nursing considerations
■ Monitor respiratory function closely.
■ Prolonged respiratory depression may occur; provide ventilatory support as needed.
■ There's no evidence that suggest change in therapy is indicated.

---

sucralfate ━━━▶◀━━━ quinolones

Carafate

ciprofloxacin, lomefloxacin, moxifloxacin, norfloxacin, ofloxacin

Risk rating: 2
Severity: Moderate   **Onset: Rapid**   **Likelihood: Probable**

Cause
Sucralfate decreases GI absorption of quinolones.

Effect
Quinolone effects decrease.

Nursing considerations
■ Avoid use together. If it's unavoidable, give sucralfate at least 6 hours after the quinolone.
■ Monitor the patient for resolving infection.
■ Help the patient develop a plan to ensure proper dosage intervals.

---

sulfadiazine ━━━▶◀━━━ cyclosporine

Gengraf, Neoral, Sandimmune

Risk rating: 2
Severity: Moderate   **Onset: Delayed**   **Likelihood: Suspected**

Cause
The mechanism of this interaction is unknown.

Effect
Effect of cyclosporine may be decreased. Oral sulfonamides such as sulfadiazine increase risk of nephrotoxicity.

Nursing considerations
■ Frequently monitor cyclosporine level.
■ Adjust cyclosporine level as needed.
■ Monitor the patient for signs and symptoms of rejection.
■ Monitor creatinine level.
■ Watch the patient for decreased urine output, increased weight, crackles, and other signs of fluid retention.

sulfadiazine 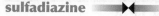 phenytoin
Dilantin

Risk rating: 2
Severity: Moderate   **Onset: Delayed**   **Likelihood: Probable**

Cause
Sulfadiazine may inhibit hepatic metabolism of phenytoin.

Effect
Phenytoin level and effects may be increased, along with risk of toxic effects.

Nursing considerations
- Monitor serum hydantoin level. Therapeutic range for phenytoin is 10 to 20 mcg/ml.
- Phenytoin dosage may need adjustment.
- **ALERT** If sulfadiazine is started during hydantoin therapy, watch for evidence of hydantoin toxicity, including drowsiness, nausea, vomiting, nystagmus, ataxia, dysarthria, tremor, slurred speech, hypotension, arrhythmias, respiratory depression, and coma.
- If sulfadiazine stops during phenytoin therapy, watch for decreased anticonvulsant effect and increased seizure activity.
- Consult the prescriber or pharmacist about other anti-infective drugs if the patient takes phenytoin.

sulfamethoxazole 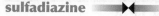 cyclosporine
Gengraf, Neoral, Sandimmune

Risk rating: 2
Severity: Moderate   **Onset: Delayed**   **Likelihood: Suspected**

Cause
The mechanism of this interaction is unknown.

Effect
Effect of cyclosporine may be decreased. Oral sulfonamides such as sulfamethoxazole increase risk of nephrotoxicity.

Nursing considerations
- Frequently monitor cyclosporine level.
- Adjust cyclosporine level as needed.
- Monitor the patient for signs and symptoms of rejection.
- Monitor creatinine level.
- Watch the patient for decreased urine output, increased weight, crackles, and other signs of fluid retention.

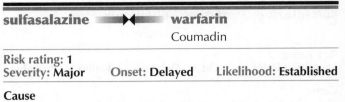

sulfasalazine ➤◄ warfarin
Coumadin

Risk rating: 1
Severity: Major   **Onset: Delayed**   **Likelihood: Established**

Cause
Hepatic metabolism of warfarin may be inhibited.

Effect
Warfarin level, effects, and risk of bleeding may increase.

Nursing considerations
- Monitor coagulation values closely.
- Tell the patient to report unusual bruising or bleeding.
- Remind the patient that warfarin interacts with many other drugs and that he should report any change in drug regimen.

sulfinpyrazone ➤◄ acetaminophen
Anturane   Acephen, Neopap, Tylenol

Risk rating: 2
Severity: Moderate   **Onset: Delayed**   **Likelihood: Suspected**

Cause
Sulfinpyrazone may induce hepatic microsomal enzymes, accelerating acetominophen metabolism.

Effect
Abnormally high rate of acetaminophen metabolism may lead to higher levels of hepatotoxic metabolites, increasing the risk of hepatic impairment.

Nursing considerations
- ◤ **ALERT** The hepatotoxic risk is greatest after acetaminophen overdose in a patient who uses sulfinpyrazone regularly.
- No special monitoring or dosage adjustment is needed at usual therapeutic dosages.
- Advise the patient taking sulfinpyrazone to avoid long-term use of acetaminophen.
- Tell the patient to notify the prescriber about abdominal pain, yellowing of skin or eyes, or dark urine.

sulfinpyrazone 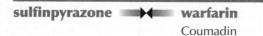 aspirin

Anturane   Bayer, Ecotrin

Risk rating: 2
Severity: Moderate   Onset: Delayed   Likelihood: Established

Cause
Salicylates such as aspirin block effect of sulfinpyrazone on tubular reabsorption of uric acid, and they displace sulfinpyrazone from plasma protein-binding sites, decreasing sulfinpyrazone level.

Effect
Uricosuric effects of sulfinpyrazone are inhibited.

Nursing considerations
◪ **ALERT** Typically, use of sulfinpyrazone with a salicylate is contraindicated.
■ Monitor serum urate level; usual goal of sulfinpyrazone therapy is about 6 mg/dl.
■ Occasional use of aspirin at low doses may not interfere with the uricosuric action of sulfinpyrazone.
◪ **ALERT** Remind the patient to carefully read labels of OTC medicines because many contain salicylates.
■ If an analgesic or antipyretic is needed during sulfinpyrazone therapy, suggest acetaminophen.
■ Advise the patient to maintain adequate fluid intake to prevent formation of uric acid kidney stones.

sulfinpyrazone ◼◼◼▶◀◼◼◼ warfarin

Coumadin

Risk rating: 1
Severity: Major   Onset: Delayed   Likelihood: Established

Cause
Hepatic metabolism of warfarin may be inhibited.

Effect
Warfarin level, effects, and risk of bleeding may increase.

Nursing considerations
■ Monitor coagulation values closely.
■ Tell the patient to report unusual bruising or bleeding.
■ Remind the patient that warfarin interacts with many other drugs and that he should report any change in drug regimen.

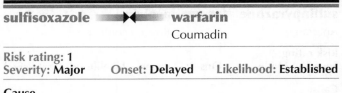

sulfisoxazole ◄► warfarin
Coumadin

Risk rating: 1
Severity: Major   **Onset: Delayed**   **Likelihood: Established**

Cause
Hepatic metabolism of warfarin may be inhibited.

Effect
Warfarin level, effects, and risk of bleeding may increase.

Nursing considerations
- Monitor coagulation values closely.
- Tell the patient to report unusual bruising or bleeding.
- Remind the patient that warfarin interacts with many other drugs and that he should report any change in drug regimen.

sumatriptan ◄► ergot derivatives
Imitrex   dihydroergotamine, ergotamine

Risk rating: 1
Severity: Major   **Onset: Rapid**   **Likelihood: Suspected**

Cause
Combined use may have additive effects.

Effect
Risk of vasospastic effects increases.

Nursing considerations
◤ **ALERT** Use of these drugs or any two selective 5-HT$_1$ receptor agonists within 24 hours of each other is contraindicated.
- Combined use may cause severe vasospastic effects, including sustained coronary artery vasospasm that triggers MI.
- Warn the patient not to mix migraine headache drugs within 24 hours of each other, but to call the prescriber if a drug isn't effective.

sumatriptan ◄► MAO inhibitors
Imitrex   isocarboxazid, phenelzine,
                           tranylcypromine

Risk rating: 1
Severity: Major   **Onset: Rapid**   **Likelihood: Suspected**

Cause
MAO inhibitors, subtype-A, may inhibit metabolism of selective 5-HT$_1$ receptor agonists such as sumatriptan.

Effect
Serum level of—and risk of cardiac toxicity from—certain selective 5-HT$_1$ receptor agonists may increase.

Nursing considerations
◼ **ALERT** Use of certain selective 5-HT$_1$ receptor agonists with or within 2 weeks of stopping an MAO inhibitor is contraindicated.
◼ If these drugs must be used together, naratriptan is less likely than sumatriptan to interact with an MAO inhibitor.
◼ Cardiac toxicity may include coronary artery vasospasm and transient myocardial ischemia.

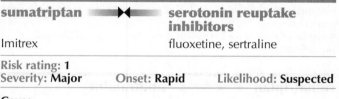

sumatriptan	serotonin reuptake inhibitors
Imitrex	fluoxetine, sertraline

Risk rating: 1
Severity: **Major**   Onset: **Rapid**   Likelihood: **Suspected**

Cause
Serotonin may accumulate rapidly in the CNS.

Effect
Risk of serotonin syndrome increases.

Nursing considerations
◼ **ALERT** If possible, avoid combined use of these drugs.
◼ Start with lowest dosages possible, and assess the patient closely.
◼ Stop the selective 5-HT$_1$ receptor agonist such as sumatriptan at the first sign of interaction, and notify the prescriber.
◼ In some patients, migraine frequency may increase and antimigraine drug efficacy may decrease when a serotonin reuptake inhibitor is started.
◼ Describe the traits of serotonin syndrome, which include CNS irritability, motor weakness, shivering, muscle twitching, and altered consciousness.
◼ Explain that serotonin syndrome can be fatal if not treated immediately.

sumatriptan	sertraline
Imitrex	Zoloft

Risk rating: 1
Severity: **Major**   Onset: **Rapid**   Likelihood: **Suspected**

Cause
Serotonin may accumulate rapidly in the CNS.

Effect
Risk of serotonin syndrome increases.

Nursing considerations
■ If possible, avoid combined use of these drugs.
■ Start with lowest dosages possible, and assess the patient closely.
■ Stop the selective 5-HT$_1$ receptor agonist at the first sign of interaction, and start an anti-serotonergic.
■ In some patients, migraine frequency may increase and antimigraine drug efficacy may decrease when an SSRI such as sertraline is started.
■ Describe the traits of serotonin syndrome, which include CNS irritability, motor weakness, shivering, muscle twitching, and altered consciousness.
■ Explain that serotonin syndrome can be fatal if not treated immediately.

---

sumatriptan ➤◄ sibutramine
Imitrex   Meridia

Risk rating: 1
Severity: Major   **Onset: Rapid**   **Likelihood: Suspected**

Cause
Sibutramine inhibits serotonin reuptake, which may have an additive effect with selective 5-HT$_1$ receptor agonists such as sumatriptan.

Effect
Risk of serotonin syndrome increases.

Nursing considerations
▣ ALERT If possible, avoid giving these drugs together.
■ Monitor the patient closely for adverse effects, which require immediate medical attention.
■ Stop the selective 5-HT$_1$ receptor agonist at the first sign of interaction, and notify the prescriber.
■ Describe the traits of serotonin syndrome, which include CNS irritability, motor weakness, shivering, muscle twitching, and altered consciousness.
■ Urge the patient to promptly report adverse effects.

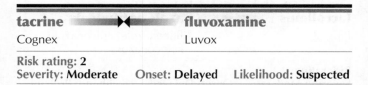

tacrine ◄►◄ fluvoxamine
Cognex   Luvox

Risk rating: 2
Severity: Moderate   Onset: Delayed   Likelihood: Suspected

Cause
Fluvoxamine may inhibit CYP1A2 metabolism of tacrine.

Effect
Tacrine level, effects, and adverse effects may increase.

Nursing considerations
- Avoid using these drugs together if possible.
- If combined use can't be avoided, watch for tacrine toxicity: nausea, vomiting, salivation, sweating, bradycardia, hypotension, and seizures.
- **⚠ ALERT** Watch for progressive muscle weakness (a symptom of tacrine toxicity), which can be fatal if respiratory muscles are involved.
- Monitor liver function tests. Urge the patient to report signs and symptoms of hepatotoxicity: abdominal pain, loss of appetite, fatigue, yellow skin or eye discoloration, and dark urine.
- Consult the prescriber or pharmacist; SSRIs that aren't metabolized by CYP1A2 metabolism, such as fluoxetine, may be safer alternatives.

tacrolimus ◄►◄ alcohol
Prograf

Risk rating: 3
Severity: Minor   Onset: Rapid   Likelihood: Suspected

Cause
The cause of this interaction is unknown.

Effect
Risk of transient facial flushing increases.

Nursing considerations
- The interaction occurs with topical tacrolimus use.
- Warn the patient of risk of increased facial flushing.
- If the patient experiences facial flushing, instruct him to avoid alcohol while using topical tacrolimus.

tacrolimus ◄►◄ azole antifungals
Prograf   fluconazole, itraconazole,
                           ketoconazole

Risk rating: 2
Severity: Moderate   Onset: Delayed   Likelihood: Probable

Cause
Azole antifungals inhibit tacrolimus metabolism in the liver and GI tract.

Effect
Tacrolimus level and risk of adverse effects may increase.

Nursing considerations
- Monitor renal function and mental status closely.
- Check tacrolimus level often. Normal trough level is 6 to 10 mcg/L.
- Tacrolimus dosage may need to be decreased when the patient takes an azole antifungal.
- Signs of toxicity commonly occur within 3 days of combined use.
- **⚠ ALERT** Watch for renal failure, nephrotoxicity, hyperkalemia, hyperglycemia, delirium, and other changes in mental status.

tacrolimus ◄►◄ diltiazem
Prograf   Cardizem

Risk rating: 2
Severity: Moderate   Onset: Delayed   Likelihood: Suspected

Cause
Tacrolimus CYP3A4 hepatic metabolism may be inhibited.

Effect
Tacrolimus level and risk of toxicity may increase.

Nursing considerations
- Monitor serum tacrolimus level; therapeutic range for liver transplants is 5 to 20 nanograms/ml; for kidney transplants, it's 7 to 20 nanograms/ml for the first 3 months of therapy and 5 to 15 nanograms/ml for months 4 through 12 of drug therapy.
- Watch for evidence of tacrolimus toxicity: delirium, confusion, agitation, tremor, adverse GI effects, and abnormal renal function tests.
- Tacrolimus dosage may need adjustment when diltiazem is started or stopped or when its dosage is changed.
- Diltiazem may have similar effects on cyclosporine and sirolimus.

tacrolimus ━━━━━▶◀━━━━━ macrolide antibiotics
Prograf   clarithromycin, erythromycin

Risk rating: 2
Severity: Moderate   Onset: Delayed   Likelihood: Suspected

Cause
Certain macrolide antibiotics inhibit CYP3A4 metabolism of
tacrolimus.

Effect
Tacrolimus level and risk of toxicity may increase.

Nursing considerations
■ If possible, use a different class of antibiotic.
■ Monitor tacrolimus level and renal function test results. Expected
trough level of tacrolimus is 6 to 10 mcg/L.
■ This effect occurs in children and adults.
■ Tacrolimus may need to be stopped temporarily because reduced
dosages may not prevent renal changes.
■ Other macrolide antibiotics may interact.

tacrolimus ━━━━━▶◀━━━━━ mycophenolate mofetil
Prograf   CellCept

Risk rating: 2
Severity: Moderate   Onset: Delayed   Likelihood: Suspected

Cause
The mechanism of this interaction is unknown.

Effect
Mycophenolate mofetil level and risk of adverse effects may increase.

Nursing considerations
■ Mycophenolate mofetil dosage may need to be adjusted when starting or stopping sirolimus therapy.
■ Monitor mycophenolate mofetil level throughout therapy.
■ Watch the patient for increased adverse effects, such as hypertension,
headache, hematuria, constipation, diarrhea, anemia, cough, and
peripheral edema.

tacrolimus ◄►► phenytoin
Prograf   Dilantin

Risk rating: 2
Severity: Moderate   Onset: Delayed   Likelihood: Suspected

Cause
CYP3A4 metabolism of tacrolimus may increase.

Effect
Tacrolimus level may decrease. Phenytoin level may increase.

Nursing considerations
■ Monitor levels of both drugs. Expected trough level of tacrolimus is 6 to 10 mcg/L; expected phenytoin level is 10 to 20 mcg/ml.
■ Watch closely for signs of neurotoxicity or syncope; adjust dosages of both drugs as needed.
■ This effect may occur with fosphenytoin as well.
■ If one drug is stopped, continue to monitor serum level of remaining drug; dosage may need to be changed.

tacrolimus ◄►► protease inhibitors
Prograf   indinavir, lopinavir/ritonavir, ritonavir, saquinavir

Risk rating: 2
Severity: Moderate   Onset: Delayed   Likelihood: Suspected

Cause
Hepatic metabolism of tacrolimus is inhibited.

Effect
Tacrolimus level and risk of toxicity may increase.

Nursing considerations
■ Monitor renal function and mental status closely.
■ Check tacrolimus level often. Normal trough level is 6 to 10 mcg/ml.
■ Tacrolimus dosage may need to be decreased when the patient takes a protease inhibitor.
◣ **ALERT** Watch for renal failure, nephrotoxicity, hyperkalemia, hyperglycemia, delirium, and other changes in mental status.

tacrolimus ━━━━▸◂━━━━ rifampin
Prograf   Rifadin, Rimactane

Risk rating: 1
Severity: Major   **Onset: Delayed**   **Likelihood: Probable**

Cause
Rifampin increases CYP3A4 metabolism of tacrolimus.

Effect
Immunosuppressive effects of tacrolimus on organ transplant recipients may decrease.

Nursing considerations
■ Monitor tacrolimus level closely when rifampin starts; it may decrease in as little as 2 days. Expected trough level is 6 to 10 mcg/L.
■ Increase tacrolimus dosage to compensate for faster metabolism.
■ Watch the patient closely and check serum level when rifampin is stopped so dosage can be adjusted upward.
■ Watch for signs of organ rejection or infection during rifampin treatment.

tacrolimus ━━━━▸◂━━━━ St. John's wort
Prograf

Risk rating: 1
Severity: Major   **Onset: Delayed**   **Likelihood: Suspected**

Cause
St. John's wort increases CYP3A4 metabolism of tacrolimus.

Effect
Tacrolimus level may decrease, increasing risk of organ transplant rejection.

Nursing considerations
■ Discourage use of tacrolimus with St. John's wort.
■ Monitor tacrolimus level closely if the patient takes St. John's wort. Dosage may need adjustment after St. John's wort is stopped.
■ It may take up to 2 weeks for this effect to fully dissipate after St. John's wort is stopped.
■ If the patient takes tacrolimus, discourage use of any herbal product without consulting the prescriber.

tacrolimus ━━━━◄━━━━ voriconazole
Prograf   Vfend

Risk rating: 2
Severity: Moderate   Onset: Delayed   Likelihood: Suspected

Cause
Voriconazole inhibits tacrolimus metabolism in the liver and GI tract.

Effect
Tacrolimus level and risk of adverse effects or toxicity may increase.

Nursing considerations
- Monitor renal function and mental status closely when using these drugs together.
- Check tacrolimus level often. Expected trough level is 6 to 10 mcg/L.
- Tacrolimus dosage may need to be decreased.
- This interaction may occur with other azole antifungals.
- **ALERT** Watch for renal failure, nephrotoxicity, hyperkalemia, hyperglycemia, delirium, and other changes in mental status.

tacrolimus ━━━━◄━━━━ ziprasidone
Prograf   Geodon

Risk rating: 1
Severity: Major   Onset: Delayed   Likelihood: Suspected

Cause
The mechanism of this interaction is unknown.

Effect
Risk of life-threatening arrhythmias, including torsades de pointes, increases.

Nursing considerations
- **ALERT** Use of ziprasidone with tacrolimus is contraindicated.
- Monitor the patient for other risk factors of torsades de pointes, including bradycardia, hypokalemia, and hypomagnesemia.
- Ask the patient if he or anyone in his family has a history of prolonged QT interval or arrhythmias.
- Monitor the patient for bradycardia.
- Measure QTc interval at baseline and throughout therapy.

tadalafil ◄►◄ alpha₁-adrenergic blockers

Cialis

alfuzosin, doxazosin, prazosin, tamsulosin, terazosin

Risk rating: 1
Severity: Major   **Onset: Rapid**   **Likelihood: Suspected**

Cause
The cause of this interaction is unknown.

Effect
The hypotensive effects of alpha₁-adrenergic blockers may be increased.

Nursing considerations
🏴 **ALERT** Administering tadalafil and an alpha₁-adrenergic blocker together is contraindicated.
■ If the patient has taken tadalafil and an alpha₁-adrenergic blocker, carefully monitor his blood pressure and cardiac output.
■ Alert the prescriber that the patient is taking tadalafil and an alpha₁-adrenergic blocker together and that their use is contraindicated.
■ Make sure the patient has readily accessible I.V. access to administer fluids if needed for hypotension.

tadalafil ◄►◄ azole antifungals

Cialis

itraconazole, ketoconazole

Risk rating: 2
Severity: Moderate   **Onset: Delayed**   **Likelihood: Suspected**

Cause
Azole antifungals inhibit CYP3A4 metabolism of phosphodiesterase-5 (PDE-5) inhibitors, such as tadalafil.

Effect
PDE-5 inhibitor level, pharmacologic effects, and risk of adverse effects may increase.

Nursing considerations
■ Dosage of PDE-5 inhibitor may need to be decreased.
■ Administer these drugs together cautiously.
■ Instruct the patient to take PDE-5 inhibitor exactly as instructed.
■ Warn the patient of adverse effects, including prolonged, painful erection.

tadalafil ◄ nitrates

Cialis

isosorbide dinitrate, isosorbide mononitrate, nitroglycerin

Risk rating: 1
Severity: Major   **Onset: Rapid**   **Likelihood: Suspected**

Cause
Tadalafil potentiates hypotensive effects of nitrates.

Effect
Risk of severe hypotension increases.

Nursing considerations
⚠ **ALERT** Use of nitrates with tadalafil is contraindicated.
■ Carefully screen the patient for tadalafil use before giving a nitrate. Even during an emergency, before giving a nitrate, find out if the patient with chest pain has taken tadalafil during the previous 48 hours.
■ Monitor the patient for orthostatic hypotension, dizziness, sweating, and headache.

tamoxifen ◄ rifampin

Nolvadex

Rifadin, Rimactane

Risk rating: 2
Severity: Moderate   **Onset: Delayed**   **Likelihood: Suspected**

Cause
Rifampin increases CYP3A4 metabolism of tamoxifen.

Effect
Tamoxifen level and antiestrogen effects may be decreased.

Nursing considerations
■ Monitor the patient's response to tamoxifen; dosage may need to be increased.
■ Warn female patients of risk of increased uterine bleeding.
■ Instruct the patient not to change dosage unless instructed by the practitioner.

tamsulosin ━━━━▶◀━━━ tadalafil

Flomax   Cialis

Risk rating: 1
Severity: Major   **Onset: Rapid**   **Likelihood: Suspected**

Cause
The cause of this interaction is unknown.

Effect
The hypotensive effects of alpha$_1$-adrenergic blockers such as tamsulosin may be increased.

Nursing considerations
◣ **ALERT** Administering tadalafil and an alpha$_1$-adrenergic blocker together is contraindicated.
■ If the patient has taken tadalafil and an alpha$_1$-adrenergic blocker, carefully monitor his blood pressure and cardiac output.
■ Alert the prescriber that the patient is taking tadalafil and an alpha$_1$-adrenergic blocker together and that their use is contraindicated.
■ Make sure the patient has readily accessible I.V. access to administer fluids if needed for hypotension.

tamsulosin ━━━━▶◀━━━ vardenafil

Flomax   Levitra

Risk rating: 2
Severity: Moderate   **Onset: Rapid**   **Likelihood: Suspected**

Cause
Vardenafil causes an additive pharmacological action.

Effect
The risk of hypotension may be increased.

Nursing considerations
◣ **ALERT** Administering vardenafil and an alpha$_1$-adrenergic blocker such as tamsulosin together is contraindicated.
■ If the patient has taken vardenafil and an alpha$_1$-adrenergic blocker, carefully monitor his blood pressure and cardiac output.
■ Alert the prescriber that the patient is taking vardenafil and an alpha$_1$-adrenergic blocker together and that their use is contraindicated.
■ Make sure the patient has readily accessible I.V. access to administer fluids if needed for hypotension.

telithromycin ▬▶◀▬ antiarrhythmic agents

Ketek

amiodarone, bretylium, disopyramide, dofetilide, procainamide, quinidine, sotalol

Risk rating: 1

Severity: Major   **Onset: Delayed**   **Likelihood: Suspected**

Cause
An additive increase in the QT interval is seen when administering macrolide antibiotics such as telithromycin and antiarrhythmic agents.

Effect
The risk of life-threatening cardiac arrhythmias, including torsades de pointes, increases.

Nursing considerations
⚑ ALERT Monitor the patient for prolonged QT interval and torsades de pointes.
■ This interaction appears to be dose related.
■ Instruct the patient to let the prescriber know if he experiences dizziness, palpitations, or light-headedness.
■ The QT interval returns to normal within 3 days of stopping the medications.

telithromycin ▬▶◀▬ benzodiazepines

Ketek

alprazolam, diazepam, midazolam, triazolam

Risk rating: 2

Severity: Moderate   **Onset: Rapid**   **Likelihood: Suspected**

Cause
Macrolide antibiotics such as telithromycin may decrease metabolism of certain benzodiazepines.

Effect
Sedative effects of benzodiazepines may be increased or prolonged.

Nursing considerations
■ Talk with the prescriber about decreasing benzodiazepine dosage during antibiotic therapy.
■ Lorazepam, oxazepam, and temazepam probably don't interact with macrolide antibiotics; substitution may be possible.
■ Urge the patient to promptly report oversedation.

telithromycin 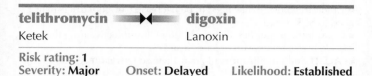 digoxin
Ketek   Lanoxin

Risk rating: 1
Severity: Major   **Onset: Delayed**   **Likelihood: Established**

Cause
Macrolide antibiotics such as telithromycin may alter GI flora and increase digoxin absorption. Telithromycin may inhibit renal clearance of digoxin.

Effect
Digoxin level and risk of toxicity may increase.

Nursing considerations
■ Monitor digoxin level. Therapeutic range is 0.8 to 2 nanograms/ml.
■ Watch for evidence of digoxin toxicity: arrhythmias (bradycardia, AV block, and ventricular ectopy), lethargy, drowsiness, confusion, hallucinations, headaches, syncope, visual disturbances, nausea, anorexia, vomiting, and diarrhea.
■ Digoxin dosage may need to be reduced.
⚑ **ALERT** Telithromycin doesn't affect the serum digoxin level given I.V. Capsule form of digoxin may increase digoxin availability and decrease risk of interaction.
■ Other macrolide antibiotics may interact with digoxin. If you suspect an interaction, consult the prescriber or pharmacist.

telithromycin 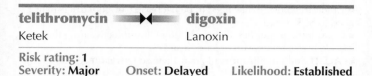 ergot derivatives
Ketek   dihydroergotamine, ergotamine

Risk rating: 1
Severity: Major   **Onset: Rapid**   **Likelihood: Probable**

Cause
Macrolide antibiotics such as telithromycin interfere with hepatic metabolism of ergotamine, although the exact mechanism of this interaction is unknown.

Effect
The patient may develop symptoms of acute ergotism.

Nursing considerations
■ Monitor the patient for evidence of peripheral ischemia, including pain in limb muscles while exercising and later at rest; numbness and tingling of fingers and toes; cool, pale, or cyanotic limbs; red or violet blisters on hands or feet; and gangrene.

- Ergot drug dosage may need to be decreased, or both drugs may need to be stopped.
- Consult the prescriber about a different anti-infective drug that's less likely to interact with ergot derivatives.
- **⚡ ALERT** Sodium nitroprusside may be used to treat macrolide-ergot–induced vasospasm.
- Explain evidence of ergot-induced peripheral ischemia. Urge the patient to report it promptly to the prescriber.

telithromycin ➤◄ HMG-CoA reductase inhibitors

Ketek

atorvastatin, lovastatin, simvastatin

Risk rating: 1
Severity: Major   **Onset: Delayed**   **Likelihood: Probable**

Cause
CYP3A4 metabolism of certain HMG-CoA reductase inhibitors may decrease.

Effect
HMG-CoA reductase inhibitor level may increase, raising risk of severe myopathy or rhabdomyolysis.

Nursing considerations
⚡ ALERT If atorvastatin, lovastatin, or simvastatin is given with a macrolide antibiotic such as telithromycin watch for evidence of rhabdomyolysis, especially 5 to 21 days after the macrolide is started. Evidence may include fatigue; muscle aches and weakness; joint pain; dark, red, or cola-colored urine; weight gain; seizures; and greatly increased serum CK level.
- Fluvastatin and pravastatin are metabolized by other enzymes and may be better choices when used with a macrolide antibiotic.
- Urge the patient to report unexplained muscle pain, tenderness, or weakness to the prescriber.

telithromycin ➤◄ pimozide

Ketek

Orap

Risk rating: 1
Severity: Major   **Onset: Delayed**   **Likelihood: Suspected**

Cause
Macrolide antibiotics such as telithromycin may inhibit CYP3A4 metabolism of pimozide.

Effect
Risk of life-threatening arrhythmias may increase.

Nursing considerations
⚠ ALERT Combined use of these drugs is contraindicated.
- Arrhythmias are related to prolonged QT interval, a known risk of pimozide.

⚠ ALERT People with normal baseline ECG and no cardiac history have died of pimozide blood levels 2.5 times the upper limit of normal from this interaction.

---

telithromycin ➤◀ rifabutin
Ketek   Mycobutin

Risk rating: 2
Severity: Moderate   **Onset: Delayed**   **Likelihood: Probable**

Cause
Rifabutin metabolism may be inhibited. Metabolism of macrolide antibiotic such as telithromycin may increase.

Effect
Adverse effects of rifabutin may increase. Antimicrobial effects of macrolide antibiotic may decrease.

Nursing considerations
- Monitor the patient for increased rifabutin adverse effects, such as abdominal pain, anorexia, nausea, vomiting, diarrhea, and rash.
- Monitor the patient for decreased response to telithromycin.
- Rifabutin and telithromycin usually cause nausea, vomiting, or diarrhea. This interaction doesn't occur with azithromycin or dirithromycin; these drugs may be better choices.
- Giving telithromycin with rifabutin may increase risk of neutropenia.

---

telithromycin ➤◀ verapamil
Ketek   Calan

Risk rating: 1
Severity: Major   **Onset: Delayed**   **Likelihood: Probable**

Cause
Certain macrolides such as telithromycin inhibit CYP3A4 metabolism of verapamil. Verapamil increases telithromycin absorption and decreases telithromycin metabolism.

Effect
Risk of cardiotoxicity is increased.

Nursing considerations
- Closely monitor cardiac function in patients taking this combination of drugs.
- Evidence of cardiotoxicity appears within 2 days to 1 week.
- Monitor the patient for dizziness, shortness of breath, weakness, profound hypotension, bradycardia, QTc prolongation, and complete AV block.
- Consult the prescriber about the possibility of using another antibiotic class.
- Tell the patient to report palpitations, dizziness, shortness of breath, unexplained weakness, and chest pain.

---

telithromycin ▶◀ warfarin
Ketek   Coumadin

Risk rating: 1
Severity: Major   **Onset: Delayed**   **Likelihood: Probable**

Cause
Warfarin clearance is reduced.

Effect
Anticoagulant effects and risk of bleeding increase.

Nursing considerations
- Monitor PT and INR closely when starting or stopping a macrolide antibiotic. PT may be prolonged within a few days.
- Warfarin dose adjustment may continue for several days after antibiotic therapy stops.
- Treat excessive anticoagulation with vitamin K.
- Tell the patient to report unusual bleeding or bruising.
- Remind the patient that warfarin interacts with many drugs and that he should report any change in drug regimen.
- Advise the patient to keep all follow-up medical appointments for proper monitoring and dosage adjustments.

---

telmisartan ▶◀ spironolactone
Micardis

Risk rating: 1
Severity: Major   **Onset: Delayed**   **Likelihood: Suspected**

Cause
Angiotensin II receptor antagonists such as telmisartan and potassium-sparing diuretics such as spironolactone may increase serum potassium level.

Effect
Risk of hyperkalemia may increase, especially among high-risk patients.

Nursing considerations
- High-risk patients include elderly people and those with renal impairment, type 2 diabetes, or decreased renal perfusion; monitor these patients closely.
- Check serum potassium, BUN, and creatinine levels regularly. If they increase, notify the prescriber.
- Advise the patient to immediately report an irregular heartbeat, slow pulse, weakness, or other evidence of hyperkalemia.
- Give the patient a list of foods high in potassium; stress the need to eat them only in moderate amounts.

---

tenofovir ▶◀ didanosine
Viread   Videx

Risk rating: 1
Severity: Major   **Onset: Delayed**   **Likelihood: Suspected**

Cause
The mechanism of this interaction is unknown.

Effect
Didanosine level and risk of adverse effects may be increased.

Nursing considerations
- Carefully monitor the patient for adverse effects, such as lactic acidosis, pancreatitis, and neuropathy.
- Monitor the patient for abdominal pain, nausea, vomiting, or diarrhea.
- Dosage of didanosine may need to be decreased.
- Instruct the patient to call the prescriber for numbness or tingling in extremities.
- The patient with renal insufficiency is at a higher risk for this interaction.

---

terazosin ▶◀ tadalafil
Hytrin   Cialis

Risk rating: 1
Severity: Major   **Onset: Rapid**   **Likelihood: Suspected**

Cause
The cause of this interaction is unknown.

Effect
The hypotensive effects of alpha$_1$-adrenergic blockers such as terazosin may be increased.

Nursing considerations

◤ **ALERT** Administering tadalafil and an alpha$_1$-adrenergic blocker together is contraindicated.

■ If the patient has taken tadalafil and an alpha$_1$-adrenergic blocker, carefully monitor his blood pressure and cardiac output.

■ Alert the prescriber that the patient is taking tadalafil and an alpha$_1$-adrenergic blocker together and that their use is contraindicated.

■ Make sure the patient has readily accessible I.V. access to administer fluids if needed for hypotension.

terazosin ▬▬▬►◄▬▬▬ vardenafil
Hytrin   Levitra

Risk rating: 2
Severity: Moderate   **Onset: Rapid**   **Likelihood: Suspected**

Cause
Vardenafil causes an additive pharmacologic action.

Effect
The risk of hypotension may be increased.

Nursing considerations

◤ **ALERT** Administering vardenafil and an alpha$_1$-adrenergic blocker together is contraindicated.

■ If the patient has taken vardenafil and an alpha$_1$-adrenergic blocker, carefully monitor his blood pressure and cardiac output.

■ Alert the prescriber that the patient is taking vardenafil and an alpha$_1$-adrenergic blocker together and that their use is contra-indicated.

■ Make sure the patient has readily accessible I.V. access to administer fluids if needed for hypotension.

terbinafine ▬▬▬►◄▬▬▬ cyclosporine
Lamisil   Gengraf, Neoral, Sandimmune

Risk rating: 2
Severity: Moderate   **Onset: Delayed**   **Likelihood: Suspected**

Cause
Terbinafine may increase cyclosporine metabolism.

Effect
Cyclosporine level may decrease.

Nursing considerations
- Monitor cyclosporine level.
- Adjust cyclosporine dose as needed.
- Closely monitor the patient for signs and symptoms of rejection when terbinafine is started or stopped.

terbinafine ━━━▶◀━━━	tricyclic antidepressants
Lamisil	amitriptyline, desipramine, imipramine, nortriptyline

Risk rating: 2
Severity: Moderate   **Onset: Delayed**   **Likelihood: Suspected**

Cause
Hepatic metabolism of tricyclic antidepressants (TCAs) may be inhibited.

Effect
Therapeutic and toxic effects of certain TCAs may increase.

Nursing considerations
- Check for toxic TCA level, and report abnormal level.
- TCA dosage may need to be decreased.
- Adverse effects or toxicity may include vertigo, fatigue, loss of appetite, ataxia, muscle twitching, or trouble swallowing.
- Describe to the patient the signs and symptoms he should look for.
- Terbinafine's inhibitory effects may take several weeks to dissipate after the drug is stopped.
- Describe signs and symptoms of toxicity the patient should look for.

tetracyclines ━━━▶◀━━━	digoxin
Sumycin	Lanoxin

Risk rating: 1
Severity: Major   **Onset: Delayed**   **Likelihood: Suspected**

Cause
Tetracycline may alter GI flora and increase digoxin absorption.

Effect
Digoxin level and risk of toxicity may increase.

Nursing considerations
- **⚑ ALERT** Effects of tetracycline on digoxin may persist for several months after antibiotic is stopped.
- Monitor digoxin level. Therapeutic range is 0.8 to 2 nanograms/ml.

- Watch for signs of digoxin toxicity: arrhythmias (bradycardia, AV block, and ventricular ectopy), lethargy, drowsiness, confusion, hallucinations, headache, syncope, visual disturbances, nausea, anorexia, vomiting, and diarrhea.
- Digoxin dosage may need to be reduced.
- Capsule form may increase digoxin availability and decrease risk of interaction.

tetracyclines ➤◄ aluminum salts

demeclocycline, doxycycline, minocycline, oxytetracycline, tetracycline

aluminum carbonate, aluminum hydroxide, magaldrate

Risk rating: 2
Severity: Moderate   Onset: Delayed   Likelihood: Probable

Cause
Formation of an insoluble chelate with aluminum may decrease tetracycline absorption.

Effect
Tetracycline level may decline more than 50%, reducing efficacy.

Nursing considerations
- Separate doses of each drug by at least 3 hours.
- If the patient must take these drugs together, notify the prescriber.
- Monitor the patient for reduced anti-infective response, including infection flare-up, fever, and malaise.
- Other tetracyclines may interact with aluminum salts. If you suspect an interaction, consult the prescriber or pharmacist.
- Help the patient develop a plan to ensure proper dosage intervals.

tetracyclines ◄ calcium salts

demeclocycline, doxycycline, minocycline, oxytetracycline, tetracycline

calcium carbonate, calcium citrate, calcium gluconate, calcium lactate, tricalcium phosphate

Risk rating: 2
Severity: Moderate   Onset: Delayed   Likelihood: Probable

Cause
Calcium salts form an insoluble complex with tetracyclines that lowers tetracycline absorption.

Effect
Tetracycline level and anti-infective efficacy decrease.

Nursing considerations
- Separate doses of tetracycline from calcium salt by at least 3 hours.
- Monitor efficacy of tetracycline in resolving infection. Notify the prescriber if infection isn't responding to treatment.
- Doxycycline is somewhat less affected by this interaction.
- Advise the patient against taking tetracycline with dairy products or calcium-fortified orange juice or within 4 hours of a calcium supplement.

---

tetracyclines ➤◄ iron salts
demeclocycline, doxycycline, minocycline, oxytetracycline, tetracycline

ferrous fumarate, ferrous gluconate, ferrous sulfate, iron polysaccharide

Risk rating: 2
Severity: Moderate   **Onset: Delayed**   **Likelihood: Probable**

Cause
Tetracyclines form insoluble chelates with iron salts, which may reduce absorption of both substances.

Effect
Tetracycline and iron salt levels and effects may decrease.

Nursing considerations
⚠ ALERT If possible, avoid giving tetracyclines with iron salts.
- Separate doses of each drug by 3 to 4 hours.
- Monitor the patient for expected response to tetracycline.
- Assess the patient for evidence of iron deficiency: fatigue, dyspnea, tachycardia, palpitations, dizziness, and orthostatic hypotension.
- If you suspect an interaction, consult the prescriber or pharmacist; an enteric-coated or sustained-release iron salt may reduce it.

tetracyclines ◄── magnesium salts

demeclocycline,
doxycycline,
minocycline,
oxytetracycline,
tetracycline

magaldrate, magnesium
carbonate, magnesium citrate,
magnesium gluconate,
magnesium hydroxide,
magnesium oxide, magnesium
sulfate, magnesium trisilicate

Risk rating: 2
Severity: Moderate   **Onset: Delayed**   **Likelihood: Probable**

Cause
Magnesium salts form an insoluble complex with tetracyclines that
lowers tetracycline absorption.

Effect
Tetracycline level and efficacy decrease.

Nursing considerations
■ Separate doses of tetracycline from magnesium salt by at least 3 hours.
■ Monitor efficacy of tetracycline in resolving infection. Notify the
prescriber if infection isn't responding to treatment.
■ Teach the patient to separate tetracycline dose from magnesium-
based antacids, laxatives, and supplements by 3 to 4 hours.

tetracyclines ◄── penicillins

demeclocycline,
doxycycline,
minocycline,
oxytetracycline,
tetracycline

amoxicillin,
ampicillin,
carbenicillin,
cloxacillin,
dicloxacillin, nafcillin,
oxacillin, penicillin G,
penicillin V, piperacillin,
ticarcillin

Risk rating: 1
Severity: Major   **Onset: Delayed**   **Likelihood: Suspected**

Cause
Tetracyclines may adversely affect bactericidal activity of penicillins.

Effect
Penicillin efficacy may be reduced.

Nursing considerations
■ If possible, avoid giving tetracycline with penicillin.
■ Monitor the patient closely for lack of penicillin effect.

theophylline ━━━►◄━━━ acyclovir
Zovirax

Risk rating: 2
Severity: Moderate   Onset: Delayed   Likelihood: Suspected

Cause
Acyclovir may inhibit oxidative metabolism of theophylline.

Effect
Theophylline level, adverse effects, and toxicity may increase.

Nursing considerations
■ Monitor serum theophylline level closely. Therapeutic range is 10 to 20 mcg/ml for adults and 5 to 15 mcg/ml for children.
■ Theophylline dosage may need to be decreased.
■ Watch for increased adverse effects of theophylline, such as tachycardia, anorexia, nausea, vomiting, diarrhea, seizures, restlessness, irritability, and headache.
■ Describe adverse effects of theophylline and signs of toxicity, and tell the patient to report them immediately.

theophylline ━━━►◄━━━ adenosine
Adenocard

Risk rating: 2
Severity: Moderate   Onset: Rapid   Likelihood: Suspected

Cause
Theophylline may antagonize cardiovascular effects of adenosine.

Effect
The exact mechanism is unknown, but it's thought that theophylline may antagonize adenosine receptors.

Nursing considerations
■ Notify the prescriber of potential of interaction.
■ Larger doses than normal of adenosine may be needed to terminate supraventricular arrhythmias.
■ Carefully monitor the patient's ECG for termination of arrhythmias after receiving adenosine.
■ If the patient is scheduled for a pharmacologic stress test with adenosine and has taken a theophylline-containing medication, the test will have to be rescheduled.

theophylline ➤◀ benzodiazepines
alprazolam, diazepam

Risk rating: 3
Severity: Minor   **Onset: Rapid**   **Likelihood: Suspected**

Cause
Theophyllines produce an antagonistic action by competitively binding to receptors.

Effect
The sedative effects of benzodiazepines may be decreased by theophylline.

Nursing considerations
■ Monitor the patient taking theophylline and benzodiazepines together for a decreased sedative effect of the benzodiazepine.
■ Consult with the prescriber and adjust benzodiazepine dose as needed.

theophylline ➤◀ cimetidine
Tagamet

Risk rating: 2
Severity: Moderate   **Onset: Delayed**   **Likelihood: Established**

Cause
Cimetidine inhibits hepatic metabolism of theophyllines.

Effect
Serum theophylline level and risk of toxicity may increase.

Nursing considerations
■ Watch for evidence of toxicity, such as tachycardia, anorexia, nausea, vomiting, diarrhea, seizures, restlessness, irritability, and headache.
■ Monitor serum theophylline level closely. Therapeutic range is 10 to 20 mcg/ml for adults and 5 to 15 mcg/ml for children.
■ Theophylline dosage may need to be decreased by 20% to 40%.
■ Describe adverse effects of theophylline and signs of toxicity, and tell the patient to report them immediately to the prescriber.
■ Giving ranitidine or famotidine instead of cimetidine for gastric hypersecretion may decrease risk of this interaction.

theophylline ➤◀ diltiazem
Cardizem

Risk rating: 2
Severity: Moderate   Onset: Delayed   Likelihood: Suspected

Cause
Theophylline metabolism may be inhibited.

Effect
Serum theophylline level and risk of toxicity may increase.

Nursing considerations
- Watch for evidence of toxicity, such as tachycardia, anorexia, nausea, vomiting, diarrhea, seizures, restlessness, irritability, and headache.
- Monitor serum theophylline level closely. Therapeutic range is 10 to 20 mcg/ml for adults and 5 to 15 mcg/ml for children.
- Describe adverse effects of theophylline and signs of toxicity, and tell the patient to report them immediately to the prescriber.

theophylline ➤◀ fluvoxamine
Luvox

Risk rating: 2
Severity: Moderate   Onset: Delayed   Likelihood: Suspected

Cause
Fluvoxamine inhibits CYP1A2 metabolism of theophylline in liver.

Effect
Theophylline level and risk of toxicity may increase.

Nursing considerations
- Monitor serum theophylline level closely. Therapeutic range is 10 to 20 mcg/ml for adults and 5 to 15 mcg/ml for children.
- If the patient taking fluvoxamine starts taking theophylline, the theophylline dosage may be reduced by 33%.
- Watch for evidence of toxicity, such as tachycardia, anorexia, nausea, vomiting, diarrhea, seizures, restlessness, irritability, and headache.
- Describe adverse effects of theophylline and signs of toxicity, and tell the patient to report them immediately to the prescriber.

theophylline 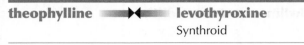 levothyroxine
Synthroid

Risk rating: 2
Severity: Moderate   Onset: Delayed   Likelihood: Suspected

Cause
Theophylline level is directly related to thyroxine level. Patients who are hyperthyroid or hypothyroid may have varying interactions.

Effect
In hypothyroidism, theophylline metabolism decreases, and serum level—and risk of toxicity—increase.

Nursing considerations
■ Monitor theophylline level and dosage carefully; adjust dosage as needed to avoid theophylline toxicity.
■ Carefully monitor serum theophylline level. Therapeutic serum levels are 10 to 20 mcg/ml; toxicity may occur at levels above 20 mcg/ml.
■ Watch for evidence of toxicity, such as tachycardia, anorexia, nausea, vomiting, diarrhea, seizures, restlessness, irritability, and headache.
■ When a patient becomes euthyroid, aminophylline clearance returns to normal.
■ Describe adverse effects of theophylline and signs of toxicity, and tell the patient to report them immediately to the prescriber.

theophylline 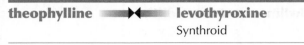 macrolide antibiotics
azithromycin, erythromycin

Risk rating: 2
Severity: Moderate   Onset: Delayed   Likelihood: Established

Cause
Certain macrolides inhibit theophylline metabolism. Theophylline increases renal clearance and decreases oral erythromycin availability.

Effect
Theophylline level and risk of toxicity may increase. Erythromycin level may decrease.

Nursing considerations
■ Monitor serum theophylline level. Therapeutic range is 10 to 20 mcg/ml for adults and 5 to 15 mcg/ml for children.
■ Consult the prescriber about possibility of using another antibiotic.
■ Watch for evidence of toxicity, such as tachycardia, anorexia, nausea, vomiting, diarrhea, seizures, restlessness, irritability, and headache.

- Describe adverse effects of theophylline and signs of toxicity, and tell the patient to report them immediately to the prescriber.
- If the patient takes theophylline, watch for decreased erythromycin efficacy; tell the prescriber promptly.

theophylline ◀▶ methimazole
Tapazole

Risk rating: 2
Severity: Moderate   Onset: Delayed   Likelihood: Suspected

Cause
Methimazole increases clearance of theophyllines in hyperthyroid patients.

Effect
Theophylline level and effects decrease.

Nursing considerations
- Watch closely for decreased theophylline efficacy while abnormal thyroid status continues.
- **⚡ ALERT** Assess the patient for return to euthyroid state, when interaction no longer occurs.
- Explain that hyperthyroidism and hypothyroidism can affect theophylline efficacy and toxicity; tell the patient to immediately report evidence of either one.
- Urge the patient to have TSH and theophylline levels tested regularly.

theophylline ◀▶ mexiletine
Mexitil

Risk rating: 2
Severity: Moderate   Onset: Delayed   Likelihood: Established

Cause
Mexiletine inhibits CYP metabolism of theophylline.

Effect
Serum theophylline level may increase, increasing risk of toxicity.

Nursing considerations
- Monitor theophylline level closely. Therapeutic range is 10 to 20 mcg/ml for adults and 5 to 15 mcg/ml for children.
- Interaction usually occurs within 2 days of combining these drugs. Theophylline dosage may be decreased when mexiletine starts.

■ Watch for evidence of toxicity, such as ventricular tachycardia, anorexia, nausea, vomiting, diarrhea, seizures, restlessness, irritability, and headache.
■ Describe adverse effects of theophylline and signs of toxicity, and tell the patient to report them immediately to the prescriber.

theophylline ➤◀ pancuronium

Risk rating: 2
Severity: Moderate   **Onset: Rapid**   **Likelihood: Suspected**

Cause
These drugs may act antagonistically.

Effect
Neuromuscular blockade may be reversed.

Nursing considerations
■ Monitor the patient closely for lack of drug effect.
■ Dosage of nondepolarizing muscle relaxant may need adjustment.
■ This interaction is dose dependent.
■ Make sure the patient is adequately sedated when receiving a non-depolarizing muscle relaxant.

theophylline ➤◀ phenytoin
Dilantin

Risk rating: 2
Severity: Moderate   **Onset: Delayed**   **Likelihood: Probable**

Cause
Metabolism of both drugs increases.

Effect
Theophylline or phenytoin efficacy may decrease.

Nursing considerations
■ Monitor levels of both drugs carefully. Expected phenytoin level is 10 to 20 mcg/ml. Expected theophylline level is 10 to 20 mcg/ml for adults and 5 to 15 mcg/ml for children.
■ Assess the patient for seizures and respiratory distress, and report findings to the prescriber promptly; dosages may need adjustment.
■ Interaction typically occurs within 5 days of combined therapy.

theophylline ━━━▶◀━━ propranolol
Inderal

Risk rating: 2
Severity: Moderate   **Onset: Rapid**   **Likelihood: Probable**

Cause
Theophylline clearance may be reduced up to 50%.

Effect
Theophylline efficacy may decrease.

Nursing considerations
- Watch for decreased theophylline efficacy.
- Monitor serum theophylline level closely, and notify the prescriber about subtherapeutic level. Therapeutic range for theophylline is 10 to 20 mcg/ml for adults and 5 to 15 mcg/ml for children.
- Selective beta-adrenergic blockers may be preferred for patients who take theophylline, but interaction still occurs with high doses of beta-adrenergic blocker.
- Other beta-adrenergic blockers may interact with theophyllines. If you suspect an interaction, consult the prescriber or pharmacist.

theophylline ━━━▶◀━━ quinolones
ciprofloxacin, norfloxacin

Risk rating: 2
Severity: Moderate   **Onset: Delayed**   **Likelihood: Established**

Cause
Hepatic metabolism of theophylline may be inhibited.

Effect
Increased theophylline level with toxicity may occur.

Nursing considerations
- Monitor theophylline level and dosage carefully; adjust dosage as needed to avoid theophylline toxicity.
- Carefully monitor serum theophylline level. Therapeutic serum level is 10 to 20 mcg/ml; toxicity may occur at a level above 20 mcg/ml.
- Watch for evidence of toxicity, such as tachycardia, anorexia, nausea, vomiting, diarrhea, seizures, restlessness, irritability, and headache.
- Describe adverse effects of theophylline and signs of toxicity, and tell the patient to report them immediately to the prescriber.

theophylline ━━━━►◄ rifampin
Rifadin, Rimactane

Risk rating: 2
Severity: Moderate   Onset: Delayed   Likelihood: Established

Cause
Rifampin may induce GI and hepatic metabolism of theophyllines.

Effect
Theophylline efficacy may decrease.

Nursing considerations
- Monitor theophylline level closely. Therapeutic range is 10 to 20 mcg/ml for adults and 5 to 15 mcg/ml for children.
- After rifampin is started, watch for increased pulmonary signs and symptoms.
- Tell the patient to immediately report all concerns about drug efficacy to the prescriber; dosage may need adjustment.

theophylline ━━━━►◄ secobarbital
Seconal

Risk rating: 2
Severity: Moderate   Onset: Delayed   Likelihood: Suspected

Cause
Barbiturates such as secobarbital may stimulate theophylline clearance by inducing the CYP pathway.

Effect
Theophylline level and efficacy may decrease.

Nursing considerations
- Monitor the patient closely to determine theophylline efficacy.
- Monitor serum theophylline level regularly. Therapeutic range is 10 to 20 mcg/ml for adults and 5 to 15 mcg/ml for children.
- When a barbiturate is added to regimen, theophylline dosage may need to be increased.
- Dyphylline undergoes renal elimination and may not be affected by this interaction.

theophylline ━━━▶◀━━━ thiabendazole
Mintezol

Risk rating: 2
Severity: Moderate   **Onset: Delayed**   **Likelihood: Suspected**

Cause
The exact cause of this interaction is unknown, but metabolic inhibition is suspected.

Effect
Theophylline level may increase with possible toxicity.

Nursing considerations
- Carefully monitor serum theophylline level. Therapeutic serum level is 10 to 20 mcg/ml; toxicity may occur at a level above 20 mcg/ml.
- Watch for evidence of toxicity, such as tachycardia, anorexia, nausea, vomiting, diarrhea, seizures, restlessness, irritability, and headache.
- Describe adverse effects of aminophylline and signs of toxicity, and tell the patient to report them immediately to the prescriber.

theophyllines ━━━▶◀━━━ ticlopidine
aminophylline,   Ticlid
theophylline

Risk rating: 2
Severity: Moderate   **Onset: Delayed**   **Likelihood: Suspected**

Cause
Theophylline elimination is impaired.

Effect
Theophylline level and risk of toxicity may increase.

Nursing considerations
- Use together cautiously. Monitor theophylline level and patient response closely.
- Watch for evidence of theophylline toxicity, including nausea, vomiting, seizures, and arrhythmias.
- If ticlopidine is stopped, theophylline dosage should be increased.
- Urge the patient to report decreasing theophylline effects.

theophyllines ▶◀ zileuton

aminophylline,   Zyflo
theophylline

Risk rating: 2
Severity: Moderate   Onset: Delayed   Likelihood: Probable

Cause
Zileuton may inhibit theophylline metabolism.

Effect
Theophylline level and risk of adverse effects may increase.

Nursing considerations
■ Monitor serum theophylline level closely. Therapeutic range is 10 to 20 mcg/ml for adults and 5 to 15 mcg/ml for children.
■ Watch for evidence of toxicity, such as tachycardia, anorexia, nausea, vomiting, diarrhea, seizures, restlessness, irritability, and headache.
■ If the patient starts zileuton while already taking theophylline, theophylline dosage should be decreased by 50%.
■ Explain common adverse effects of theophylline and signs of toxicity, and tell the patient to report them immediately to the prescriber.

thiabendazole ▶◀ theophyllines

Mintezol   aminophylline, theophylline

Risk rating: 2
Severity: Moderate   Onset: Delayed   Likelihood: Suspected

Cause
The exact cause of this interaction is unknown, but metabolic inhibition is suspected.

Effect
Theophylline level may increase with possible toxicity.

Nursing considerations
■ Carefully monitor serum theophylline level. Therapeutic serum level is 10 to 20 mcg/ml; toxicity may occur at a level above 20 mcg/ml.
■ Watch for evidence of toxicity, such as tachycardia, anorexia, nausea, vomiting, diarrhea, seizures, restlessness, irritability, and headache.
■ Describe adverse effects of theophyllines and signs of toxicity, and tell the patient to report them immediately to the prescriber.

thioridazine ➤◄ alcohol

Risk rating: 2
Severity: Moderate   **Onset: Rapid**   **Likelihood: Probable**

Cause
The mechanism of this interaction is unknown. These substances may produce CNS depression by working on different sites in the brain. Also, alcohol may lower resistance to neurotoxic effects of phenothiazines such as thioridazine.

Effect
CNS depression may increase.

Nursing considerations
■ Watch for extrapyramidal reactions, such as dystonic reactions and acute akathisia or restlessness.
■ If the patient takes a phenothiazine, warn that alcohol may worsen CNS depression and impair psychomotor skills.
■ Discourage alcohol consumption during phenothiazine therapy.

thioridazine ➤◄ antiarrhythmics
amiodarone, disopyramide, procainamide, quinidine, sotalol

Risk rating: 1
Severity: Major   **Onset: Delayed**   **Likelihood: Suspected**

Cause
Thioridazine may have additive effects on prolongation of the QTc interval.

Effect
Risk of life-threatening arrhythmias may increase.

Nursing considerations
◨ **ALERT** Use of these drugs together is contraindicated.
■ Life-threatening torsades de pointes may result.
■ Bradycardia, hypokalemia, and congenital prolongation of the QTc interval are added risk factors for torsades de pointes or sudden death.
■ Prolongation of the QTc interval depends on the dose of thioridazine, becoming more pronounced as the dose increases.

thioridazine ▰▰▰►◄▰▰▰ anticholinergics
benztropine, orphenadrine,
procyclidine, trihexyphenidyl

Risk rating: 2
Severity: Moderate   Onset: Delayed   Likelihood: Suspected

Cause
Anticholinergics may antagonize phenothiazines such as thioridazine.
Also, phenothiazine metabolism may increase.

Effect
Phenothiazine efficacy may decrease.

Nursing considerations
- Data regarding this interaction conflict.
- Monitor the patient for decreased phenothiazine efficacy.
- Phenothiazine dosage may need adjustment.
- Anticholinergic adverse effects may increase.
- Monitor the patient for adynamic ileus, hyperpyrexia, hypoglycemia,
and neurologic changes.

thioridazine ▰▰▰►◄▰▰▰ beta-adrenergic blockers
pindolol, propranolol

Risk rating: 1
Severity: Major   Onset: Delayed   Likelihood: Probable

Cause
Pindolol and propranolol inhibit thioridazine metabolism.

Effect
The effects of both drugs and risk of serious adverse reactions may
increase.

Nursing considerations
- **◳ ALERT** Use of thioridazine with pindolol or propranolol is contraindicated.
- Assess the patient for fatigue, lethargy, dizziness, nausea, heart failure,
and agranulocytosis, all of which are adverse reactions to propranolol.
- Explain expected and adverse effects of these drugs and risk of
interaction.
- Other beta-adrenergic blockers may interact with thioridazine. If
you suspect an interaction, consult the prescriber or pharmacist.

thioridazine ━━━▶◀━━━ duloxetine
Cymbalta

Risk rating: 1
Severity: Major   **Onset: Delayed**   **Likelihood: Suspected**

Cause
Thioridazine metabolism is inhibited.

Effect
Thioridazine level and risk of life-threatening arrhythmias and sudden death increases.

Nursing considerations
⚠ **ALERT** Don't use these drugs together.
■ Thioridazine may increase QT interval, causing serious ventricular arrhythmias and sudden death.
■ Because of the seriousness of the interaction, this information is based on pharmacodynamics, not actual patient studies.

thioridazine ━━━▶◀━━━ fluoxetine
Prozac

Risk rating: 1
Severity: Major   **Onset: Delayed**   **Likelihood: Suspected**

Cause
Thioridazine metabolism may be inhibited by fluoxetine.

Effect
Risk of life-threatening arrhythmias may increase.

Nursing considerations
⚠ **ALERT** Use of these drugs together is contraindicated.
■ Life-threatening torsades de pointes may result.
■ Prolonging QTc interval depends on thioridazine dose, becoming more pronounced as dose increases.
■ The CYP2D6 pathway is implicated in the slowed metabolism of thioridazine when given with fluoxetine.

thioridazine ━━━▶◀━━━ fluvoxamine
Luvox

Risk rating: 1
Severity: Major   **Onset: Delayed**   **Likelihood: Suspected**

Cause
Thioridazine metabolism may be inhibited by fluvoxamine.

Effect
Risk of life-threatening arrhythmias and other adverse effects may increase.

Nursing considerations
◤ **ALERT** Use of these drugs together is contraindicated.
- Life-threatening torsades de pointes may result.
- This interaction continues for more than 2 weeks after fluvoxamine is stopped.
- Other possible adverse effects include tardive dyskinesia, neuroleptic malignant syndrome, constipation, orthostatic hypotension, and urine retention.

thioridazine ━━━▶◀━━━ pimozide
Orap

Risk rating: 1
Severity: Major   **Onset: Delayed**   **Likelihood: Suspected**

Cause
Thioridazine may have additive effects on prolonging QTc interval.

Effect
Risk of life-threatening arrhythmias may increase.

Nursing considerations
◤ **ALERT** Use of these drugs together is contraindicated.
- Life-threatening torsades de pointes may result.
- Bradycardia, hypokalemia, and congenital prolonged QTc interval are added risk factors for torsades de pointes or sudden death.
- Prolonging the QTc interval depends on the thioridazine dose, becoming more pronounced as the dose increases.

thioridazine 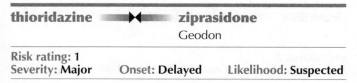 ziprasidone
Geodon

Risk rating: 1
Severity: Major   **Onset: Delayed**   **Likelihood: Suspected**

Cause
The mechanism of this interaction is unknown.

Effect
Risk of life-threatening arrhythmias, including torsades de pointes, increases.

Nursing considerations
⚠ ALERT Use of ziprasidone with a phenothiazine is contraindicated.
■ Monitor the patient for other risk factors for torsades de pointes, including bradycardia, hypokalemia, and hypomagnesemia.
■ Ask the patient if he or anyone in his family has a history of prolonged QT interval or arrhythmias.
■ Monitor the patient for bradycardia.
■ Measure QTc interval at baseline and throughout therapy.

ticarcillin 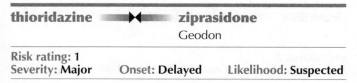 aminoglycosides
Ticar   amikacin, gentamicin,
                               tobramycin

Risk rating: 2
Severity: Moderate   **Onset: Delayed**   **Likelihood: Probable**

Cause
The mechanism of this interaction is unknown.

Effect
Ticarcillin and other penicillins may inactivate certain aminoglycosides, decreasing their effects.

Nursing considerations
⚠ ALERT Check peak and trough aminoglycoside level after third dose. For peak level, draw blood 30 minutes after I.V. or 60 minutes after I.M. dose. For trough level, draw blood just before a dose.
■ Monitor the patient's renal function.
■ Other aminoglycosides may interact with penicillins. If you suspect an interaction, consult the prescriber or pharmacist.
■ Penicillin affects gentamicin and tobramycin more than amikacin.

ticarcillin ━━━━▶◀━━━ warfarin

Ticar   Coumadin

Risk rating: 2
Severity: Moderate   Onset: Delayed   Likelihood: Suspected

Cause
Warfarin induces hypoprothrombinemia, and ticarcillin inhibits platelet aggregation.

Effect
Bleeding time is prolonged. Warfarin resistance may also occur.

Nursing considerations
- Monitor PT and INR closely during combined use.
- Risk of interaction increases with large doses of I.V. penicillins.
- Monitor coagulation values before starting ticarcillin and for at least 3 weeks after stopping to check for warfarin resistance.
- Tell the patient to report unusual bleeding or bruising.
- Remind the patient that warfarin interacts with many drugs and that he should report any change in drug regimen.
- Advise the patient to keep all follow-up medical appointments for proper monitoring and dosage adjustments.

ticlopidine ━━━━▶◀━━━ cyclosporine

Ticlid   Gengraf, Neoral, Sandimmune

Risk rating: 2
Severity: Moderate   Onset: Delayed   Likelihood: Suspected

Cause
The mechanism of this interaction is unknown.

Effect
Cyclosporine level may decrease.

Nursing considerations
- Monitor cyclosporine level.
- Adjust cyclosporine dose as needed.
- Closely monitor the patient for signs and symptoms of rejection when ticlopidine is started or stopped.

ticlopidine ━━━▶◀━━━ phenytoin
Ticlid   Dilantin

Risk rating: 2
Severity: Moderate   Onset: Delayed   Likelihood: Probable

Cause
Ticlopidine may inhibit hepatic metabolism of hydantoins.

Effect
Hydantoin level and risk of adverse effects may increase.

Nursing considerations
- Monitor serum hydantoin level. Therapeutic range for phenytoin is 10 to 20 mcg/ml.
- Hydantoin level may increase gradually over 1 month, and hydantoin dosage may need adjustment.
- If ticlopidine starts during hydantoin therapy, monitor the patient for adverse CNS effects of hydantoins, including vertigo, ataxia, and somnolence. If ticlopidine stops during hydantoin therapy, watch for decreased anticonvulsant effect and increased seizure activity.

ticlopidine ━━━━▶◀━━━ theophylline
Ticlid

Risk rating: 2
Severity: Moderate   Onset: Delayed   Likelihood: Suspected

Cause
Theophylline elimination is impaired.

Effect
Theophylline level and risk of toxicity may increase.

Nursing considerations
- Combine cautiously. Monitor theophylline level and patient response.
- Watch for evidence of theophylline toxicity, including nausea, vomiting, seizures, and arrhythmias.
- If ticlopidine is stopped, theophylline dosage should be increased.
- Urge the patient to report decreased theophylline effects.

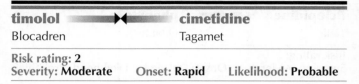

timolol ◄ cimetidine
Blocadren   Tagamet

Risk rating: 2
Severity: Moderate   **Onset: Rapid**   **Likelihood: Probable**

Cause
By inhibiting the CYP pathway, cimetidine reduces the first-pass metabolism of certain beta-adrenergic blockers, such as timolol.

Effect
Timolol clearance decreases and its action increases.

Nursing considerations
■ Monitor the patient for severe bradycardia and hypotension.
■ If interaction occurs, beta-adrenergic blocker dosage may be decreased.
■ Teach the patient to monitor his pulse rate. If it's significantly lower than usual, tell him to withhold the beta-adrenergic blocker and to contact his prescriber.
■ Instruct the patient to change positions slowly to reduce effects of orthostatic hypotension.
■ Other beta-adrenergic blockers may interact with cimetidine. If you suspect an interaction, consult the prescriber or pharmacist.

timolol ◄ clonidine
Blocadren   Catapres

Risk rating: 1
Severity: Major   **Onset: Delayed**   **Likelihood: Suspected**

Cause
The mechanism of this interaction is unclear.

Effect
Potentially life-threatening hypertension may occur.

Nursing considerations
■ Life-threatening hypertension may occur after simultaneously stopping clonidine and a beta-adrenergic blocker such as timolol.
■ It's unknown whether hypertension is caused by an interaction or withdrawal syndrome linked to each drug.
■ Closely monitor blood pressure after starting or stopping timolol or clonidine.
■ When stopping combined therapy, gradually withdraw timolol first to minimize adverse reactions.

timolol ━━━━▶◀━━━━ quinidine
Blocadren

Risk rating: 2
Severity: Moderate   **Onset: Rapid**   **Likelihood: Suspected**

Cause
Quinidine may inhibit metabolism of certain beta-adrenergic blockers, such as timolol, in patients who are extensive metabolizers of debrisoquin.

Effect
Beta-adrenergic blocker effects may increase.

Nursing considerations
- Monitor pulse and blood pressure more often than usual during combined use.
- If pulse slows or blood pressure falls, consult the prescriber. Beta-adrenergic blocker dosage may need to be decreased.
- Instruct the patient to check blood pressure and pulse rate regularly.
- If the patient uses timolol eyedrops, warn about possible systemic effects, including slow pulse and low blood pressure; urge the patient to notify the prescriber promptly if they occur.

timolol ━━━━▶◀━━━━ verapamil
Blocadren   Calan

Risk rating: 1
Severity: Major   **Onset: Rapid**   **Likelihood: Probable**

Cause
Verapamil may inhibit metabolism of beta-adrenergic blockers such as timolol.

Effect
Effects of both drugs may increase.

Nursing considerations
- Combined use is common in hypertension with unstable angina.
- **◀ ALERT** Risk of adverse effects increases, including heart failure, conduction disturbances, arrhythmias, and hypotension.
- Assess the patient for adverse effects, including left ventricular dysfunction and AV conduction defects.
- Risk of interaction is greater when drugs are given I.V.
- Dosages of both drugs may need to be decreased.

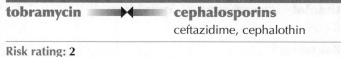

tobramycin ◀▶ cephalosporins
ceftazidime, cephalothin

Risk rating: 2
Severity: Moderate   Onset: Delayed   Likelihood: Suspected

Cause
The mechanism of this interaction is unknown.

Effect
Bactericidal activity may increase against some organisms, but the risk of nephrotoxicity also may increase.

Nursing considerations
■ **ALERT** Check peak and trough tobramycin levels after third dose. For peak level, draw blood 30 minutes after I.V. or 60 minutes after I.M. dose. For trough level, draw blood just before a dose.
■ Assess BUN and creatinine levels.
■ Monitor urine output, and check urine for increased protein, cell, or cast levels.
■ If renal insufficiency develops, notify the prescriber. Dosage may need to be reduced, or drug may need to be stopped.
■ Aminoglycosides other than tobramycin may interact with cephalosporins. If you suspect an interaction, consult the prescriber or pharmacist.

tobramycin ◀▶ loop diuretics
ethacrynic acid, furosemide

Risk rating: 1
Severity: Major   Onset: Rapid   Likelihood: Suspected

Cause
The mechanism of this interaction is unknown.

Effect
Synergistic ototoxicity may cause hearing loss of varying degrees, possibly permanent.

Nursing considerations
■ **ALERT** Renal insufficiency increases the risk of ototoxicity.
■ Perform baseline and periodic hearing function tests.
■ Aminoglycosides other than tobramycin may interact with loop diuretics. If you suspect an interaction, consult the prescriber or pharmacist.

- Tell the patient to immediately report ringing or roaring in the ears, muffled sounds, or any noticeable changes in hearing.
- Advise family members to stay alert for evidence of hearing loss.

tobramycin ━━━▶◀━━━ nondepolarizing muscle relaxants

atracurium, pancuronium, rocuronium

Risk rating: 1

| Severity: **Major** | Onset: **Rapid** | Likelihood: **Probable** |

Cause
These drugs may be synergistic.

Effect
Effects of nondepolarizing muscle relaxants may increase.

Nursing considerations
- Give these drugs together only when needed.
- The nondepolarizing muscle relaxant dose may need adjustment based on neuromuscular response.
- Monitor the patient for prolonged respiratory depression.
- Provide ventilatory support as needed.

tobramycin ━━━▶◀━━━ penicillins

ampicillin, penicillin G, piperacillin, ticarcillin

Risk rating: 2

| Severity: **Moderate** | Onset: **Delayed** | Likelihood: **Probable** |

Cause
The mechanism of this interaction is unknown.

Effect
Penicillins may inactivate certain aminoglycosides, such as tobramycin, decreasing their effects.

Nursing considerations
- **⚡ ALERT** Check peak and trough tobramycin levels after third dose. For peak level, draw blood 30 minutes after I.V. or 60 minutes after I.M. dose. For trough level, draw blood just before a dose.
- Monitor the patient's renal function.

tolbutamide ▰▰▰►◄▰▰▰ aspirin

Orinase   Ecotrin, Bayer

Risk rating: 2
Severity: Moderate   Onset: Delayed   Likelihood: Probable

Cause
Salicylates such as aspirin reduce blood glucose level and prompt insulin secretion.

Effect
Hypoglycemic effects of tolbutamide and other sulfonylureas increase.

Nursing considerations
■ Monitor the patient for hypoglycemia.
■ Consult the prescriber and the patient about possibly replacing a salicylate with acetaminophen or an NSAID.
■ Describe signs and symptoms of hypoglycemia, including diaphoresis, fatigue, headache, hunger, irritability, malaise, nervousness, rapid heart rate, tension, and trembling.
■ Instruct the patient to eat a small carbohydrate snack or meal if hypoglycemia develops, preferably after checking blood glucose level.

tolbutamide ▰▰▰►◄▰▰▰ chloramphenicol

Orinase   Chloromycetin

Risk rating: 2
Severity: Moderate   Onset: Delayed   Likelihood: Suspected

Cause
Chloramphenicol reduces hepatic clearance of sulfonylureas such as tolbutamide.

Effect
Because sulfonylurea level is prolonged, hypoglycemia may occur.

Nursing considerations
■ If the patient takes a sulfonylurea, start chloramphenicol carefully, and monitor the patient for hypoglycemia.
■ Describe signs and symptoms of hypoglycemia, including diaphoresis, fatigue, headache, hunger, irritability, malaise, nervousness, rapid heart rate, tension, and trembling.
■ Instruct the patient to eat a small carbohydrate snack or meal if hypoglycemia develops, preferably after checking blood glucose level.

tolbutamide ▬▶◀▬ fluconazole
Orinase   Diflucan

Risk rating: 2
Severity: Moderate   **Onset: Delayed**   **Likelihood: Suspected**

Cause
Fluconazole may inhibit CYP2C9 metabolism of certain sulfonylureas such as tolbutamide.

Effect
Hypoglycemic effect may increase.

Nursing considerations
■ Monitor blood glucose level.
■ Watch for evidence of hypoglycemia: tingling of lips and tongue, nausea, vomiting, epigastric pain, lethargy, confusion, agitation, tachycardia, diaphoresis, tremor, seizures, and coma.
■ Other sulfonylureas may interact with fluconazole. If you suspect an interaction, consult the prescriber or pharmacist.
■ If the patient takes a sulfonylurea, consult the prescriber about a different antifungal.
■ Urge the patient to monitor blood glucose level at home and to report increased episodes of hypoglycemia.

tolbutamide ▬▶◀▬ MAO inhibitors
Orinase   phenelzine, tranylcypromine

Risk rating: 2
Severity: Moderate   **Onset: Rapid**   **Likelihood: Suspected**

Cause
The mechanism of this interaction is unknown.

Effect
MAO inhibitors increase the hypoglycemic effects of sulfonylureas such as tolbutamide.

Nursing considerations
■ If the patient takes a sulfonylurea, start an MAO inhibitor carefully, monitoring the patient for hypoglycemia.
■ Consult the prescriber about adjusting either drug, if needed to better control glucose level and mental state.
■ Make the patient aware of the signs and symptoms of hypoglycemia, including diaphoresis, fatigue, headache, hunger, irritability, malaise, nervousness, rapid heart rate, tension, and trembling.
■ Instruct the patient to eat a small carbohydrate snack or meal if hypoglycemia develops, preferably after checking blood glucose level.

tolbutamide ▰▰▰◀ rifampin

Orinase   Rifadin, Rimactane

Risk rating: 2
Severity: Moderate   Onset: Delayed   Likelihood: Probable

Cause
Rifampin may increase hepatic metabolism of certain sulfonylureas, such as tolbutamide.

Effect
The risk of hyperglycemia increases.

Nursing considerations
- Use these drugs together cautiously.
- Monitor the patient's blood glucose level regularly; consult the prescriber about adjustments to either drug to maintain stable glucose level.
- Teach the patient to use a self-monitoring glucose meter and to report significant changes to the prescriber.
- Tell the patient to stay alert for increased fatigue, thirst, eating, or urination and possible blurred vision or dry skin and mucous membranes as evidence of high blood glucose level.

tolbutamide ▰▰▰◀ thiazide diuretics

Orinase   chlorothiazide,
                                 hydrochlorothiazide

Risk rating: 2
Severity: Moderate   Onset: Delayed   Likelihood: Probable

Cause
Thiazide diuretics may decrease insulin secretion and tissue sensitivity to insulin, and they may increase sodium loss.

Effect
The risk of hyperglycemia and hyponatremia may increase.

Nursing considerations
- Use these drugs together cautiously.
- Monitor the patient's blood glucose and sodium levels regularly; consult the prescriber about adjustments to either drug to maintain stable levels.
- This interaction may occur several days to many months after dual therapy starts but is readily reversible when the diuretic stops.

- Describe signs and symptoms of hypoglycemia, including diaphoresis, fatigue, headache, hunger, irritability, malaise, nervousness, rapid heart rate, tension, and trembling.
- Instruct the patient to eat a small carbohydrate snack or meal if hypoglycemia develops, preferably after checking blood glucose level.

tolterodine ➤◄ ketoconazole
Detrol   Nizoral

Risk rating: 2
Severity: Moderate   Onset: Delayed   Likelihood: Suspected

Cause
Azole antifungals such as ketoconazole inhibit CYP3A4, which is needed for tolterodine metabolism.

Effect
Tolterodine level, effects, and risk of adverse effects may increase.

Nursing considerations
- Notify the prescriber if the patient takes both drugs; an alternative may be available.
- Watch for evidence of tolterodine overdose, such as dry mouth, urine retention, constipation, dizziness, and headache.
- Explain adverse tolterodine effects, and tell the patient to report them promptly.
- Other CYP3A4 inhibitors may interact with tolterodine. If you suspect an interaction, consult the prescriber or pharmacist.

topiramate ➤◄ estrogens
Topamax

Risk rating: 2
Severity: Moderate   Onset: Delayed   Likelihood: Suspected

Cause
Topiramate may increase estrogen metabolism.

Effect
Estrogen efficacy may decrease.

Nursing considerations
- Watch for worsening of menopausal vasomotor symptoms, including hot flashes, diaphoresis, headache, nausea, palpitations, dizziness, and a skin-crawling sensation.
- If the patient takes topiramate, estrogen dosage may need to be increased; consult the prescriber or pharmacist.

■ Tell the patient that estrogen may be less effective when taken with topiramate. Suggest a nonhormonal contraceptive.
■ Urge the patient to report loss of drug effect—such as spotting, breakthrough bleeding, and amenorrhea—or increased adverse effects.

---

tramdol ◄► serotonin reuptake inhibitors

Ultram

citalopram, fluoxetine, sertraline, venlafaxine

Risk rating: 1
Severity: Major   **Onset: Delayed**   **Likelihood: Suspected**

Cause
Additive serotonergic effects.

Effect
Serotonin syndrome may occur.

Nursing considerations
■ Watch closely for increased CNS effects, such as anxiety, jitteriness, agitation, and restlessness.
■ If serotonin syndrome occurs, stop the serotonin reuptake inhibitor and obtain immediate medical attention for patient.
■ Describe traits of serotonin syndrome: CNS irritability, motor weakness, shivering, myoclonus, and altered consciousness.
■ Urge the patient to promptly report adverse effects.

---

tranylcypromine ◄► anorexiants

Parnate

amphetamine, dextroamphet-amine, methamphetamine

Risk rating: 1
Severity: Major   **Onset: Rapid**   **Likelihood: Suspected**

Cause
This interaction probably stems from increased norepinephrine level at the synaptic cleft.

Effect
Anorexiant effects increase.

Nursing considerations
■ If possible, avoid giving these drugs together.
■ Headache and severe hypertension may occur rapidly if amphetamine is given with an MAO inhibitor, such as tranylcypromine.

⚡ ALERT Several deaths have resulted from hypertensive crisis and resulting cerebral hemorrhage.
■ Monitor the patient for hypotension, hyperpyrexia, and seizures.
■ Hypertensive reaction may occur for several weeks after stopping an MAO inhibitor.

---

tranylcypromine ➡◀ atomoxetine
Parnate   Strattera

Risk rating: 1
Severity: Major   **Onset: Rapid**   **Likelihood: Suspected**

Cause
Level of monoamine in the brain may change.

Effect
Serious or fatal reaction resembling neuroleptic malignant syndrome may occur.

Nursing considerations
⚡ ALERT Use of atomoxetine and an MAO inhibitor together or within 2 weeks of each other is contraindicated.
■ Before starting atomoxetine, ask the patient when he last took an MAO inhibitor such as tranylcypromine. Before starting an MAO inhibitor, ask the patient when he last took atomoxetine.
■ Monitor the patient for hyperthermia, rapid changes in vital signs, rigidity, muscle twitching, and mental status changes.

---

tranylcypromine ➡◀ bupropion
Parnate   Wellbutrin, Zyban

Risk rating: 1
Severity: Major   **Onset: Delayed**   **Likelihood: Suspected**

Cause
The cause of this interaction is unknown.

Effect
Risk of acute bupropion toxicity is increased.

Nursing considerations
⚡ ALERT Coadministration of bupropion and MAO inhibitors, such as tranylcypromine, is contraindicated.
■ Allow at least 14 days between discontinuing an MAO inhibitor and starting bupropion.
■ Interaction warning is based on animal trials, not actual patient studies.

tranylcypromine ➡◀ carbamazepine

Parnate

Carbatrol, Epitol, Equetro, Tegretol

Risk rating: 1

Severity: Major   **Onset: Delayed**   **Likelihood: Suspected**

Cause
The mechanism of this interaction is unknown.

Effect
Risk of severe adverse effects, including hyperpyrexia, hyperexcitability, muscle rigidity, and seizures, may increase.

Nursing considerations
▪ **ALERT** Use of carbamazepine with an MAO inhibitor is contraindicated.
▪ **ALERT** Carbamazepine is structurally related to tricyclic antidepressants, which may cause hypertensive crisis, seizures, and death when given with MAO inhibitors such as tranylcypromine.
■ MAO inhibitor should be stopped at least 14 days before carbamazepine starts.
■ Urge the patient to tell the prescriber about all drugs and supplements he takes and about any increase in adverse effects.

tranylcypromine ➡◀ foods that contain amines

Parnate

aged, fermented, and overripe foods and drinks: broad beans, caviar, fermented sausage, liver, pickled herring, red wine, some cheeses, yeast extract

Risk rating: 2

Severity: Major   **Onset: Rapid**   **Likelihood: Established**

Cause
MAO inhibition interferes with metabolism of tyramine and other amines in certain foods.

Effect
Risk of marked hypertension increases.

Nursing considerations
■ Give the patient a list of foods to avoid while taking an MAO inhibitor such as tranylcypromine.

■ Urge the patient to avoid high-amine foods for 4 or more weeks after stopping an MAO inhibitor.

∾ ALERT Monitor blood pressure closely because marked hypertension, hypertensive crisis, and hemorrhagic stroke are possible.

■ Explain that dietary supplements containing yeast, and chocolates containing cocoa, may cause this interaction.

---

tranylcypromine ➡◀ insulin
Parnate

Risk rating: 2
Severity: Moderate   **Onset: Delayed**   **Likelihood: Established**

Cause
MAO inhibitors such as tranylcypromine stimulate insulin secretion and inhibit gluconeogenesis (glucose formation).

Effect
Hypoglycemic response to insulin may be increased and prolonged.

Nursing considerations
■ Monitor glucose level closely if MAO inhibitor starts or dosage changes.
■ The extent of MAO inhibitor effect on glucose level may not be known for several weeks.
■ Watch for evidence of hypoglycemia: tachycardia, palpitations, anxiety, diaphoresis, nausea, hunger, dizziness, restlessness, headache, confusion, tremors, and speech and motor dysfunction.
■ Consult the prescriber if the patient experiences hypoglycemia; insulin dosage may need to be decreased.
■ Treat hypoglycemia as needed, such as with fast-acting oral carbohydrates, parenteral glucagon, or I.V. $D_{50}W$ bolus.
■ Make sure the patient and his family can recognize hypoglycemia and respond appropriately.

---

tranylcypromine ➡◀ levodopa
Parnate   Larodopa

Risk rating: 1
Severity: Major   **Onset: Rapid**   **Likelihood: Established**

Cause
Peripheral metabolism of levodopa-derived dopamine is inhibited, increasing level at dopamine receptors.

Effect
Risk of hypertensive reaction increases.

Nursing considerations
- If possible, avoid giving these drugs together.
- Interaction occurs within 1 hour and appears to be dose related.
- Monitor the patient for flushing, light-headedness, and palpitations.
- The MAO selegiline doesn't cause hypertensive reaction and may be used instead of tranylcypromine and other MAO inhibitors in patients who are taking levodopa.

tranylcypromine ➤◀ L-tryptophan
Parnate

Risk rating: 1
Severity: Major   **Onset: Rapid**   **Likelihood: Suspected**

Cause
Additive serotonergic effects may occur.

Effect
Risk of serotonin syndrome increases.

Nursing considerations
🖎 **ALERT** Combined use of these drugs is contraindicated.
- They may cause CNS irritability, motor weakness, shivering, muscle twitching, and altered consciousness.

tranylcypromine ➤◀ meperidine
Parnate   Demerol

Risk rating: 1
Severity: Major   **Onset: Rapid**   **Likelihood: Probable**

Cause
The mechanism of this interaction is unknown.

Effect
Risk of severe adverse reactions increases.

Nursing considerations
- If possible, avoid giving these drugs together.
- Monitor the patient; report agitation, seizures, diaphoresis, and fever.
🖎 **ALERT** Reaction may progress to coma, apnea, and death.
- Reaction may occur several weeks after stopping the MAO inhibitor.
- Give opioid analgesics other than meperidine cautiously. It isn't known if similar reactions occur.

tranylcypromine ➤◄ methylphenidates

Parnate

dexmethylphenidate,
methylphenidate

Risk rating: 1
Severity: Major   **Onset: Delayed**   **Likelihood: Suspected**

Cause
The mechanism of this interaction is unknown.

Effect
Risk of hypertensive crisis increases.

Nursing considerations
▣ **ALERT** Use of dexmethylphenidate with an MAO inhibitor, such as tranylcypromine, is contraindicated.
▪ Don't use dexmethylphenidate within 14 days after stopping an MAO inhibitor.
▪ Monitor blood pressure closely.
▪ Teach the patient and responsible family members to monitor blood pressure at home.

tranylcypromine ➤◄ selective 5-HT$_1$ receptor agonists

Parnate

rizatriptan, sumatriptan,
zolmitriptan

Risk rating: 1
Severity: Major   **Onset: Rapid**   **Likelihood: Suspected**

Cause
Tranylcypromine and other MAO inhibitors, subtype-A, may inhibit the metabolism of selective 5-HT$_1$ receptor agonists.

Effect
Selective 5-HT$_1$ receptor agonist level and risk of cardiac toxicity may increase.

Nursing considerations
▣ **ALERT** Use of certain selective 5-HT$_1$ receptor agonists with or within 2 weeks of stopping an MAO inhibitor is contraindicated.
▪ Naratriptan is less likely to interact with an MAO inhibitor.
▪ Cardiac toxicity may include coronary artery vasospasm and transient myocardial ischemia.

tranylcypromine ➤◀ serotonin reuptake inhibitors

Parnate

citalopram, duloxetine, fluoxetine, sertraline, venlafaxine

Risk rating: 1
Severity: Major   **Onset: Rapid**   **Likelihood: Probable**

Cause
Serotonin may accumulate rapidly in the CNS.

Effect
Risk of serotonin syndrome increases.

Nursing considerations
⚠ **ALERT** Don't use these drugs together.
■ Allow 1 week after stopping venlafaxine (2 weeks after stopping citalopram, or sertraline; 5 weeks after stopping fluoxetine) before giving an MAO inhibitor such as tranylcypromine.
■ Wait 2 weeks after stopping an MAO inhibitor before giving a serotonin reuptake inhibitor.
■ The selective MAO type-B inhibitor selegiline has been given with fluoxetine, paroxetine, or sertraline to patients with Parkinson's disease without negative effects.
■ Make the patient aware of the traits of serotonin syndrome: CNS irritability, motor weakness, shivering, myoclonus, and altered consciousness.
■ Urge the patient to promptly report adverse effects to the prescriber.

tranylcypromine ➤◀ sulfonylureas

Parnate

chlorpropamide, tolbutamide

Risk rating: 2
Severity: Moderate   **Onset: Rapid**   **Likelihood: Suspected**

Cause
The mechanism of this interaction is unknown.

Effect
Tranylcypromine and other MAO inhibitors increase the hypoglycemic effects of sulfonylureas.

Nursing considerations
■ Monitor the patient for hypoglycemia.
■ Consult the prescriber about adjustments to either drug, if needed, to control glucose level and mental state.

- Describe signs and symptoms of hypoglycemia, including diaphoresis, fatigue, headache, hunger, irritability, malaise, nervousness, rapid heart rate, tension, and trembling.
- Instruct the patient to eat a small carbohydrate snack or meal if hypoglycemia develops, preferably after checking blood glucose level.

tranylcypromine ➤◀ sympathomimetics

Parnate

dopamine, ephedrine,
phenylephrine,
pseudoephedrine

Risk rating: 1
Severity: Major   **Onset: Rapid**   **Likelihood: Established**

Cause
When MAO is inhibited, norepinephrine accumulates and is released by indirect and mixed-acting sympathomimetics, increasing the pressor response at receptor sites.

Effect
Risk of severe headaches, hypertension, high fever, and hypertensive crisis increases.

Nursing considerations
- Avoid giving indirect or mixed-acting sympathomimetics with an MAO inhibitor such as tranylcypromine.
- Phentolamine can be administered to block epinephrine- and norepinephrine-induced vasoconstriction and reduce blood pressure.
- Direct-acting sympathomimetics interact minimally.
⚠ **ALERT** Warn the patient that decongestants and other OTC medicines may cause this interaction.

tranylcypromine ➤◀ tricyclic antidepressants

Parnate

amitriptyline, clomipramine,
desipramine, doxepin,
imipramine

Risk rating: 1
Severity: Major   **Onset: Rapid**   **Likelihood: Suspected**

Cause
The mechanism of this interaction is unknown.

Effect
Risk of hyperpyretic crisis, seizures, and death increase.

Nursing considerations
⚡ ALERT Don't give a tricyclic antidepressant with or within 2 weeks of an MAO inhibitor such as tranylcypromine.
- Imipramine and clomipramine may be more likely to interact with MAO inhibitors.
- Watch for adverse effects, including confusion, hyperexcitability, rigidity, seizures, increased temperature, increased pulse, increased respiration, sweating, mydriasis, flushing, headache, coma, and DIC.

---

triamcinolone ▰▰▰◀▶ salicylates
Aristocort   aspirin, choline salicylate, sodium salicylate

Risk rating: 2
Severity: Moderate   Onset: Delayed   Likelihood: Probable

Cause
Triamcinolone and other corticosteroids stimulate hepatic metabolism of salicylates and may increase renal excretion.

Effect
Salicylate level and effects decrease.

Nursing considerations
- Monitor salicylate level and efficacy; dosage may need adjustment.
⚡ ALERT Giving a salicylate while tapering a corticosteroid may result in salicylate toxicity.
- Watch for evidence of salicylate toxicity, including diaphoresis, nausea, vomiting, tinnitus, hyperventilation, and CNS depression.
- Patients with renal impairment may be at greater risk.

---

triamterene ▰▰▰◀▶ eplerenone
Dyrenium   Inspra

Risk rating: 1
Severity: Major   Onset: Delayed   Likelihood: Suspected

Cause
Potassium-sparing diuretics, such as triamterene, decrease renal elimination of potassium ions.

Effect
Serum potassium levels increase.

Nursing considerations
⚡ ALERT Taking eplerenone and potassium-sparing diuretics together is contraindicated.

■ If the patient is taking eplerenone and triamterene together, notify the prescriber that this combination is contraindicated.
■ Monitor the patient for signs of hyperkalemia, such as muscle weakness and cardiac arrhythmias.
■ Monitor serum potassium levels closely.
■ Urge the patient to immediately report an irregular heartbeat, a slow pulse, weakness, and other evidence of hyperkalemia.

triamterene ◄► potassium preparations

Dyrenium

potassium acetate, potassium bicarbonate, potassium chloride, potassium citrate, potassium gluconate, potassium iodine, potassium phosphate

Risk rating: 1
Severity: Major   **Onset: Delayed**   **Likelihood: Established**

Cause
This interaction reduces renal elimination of potassium ions.

Effect
Risk of severe hyperkalemia increases.

Nursing considerations
◤ ALERT Don't use this combination unless the patient has severe hypokalemia that isn't responding to either drug class alone.
■ To avoid hyperkalemia, monitor potassium level often.
■ Tell the patient to avoid high-potassium foods, such as citrus juices, bananas, spinach, broccoli, beans, potatoes, and salt substitutes.
■ Urge the patient to immediately report palpitations, chest pain, nausea, vomiting, paresthesia, muscle weakness, and other signs of potassium overload.

triazolam ◄► alcohol

Halcion

Risk rating: 2
Severity: Moderate   **Onset: Rapid**   **Likelihood: Established**

Cause
Alcohol inhibits hepatic enzymes, which decreases clearance and increases peak level of triazolam and other benzodiazepines.

Effect
Additive or synergistic effects may occur.

Nursing considerations
■ Advise patient against consuming alcohol while taking a benzodiazepine.
■ Before benzodiazepine therapy starts, assess the patient thoroughly for history or evidence of alcohol use.
■ Watch for additive CNS effects, which may suggest benzodiazepine overdose.

---

triazolam ━━━━▶◀ azole antifungals
Halcion   fluconazole, itraconazole, ketoconazole, voriconazole

---

Risk rating: 2
Severity: Moderate   Onset: Delayed   Likelihood: Established

Cause
Azole antifungals decrease CYP3A4 metabolism of certain benzodiazepines, such as triazolam.

Effect
Benzodiazepine effects are increased and prolonged.

Nursing considerations
◪ **ALERT** Use of triazolam with itraconazole or ketoconazole is contraindicated.
■ If the patient takes fluconazole or miconazole, consult the prescriber about giving a lower benzodiazepine dose or a drug not metabolized by CYP3A4, such as temazepam or lorazepam.
■ Caution that the effects of this interaction may last several days after stopping the azole antifungal.
■ Explain that taking these drugs together may increase sedative effects; tell the patient to report such effects promptly.
■ Explain alternative methods of inducing sleep or relieving anxiety.
■ Various benzodiazepine–azole antifungal combinations may interact. If you suspect an interaction, consult the prescriber or pharmacist.

---

triazolam ━━━━▶◀ cimetidine
Halcion   Tagamet

Risk rating: 3
Severity: Minor   Onset: Rapid   Likelihood: Probable

Cause
Hepatic metabolism of benzodiazepines, such as triazolam, may be decreased.

Effect
Serum levels of triazolam may be increased, causing increased sedation.

Nursing considerations
◪ **ALERT** Carefully monitor the patient for increased sedation after taking cimetidine and a benzodiazepine.
- Warn the patient about the risk of increased sedation when taking cimetidine and triazolam together.
- If the patient has increased sedation, discuss the possibility of decreasing the dose of triazolam with the prescriber.
- Monitor serum benzodiazepine levels while the patient is taking cimetidine and a benzodiazepine together.

◪ **ALERT** Elderly patients are at a higher risk for increased levels of sedation.

---

triazolam ━━━▶◀ diltiazem
Halcion   Cardizem

Risk rating: 2
Severity: Moderate   **Onset: Rapid**   **Likelihood: Probable**

Cause
Diltiazem may decrease metabolism of some benzodiazepines, such as triazolam.

Effect
Benzodiazepine effects may increase.

Nursing considerations
- Watch for signs of increased CNS depression: sedation, dizziness, confusion, asthenia, ataxia, altered level of consciousness, hypoactive reflexes, hypotension, bradycardia, and respiratory depression.
- Lower triazolam dose may be needed.
- Explain the risk of increased and prolonged CNS effects.
- Warn the patient to avoid hazardous activities until effects of this combination are clear.
- Other benzodiazepines may interact with diltiazem. If you suspect an interaction, consult the prescriber or pharmacist.

---

triazolam ━━━▶◀ grapefruit juice
Halcion

Risk rating: 2
Severity: Moderate   **Onset: Rapid**   **Likelihood: Probable**

Cause
Grapefruit juice inhibits first-pass CYP3A4 metabolism of certain benzodiazepines, such as triazolam.

Effect
Benzodiazepine onset is delayed and effects are increased.

Nursing considerations
■ **ALERT** Tell the patient not to take the drug with grapefruit juice.
■ If he does, explain that oversedation may last up to 72 hours.
■ This interaction is increased in patients with cirrhosis of the liver.
■ Instruct the patient to tell the prescriber if he experiences increased sedation or has trouble walking or using his limbs.

---

triazolam ◄──►► macrolide antibiotics
Halcion   clarithromycin, erythromycin, telithromycin

Risk rating: 2
Severity: Moderate   **Onset: Rapid**   **Likelihood: Suspected**

Cause
Macrolide antibiotics may decrease metabolism of certain benzodiazepines, such as triazolam.

Effect
Sedative effects of benzodiazepines may be increased or prolonged.

Nursing considerations
■ Consult the prescriber about decreasing benzodiazepine dosage during antibiotic therapy.
■ Urge the patient to promptly report oversedation.
■ Lorazepam, oxazepam, and temazepam probably don't interact with macrolide antibiotics; substitution for triazolam may be possible.

---

triazolam ◄──►► modafinil
Halcion   Provigil

Risk rating: 2
Severity: Moderate   **Onset: Delayed**   **Likelihood: Suspected**

Cause
Modafinil may induce the GI and hepatic (CYP3A4/5) metabolism of triazolam.

Effect
Triazolam level and effects may decrease.

Nursing considerations
- Observe the patient for quality and quantity of sleep.
- Triazolam dosage may need to be adjusted.
- Discuss the possible effects of this combination on the sleep-wake cycle.

triazolam ███████◄► nonnucleoside reverse-transcriptase inhibitors

Halcion

delavirdine, efavirenz

Risk rating: 2
Severity: Moderate   **Onset: Delayed**   **Likelihood: Suspected**

Cause
Nonnucleoside reverse-transcriptase inhibitors may inhibit CYP3A4 metabolism of certain benzodiazepines, such as triazolam.

Effect
Sedative effects of benzodiazepines may be increased or prolonged.

Nursing considerations
⚠ ALERT Don't combine triazolam with delavirdine or efavirenz.
- Explain the risk of oversedation and respiratory depression.
- Urge the patient to promptly report any suspected interaction.
- Other benzodiazepines and nonnucleoside reverse-transcriptase inhibitors may interact. If you suspect an interaction, consult the prescriber or pharmacist.

triazolam ███████◄► omeprazole

Halcion

Prilosec

Risk rating: 3
Severity: Minor   **Onset: Delayed**   **Likelihood: Suspected**

Cause
Metabolism of benzodiazepines, such as triazolam, may be decreased.

Effect
Half-life of triazolam may be increased, leading to increased levels. Sedation or ataxia may be enhanced.

Nursing considerations
- Monitor the patient for increased sedation or CNS impairment.
- Consult the prescriber about reducing diazepam dosage.
- Other benzodiazepines may not have this interaction.

triazolam ━━━━▶◀━━━ protease inhibitors
Halcion

atazanavir, darunavir indinavir, nelfinavir, ritonavir, saquinavir

Risk rating: 1
Severity: Major   **Onset: Delayed**   **Likelihood: Suspected**

Cause
Protease inhibitors may inhibit CYP3A4 metabolism of certain benzodiazepines, such as triazolam.

Effect
Sedative effects of benzodiazepines may be increased or prolonged.

Nursing considerations
◼ **ALERT** Use of triazolam with a protease inhibitor is contraindicated.
▪ If the patient takes any benzodiazepine–protease inhibitor combination, notify the prescriber. Interaction also involves other drugs in the class.
▪ Watch for evidence of oversedation and respiratory depression.
▪ Explain the risks of using these drugs together.

triazolam ━━━━▶◀━━━ rifampin
Halcion

Rifadin, Rimactane

Risk rating: 2
Severity: Moderate   **Onset: Delayed**   **Likelihood: Suspected**

Cause
Rifampin may increase CYP3A4 metabolism of benzodiazepines such as triazolam.

Effect
Antianxiety, sedative, and sleep-inducing effects may decrease.

Nursing considerations
▪ Watch for expected benzodiazepine effects and lack of efficacy.
▪ If benzodiazepine efficacy decreases, dosage may be changed.
▪ Other benzodiazepines may interact with rifampin. If you suspect an interaction, consult the prescriber or pharmacist.
▪ For insomnia, temazepam may be more effective than triazolam because it doesn't undergo CYP3A4 metabolism.

trihexyphenidyl 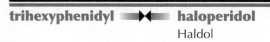 haloperidol
Haldol

Risk rating: 2
Severity: Moderate   Onset: Delayed   Likelihood: Suspected

Cause
The mechanism of this interaction is unknown. It may involve central cholinergic pathways rather than a true pharmacokinetic interaction.

Effect
Effects may vary and include decreased haloperidol level, worsened schizophrenic symptoms, and development of tardive dyskinesia.

Nursing considerations
■ **ALERT** If the patient takes haloperidol, avoid anticholinergics such as trihexyphenidyl if possible.

■ Watch for signs of worsening schizophrenia, including delusions, hallucinations, disorganized speech or behavior, inappropriate affect, and abnormal psychomotor activity.

■ Watch for the development of tardive dyskinesia: involuntary abnormal repetitive movements, including lip smacking, cheek puffing, chewing motions, tongue thrusting, finger flicking, and trunk twisting.

■ Consult the prescriber if adverse effects occur. Trihexyphenidyl may need to be stopped, or haloperidol dosage may need adjustment.

trihexyphenidyl 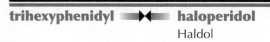 phenothiazines
chlorpromazine, per-
phenazine, thioridazine

Risk rating: 2
Severity: Moderate   Onset: Delayed   Likelihood: Suspected

Cause
Anticholinergics, such as trihexyphenidyl, may antagonize phenothiazines. Also, phenothiazine metabolism may increase.

Effect
Phenothiazine efficacy may decrease.

Nursing considerations
- Data regarding this interaction conflict.
- Monitor the patient for decreased phenothiazine efficacy.
- The phenothiazine dosage may need adjustment.
- Anticholinergic adverse effects may increase.
- Monitor the patient for adynamic ileus, hyperpyrexia, hypoglycemia, and neurologic changes.
- Other anticholinergics may interact with phenothiazines. If you suspect an interaction, consult the prescriber or pharmacist.

---

trimethoprim ➤◀ methotrexate
Proloprim   Rheumatrex, Trexall

Risk rating: 1
Severity: Major   **Onset: Delayed**   **Likelihood: Suspected**

Cause
Combination may have a synergistic effect on folate metabolism.

Effect
Risk of methotrexate toxicity increases.

Nursing considerations
- Avoid using methotrexate with trimethoprim if possible.
- **◖ ALERT** Monitor the patient for methotrexate-induced bone marrow suppression and megaloblastic anemia.
- Consider leucovorin to treat megaloblastic anemia and neutropenia resulting from folic acid deficiency.

---

trimethoprim- ➤◀ cyclosporine
sulfamethoxazole
Proloprim, Septra   Gengraf, Neoral, Sandimmune

Risk rating: 2
Severity: Moderate   **Onset: Delayed**   **Likelihood: Suspected**

Cause
The mechanism of this interaction is unknown.

Effect
Effect of cyclosporine may be decreased. Oral sulfonamides increase the risk of nephrotoxicity.

Nursing considerations
- Frequently monitor cyclosporine levels.
- Adjust cyclosporine level as needed.
- Monitor the patient for signs and symptoms of transplant rejection.

- Monitor creatinine level.
- Watch the patient for decreased urine output, increased weight, crackles, and other signs of fluid retention.

trimethoprim-sulfamethoxazole ➤◄ warfarin

Proloprim, Septra   Coumadin

Risk rating: 1
Severity: Major   **Onset: Delayed**   **Likelihood: Established**

Cause
Hepatic metabolism of warfarin may be inhibited.

Effect
Warfarin level, effects, and risk of bleeding may increase.

Nursing considerations
- Monitor coagulation values closely.
- Tell the patient to report unusual bruising or bleeding.
- Remind the patient that warfarin interacts with many other drugs, and tell the patient to report any change in drug regimen.

trimethoprim, trimethoprim-sulfamethoxazole ➤◄ dapsone

Proloprim, Septra

Risk rating: 2
Severity: Moderate   **Onset: Delayed**   **Likelihood: Suspected**

Cause
Mechanism is unknown; it's possible that dapsone and trimethoprim decrease the elimination of each other.

Effect
Levels of dapsone and trimethoprim, along with pharmacologic and toxic effects, may occur.

Nursing considerations
- Monitor the patient for dapsone toxicity.
- Watch the patient for signs and symptoms of toxicity, including shortness of breath, cyanosis, mental status changes, headache, fatigue, and dizziness.
- No adverse effects from increased trimethoprim levels were noted.
- Patients taking trimethoprim-sulfamethoxazole had increased toxicity compared to trimethoprim.

trimethoprim, trimethoprim-sulfamethoxazole   ◾️◀ dofetilide

Proloprim, Septra   Tikosyn

Risk rating: 1
Severity: Major   **Onset: Delayed**   **Likelihood: Suspected**

Cause
Dofetilide renal elimination may be inhibited.

Effect
Dofetilide level and risk of ventricular arrhythmias, including torsades de pointes, increase.

Nursing considerations
▶ **ALERT** Use of dofetilide with trimethoprim or trimethoprim-sulfamethoxazole is contraindicated.
■ Monitor ECG for excessive prolongation of the QTc interval or the development of ventricular arrhythmias.
■ Monitor renal function and the QTc interval every 3 months during dofetilide therapy.
■ Monitor the patient for prolonged diarrhea, sweating, and vomiting during dofetilide therapy. Alert the prescriber because electrolyte imbalance may increase the risk of arrhythmias.
■ Consult the prescriber about alternative anti-infective therapy.

trimipramine   ◾️◀ fluvoxamine

Surmontil   Luvox

Risk rating: 2
Severity: Moderate   **Onset: Delayed**   **Likelihood: Probable**

Cause
Fluvoxamine may inhibit oxidative metabolism of tricyclic antidepressants (TCAs), such as trimipramine, via the CYP2D6 pathway.

Effect
TCA level and risk of toxicity increase.

Nursing considerations
■ If combined use can't be avoided, TCA dosage may be decreased.
■ When starting or stopping fluvoxamine, monitor serum TCA level.
■ Report evidence of toxicity or increased TCA level.
■ Inhibitory effects of fluvoxamine may take up to 2 weeks to dissipate after drug is stopped.
■ Using desipramine instead of trimipramine may avoid this interaction.
■ Urge the patient and family to watch for and report increased anti-cholinergic effects, dizziness, drowsiness, and psychosis.

valproate sodium ⬛▶◀⬛ tricyclic antidepressants
Depacon   amitriptyline, clomipramine

Risk rating: 2
Severity: Moderate   Onset: Delayed   Likelihood: Suspected

Cause
Valproate sodium may inhibit hepatic metabolism of tricyclic anti-depressants (TCAs).

Effect
Level and adverse effects of TCAs may increase.

Nursing considerations
- Use these drugs together cautiously.
- If the patient is stable on valproate sodium, start TCA at reduced dosage and adjust upward slowly to address symptoms and serum level.
- If the patient is stable on a TCA, monitor serum level and patient status closely when starting or stopping valproate sodium.
- Explain signs and symptoms to watch for.
- Other TCAs may interact with valproate sodium. If you suspect an interaction, consult the prescriber or pharmacist.

valproic acid ⬛▶◀⬛ aspirin
Depakene   Bayer, Ecotrin

Risk rating: 2
Severity: Moderate   Onset: Delayed   Likelihood: Suspected

Cause
Salicylates such as aspirin displace valproic acid from its usual binding sites and may alter valproic acid metabolic pathways.

Effect
Toxicity of valproic acid may increase.

Nursing considerations
- Check serum free fraction and serum valproic acid level.
- Hepatotoxic metabolites of valproic acid may be more likely to form.
- Watch for evidence of valproic acid toxicity, such as tremor, drowsiness, ataxia, nystagmus, and personality changes.
- Explain risks of combined use and signs of toxicity.

valproic acid ➤◀ carbamazepine

divalproex
sodium,
valproic acid

Carbatrol,
Epitol, Equetro,
Tegretol

Risk rating: 2
Severity: Moderate   Onset: Delayed   Likelihood: Established

Cause
Metabolism of valproic acid may be altered by carbamazepine. Conversion of valproic acid to a hepatotoxic and teratogenic metabolite may increase.

Effect
Valproic acid level decreases, with possible loss of seizure control. Also, carbamazepine level may change.

Nursing considerations
■ These drugs have been used safely together in many patients to manage epilepsy and psychiatric disorders.
■ Monitor seizure control and toxicity for at least 1 month after starting or stopping combined use.
■ Check levels of both drugs during use and for 1 month after either drug is stopped.
■ Although rare, pancreatitis and acute psychosis may arise because of slow excretion after combined use has stopped.

valproic acid ➤◀ carbapenem antibiotics

Depakote

imipenem-cilastatin,
meropenem

Risk rating: 2
Severity: Moderate   Onset: Delayed   Likelihood: Suspected

Cause
The mechanism of this interaction is unknown.

Effect
Valproic acid plasma levels may be decreased.

Nursing considerations
■ Monitor the patient's valproic acid levels and observe the patient for seizure activity when starting a carbapenem antibiotic.
■ Consider giving an alternative antibiotic if an interaction is suspected.
■ If carbapenem antibiotic is stopped, you may have to decrease the dose of valproic acid.

valproic acid ◀▶ cholestyramine

Depakote

Locholest, Prevalite, Questran

Risk rating: 2
Severity: Moderate   **Onset: Rapid**   **Likelihood: Suspected**

Cause
Cholestyramine may prevent GI absorption of valproic acid.

Effect
Valproic acid effects may decrease.

Nursing considerations
- Give valproic acid at least 3 hours before or after cholestyramine.
- Watch for loss of therapeutic effects (loss of seizure control).
- Valproic acid dosage may need adjustment during combined use.
- Consult the prescriber about other antihyperlipidemic drugs as alternatives to cholestyramine.

valproic acid ◀▶ felbamate

divalproex
sodium, valproic
acid

Felbatol

Risk rating: 2
Severity: Moderate   **Onset: Delayed**   **Likelihood: Probable**

Cause
Felbamate inhibits metabolism of valproic acid.

Effect
Valproic acid level and risk of toxicity may increase.

Nursing considerations
- Monitor serum valproic acid level when starting or stopping felbamate or adjusting its dose. Valproic acid dosage may need adjustment.
- If the patient takes valproic acid, start felbamate slowly if possible.
- If felbamate must start quickly, valproic acid dosage may need to be reduced. Watch the patient closely.
- Watch for valproic acid toxicity: sedation, nausea, vomiting, pancreatitis, hepatitis, hemorrhage, emotional changes, and serious rash.
- Teach signs and symptoms to watch for.

valproic acid ▰▰▶◀ lamotrigine
divalproex
sodium, valproic
acid

Lamictal

Risk rating: 2
Severity: Moderate   **Onset: Delayed**   **Likelihood: Probable**

Cause
Valproic acid may inhibit lamotrigine metabolism.

Effect
Both drugs may have increased effects and toxicity.

Nursing considerations
■ Observe the patient closely for Stevens-Johnson rash, disabling tremor, and other signs of toxicity when starting the second anticonvulsant.
■ Monitor serum valproic acid and lamotrigine levels, and report increasing level of either drug.
■ Explain that combined use may improve seizure control; instruct the patient to be alert for adverse effects and toxicity.
■ Lamotrigine level decreases readily when valproic acid is stopped.

valproic acid ▰▰▶◀ phenytoin
Depakote

Dilantin

Risk rating: 2
Severity: Moderate   **Onset: Delayed**   **Likelihood: Suspected**

Cause
Valproic acid metabolism increases; phenytoin metabolism decreases.

Effect
Phenytoin effects may increase. Valproic acid effects may decrease. Phenytoin toxicity may occur despite therapeutic total serum level.

Nursing considerations
■ Watch for altered seizure control and evidence of toxicity: tremor, drowsiness, ataxia, nystagmus, slurred speech, and personality changes.
■ Monitor serum levels of free phenytoin and valproic acid. The amount of free phenytoin may be more important than the therapeutic range of 10 to 20 mcg/ml.
■ Be prepared to alter the dosage of either drug as needed.
■ Other hydantoins may interact with valproic acid. If you suspect an interaction, consult the prescriber or pharmacist.

valproic acid ►◄ tricyclic antidepressants

divalproex sodium,
valproate sodium

amitriptyline, clomipramine

Risk rating: 2
Severity: Moderate **Onset: Delayed** **Likelihood: Suspected**

Cause
Valproic acid may inhibit hepatic metabolism of tricyclic antidepressants (TCAs).

Effect
Level and adverse effects of TCA may increase.

Nursing considerations
- Use these drugs together cautiously.
- If the patient is stable on valproic acid, start a TCA at reduced dosage and adjust upward slowly to address symptoms and serum level.
- If the patient is stable on a TCA, monitor serum level and patient status closely when starting or stopping valproic acid.
- Explain signs and symptoms to watch for.
- Other TCAs may interact with valproic acid. If you suspect an interaction, consult the prescriber or pharmacist.

valsartan ►◄ lithium

Diovan

Eskalith

Risk rating: 2
Severity: Moderate **Onset: Delayed** **Likelihood: Suspected**

Cause
Angiotensin II receptor antagonists, such as valsartan, may decrease lithium excretion.

Effect
Lithium level, effects, and risk of toxicity may increase.

Nursing considerations
- If the patient takes lithium, consider an antihypertensive other than an angiotensin II receptor antagonist.
- Monitor lithium level. Steady state lithium level should be 0.6 to 1.2 mEq/L.
- Adjust lithium dose as needed.
- Monitor the patient for evidence of lithium toxicity, such as diarrhea, vomiting, dehydration, drowsiness, muscle weakness, tremor, fever, and ataxia.

vancomycin ━━━▶◀━━━ nondepolarizing muscle relaxants

Vancocin

atracurium, pancuronium, vecuronium

Risk rating: 2
Severity: Moderate   **Onset: Rapid**   **Likelihood: Probable**

Cause
Vancomycin and other polypeptide antibiotics may act synergistically with nondepolarizing muscle relaxants.

Effect
Neuromuscular blockade may increase.

Nursing considerations
- If possible, avoid using polypeptide antibiotics with nondepolarizing muscle relaxants.
- Monitor neuromuscular function closely.
- Dosage of nondepolarizing muscle relaxant may need adjustment.
- Provide ventilatory support as needed.
- Make sure the patient is adequately sedated when receiving a nondepolarizing muscle relaxant.

vardenafil ━━━▶◀━━━ alpha$_1$-adrenergic blockers

Levitra

alfuzosin, doxasozin, prazosin, tamsulosin, terasozin

Risk rating: 2
Severity: Moderate   **Onset: Rapid**   **Likelihood: Suspected**

Cause
Vardenafil causes an additive pharmacologic action.

Effect
The risk of hypotension may be increased.

Nursing considerations
⚡ **ALERT** Administering vardenafil and an alpha$_1$-adrenergic blocker together is contraindicated.
- If the patient has taken vardenafil and an alpha$_1$-adrenergic blocker, carefully monitor his blood pressure and cardiac output.
- Alert the prescriber that the patient is taking vardenafil and an alpha$_1$-adrenergic blocker together and their use is contraindicated.
- Make sure the patient has readily accessible I.V. access to administer fluids if needed for hypotension.

vardenafil ━━━━▶◀━━━━ antiarrhythmics

Levitra

amiodarone, bretylium, disopyramide, moricizine, procainamide, sotalol

Risk rating: 1
Severity: Major   **Onset: Rapid**   **Likelihood: Suspected**

Cause
The mechanism of this interaction is unknown.

Effect
QTc interval may be prolonged, particularly in patients with previous QT-interval prolongation, increasing the risk of such life-threatening arrhythmias as torsades de pointes.

Nursing considerations
⚑ **ALERT** Use of vardenafil with a class IA or class III antiarrhythmic is contraindicated.
■ Monitor ECG before and during vardenafil use.
■ Urge the patient to report light-headedness, faintness, palpitations, and chest pain or pressure while taking vardenafil.
■ To reduce risk of adverse effects, patients age 65 and older should start with 5 mg vardenafil, one-half of the usual starting dose.

vardenafil ━━━━▶◀━━━━ azole antifungal agents

Levitra

itraconazole, ketoconazole

Risk rating: 2
Severity: Moderate   **Onset: Delayed**   **Likelihood: Suspected**

Cause
Azole antifungals inhibit CYP3A4 metabolism of phosphodiesterase type 5 (PDE-5) inhibitors such as vardenafil.

Effect
PDE5 inhibitor levels, pharmacologic effects, and risk of adverse effects may increase.

Nursing considerations
■ Dosage of PDE5 inhibitor may need to be decreased.
■ Administer these drugs together cautiously.
■ Instruct the patient to take PDE5 exactly as instructed.
■ Warn the patient of adverse effects, including prolonged, painful erection.

vardenafil ━━━►◄━━━ nitroglycerin
Levitra   NitroBid, NitroDur

Risk rating: 1

Severity: **Major**   Onset: **Rapid**   Likelihood: **Suspected**

Cause
Vardenafil potentiates the hypotensive effects of nitrates.

Effect
Risk of severe hypotension increases.

Nursing considerations
◩ **ALERT** Use of vardenafil with nitrates or nitric oxide donors is contraindicated.
■ Carefully screen the patient for vardenafil use before giving a nitrate.
■ Watch for orthostatic hypotension, dizziness, sweating, and headache.
■ This interaction may not occur if vardenafil is taken 24 hours or more before the patient receives a nitrate.

vecuronium ━━━►◄━━━ carbamazepine
                                 Carbatrol, Epitol, Equetro,
                                 Tegretol

Risk rating: 2

Severity: **Moderate**   Onset: **Rapid**   Likelihood: **Probable**

Cause
The mechanism of this interaction is unknown.

Effect
Effects or duration of a nondepolarizing muscle relaxant, such as vecuronium, may decrease.

Nursing considerations
■ Monitor the patient for decreased efficacy of muscle relaxant.
■ Dosage of nondepolarizing muscle relaxant may be increased.
■ Make sure the patient is adequately sedated when receiving a non-depolarizing muscle relaxant.

vecuronium ━━▶◀━━ inhalation anesthetics

enflurane, isoflurane,
nitrous oxide

Risk rating: 1
Severity: Major   **Onset: Rapid**   **Likelihood: Established**

Cause
These drugs potentiate pharmacologic actions.

Effect
The actions of nondepolarizing muscle relaxants, such as vecuronium, are potentiated.

Nursing considerations
- Closely monitor respiratory function.
- The dose of both the inhalation anesthetic and vecuronium may need to be adjusted.
- Provide ventilatory support as needed.
- The interaction is dose-dependant.
- If the patient is receiving vecuronium continuously, the maintenance dose may need to be decreased 25% to 30%.

vecuronium ━━▶◀━━ magnesium sulfate

Risk rating: 2
Severity: Moderate   **Onset: Rapid**   **Likelihood: Suspected**

Cause
Magnesium probably potentiates the action of nondepolarizing muscle relaxants, such as vecuronium.

Effect
Vecuronium effects may increase.

Nursing considerations
- Use these drugs together cautiously.
- The nondepolarizing muscle relaxant dosage may need adjustment.
- Monitor the patient for respiratory depression, which may be profound.
- Provide ventilatory support as needed.
- Make sure the patient is adequately sedated when receiving a nondepolarizing muscle relaxant.

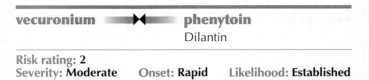

vecuronium → phenytoin
Dilantin

Risk rating: 2
Severity: Moderate   **Onset: Rapid**   **Likelihood: Established**

Cause
Phenytoin effects at prejunctional sites are similar to those of non-depolarizing muscle relaxants such as vecuronium.

Effect
Nondepolarizing muscle relaxant effects or duration may decrease.

Nursing considerations
■ Monitor the patient for decreased efficacy of the muscle relaxant.
■ Dosage of nondepolarizing muscle relaxant may be increased.
■ Atracurium may be a suitable alternative to vecuronium because this interaction may not occur in all the patients.
■ Make sure the patient is adequately sedated when receiving a nondepolarizing muscle relaxant.

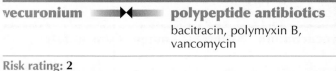

vecuronium → polypeptide antibiotics
bacitracin, polymyxin B, vancomycin

Risk rating: 2
Severity: Moderate   **Onset: Rapid**   **Likelihood: Probable**

Cause
Polypeptide antibiotics may act synergistically with nondepolarizing muscle relaxants such as vecuronium.

Effect
Neuromuscular blockade may increase.

Nursing considerations
■ If possible, avoid using polypeptide antibiotics with nondepolarizing muscle relaxants.
■ Monitor neuromuscular function closely.
■ Dosage of nondepolarizing muscle relaxant may need adjustment.
■ Provide ventilatory support as needed.
■ Make sure the patient is adequately sedated when receiving a nondepolarizing muscle relaxant.

vecuronium ▶◀ verapamil
Calan

Risk rating: 2
Severity: **Moderate**   Onset: **Rapid**   Likelihood: **Suspected**

Cause
This interaction may stem from a blockade of calcium channels in the skeletal muscle.

Effect
Effects of nondepolarizing muscle relaxants, such as vecuronium, may increase.

Nursing considerations
■ If possible, avoid using verapamil and nondepolarizing muscle relaxants together.
■ Monitor the patient for prolonged respiratory depression.
■ Provide ventilatory support as needed.
■ Dosage of nondepolarizing muscle relaxant may be decreased.

venlafaxine ▶◀ linezolid
Effexor   Zyvox

Risk rating: 1
Severity: **Major**   Onset: **Delayed**   Likelihood: **Suspected**

Cause
Serotonin may accumulate rapidly in the CNS.

Effect
The risk of serotonin syndrome increases.

Nursing considerations
⚑ ALERT Don't use these drugs together.
■ Allow 2 weeks between stopping linezolid and administering venlafaxine.
■ Allow 2 weeks between stopping an SSRI such as venlafaxine and administering linezolid.
■ Describe the traits of serotonin syndrome, including confusion, restlessness, incoordination, muscle tremors and rigidity, fever, and sweating.
■ Explain that serotonin-induced symptoms can be fatal if not treated immediately.

venlafaxine ▬▬►◄▬▬ MAO inhibitors

Effexor

isocarboxazid, phenelzine,
selegiline, tranylcypromine

Risk rating: 1
Severity: Major   **Onset: Rapid**   **Likelihood: Probable**

Cause
Serotonin may accumulate rapidly in the CNS.

Effect
Risk of serotonin syndrome increases.

Nursing considerations
◪ **ALERT** Don't use these drugs together.
■ Allow 1 week after stopping venlafaxine before giving an MAO
inhibitor.
■ The selective MAO type-B inhibitor selegiline has been given with
fluoxetine, paroxetine, or sertraline to patients with Parkinson's disease
without negative effects.
■ Describe the traits of serotonin syndrome, including CNS irritability,
motor weakness, shivering, myoclonus, and altered consciousness.
■ Urge the patient to promptly report adverse effects to the prescriber.

venlafaxine ▬▬►◄▬▬ sibutramine

Effexor

Meridia

Risk rating: 1
Severity: Major   **Onset: Rapid**   **Likelihood: Suspected**

Cause
Serotonin may accumulate rapidly in the CNS.

Effect
Risk of serotonin syndrome increases.

Nursing considerations
◪ **ALERT** If possible, don't give these drugs together.
■ Watch carefully for adverse effects; they need immediate attention.
■ Describe the traits of serotonin syndrome: CNS irritability, motor
weakness, shivering, muscle twitching, and altered consciousness.
■ Explain that serotonin syndrome can be fatal if not treated
immediately.

venlafaxine ■■■■►◄ sympathomimetics

Effexor

amphetamine, dextroamphetamine, phentermine

Risk rating: 2
Severity: Moderate   **Onset: Rapid**   **Likelihood: Suspected**

Cause
The mechanism of this interaction is unknown.

Effect
Sympathomimetic effects and risk of serotonin syndrome increase.

Nursing considerations
- Watch closely for increased CNS effects, such as anxiety, jitteriness, agitation, and restlessness.
- Mild serotonin-like symptoms may develop, including anxiety, dizziness, restlessness, nausea, and vomiting.
- Explain risk of interaction and need to avoid sympathomimetics.
- Describe traits of serotonin syndrome: CNS irritability, motor weakness, shivering, myoclonus, and altered consciousness.

venlafaxine ■■■■►◄ tramadol

Effexor

Ultram

Risk rating: 1
Severity: Major   **Onset: Delayed**   **Likelihood: Suspected**

Cause
Additive serotonergic effects.

Effect
Serotonin syndrome may occur.

Nursing considerations
- Watch closely for increased CNS effects, such as anxiety, jitteriness, agitation, and restlessness.
- If serotonin syndrome occurs, stop the venlafaxine and obtain immediate medical attention for the patient.
- Describe the traits of serotonin syndrome: CNS irritability, motor weakness, shivering, myoclonus, and altered consciousness.
- Urge the patient to promptly report adverse effects.

verapamil ━━━━▶◀ beta-adrenergic blockers

Calan

atenolol, metoprolol, pindolol, propranolol, timolol

Risk rating: 1
Severity: Major   **Onset: Rapid**   **Likelihood: Probable**

Cause
Verapamil may inhibit metabolism of beta-adrenergic blockers.

Effect
Effects of both drugs may increase.

Nursing considerations
■ Combined use is common in hypertension with unstable angina.
◤ **ALERT** Risk of adverse effects increases, including heart failure, conduction disturbances, arrhythmias, and hypotension.
■ Assess the patient for adverse effects, including left ventricular dysfunction and AV conduction defects.
■ Risk of interaction is greater when drugs are given I.V.
■ Dosages of both drugs may need to be decreased.

verapamil ━━━━▶◀ buspirone

Calan

BuSpar

Risk rating: 2
Severity: Moderate   **Onset: Delayed**   **Likelihood: Suspected**

Cause
Buspirone level may increase from reduced CYP3A4 metabolism.

Effect
Buspirone level and adverse effects may increase.

Nursing considerations
■ Watch closely if verapamil is started or stopped or if its dosage is changed.
■ Watch for evidence of buspirone toxicity, including increased CNS effects (dizziness, drowsiness, headache), vomiting, and diarrhea.
■ Buspirone dose may need to be adjusted.
■ An antianxiety drug not metabolized by CYP3A4 (such as lorazepam) should be considered if the patient takes verapamil.
■ Calcium channel blockers other than verapamil may interact with buspirone. If you suspect an interaction, consult the prescriber or pharmacist.

■ Dihydropyridine calcium channel blockers that don't inhibit
CYP3A4 metabolism (such as amlodipine and felodipine) probably
don't disrupt buspirone metabolism. Consult the prescriber.

verapamil ➤◄	calcium salts
Calan	calcium acetate, calcium carbonate, calcium chloride, calcium citrate, calcium gluceptate, calcium gluconate, calcium lactate, tricalcium phosphate

Risk rating: 2
Severity: Moderate   **Onset: Rapid**   **Likelihood: Suspected**

Cause
Calcium salts antagonize certain of verapamil's effects.

Effect
Calcium can reverse changes in cardiac output, blood pressure, and
AV intervals without slowing the sinus rate or causing AV block.

Nursing considerations
■ Calcium can be useful in verapamil overdose and in reversing or
preventing hypotension when verapamil starts.
■ The beneficial effects of calcium with verapamil are dose dependent.
If too much calcium is used, verapamil may be ineffective.
■ Obtain a complete drug history to detect calcium consumption in
any patient who takes verapamil.
■ Teach the patient taking verapamil to always consult the prescriber
before consuming anything that contains calcium.

verapamil ➤◄	carbamazepine
Calan	Carbatrol, Epitol, Equetro, Tegretol

Risk rating: 2
Severity: Moderate   **Onset: Delayed**   **Likelihood: Suspected**

Cause
Verapamil may decrease hepatic metabolism of carbamazepine.

Effect
Carbamazepine level and toxic effects may increase.

Nursing considerations
- Monitor carbamazepine level; therapeutic range is 4 to 12 mcg/ml.
- Watch for evidence of carbamazepine toxicity: dizziness, ataxia, respiratory depression, tachycardia, arrhythmias, blood pressure changes, impaired consciousness, abnormal reflexes, nystagmus, seizures, nausea, vomiting, and urine retention.
- Carbamazepine dose may need to be reduced by 40% to 50%.
- If verapamil is stopped, watch for loss of carbamazepine effect.
- Calcium channel blockers other than verapamil may interact with carbamazepine. If you suspect an interaction, consult the prescriber or pharmacist.

---

verapamil ▶◀ cyclosporine
Calan   Gengraf, Neoral, Sandimmune

Risk rating: 2
Severity: Moderate   **Onset: Delayed**   **Likelihood: Established**

Cause
Hepatic and gut wall metabolism of cyclosporine is inhibited.

Effect
Cyclosporine levels, and risk of nephrotoxicity, may increase.

Nursing considerations
- Monitor cyclosporine level.
- Decrease cyclosporine dose as needed.
- Assess renal function.
- Signs and symptoms of toxicity may include shakiness, headaches, tremor, hypertension, and fatigue.
- Administering verapamil before cyclosporine may be nephroprotective.
- This interaction is generally seen within 7 days of starting verapamil and decreases within 1 week of discontinuation.

---

verapamil ▶◀ digoxin
Calan   Lanoxin

Risk rating: 1
Severity: Major   **Onset: Delayed**   **Likelihood: Established**

Cause
Verapamil decreases digoxin elimination. Verapamil and digoxin have additive effects in decreasing AV conduction.

Effect
Digoxin level, effects, and risk of toxicity may increase.

Nursing considerations
- Monitor digoxin level. Therapeutic range is 0.8 to 2 nanograms/ml.
- Watch for evidence of digoxin toxicity, including arrhythmias (bradycardia, AV block, and ventricular ectopy), lethargy, drowsiness, confusion, hallucinations, headaches, syncope, vision disturbances, nausea, anorexia, vomiting, and diarrhea.
- Digoxin dosage may need reduction.
- Advise the patient to report adverse reactions, such as nausea, vomiting, diarrhea, appetite loss, and vision disturbances, which may be early indicators of toxicity.

---

verapamil ◄─── **dofetilide**
Calan   Tikosyn

Risk rating: 1
Severity: Major   **Onset: Delayed**   **Likelihood: Suspected**

Cause
Verapamil may increase dofetilide absorption.

Effect
Dofetilide level and risk of ventricular arrhythmias, including torsades de pointes, may increase.

Nursing considerations
⚠ **ALERT** Use of dofetilide with verapamil is contraindicated.
- Monitor ECG for excessive prolongation of the QTc interval and development of ventricular arrhythmias.
- Monitor renal function and QTc interval every 3 months during dofetilide therapy.

---

verapamil ◄─── **macrolide antibiotics**
Calan   erythromycin, telithromycin

Risk rating: 1
Severity: Major   **Onset: Delayed**   **Likelihood: Probable**

Cause
Certain macrolides inhibit CYP3A4 metabolism of verapamil. Verapamil increases macrolide absorption and decreases macrolide metabolism.

Effect
Risk of cardiotoxicity increases.

Nursing considerations
- Closely monitor cardiac function in patients taking this combination of drugs.
- Evidence of cardiotoxicity appears in 2 days to 1 week.
- Monitor the patient for dizziness, shortness of breath, weakness, profound hypotension, bradycardia, QTc prolongation, and complete AV heart block.
- Consult the prescriber about the possibility of using another antibiotic class.
- Tell the patient to report palpitations, dizziness, shortness of breath, unexplained weakness, and chest pain.

---

verapamil ▶◀ nondepolarizing muscle relaxants
Calan   pancuronium, vecuronium

Risk rating: 2
Severity: Moderate   **Onset: Rapid**   **Likelihood: Suspected**

Cause
This interaction may stem from a blockade of calcium channels in the skeletal muscle.

Effect
Nondepolarizing muscle relaxant effects may increase.

Nursing considerations
- Avoid using verapamil with nondepolarizing muscle relaxants.
- Monitor the patient for prolonged respiratory depression.
- Provide ventilatory support as needed.
- The dosage of nondepolarizing muscle relaxant may need to be decreased.

---

verapamil ▶◀ quinidine
Calan

Risk rating: 1
Severity: Major   **Onset: Rapid**   **Likelihood: Suspected**

Cause
Verapamil may interfere with quinidine clearance and prolong its half-life.

Effect
Serious cardiac events may result.

Nursing considerations
- Use together only when there are no other alternatives.
- Monitor the patient for hypotension, bradycardia, ventricular tachycardia, and AV block.
- Tell the patient to report diaphoresis, dizziness or fainting, blurred vision, palpitations, shortness of breath, and chest pain.
- Notify the prescriber if arrhythmias occur. One or both drugs may need to be stopped.
- The complications of this interaction may be noticed in as little as 1 day or after as long as 5 months of combined use.

---

verapamil ◄► simvastatin
Calan   Zocor

Risk rating: 2
Severity: Moderate   **Onset: Delayed**   **Likelihood: Probable**

Cause
CYP3A4 metabolism of certain HMG-CoA reductase inhibitors such as simvastatin may decrease.

Effect
HMG-CoA reductase inhibitor level and risk of adverse effects may increase.

Nursing considerations
- Avoid giving an HMG-CoA reductase inhibitor with verapamil.
- Consult the prescriber; HMG-CoA reductase inhibitor dosage may be decreased.
- **ALERT** Watch for evidence of rhabdomyolysis, including fatigue; muscle aches and weakness; joint pain; dark, red, or cola-colored urine; weight gain; seizures; and greatly increased serum CK level.
- Fluvastatin and pravastatin are metabolized by other enzymes and may be better choices for combined use with verapamil.
- Urge the patient to report muscle pain, tenderness, or weakness.

---

vinblastine ◄► erythromycin
Velban   E-mycin, Eryc

Risk rating: 1
Severity: Major   **Onset: Delayed**   **Likelihood: Suspected**

Cause
Erythromycin inhibits metabolism of vinblastine.

Effect
Risk of vinblastine toxicity increases.

Nursing considerations
■ If possible, avoid this drug combination.
■ If erythromycin and vinblastine must be given together, a conservative dose of vinblastine should be given.
■ Watch for evidence of toxicity, such as constipation, myalgia, hypertension, hyponatremia, and neutropenia.
■ If erythromycin is stopped because of adverse reactions when coadministered with vinblastine, the patient's myalgia and neutropenia may resolve, decrease, or recur.
■ Explain adverse reactions of vinblastine to the patient. Tell the patient to report them.

---

vinblastine ➤◀ phenytoin
Velban   Dilantin

Risk rating: 2
Severity: Moderate   **Onset: Delayed**   **Likelihood: Suspected**

Cause
Phenytoin absorption may be decreased or metabolism may be increased.

Effect
Phenytoin level and effects may decrease.

Nursing considerations
■ Monitor phenytoin level closely. Dosage may need to be adjusted.
■ Therapeutic range for phenytoin is 10 to 20 mcg/ml.
■ Toxic effects can occur at therapeutic level. Adjust the measured level for hypoalbuminemia or renal impairment, which can increase free drug level.
■ Monitor the patient for seizure activity.
■ Carefully monitor phenytoin level between courses of chemotherapy. Phenytoin dose may need to be reduced.
■ Signs and symptoms of phenytoin toxicity include nystagmus, slurred speech, ataxia, blurred or double vision, confusion, drowsiness, and lethargy.

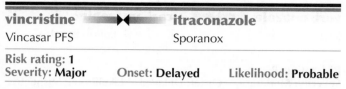

vincristine ▶◀ itraconazole

Vincasar PFS   Sporanox

Risk rating: 1
Severity: **Major**   Onset: **Delayed**   Likelihood: **Probable**

Cause
Itraconazole inhibits CYP3A4, which is needed for vincristine metabolism.

Effect
Risk of vincristine toxicity increases.

Nursing considerations
- If possible, avoid giving these drugs together.
- Watch for evidence of toxicity, such as constipation, myalgia, hypertension, hyponatremia, and neutropenia.
- Explain adverse vincristine effects; tell the patient to report them.
- Stop itraconazole as soon as possible.

voriconazole ▶◀ benzodiazepines

Vfend   alprazolam, chlordiazepoxide, midazolam, quazepam, triazolam

Risk rating: 2
Severity: **Moderate**   Onset: **Delayed**   Likelihood: **Established**

Cause
Azole antifungals, such as voriconazole, decrease CYP3A4 metabolism of certain benzodiazepines.

Effect
Benzodiazepine effects are increased and prolonged, which may cause CNS depression and psychomotor impairment.

Nursing considerations
- If the patient takes voriconazole, talk with the prescriber about giving a lower benzodiazepine dose or a drug not metabolized by CYP3A4, such as temazepam or lorazepam.
- Caution that the effects of this interaction may last several days after stopping the azole antifungal.
- Explain the risk of sedation; tell the patient to report it promptly.
- Explain alternative methods of inducing sleep or relieving anxiety during antifungal therapy.
- Various azole antifungal–benzodiazepine combinations may interact. If you suspect an interaction, consult the prescriber or pharmacist.

voriconazole ▸◀ carbamazepine
Vfend

Carbatrol, Epitol, Equetro, Tegretol

Risk rating: 2
Severity: Moderate   **Onset: Delayed**   **Likelihood: Suspected**

Cause
Carbamazepine may increase CYP3A4 metabolism of voriconazole.

Effect
Voriconazole effects may decrease.

Nursing considerations
⚠ ALERT Use of these drugs together is contraindicated.
- Instruct the patient to avoid carbamazepine while taking voriconazole; consult the prescriber about alternative therapies.

voriconazole ▸◀ cyclosporine
Vfend

Sandimmune, Neoral, Gengraf

Risk rating: 2
Severity: Moderate   **Onset: Delayed**   **Likelihood: Established**

Cause
Voriconazole decreases cyclosporine metabolism.

Effect
Cyclosporine level and toxicity may increase.

Nursing considerations
- Cyclosporine level may increase 1 to 3 days after starting an azole antifungal and persist for more than 1 week after stopping it.
- Monitor cyclosporine level.
- Adjust cyclosporine dosage to maintain therapeutic level.
- Cyclosporine dose may need to be decreased by 68% to 97%.
- Monitor the patient for hepatotoxicity and nephrotoxicity.

voriconazole ▸◀ efavirenz
Vfend

Sustiva

Risk rating: 1
Severity: Major   **Onset: Delayed**   **Likelihood: Suspected**

Cause
Efavirenz increases the CYP3A4 metabolism of voriconazole.
Voriconazole may inhibit the CYP3A4 metabolism of efavirenz.

Effect
Voriconazole plasma levels and efficacy may be reduced. Efavirenz levels and adverse effects may be increased.

Nursing considerations
◼ ALERT Use of voriconazole with efavirenz is contraindicated.
▪ This interaction is based on pharmacodynamics. Due to the seriousness, it hasn't been studied in humans.

---

voriconazole ━━▶◀━━ ergot derivatives
Vfend   dihydroergotamine, ergotamine

Risk rating: 1
Severity: **Major**   Onset: **Delayed**   Likelihood: **Suspected**

Cause
Voriconazole may inhibit CYP3A4 metabolism of ergot derivatives.

Effect
Risk of ergot toxicity may increase.

Nursing considerations
◼ ALERT Use of these drugs together is contraindicated.
▪ Signs of ergot toxicity include peripheral vasospasm and ischemia of the extremities.
▪ Instruct the patient to avoid taking ergot derivatives, as for migraine, while taking voriconazole.

---

voriconazole ━━▶◀━━ NSAIDs
Vfend   flurbiprofen, ibuprofen

Risk rating: 2
Severity: **Moderate**   Onset: **Delayed**   Likelihood: **Suspected**

Cause
Voriconazole inhibits metabolism of NSAIDs.

Effect
NSAID levels, pharmacologic effects, and adverse reactions increase.

Nursing considerations
▪ Observe the patient for increase in NSAID adverse reactions and adjust NSAID dose as needed.
▪ Monitor the patient for NSAID adverse reactions including: dizziness, fluid retention, tinnitus, abdominal pain, heartburn, acute renal failure, leukopenia, prolonged bleeding time, and thrombocytopenia.

- Tell the patient to watch for and report signs and symptoms of GI bleeding, including blood in vomit, urine, or stools; coffee-ground vomitus; and black, tarry stools.
- Maximum daily NSAID dose shouldn't exceed 1200 mg for adults.

voriconazole ◢◣◤ opioid analgesics
Vfend   fentanyl, alfentanil

Risk rating: 1
Severity: Major   **Onset: Rapid**   **Likelihood: Suspected**

Cause
Azole antifungals, such as voriconazole, inhibit CYP3A4 metabolism of opioid analgesics.

Effect
Opioid pharmacologic and adverse effects may increase.

Nursing considerations
⚠ ALERT Carefully monitor the patient for increased effects of opioid analgesics, including respiratory depression, decreased level of consciousness, and bradycardia.
- Alert the prescriber about the risk of interaction between the opioid analgesic and the azole antifungal and discuss a possible decrease in opioid dosage.
- Keep naloxone available to treat respiratory depression.
- Monitor the patient's pain level and administer pain medication as needed to keep him comfortable, but without significant adverse effects.

voriconazole ◢◣◤ phenobarbital
Vfend

Risk rating: 1
Severity: Major   **Onset: Delayed**   **Likelihood: Suspected**

Cause
Long-acting barbiturates, such as phenobarbital, may increase CYP3A4 metabolism of voriconazole.

Effect
Voriconazole level and efficacy may decrease.

Nursing considerations
⚠ ALERT Use of these drugs together is contraindicated.
■ Voriconazole efficacy in treating fungal infections may decrease.
■ Other barbiturates and voriconazole may interact. If you suspect an interaction, consult the prescriber or pharmacist.

voriconazole ➤◄ pimozide
Vfend   Orap

Risk rating: 1
Severity: Major   **Onset: Delayed**   **Likelihood: Suspected**

Cause
Azole antifungals, such as voriconazole, may inhibit CYP3A4 metabolism of pimozide.

Effect
Risk of life-threatening arrhythmias may increase.

Nursing considerations
⚠ ALERT Combined use of these drugs is contraindicated.
■ Arrhythmias are related to prolonged QT interval, a known risk of pimozide.
■ Interaction warning is based on pharmacokinetics of these drugs, not actual patient studies.

voriconazole ➤◄ sirolimus
Vfend   Rapamune

Risk rating: 2
Severity: Moderate   **Onset: Delayed**   **Likelihood: Suspected**

Cause
Voriconazole may increase CYP3A4 metabolism of sirolimus.

Effect
Sirolimus level and adverse effects may increase.

Nursing considerations
⚠ ALERT Use of these drugs together is contraindicated.
■ The immunosuppressant benefits of sirolimus may be compromised by increased adverse effects, such as heart failure, toxic nephropathy, thrombocytopenia with hemorrhage, sepsis, and lung edema.

voriconazole ■■■►◄ tacrolimus
Vfend   Prograf

Risk rating: 2
Severity: Moderate   Onset: Delayed   Likelihood: Suspected

Cause
Voriconazole inhibits tacrolimus metabolism in the liver and GI tract.

Effect
Tacrolimus level and risk of adverse effects or toxicity may increase.

Nursing considerations
- Monitor renal function and mental status closely when using these drugs together.
- Check tacrolimus level often. Expected trough level is 6 to 10 mcg/L.
- Tacrolimus dosage may need to be decreased.
- This interaction may occur with other azole antifungals.
- **⧈ ALERT** Watch for renal failure, nephrotoxicity, hyperkalemia, hyperglycemia, delirium, and other changes in mental status.

voriconazole ■■■►◄ warfarin
Vfend   Coumadin

Risk rating: 1
Severity: Major   Onset: Delayed   Likelihood: Established

Cause
Warfarin metabolism is inhibited.

Effect
Anticoagulant effects may increase.

Nursing considerations
- Monitor PT and INR at least every 2 days.
- Patients with renal insufficiency may be at greater risk.
- Although all azole antifungals interact with warfarin, some interactions may be more significant than others.
- Watch for evidence of bleeding.
- Tell the patient to report unusual bruising or bleeding.
- Remind the patient that warfarin interacts with many drugs and that he should report any change in drug regimen.

voriconazole ━━▶◀━━ zolpidem
Vfend   Ambien

Risk rating: 2
Severity: Moderate   **Onset: Delayed**   **Likelihood: Suspected**

Cause
Voriconazole inhibits CYP3A4 metabolism of zolpidem.

Effect
Zolpidem levels and therapeutic effects may increase.

Nursing considerations
■ If coadministration of voriconazole and zolpidem is given, monitor the patient's response. Zolpidem dosage may need to be decreased.
■ Instruct the patient about the signs and symptoms of increased effects of zolpidem, including headache, daytime drowsiness, hangover, lethargy, light-headedness, palpitations, abdominal pain, nausea, myalgia, and back or chest pain.
■ Caution the patient to avoid performing activities that require mental alertness or physical coordination during therapy.

warfarin ━━▶◀━━ acetaminophen
Coumadin   Acephen, Neopap, Tylenol

Risk rating: 2
Severity: Moderate   **Onset: Delayed**   **Likelihood: Suspected**

Cause
Acetaminophen or one of its metabolites may enhance vitamin K antagonism.

Effect
Antithrombotic effect of warfarin may increase.

Nursing considerations
◣ **ALERT** Effects of this interaction seem to be dose related. Daily acetaminophen use at 325 to 650 mg causes a 3.5-fold INR elevation. Daily use of 1,250 mg increases this risk 10-fold.
■ This interaction may be of little significance with low-dose acetaminophen or up to six 325-mg tablets weekly.
■ Monitor coagulation values once or twice weekly when starting or stopping acetaminophen.

- Other risk factors may be present that place the patient at higher risk, such as diarrheal illness or medical conditions that affect acetaminophen metabolism.
- Tell the patient to report unusual bruising or bleeding.
- Remind the patient that warfarin interacts with many drugs; caution him to report any change in drug regimen.

---

warfarin ▶◀ alteplase
Coumadin   Activase, tPA

Risk rating: 1
Severity: Major   **Onset: Rapid**   **Likelihood: Suspected**

Cause
The combined effect of this interaction may be greater than the sum of each individual effect.

Effect
Risk of serious bleeding increases.

Nursing considerations
⚠ **ALERT** Using alteplase in a patient with acute ischemic stroke is contraindicated if the patient has a bleeding diathesis, which can be a result of many different factors, including the use of oral anticoagulants. Administering alteplase to such patients increases the risk of bleeding and may cause disability or death.
- Oral anticoagulants other than warfarin may interact with alteplase. Consult the prescriber or pharmacist.
- Alert the prescriber that the patient takes warfarin.
- Tell the patient to report unusual bruising or bleeding.
- Remind the patient that warfarin interacts with many drugs, and tell the patient to report any change in drug regimen.

---

warfarin ▶◀ aminoglutethimide
Coumadin   Cytadren

Risk rating: 2
Severity: Moderate   **Onset: Delayed**   **Likelihood: Suspected**

Cause
Liver enzyme activity is increased, resulting in increased warfarin metabolism.

Effect
Warfarin's ability to increase PT may be reduced.

Nursing considerations
- Carefully monitor the patient's PT when starting or stopping aminoglutethimide.
- Consult with the prescriber and adjust the dose of warfarin as needed.

---

warfarin ━━━━▶◀ amiodarone
Coumadin   Cordarone, Pacerone

Risk rating: 1
Severity: Major   **Onset: Delayed**   **Likelihood: Established**

Cause
Amiodarone inhibits CYP1A2 and CYP2C9 metabolism of warfarin.

Effect
Anticoagulant effects increase.

Nursing considerations
- Monitor the patient closely for bleeding. Urge compliance with required blood tests.
- ⚠ **ALERT** Check INR closely during the first 6 to 8 weeks of amiodarone use. Warfarin dose reduction depends on escalating amiodarone dose. Typically, warfarin needs a 30% to 50% reduction.
- If amiodarone is stopped, the effects of the interaction may persist up to 4 months, requiring continual warfarin adjustment.
- Tell the patient to report unusual bruising or bleeding.
- Remind the patient that warfarin interacts with many drugs, and tell the patient to report any change in drug regimen.

---

warfarin ━━━━▶◀ androgens (17-alkyl)
Coumadin   danazol, methyltestosterone, oxandrolone

Risk rating: 1
Severity: Major   **Onset: Delayed**   **Likelihood: Probable**

Cause
The mechanism of this interaction is unknown.

Effect
Anticoagulant effects increase.

Nursing considerations
- If possible, avoid this combination.
- Monitor coagulation values carefully. It may be necessary to decrease warfarin dosage.

- Tell the patient to report unusual bruising or bleeding.
- Remind the patient that warfarin interacts with many drugs, and tell the patient to report any change in drug regimen.

warfarin ◄►►◄	antineoplastics
Coumadin	capecitabine, carboplatin, cyclophosphamide, etoposide, fluorouracil, gemcitabine, paclitaxel

Risk rating: 1
Severity: Major   **Onset: Delayed**   **Likelihood: Suspected**

Cause
Warfarin metabolism, clotting factor synthesis, and possibly protein displacement may be inhibited.

Effect
Anticoagulant effects increase.

Nursing considerations
- Monitor PT and INR closely during and after chemotherapy.
- Tell the patient to report unusual bruising or bleeding.
- Remind the patient that warfarin interacts with many drugs, and tell the patient to report any change in drug regimen.

warfarin ◄►►◄	azole antifungals
Coumadin	fluconazole, itraconazole, ketoconazole, voriconazole

Risk rating: 1
Severity: Major   **Onset: Delayed**   **Likelihood: Established**

Cause
Warfarin metabolism is inhibited.

Effect
Anticoagulant effects may increase.

Nursing considerations
- Monitor PT and INR at least every 2 days.
- Patients with renal insufficiency may be at greater risk.
- Although all azole antifungals interact with warfarin, some interactions may be more significant than others.
- Watch for evidence of bleeding.
- Tell the patient to report unusual bruising or bleeding.
- Remind the patient that warfarin interacts with many drugs, and tell the patient to report any change in drug regimen.

warfarin ▶◀ bosentan

Coumadin   Tracleer

Risk rating: 2
Severity: Moderate   Onset: Delayed   Likelihood: Suspected

Cause
Bosentan induces CYP3A4 and CYP2C9 metabolism of warfarin.

Effect
Effects of warfarin may be decreased.

Nursing considerations
■ Monitor PT and INR when starting, changing, or stopping bosentan therapy in patients who take warfarin.
■ Maintain INR at 2 to 3 for an acute MI, atrial fibrillation, treatment of pulmonary embolism, prevention of systemic embolism, tissue heart valves, valvular heart disease, or prophylaxis or treatment of venous thrombosis. Maintain INR at 3 to 4.5 for mechanical prosthetic valves or recurrent systemic embolism.
■ Warfarin dose may need to be adjusted.
■ Tell the patient to report unusual bruising or bleeding.
■ Remind the patient that warfarin interacts with many drugs, and tell the patient to report any change in drug regimen.

warfarin ▶◀ carbamazepine

Coumadin   Carbatrol, Epitol, Equetro, Tegretol

Risk rating: 2
Severity: Moderate   Onset: Delayed   Likelihood: Probable

Cause
Carbamazepine may increase hepatic metabolism of warfarin.

Effect
Anticoagulant effects decrease.

Nursing considerations
■ Monitor PT and INR when starting, changing, or stopping carbamazepine therapy in patients who take warfarin.
■ Maintain INR at 2 to 3 for an acute MI, atrial fibrillation, treatment of pulmonary embolism, prevention of systemic embolism, tissue heart valves, valvular heart disease, or prophylaxis or treatment of venous thrombosis. Maintain INR at 3 to 4.5 for mechanical prosthetic valves or recurrent systemic embolism.
■ Warfarin dose may need to be adjusted.

■ Tell the patient to report unusual bruising or bleeding.
■ Remind the patient that warfarin interacts with many drugs, and tell him to report any change in drug regimen to the prescriber or pharmacist.

---

warfarin ▶◀ cephalosporins

Coumadin

cefazolin, cefoperazone, cefotetan, cefoxitin, ceftriaxone

Risk rating: 2
Severity: Moderate   **Onset: Delayed**   **Likelihood: Suspected**

Cause
The mechanism of this interaction is unknown.

Effect
Anticoagulant effects increase.

Nursing considerations
■ If given with a parenteral cephalosporin, warfarin dose may need to be reduced.
■ Monitor PT and INR closely.
■ Patients with renal insufficiency may be at greater risk.
■ Monitor the patient for signs of bleeding.
■ Tell the patient to report unusual bruising or bleeding.
■ Remind the patient that warfarin interacts with many drugs, and tell the patient to report any change in drug regimen.

---

warfarin ▶◀ chloramphenicol

Coumadin

Chloromycetin

Risk rating: 2
Severity: Moderate   **Onset: Delayed**   **Likelihood: Suspected**

Cause
Hepatic metabolism of warfarin is inhibited.

Effect
Anticoagulant effects may increase.

Nursing considerations
■ Monitor coagulation values carefully.
■ A lower warfarin dose may be needed if the patient is taking chloramphenicol.
■ Tell the patient to report unusual bleeding or bruising.
■ Remind the patient that warfarin interacts with many drugs, and tell the patient to report any change in drug regimen.

warfarin ▶◀ cholestyramine

Coumadin   Locholest, Prevalite, Questran

Risk rating: 2
Severity: Moderate   **Onset: Delayed**   **Likelihood: Probable**

Cause
Warfarin absorption may decrease and elimination increase.

Effect
Anticoagulant effects may decrease.

Nursing considerations
- Tell the patient to separate warfarin dose from cholestyramine by at least 3 hours.
- Advise the patient of the risks of reduced anticoagulant effects.
- Help the patient develop a plan to ensure proper dosage intervals.
- Tell the patient to report unusual bruising or bleeding.
- Remind the patient that warfarin interacts with many drugs, and tell the patient to report any change in drug regimen.

warfarin ▶◀ cimetidine

Coumadin   Tagamet

Risk rating: 1
Severity: Major   **Onset: Delayed**   **Likelihood: Established**

Cause
Hepatic metabolism of warfarin is inhibited.

Effect
Anticoagulant effects increase.

Nursing considerations
- Suggest the use of an H_2 antagonist other than cimetidine because famotidine, ranitidine, and nizatidine are unlikely to interact with warfarin.
- Avoid using these drugs together. If unavoidable, monitor coagulation values closely.
- Tell the patient to report unusual bruising or bleeding.
- Remind the patient that warfarin interacts with many drugs, and tell the patient to report any change in drug regimen.

warfarin ◗◖ cranberry juice
Coumadin

Risk rating: 1
Severity: Major   **Onset: Delayed**   **Likelihood: Suspected**

Cause
The mechanism of this interaction is unknown.

Effect
Risk of serious bleeding increases.

Nursing considerations
- Tell the patient to take warfarin with liquid other than cranberry juice.
- If warfarin dose has been stabilized with a patient consuming cranberry juice, the patient's coagulation status may need to be monitored if he switches to another beverage.
- Tell the patient to report unusual bruising or bleeding.
- Remind the patient that warfarin interacts with many drugs, and tell the patient to report any change in drug regimen.

warfarin ◗◖ danshen root
Coumadin

Risk rating: 2
Severity: Moderate   **Onset: Delayed**   **Likelihood: Suspected**

Cause
The mechanism of this interaction is unknown.

Effect
Risk of bleeding may increase.

Nursing considerations
- Monitor coagulation values.
- Monitor the patient for signs of bleeding.
- Caution the patient to consult the prescriber before taking OTC drugs or herbal supplements.
- Tell the patient to report unusual bruising or bleeding.

warfarin ━━━━▶◀━━━━ disulfiram
Coumadin   Antabuse

Risk rating: 2
Severity: Moderate   **Onset: Delayed**   **Likelihood: Probable**

Cause
The mechanism of this interaction is unknown.

Effect
Anticoagulant effects may increase.

Nursing considerations
- Monitor coagulation values.
- Disulfiram's effects on warfarin may be dose dependent. If disulfiram dose decreases, warfarin dose may need to be increased.
- Monitor the patient for signs of bleeding.
- Tell the patient to report unusual bruising or bleeding.
- Remind the patient that warfarin interacts with many drugs, and tell the patient to report any change in drug regimen.

warfarin ━━━━▶◀━━━━ fibric acids
Coumadin   fenofibrate, gemfibrozil

Risk rating: 1
Severity: Major   **Onset: Delayed**   **Likelihood: Established**

Cause
Coagulation factor synthesis may be altered.

Effect
Hypoprothrombinemic effects of warfarin may increase.

Nursing considerations
- Avoid use together if possible. If unavoidable, INR should be checked often.
- ⚠ ALERT Plasma warfarin level isn't affected by this interaction, but INR will increase. Hemorrhage and death may occur.
- Tell the patient to report unusual bruising or bleeding.
- Remind the patient that warfarin interacts with many drugs, and tell the patient to report any change in drug regimen.
- Advise the patient to keep all follow-up medical appointments for proper monitoring and dosage adjustments.

warfarin 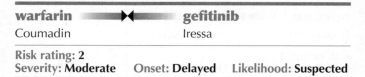 gefitinib
Coumadin   Iressa

Risk rating: 2
Severity: Moderate   **Onset: Delayed**   **Likelihood: Suspected**

Cause
The mechanism of this interaction is unknown.

Effect
Anticoagulant effects and risk of bleeding may be increased.

Nursing considerations
- Monitor coagulation values closely when starting or stopping gefitinib.
- Adjust the warfarin dose as needed.
- Tell the patient to report unusual bruising or bleeding.
- Remind the patient that warfarin interacts with many other drugs, and tell the patient to report any change in drug regimen.
- **ALERT** The FDA has limited the use of gefitinib to certain patient populations. New clinical trials are being developed to determine future benefits of this drug.

warfarin 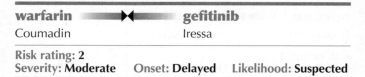 griseofulvin
Coumadin   Grisactin

Risk rating: 2
Severity: Moderate   **Onset: Delayed**   **Likelihood: Suspected**

Cause
The mechanism of this interaction is unknown.

Effect
Anticoagulant effects decrease.

Nursing considerations
- Monitor the patient for inadequate response to warfarin.
- If the patient's INR is stabilized while taking griseofulvin, monitor closely when griseofulvin is stopped. The warfarin dose may need to be reduced to avoid serious bleeding.
- Urge the patient to keep all follow-up medical appointments for monitoring and dosage adjustments. Monitoring may take several weeks.
- Tell the patient to report unusual bruising or bleeding.
- Remind the patient that warfarin interacts with many drugs, and tell the patient to report any change in drug regimen.

warfarin ▶◀ HMG-CoA reductase inhibitors

Coumadin

fluvastatin, lovastatin, rosuvastatin, simvastatin

Risk rating: 2
Severity: Moderate   **Onset: Delayed**   **Likelihood: Probable**

Cause
Hepatic metabolism of warfarin may be inhibited.

Effect
Anticoagulant effects may increase.

Nursing considerations
- Monitor PT and INR closely when starting or stopping an HMG-CoA inhibitor.
- Atorvastatin and pravastatin don't appear to have this interaction with warfarin.
- Tell the patient to report unusual bruising or bleeding.
- Remind the patient that warfarin interacts with many drugs, and tell the patient to report any change in drug regimen.
- Advise the patient to keep all follow-up medical appointments for proper monitoring and dosage adjustments.

warfarin ▶◀ macrolide antibiotics

Coumadin

azithromycin, clarithromycin, erythromycin, telithromycin

Risk rating: 1
Severity: Major   **Onset: Delayed**   **Likelihood: Probable**

Cause
Warfarin clearance is reduced.

Effect
Anticoagulant effects and risk of bleeding increase.

Nursing considerations
- Monitor PT and INR closely during, or when starting or stopping, a macrolide antibiotic. The PT may be prolonged within a few days.
- Warfarin dose adjustment may continue for several days after antibiotic therapy stops.
- Treat excessive anticoagulation with vitamin K.
- Tell the patient to report unusual bruising or bleeding.

■ Remind the patient that warfarin interacts with many drugs, and tell the patient to report any change in drug regimen.
■ Advise the patient to keep all follow-up medical appointments for proper monitoring and dosage adjustments.

warfarin ➤◄ methimazole
Coumadin   Tapazole

Risk rating: 1
Severity: Major   **Onset: Delayed**   **Likelihood: Suspected**

Cause
The mechanism of this interaction is unknown.

Effect
Anticoagulant effects may be altered.

Nursing considerations
■ Monitor coagulation values closely.
■ Monitor the patient for inadequate response to anticoagulant.
■ Tell the patient to report unusual bruising or bleeding.
■ Remind the patient that warfarin interacts with many other drugs, and tell the patient to report any change in drug regimen.

warfarin ➤◄ metronidazole
Coumadin   Flagyl

Risk rating: 1
Severity: Major   **Onset: Delayed**   **Likelihood: Established**

Cause
Metronidazole may decrease hepatic metabolism of warfarin.

Effect
Anticoagulant effects and risk of bleeding increase.

Nursing considerations
■ Monitor the patient for signs of bleeding.
■ Warfarin dose may need to be reduced during metronidazole use.
■ Tell the patient to report unusual bruising or bleeding.
■ Remind the patient that warfarin interacts with many drugs, and tell the patient to report any change in drug regimen.

warfarin ➤◄ NSAIDs

Coumadin

diclofenac, etodolac, fenopro-
fen, flurbiprofen, ibuprofen,
indomethacin, ketoprofen,
ketorolac, nabumetone,
naproxen, oxaprozin, piroxicam, sulindac, tolmetin

Risk rating: 1
Severity: Major   **Onset: Delayed**   **Likelihood: Probable**

Cause
Platelet function is decreased and GI irritation increased.

Effect
Anticoagulant effects and risk of bleeding increase.

Nursing considerations
■ Monitor PT and INR closely during combined use and when starting
or stopping an NSAID.
■ Tell the patient to report unusual bruising or bleeding.
■ Remind the patient that warfarin interacts with many drugs; tell him
to report any change in drug regimen.
■ Advise the patient to keep all follow-up medical appointments for
proper monitoring and dosage adjustments.

warfarin ➤◄ penicillins

Coumadin

dicloxacillin, nafcillin,
ticarcillin

Risk rating: 2
Severity: Moderate   **Onset: Delayed**   **Likelihood: Suspected**

Cause
Warfarin induces hypoprothrombinemia, and penicillin inhibits
platelet aggregation.

Effect
Bleeding time is prolonged.

Nursing considerations
■ Monitor PT and INR closely during combined use.
■ Risk of interaction increases with large doses of I.V. penicillins.
Nafcillin and dicloxacillin may cause warfarin resistance.

- Monitor coagulation values before starting nafcillin or dicloxacillin and for at least 3 weeks after stopping to check for warfarin resistance.
- Tell the patient to report unusual bruising or bleeding.
- Remind the patient that warfarin interacts with many drugs, and tell the patient to report any change in drug regimen.
- Advise the patient to keep all follow-up medical appointments for proper monitoring and dosage adjustments.

warfarin ▶◀ phenytoin
Coumadin   Dilantin

Risk rating: 2
Severity: Moderate   Onset: Delayed   Likelihood: Suspected

Cause
Phenytoin level may increase and half-life lengthen. Phenytoin may increase PT when added to warfarin therapy.

Effect
Risk of phenytoin toxicity and severe bleeding increases.

Nursing considerations
- Monitor the patient for signs or symptoms of phenytoin toxicity or for altered anticoagulant effects.
- Therapeutic range for phenytoin is 10 to 20 mcg/ml.
- Toxic effects can occur at therapeutic level. Adjust the measured level for hypoalbuminemia or renal impairment, which can increase free drug level.
- Signs and symptoms of phenytoin toxicity include nystagmus, slurred speech, ataxia, blurred or double vision, confusion, drowsiness, and lethargy.
- Monitor phenytoin level 7 to 10 days after therapy starts or changes.
- Tell the patient to report unusual bruising or bleeding.

warfarin ▶◀ quinine derivatives
Coumadin   quinidine, quinine

Risk rating: 1
Severity: Major   Onset: Delayed   Likelihood: Suspected

Cause
Quinidine derivatives may inhibit clotting factors synthesized in the liver.

Effect
Anticoagulant effects and risk of bleeding may increase.

Nursing considerations
- Monitor PT and INR closely.
- Tell the patient to report unusual bruising or bleeding.
- Remind the patient that warfarin interacts with many drugs, and tell the patient to report any change in drug regimen.

---

warfarin ▶◀ quinolones
Coumadin   ciprofloxacin, levofloxacin, moxifloxacin norfloxacin, ofloxacin

Risk rating: 1
Severity: Major   **Onset: Delayed**   **Likelihood: Probable**

Cause
The mechanism of this interaction is unknown.

Effect
Anticoagulant effects may increase.

Nursing considerations
- Monitor PT and INR closely.
- Tell the patient to report unusual bruising or bleeding.
- Remind the patient that warfarin interacts with many drugs, and tell the patient to report any change in drug regimen.

---

warfarin ▶◀ rifamycins
Coumadin   rifampin, rifapentine

Risk rating: 2
Severity: Moderate   **Onset: Delayed**   **Likelihood: Established**

Cause
Hepatic metabolism of warfarin is increased by rifamycins.

Effect
Anticoagulant effects decrease.

Nursing considerations
- Monitor the patient for inadequate response to warfarin.
- Warfarin dose may need to be increased during rifamycin therapy; monitor PT and INR often.
- Blood tests may be needed for several weeks after stopping a rifamycin.
- Tell the patient to report unusual bruising or bleeding.
- Remind the patient that warfarin interacts with many drugs, and tell the patient to report any change in drug regimen.
- Explain importance of following up with the prescriber for proper monitoring and dosage adjustments.

warfarin ▶◀ salicylates
Coumadin   aspirin, methyl salicylate

Risk rating: 1
Severity: Major   **Onset: Delayed**   **Likelihood: Established**

Cause
Anticoagulant activity increases; platelet aggregation decreases.

Effect
Risk of significant bleeding may increase.

Nursing considerations
- Use together should be avoided.
- Monitor coagulation values closely.
- Aspirin doses of 500 mg or more daily increase risk of bleeding.
- Explain that interaction can happen with topical and oral salicylates.
- Tell the patient to report unusual bruising or bleeding.
- Remind the patient that warfarin interacts with many drugs, and tell the patient to report any change in drug regimen.
- **ALERT** Warfarin dose should be adjusted when aspirin is stopped.

warfarin ▶◀ sulfinpyrazone
Coumadin   Anturane

Risk rating: 1
Severity: Major   **Onset: Delayed**   **Likelihood: Established**

Cause
Hepatic metabolism of warfarin decreases.

Effect
Warfarin level, effects, and risk of bleeding may increase.

Nursing considerations
- Monitor coagulation values closely.
- **ALERT** Warfarin dose may decrease when sulfinpyrazone is started and increase when sulfinpyrazone is stopped.
- Tell the patient to report unusual bruising or bleeding.
- Remind the patient that warfarin interacts with many other drugs, and tell the patient to report any changes in drug regimen.

warfarin ▶◀ sulfonamides
Coumadin sulfasalazine, sulfisoxazole
trimethoprim-sulfamethoxazole

Risk rating: 1
Severity: Major **Onset: Delayed** **Likelihood: Established**

Cause
Hepatic metabolism of warfarin may be inhibited.

Effect
Warfarin level, effects, and risk of bleeding may increase.

Nursing considerations
- Monitor coagulation values closely.
- Tell the patient to report unusual bruising or bleeding.
- Remind the patient that warfarin interacts with many other drugs, and tell the patient to report any change in drug regimen.

warfarin ▶◀ thiopurines
Coumadin azathioprine, mercaptopurine

Risk rating: 2
Severity: Moderate **Onset: Delayed** **Likelihood: Suspected**

Cause
The mechanism of the interaction is unknown. Thiopurines may increase the synthesis of prothrombin and decrease plasma warfarin levels.

Effect
The effects of warfarin may be decreased.

Nursing considerations
- Monitor PT and INR when starting, changing, or stopping azathioprine therapy in the patient who takes warfarin.
- Maintain INR at 2 to 3 for an acute MI, atrial fibrillation, treatment of pulmonary embolism, prevention of systemic embolism, tissue heart valves, valvular heart disease, or prophylaxis or treatment of venous thrombosis. Maintain INR at 3 to 4.5 for mechanical prosthetic valves or recurrent systemic embolism.
- Warfarin dose may need to be adjusted.
- Tell the patient to report unusual bruising or bleeding.
- Remind the patient that warfarin interacts with many drugs, and tell the patient to report any change in drug regimen.

warfarin ━━━▶◀━━━ thyroid hormones
Coumadin   levothyroxine, liothyronine

Risk rating: 1
Severity: Major   **Onset: Delayed**   **Likelihood: Probable**

Cause
Thyroid hormones increase the breakdown of vitamin K–dependent clotting factors.

Effect
Anticoagulant effects and risk of bleeding may increase.

Nursing considerations
- Monitor coagulation values carefully.
- A lower warfarin dose may be needed.
- If the patient's anticoagulant values are stabilized during combined therapy and the thyroid hormones are stopped, warfarin dose may need to be increased.
- Tell the patient to report unusual bruising or bleeding.
- Remind the patient that warfarin interacts with many drugs, and tell the patient to report any change in drug regimen.

warfarin ━━━▶◀━━━ vitamin E
Coumadin

Risk rating: 1
Severity: Major   **Onset: Delayed**   **Likelihood: Suspected**

Cause
Vitamin E may interfere with vitamin K–dependent clotting factors.

Effect
Anticoagulant effects may increase.

Nursing considerations
- Monitor coagulation values carefully.
- A lower warfarin dose may be needed if the patient is taking vitamin E.
- Less than 400 mg of vitamin E daily may not affect anticoagulation.
- Tell the patient to report unusual bruising or bleeding.
- Remind the patient that warfarin interacts with many drugs, and tell the patient to report any change in drug regimen.

warfarin ━━━━▶◀━━━━ vitamin K

Coumadin

Risk rating: 2
Severity: Moderate   Onset: Delayed   Likelihood: Established

Cause
Warfarin interferes with activation of vitamin K–dependent clotting factors in blood, an action overcome by vitamin K.

Effect
Anticoagulant effects are reversed and risk of thrombus is increased.

Nursing considerations
■ Monitor PT and INR closely.
■ Tell the patient to avoid or minimize variations in vitamin K consumption, including green, leafy vegetables, green tea, and supplements.
▨ **ALERT** Watch for signs of thrombus formation, including dyspnea, mottled extremities, and impaired thinking or coordination.
■ Tell the patient to report a change in dietary habits if he has been stabilized on warfarin. Coagulation values may have to be monitored and warfarin dose adjusted.
■ Tell the patient to report unusual bruising or bleeding.
■ Remind the patient that warfarin interacts with many drugs, and tell the patient to report any change in drug regimen.

zidovudine ━━━━▶◀━━━━ atovaquone

AZT, Retrovir   Mepron

Risk rating: 2
Severity: Moderate   Onset: Delayed   Likelihood: Suspected

Cause
Excretion of zidovudine may be decreased.

Effect
Risk of zidovudine toxicity is increased.

Nursing considerations
■ Monitor the patient for toxic effects of zidovudine, including agranulocytosis, bone marrow suppression, and thrombocytopenia.
■ If an interaction is suspected, a lower dose of zidovudine may be needed.
■ Instruct the patient to notify the prescriber immediately if he notices new or increased bruising or bleeding.
■ Tell the patient not to change his HIV therapy before discussing it with the prescriber.

zidovudine ▰▰▰►◄▰▰▰ ganciclovir

AZT, Retrovir   Cytovene

Risk rating: 1
Severity: Major   **Onset: Delayed**   **Likelihood: Probable**

Cause
Ganciclovir may increase zidovudine level.

Effect
The risk of severe hematologic toxicities, including anemia, neutropenia, and leukopenia, increases.

Nursing considerations
■ Use together should be avoided. Foscarnet (Foscavir) may be an adequate substitute for ganciclovir.
■ Monitor CBC with differential.
■ Use together may warrant reduction of ganciclovir dosage.
■ Explain that adverse hematologic effects may not appear for 3 to 5 weeks; tell the patient to report symptoms of infection, such as fever, sore throat, and unexplained tiredness.

zidovudine ▰▰▰►◄▰▰▰ methadone

AZT, Retrovir   Methadose

Risk rating: 2
Severity: Moderate   **Onset: Delayed**   **Likelihood: Probable**

Cause
The mechanism of this interaction is unknown.

Effect
Zidovudine levels—and risk of adverse effects—increases.

Nursing considerations
■ Monitor clinical response to zidovudine therapy.
■ If adverse effects to zidovudine increase, discuss a lower dosage with the prescriber.
■ Monitor the patient for anemia, neutropenia, leukopenia, muscle aches, and fever.

zidovudine ━━━━▶◀━━━━ probenecid
AZT, Retrovir

Risk rating: 2
Severity: Moderate   **Onset: Delayed**   **Likelihood: Suspected**

Cause
Zidovudine glucuronidation decreases and level increases.

Effect
Risk of rash increases, possibly with malaise, myalgia, and fever.

Nursing considerations
- Monitor the patient for rash.
- Zidovudine dosage interval may need to be doubled.
- Tell the patient to report muscle aches, fever, and general illness.

zileuton ━━━━▶◀━━━━ pimozide
Zyflo   Orap

Risk rating: 1
Severity: Major   **Onset: Delayed**   **Likelihood: Suspected**

Cause
Zileuton may inhibit CYP3A4 metabolism of pimozide.

Effect
Risk of life-threatening arrhythmias may increase.

Nursing considerations
⚑ **ALERT** Combined use of these drugs is contraindicated.
- Arrhythmias are related to prolonged QT interval, a known risk of pimozide.
- Interaction warning is based on known pharmacokinetics of these drugs, not actual patient studies.

zileuton ━━━━▶◀━━━━ theophyllines
Zyflo   aminophylline, theophylline

Risk rating: 2
Severity: Moderate   **Onset: Delayed**   **Likelihood: Probable**

Cause
Zileuton may inhibit theophylline metabolism.

Effect

Theophylline level and risk of adverse effects may increase.

Nursing considerations

- Monitor theophylline level closely. Therapeutic range is 10 to 20 mcg/ml for adults and 5 to 15 mcg/ml for children.
- Watch for evidence of toxicity, such as tachycardia, anorexia, nausea, vomiting, diarrhea, seizures, restlessness, irritability, and headache.
- If the patient starts zileuton while taking theophylline, theophylline dosage should be decreased by 50%.
- Explain common adverse effects of theophylline and signs of toxicity, and tell the patient to report them immediately to the prescriber.

---

ziprasidone ▆▆▆▆▶◀▆▆▆ **antiarrhythmics**

Geodon   amiodarone, bretylium,
                                disopyramide, procainamide,
                                quinidine, sotalol

Risk rating: 1
Severity: Major   **Onset: Delayed**   **Likelihood: Suspected**

Cause

The mechanism of this interaction is unknown.

Effect

Risk of life-threatening arrhythmias, including torsades de pointes, increases.

Nursing considerations

⚑ **ALERT** Use of ziprasidone with certain antiarrhythmics is contraindicated.

- Monitor the patient for other risk factors for torsades de pointes, including bradycardia, hypokalemia, and hypomagnesemia.
- Ask the patient if he or anyone in his family has a history of prolonged QT interval or arrhythmias.
- Monitor the patient for bradycardia.
- Measure the QTc interval at baseline and throughout therapy.

---

ziprasidone ▆▆▆▆▶◀▆▆▆ **arsenic trioxide**

Geodon   Trisenox

Risk rating: 1
Severity: Major   **Onset: Delayed**   **Likelihood: Suspected**

Cause

The mechanism of this interaction is unknown.

Effect

Risk of life-threatening arrhythmias, including torsades de pointes, increases.

Nursing considerations

⚠ **ALERT** Use of ziprasidone with arsenic trioxide is contraindicated.

■ Monitor the patient for other risk factors for torsades de pointes, including bradycardia, hypokalemia, and hypomagnesemia.

■ Ask the patient if he or anyone in his family has a history of prolonged QT interval or arrhythmias.

■ Monitor the patient for bradycardia.

■ Measure the QTc interval at baseline and throughout therapy.

---

ziprasidone ➤◀ **carbamazepine**

Geodon   Carbatrol, Epitol, Equetro, Tegretol

Risk rating: 2

Severity: Moderate   Onset: Delayed   Likelihood: Suspected

Cause

Carbamazepine induces increased CYP3A4 metabolism of ziprasidone.

Effect

Ziprasidone levels and effects may be decreased.

Nursing considerations

■ Monitor the patient's response to ziprasidone when starting, stopping, or changing the dose of carbamazepine.

■ Be prepared to change the dose of ziprasidone as needed.

■ Monitor the patient for increased schizophrenic symptoms, agitation, mania, or acute depression.

---

ziprasidone ➤◀ **dofetilide**

Geodon   Tikosyn

Risk rating: 2

Severity: Major   Onset: Delayed   Likelihood: Suspected

Cause

Interaction may cause additive prolongation of the QTc interval.

Effect

Risk of ventricular arrhythmias, including torsades de pointes, increases.

Nursing considerations
⚠ **ALERT** Use of dofetilide with ziprasidone is contraindicated.
- Monitor ECG for excessive prolongation of QTc interval and development of ventricular arrhythmias.
- Monitor renal function and QTc interval every 3 months during dofetilide therapy.
- If the patient takes dofetilide, consult the prescriber or pharmacist about antipsychotics other than ziprasidone.
- Urge the patient to tell the prescriber about increased adverse effects, including lightheadedness, palpitations, and dizziness.

---

ziprasidone ▶◀ dolasetron
Geodon   Anzemet

Risk rating: 1
Severity: Major   **Onset: Delayed**   **Likelihood: Suspected**

Cause
The mechanism of this interaction is unknown.

Effect
Risk of life-threatening arrhythmias, including torsades de pointes, increases.

Nursing considerations
⚠ **ALERT** Use of ziprasidone with dolasetron is contraindicated.
- Ask the patient if he or anyone in his family has a history of prolonged QT interval or arrhythmias.
- Monitor the patient for other risk factors for torsades de pointes, including bradycardia, hypokalemia, and hypomagnesemia.
- Measure the QTc interval at baseline and throughout therapy.
- Monitor the patient for bradycardia.

---

ziprasidone ▶◀ droperidol
Geodon   Inapsine

Risk rating: 1
Severity: Major   **Onset: Delayed**   **Likelihood: Suspected**

Cause
The mechanism of this interaction is unknown.

Effect
Risk of life-threatening arrhythmias, including torsades de pointes, increases.

Nursing considerations
⚠ **ALERT** Use of ziprasidone with droperidol is contraindicated.
- Ask the patient if he or anyone in his family has a history of prolonged QT intervals or arrhythmias.
- Monitor the patient for other risk factors for torsades de pointes, including bradycardia, hypokalemia, and hypomagnesemia.
- Monitor the patient for bradycardia.
- Measure the QTc interval at baseline and throughout therapy.

---

ziprasidone ◀▶ mefloquine
Geodon   Lariam

Risk rating: 1
Severity: Major   **Onset: Delayed**   **Likelihood: Suspected**

Cause
The combination may give rise to synergistic or additive prolongation of the QT interval.

Effect
Risk of life-threatening arrhythmias, including torsades de pointes, increases.

Nursing considerations
⚠ **ALERT** Use of mefloquine with ziprasidone is contraindicated.
- Monitor the patient for other risk factors for torsades de pointes, including bradycardia, hypokalemia, and hypomagnesmia.
- Ask the patient if he or anyone in his family has a history of prolonged QT interval or arrhythmias.
- Monitor the patient for bradycardia.
- Measure the QTc interval at baseline and throughout therapy.

---

ziprasidone ◀▶ phenothiazines
Geodon   chlorpromazine, thioridazine

Risk rating: 1
Severity: Major   **Onset: Delayed**   **Likelihood: Suspected**

Cause
The mechanism of this interaction is unknown.

Effect
Risk of life-threatening arrhythmias, including torsades de pointes, increases.

Nursing considerations

ALERT Use of ziprasidone with a phenothiazine is contraindicated.

- Monitor the patient for other risk factors for torsades de pointes, including bradycardia, hypokalemia, and hypomagnesemia.
- Ask the patient if he or anyone in his family has a history of prolonged QT interval or arrhythmias.
- Monitor the patient for bradycardia.
- Measure the QTc interval at baseline and throughout therapy.

ziprasidone ⧓ pimozide

Geodon — Orap

Risk rating: 1
Severity: Major **Onset: Delayed** **Likelihood: Suspected**

Cause

Ziprasidone may have additive effects on QT-interval prolongation.

Effect

Risk of life-threatening arrhythmias, including torsades de pointes, may increase.

Nursing considerations

ALERT Combined use of these drugs is contraindicated.

- Arrhythmias are related to prolonged QT interval, a known risk of pimozide.
- Interaction warning is based on known pharmacokinetics of these drugs, not actual patient studies.

ziprasidone ⧓ quinolones

Geodon — gatifloxacin, levofloxacin, moxifloxacin

Risk rating: 1
Severity: Major **Onset: Delayed** **Likelihood: Suspected**

Cause

The mechanism of this interaction is unknown.

Effect

Risk of life-threatening arrhythmias, including torsades de pointes, increases.

Nursing considerations

ALERT Use of ziprasidone with a quinolone is contraindicated.

- Monitor the patient for other risk factors for torsades de pointes, including bradycardia, hypokalemia, and hypomagnesemia.

- Ask the patient if he or anyone in his family has a history of prolonged QT interval or arrhythmias.
- Monitor the patient for bradycardia.
- Measure the QTc interval at baseline and throughout therapy.

ziprasidone ▶◀ tacrolimus

Geodon   Prograf

Risk rating: 1
Severity: Major   **Onset: Delayed**   **Likelihood: Suspected**

Cause
The mechanism of this interaction is unknown.

Effect
Risk of life-threatening arrhythmias, including torsades de pointes, increases.

Nursing considerations
⚠ ALERT Use of ziprasidone with tacrolimus is contraindicated.
- Monitor the patient for other risk factors for torsades de pointes, including bradycardia, hypokalemia, and hypomagnesemia.
- Ask the patient if he or anyone in his family has a history of prolonged QT interval or arrhythmias.
- Monitor the patient for bradycardia.
- Measure the QTc interval at baseline and throughout therapy.

zolmitriptan ▶◀ ergot derivatives

Zomig   dihydroergotamine, ergotamine

Risk rating: 1
Severity: Major   **Onset: Rapid**   **Likelihood: Suspected**

Cause
Combined use may have additive effects.

Effect
Risk of vasospastic effects increases.

Nursing considerations
⚠ ALERT Use of these drugs within 24 hours of each other is contraindicated.
- Combined use may cause severe vasospastic effects, including sustained coronary artery vasospasm that triggers MI.
⚠ ALERT Use of two selective 5-HT$_1$ receptor agonists within 24 hours of each other is contraindicated. Warn the patient not to mix migraine headache drugs within 24 hours of each other, but to call the prescriber if a drug isn't effective.

zolmitriptan ▰▶◀▰ MAO inhibitors

Zomig

isocarboxazid, phenelzine, tranylcypromine

Risk rating: 1
Severity: **Major**   Onset: **Rapid**   Likelihood: **Suspected**

Cause
MAO inhibitors, subtype-A, may inhibit metabolism of selective $5-HT_1$ receptor agonists, such as zolmitriptan.

Effect
Zolmitriptan level and risk of cardiac toxicity may increase.

Nursing considerations
◼ **ALERT** Use of certain selective $5-HT_1$ receptor agonists with or within 2 weeks of stopping an MAO inhibitor is contraindicated.
◼ If these drugs must be used together, naratriptan is less likely than zolmitriptan to interact with an MAO inhibitor.
◼ Cardiac toxicity may include coronary artery vasospasm and transient myocardial ischemia.

zolpidem ▰▶◀▰ fluconazole

Ambien

Diflucan

Risk rating: 2
Severity: **Moderate**   Onset: **Delayed**   Likelihood: **Suspected**

Cause
Fluconazole inhibits CYP3A4 metabolism of zolpidem.

Effect
Zolpidem levels and therapeutic effects may increase.

Nursing considerations
◼ If coadministration of fluconazole and zolpidem is given, monitor the patient's response. Zolpidem dosage may need to be decreased.
◼ Instruct the patient on signs and symptoms of increased effects of zolpidem, including headache, daytime drowsiness, hangover, lethargy, light-headedness, palpitations, abdominal pain, nausea, myalgia, and back or chest pain.
◼ Caution the patient to avoid performing activities that require mental alertness or physical coordination during therapy.

zolpidem ▶◀ rifampin
Ambien   Rifadin, Rimactane

Risk rating: 3
Severity: Minor   **Onset: Delayed**   **Likelihood: Suspected**

Cause
Rifampin increases CYP3A4 metabolism of zolpidem.

Effect
Zolpidem levels and therapeutic effects may be decreased.

Nursing considerations
- Monitor the patient's response to zolpidem.
- Dose of zolpidem may need to be increased while the patient is taking rifampin.
- Instruct the patient to notify the prescriber for increased sleeplessness or insomnia.
- Tell the patient not to increase zolpidem dose before discussing it with the prescriber.

zolpidem ▶◀ ritonavir
Ambien   Norvir

Risk rating: 2
Severity: Moderate   **Onset: Delayed**   **Likelihood: Suspected**

Cause
Hepatic metabolism of zolpidem is inhibited.

Effect
Severe sedation and respiratory depression may occur.

Nursing considerations
- **⚠ ALERT** Concurrent use of these drugs together is contraindicated.
- Monitor the patient's respiratory status closely.
- Have emergency respiratory equipment available.

zolpidem ━━━▶◀━━━ sertraline
Ambien   Zoloft

Risk rating: 3
Severity: Minor   **Onset: Delayed**   **Likelihood: Suspected**

Cause
Sertraline inhibits the metabolism of zolpidem.

Effect
Onset of action of zolpidem is decreased and the pharmacologic effect is increased.

Nursing considerations
- Monitor the patient for increased response to zolpidem.
- Watch the patient for excessive daytime sleepiness and sedation.

Appendix and index

Cytochrome P-450 enzymes and common drug interactions

Cytochrome P-450 enzymes, identified by "CYP" followed by numbers and letters identifying the enzyme families and subfamilies, are found throughout the body (primarily in the liver) and are important in the metabolism of many drugs. This table lists common drug-drug interactions based on substrates, inducers, and inhibitors that can influence drug metabolism.

CYP enzyme	Substrates
1A2	acetaminophen, aminophylline, amitriptyline, betaxolol, caffeine, chlordiazepoxide, clomipramine, clozapine, cyclobenzaprine, desipramine, diazepam, doxepin, flutamide, fluvoxamine, haloperidol, imipramine, mirtazapine, naproxen, olanzapine, pimozide, ropinirole, tacrine, theophylline, verapamil, warfarin, zileuton, zolmitriptan
2C9	alosetron, amiodarone, amitriptyline, bosentan, carvedilol, clomipramine, dapsone, diazepam, diclofenac, flurbiprofen, fluvastatin, glimepiride, glipizide, ibuprofen, imipramine, indomethacin, losartan, mirtazapine, montelukast, naproxen, omeprazole, phenytoin, pioglitazone, piroxicam, ritonavir, sildenafil, tolbutamide, torsemide, vardenafil, voriconazole, warfarin, zafirlukast, zileuton
2C19	amitriptyline, carisoprodol, celecoxib, citalopram, clomipramine, cyclophosphamide, diazepam, doxepin, escitalopram, esomeprazole, fenofibrate, fluoxetine, glyburide, imipramine, irbesartan, lansoprazole, mephenytoin, omeprazole, pantoprazole, pentamidine, phenytoin, phenobarbital, rabeprazole, voriconazole, warfarin
2D6	amitriptyline, amphetamine, aripiprazole, atomoxetine, betaxolol, captopril, carvedilol, chlorpheniramine, chlorpromazine, clomipramine, clozapine, codeine, cyclobenzaprine, delavirdine, desipramine, dextromethorphan, donepezil, doxepin, fentanyl, flecainide, fluoxetine, fluphenazine, fluvoxamine, haloperidol, hydrocodone, imipramine, labetalol, loratadine, maprotiline, meperidine, methadone, methamphetamine, metoprolol, mexiletine, mirtazapine, morphine, nefazodone, nortriptyline, oxycodone, paroxetine, perphenazine, procainamide, propafenone, propoxyphene, propranolol, risperidone, tamoxifen, thioridazine, timolol, tolterodine, tramadol, trazodone, venlafaxine
3A	albuterol, alfentanil, alprazolam, amiodarone, amitriptyline, amlodipine, amprenavir, aripiprazole, atazanavir, atorvastatin, bosentan, bromocriptine, buspirone, busulfan, carbamazepine, chlordiazepoxide, chlorpheniramine, citalopram, clarithromycin, clomipramine, clonazepam, clorazepate, cocaine, colchicine, corticosteroids, cyclophosphamide, cyclosporine (neural), dapsone, delavirdine, dexamethasone, diazepam, diltiazem, disopyramide, docetaxel, doxepin, doxorubicin, doxycycline, efavirenz, enalapril, eplerenone, ergotamine, erythromycin, escitalopram, esomeprazole, estrogens, ethosuximide, etoposide, felodipine, fentanyl, fexofenadine, finasteride, flurazepam, flutamide, fluvastatin, haloperidol, ifosfamide, imatinib, imipramine, indinavir, isosorbide, isradipine, itraconazole, ketamine, ketoconazole, lansoprazole, lidocaine, loratadine, losartan, lovastatin, methadone, methylprednisolone, miconazole, midazolam, mirtazapine, montelukast, nefazodone, nevirapine, nicardipine, nifedipine, nimodipine, nisoldipine, ondansetron, paclitaxel, pantoprazole, pioglitazone, pravastatin, prednisone, quinidine, quinine, rabeprazole, rifabutin, ritonavir, saquinavir, sertraline, sildenafil, simvastatin, tacrolimus, tamoxifen, teniposide, testosterone, tolterodine, trazodone, triazolam, troleandomycin, vardenafil, verapamil, vinca alkaloids, voriconazole, warfarin, zileuton, zolpidem

Inducers	Inhibitors
carbamazepine, cigarette smoking, insulin, omeprazole, phenobarbital, phenytoin, primidone, rifampin, ritonavir	atazanavir, caffeine, cimetidine, ciprofloxacin, clarithromycin, enoxacin, erythromycin, fluvoxamine, grapefruit juice, interferon, isoniazid, ketoconazole, levofloxacin, mexiletine, norethindrone, norfloxacin, omeprazole, paroxetine, tacrine, ticlopidine, zileuton
carbamazepine, phenobarbital, phenytoin, primidone, rifampin	amiodarone, atazanavir, chloramphenicol, cimetidine, cotrimoxazole, delavirdine, disulfiram, fluconazole, fluoxetine, fluvastatin, fluvoxamine, isoniazid, itraconazole, ketoconazole, lovastatin, metronidazole, omeprazole, ritonavir, sertraline, sulfinpyrazone, ticlopidine, trimethoprime, zafirlukast
carbamazepine, phenytoin, prednisone, rifampin	cimetidine, delavirdine, esomeprazole, felbamate, fluconazole, fluoxetine, fluvoxamine, ketoconazole, lansoprazole, omeprazole, sertraline, ticlopidine, topiramate
carbamazepine, dexamethasone, phenobarbital, phenytoin, primidone	amiodarone, bupropion, celecoxib, chloroquine, chlorpheniramine, cimetidine, citalopram, cocaine, delavirdine, fluoxetine, fluphenazine, fluvoxamine, haloperidol, methadone, nefazodone, paroxetine, perphenazine, propafenone, propoxyphene, quinidine, quinine, ritonavir, rosiglitazone, sertraline, terbinafine, thioridazine, venlafaxine
barbiturates, carbamazepine, glucocorticoids, griseofulvin, nafcillin, nevirapine, oxcarbazepine, phenytoin, primidone, rifabutin, rifampin	amprenavir, atazanavir, bromocriptine, clarithromycin, cimetidine, cyclosporine (neural), danazol, delavirdine, diltiazem, erythromycin, fluconazole, fluoxetine, fluvoxamine, fosamprenavir, grapefruit juice, imatinib, indinavir, isoniazid, itraconazole, ketoconazole, metronidazole, miconazole, nefazodone, nelfinavir, nicardipine, nifedipine, norfloxacin, omeprazole, prednisone, quinidine, quinine, rifabutin, ritonavir, saquinavir, sertraline, troleandomycin, verapamil, zafirlukast

Index

carmustine, 125, 149–150
chloroquine, 132, 150
clorazepate, 148, 178–179
desipramine, 155, 214
diazepam, 148, 225
dofetilide, 150–151, 262
doxepin, 155, 269
flurazepam, 148, 340
hydantoins, 152, 591–592
imipramine, 155, 382
itraconazole, 147, 424
ketoconazole, 147
lidocaine, 151, 460
metoprolol, 148–149, 505
midazolam, 148, 514
nifedipine, 151–152, 544
nortriptyline, 155, 553
phenytoin, 152, 591–592
praziquantel, 153, 629–630
procainamide, 153, 629–630
propranolol, 148–149, 640
quinidine, 154, 654
theophylline, 154, 764
theophyllines, 21, 154, 764
timolol, 148–149, 780
triazolam, 148, 798–799
tricyclic antidepressants, 36,
    155, 214, 269, 382, 553
warfarin, 155, 839
Cipro. See ciprofloxacin.
ciprofloxacin
aminophylline, 26, 159
didanosine, 156, 231
ferrous fumarate, 156
ferrous gluconate, 156
ferrous sulfate, 156
iron salts, 156, 405
milk, 157
procainamide, 157, 631
sevelamer, 158, 714
sucralfate, 158, 736
theophylline, 159, 769
theophyllines, 26, 159
warfarin, 159, 847
cisatracurium
carbamazepine, 116, 160
phenytoin, 160, 603

cisplatin
bumetanide, 91, 161
ethacrynic acid, 161, 308
furosemide, 161, 352
loop diuretics, 91, 161, 308, 352
phenytoin, 161–162, 590
citalopram
amphetamine, 42–43, 164, 222
clozapine, 162, 180–181
dextroamphetamine, 164, 222
isocarboxazid, 163, 409–410
linezolid, 162–163, 461
MAO inhibitors, 163, 409–410,
    585, 707–708, 794
phenelzine, 163, 585
phentermine, 164, 587
pimozide, 163–164, 611
selegiline, 163, 707–708
sympathomimetics, 164, 587
tramadol, 164–165, 788
tranylcypromine, 163, 794
clarithromycin
alprazolam, 11, 165–166
amiodarone, 29–30, 165
antiarrhythmics, 29–30, 88, 165,
    254, 263, 630, 655–656,
    727
atorvastatin, 71–72, 170–171
benzodiazepines, 11, 165–166,
    226, 515–516, 800
bretylium, 88, 165
cabergoline, 166
carbamazepine, 114–115, 166–167
colchicine, 167, 181–182
conivaptan, 167, 184
cyclosporine, 168, 195
diazepam, 165–166, 226
digoxin, 168–169, 237
dihydroergotamine, 169–170,
    243
disopyramide, 165, 254
dofetilide, 165, 263
eplerenone, 169, 284
ergotamine, 169–170, 288
ergot derivatives, 169–170, 243,
    288

erythromycin, 181–182, 294–295
macrolide antibiotics, 181–182,
    294–295
Colestid. *See* colestipol.
colestipol
    digoxin, 182, 234–235
    furosemide, 182–183, 353
    hydrocortisone, 183, 376–377
Compazine. *See* prochlorperazine.
Concerta. *See* methylphenidate.
conivaptan
    azole antifungals, 183–184, 418,
        435–436
    clarithromycin, 167, 184
    indinavir, 184, 390
    itraconazole, 183–184, 418
    ketoconazole, 183–184, 435–436
    macrolide antibiotics, 167, 184
    protease inhibitors, 184, 685
    ritonavir, 184, 685
conjugated estrogens
    corticosteroids, 305, 623
    hydantoins, 595–596
    phenytoin, 306, 595–596
    prednisolone, 305, 623
    prednisone, 305, 623
    rifampin, 668–669
Cordarone. *See* amiodarone.
Coreg. *See* carvedilol.
Corgard. *See* nadolol.
Cortef. *See* hydrocortisone.
Corticosteroids
    aminoglutethimide, 218
    anticholinergics, 375–376
    aprepitant, 49, 218, 497–498
    aspirin, 53–54, 220, 378, 622, 796
    azole antifungals, 90, 219,
        341–342, 498
    barbiturates, 219, 376, 498–499,
        623, 625
    choline salicylate, 220, 378, 622,
        796
    cholinesterase inhibitors,
        185–186, 499, 541–542,
        624, 649
    conjugated estrogens, 305

diltiazem, 499–500
esterified estrogens, 305
estradiol, 305
estrogens, 305
estrone, 305
estropipate, 305
ethinyl estradiol, 305
hydantoins, 220, 377, 500–501,
    592–593, 621
itraconazole, 90, 219, 341–342,
    418, 498
ketoconazole, 90, 219, 341–342,
    436, 498
neostigmine, 185–186, 375–376,
    499, 541–542, 624
pentobarbital, 219, 376
phenobarbital, 219, 498–499
phenytoin, 220, 329, 377,
    592–593, 621
primidone, 219, 376, 498–499,
    501, 625
pyridostigmine, 185–186,
    375–376, 499, 624, 649
rifampin, 186, 330, 377–378,
    501–502, 667
rifamycins, 186
salicylates, 53–54, 220, 378,
    622, 796
sodium salicylate, 220, 378, 622,
    796
corticotropin
    cholinesterase inhibitors, 185,
        541–542, 649
    neostigmine, 185, 541–542
    pyridostigmine, 185, 649
cortisone
    cholinesterase inhibitors,
        185–186, 541–542, 649
    neostigmine, 185–186, 541–542
    pyridostigmine, 185–186, 649
    rifampin, 186, 667
Coumadin. *See* warfarin.
Cozaar. *See* losartan.
cranberry juice, warfarin, 840
Crestor. *See* rosuvastatin.
Crixivan. *See* indinavir.

H

phenelzine, 452, 583
phenytoin, 451–452, 601
pyridoxine, 452–453, 649–650
tranylcypromine, 452, 791–792
vitamin B_6, 452–453, 649–650
levofloxacin
    amiodarone, 32, 453–454
    antiarrhythmics, 32, 88, 255,
        453–454, 631, 657, 728
    bretylium, 88, 453–454
    disopyramide, 255, 453–454
    erythromycin, 299–300, 454
    imipramine, 385, 454–455
    macrolide antibiotics, 299–300
    procainamide, 453–454, 631
    quinidine, 453–454, 657
    sotalol, 453–454, 728
    tricyclic antidepressants, 385
    warfarin, 455, 847
    ziprasidone, 455, 858–859
Levophed. See norepinephrine.
levothyroxine
    aminophylline, 23, 458–459
    cholestyramine, 144–145, 456
    digoxin, 242, 456–457
    ferrous fumarate, 458
    ferrous gluconate, 458
    ferrous sulfate, 458
    food, 457
    grapefruit juice, 457
    imatinib, 379, 457–458
    iron polysaccharide, 458
    iron salts, 404, 458
    theophylline, 458–459, 766
    theophyllines, 23, 458–459
    warfarin, 459, 850
Levoxyl. See levothyroxine.
Lexiva. See fosamprenavir.
Librium. See chlordiazepoxide.
lidocaine
    atenolol, 65–66, 459–460
    beta blockers, 65–66, 459–460,
        506, 529, 613, 643
    cimetidine, 151, 460
    histamine$_2$–receptor antagonists,
        151, 460

metoprolol, 459–460, 506
nadolol, 459–460, 529
pindolol, 459–460, 613
propranolol, 459–460, 643
succinylcholine, 460–461,
    735–736
Lincosamides
    nondepolarizing muscle relaxants,
        567
    pancuronium, 175
linezolid
    citalopram, 162–163, 461
    fluoxetine, 333, 461
    paroxetine, 461, 573
    serotonin reuptake inhibitors,
        333, 461, 573, 709, 817
    sertraline, 461, 708–709
    venlafaxine, 461, 817
liothyronine
    digoxin, 242, 461–462
    warfarin, 462, 850
Lipitor. See atorvastatin.
lisinopril
    amiloride, 16, 463–464
    aspirin, 51, 462–463
    lithium, 463, 464
    potassium-sparing diuretics, 16,
        463–464
    salicylates, 51, 462–463
    spironolactone, 463–464, 730
lithium
    ACE inhibitors, 280, 463, 464
    angiotensin II receptor antago-
        nists, 464–465, 474, 811
    bumetanide, 92, 466
    candesartan, 464–465
    carbamazepine, 114, 465
    celecoxib, 467
    chlorothiazide, 132–133, 468
    chlorthalidone, 140, 468
    diclofenac, 467
    enalapril, 280, 464
    ethacrynic acid, 309, 466
    furosemide, 354, 466
    haloperidol, 371, 465–466
    hydrochlorothiazide, 374, 468

M

Macrolide antibiotics
alprazolam, 11, 165–166, 292, 752
aminophylline, 23–24, 81,
300–301
amiodarone, 29–30, 79–80, 165,
291–292, 752
antiarrhythmics, 29–30, 79–80,
88, 165, 254, 263,
291–292, 630, 655–656,
727, 752
atorvastatin, 71–72, 170–171,
298, 754
benzodiazepines, 11, 165–166,
226, 292, 515–516, 752,
800
bretylium, 79–80, 88, 165, 752
buspirone, 96–97, 293
carbamazepine, 114–115,
166–167, 293–294
cilostazol, 146–147, 294
clarithromycin, 168
colchicine, 181–182, 294–295
conivaptan, 167, 184
cyclosporine, 80, 195, 295
diazepam, 165–166, 226, 292, 752
digoxin, 237, 295–296, 753
dihydroergotamine, 169–170,
243, 296, 753–754
disopyramide, 79–80, 165, 254,
752
dofetilide, 79–80, 165, 263, 752
eplerenone, 169, 284
ergotamine, 169–170, 288, 296,
753–754
ergot derivatives, 169–170, 243,
288, 296, 753–754
food, 297–298
gatifloxacin, 299–300
grapefruit juice, 170, 297–298
HMG-CoA reductase inhibitors,
71–72, 170–171, 298,
477–478, 722, 754
levofloxacin, 299–300
lovastatin, 170–171, 298,
477–478, 754

methylprednisolone, 500
midazolam, 165–166, 292,
515–516, 752
moxifloxacin, 299–300
pimozide, 80–81, 172, 299, 609,
754–755
procainamide, 79–80, 165, 630,
752
quinidine, 79–80, 165, 655–656,
752
quinolones, 299–300
repaglinide, 173, 663
rifabutin, 173–174, 665, 755
simvastatin, 170–171, 298, 722,
754
sotalol, 79–80, 165, 727, 752
tacrolimus, 174, 300, 745
theophylline, 81, 300–301,
766–767
theophyllines, 23–24, 81,
300–301
triazolam, 165–166, 292, 752, 800
verapamil, 301, 755–756,
823–824
warfarin, 81–82, 174–175, 302,
843–844
magaldrate
demeclocycline, 760, 762
doxycycline, 479–480, 760, 762
minocycline, 479–480, 760, 762
oxytetracycline, 479–480, 760,
762
penicillamine, 575–576
tetracycline, 479–480, 760, 762
tetracyclines, 479–480, 760, 762
magnesium carbonate
demeclocycline, 762
doxycycline, 479–480, 762
minocycline, 479–480, 762
oxytetracycline, 479–480, 762
tetracycline, 479–480, 762
tetracyclines, 479–480, 762
magnesium citrate
demeclocycline, 762
doxycycline, 479–480, 762
minocycline, 479–480, 762

rifampin (*cont.*)
  theophylline, 676, 770
  theophyllines, 26–27, 676, 770
  tolbutamide, 674–675, 786
  triazolam, 666, 802
  tricyclic antidepressants, 555, 673
  warfarin, 680, 847
  zolpidem, 676, 861
Rifamycins
  amprenavir, 47–48, 677
  azole antifungals, 326, 429, 443, 677
  buspirone, 98, 667
  corticosteroids, 186, 624
  cortisone, 186
  cyclosporine, 199–200, 678
  dapsone, 206, 678
  delavirdine, 212, 679
  erlotinib, 291, 679
  fluconazole, 326, 677
  gefitinib, 358–359, 669–670
  haloperidol, 371–372
  indinavir, 394, 680
  itraconazole, 429, 677
  ketoconazole, 443, 677
  prednisolone, 624
  prednisone, 624
  protease inhibitors, 394
  warfarin, 680, 847
rifapentine
  azole antifungals, 443, 677
  erlotinib, 291
  corticosteroids, 624
  indinavir, 394
  ketoconazole, 443
  prednisolone, 624
  prednisone, 624
  protease inhibitors, 394
  warfarin, 847
rifaximin, buspirone, 98
Rimactane. *See* rifampin.
Risperdal. *See* risperidone.
risperidone
  fluoxetine, 336, 681
  paroxetine, 573, 681

  serotonin reuptake inhibitors, 336, 573, 681, 711
  sertraline, 681, 711
Ritalin. *See* methylphenidate.
ritonavir
  alprazolam, 12, 683
  amiodarone, 31, 681
  atorvastatin, 72, 682
  azole antifungals, 325, 428, 442, 682
  benzodiazepines, 12, 179, 228, 304, 341, 517, 683, 802
  buprenorphine, 94, 691
  bupropion, 95, 683
  carbamazepine, 119, 684
  clonazepam, 683
  clorazepate, 179
  clozapine, 180, 684
  conivaptan, 184, 685
  diazepam, 228, 683
  digoxin, 240, 685
  dihydroergotamine, 245–246, 686
  efavirenz, 277, 690
  eplerenone, 286, 686
  ergonovine, 287, 686
  ergotamine, 290, 686
  ergot derivatives, 245–246, 287, 290, 496–497, 686
  estazolam, 304, 683
  fentanyl, 318, 691
  flecainide, 320, 687
  fluconazole, 325, 682
  fluoxetine, 336–337, 687–688
  flurazepam, 341, 683
  indinavir, 395, 688
  itraconazole, 428, 682
  ketoconazole, 442, 682
  loperamide, 469, 688
  lovastatin, 478, 689
  meperidine, 482, 689
  methadone, 487, 690
  methylergonovine, 496–497, 686
  midazolam, 517, 683
  nevirapine, 543, 690